C000088765

1,000,000 Books
are available to read at

Forgotten Books

www.ForgottenBooks.com

Read online
Download PDF
Purchase in print

ISBN 978-1-5279-4115-1
PIBN 10921655

This book is a reproduction of an important historical work. Forgotten Books uses state-of-the-art technology to digitally reconstruct the work, preserving the original format whilst repairing imperfections present in the aged copy. In rare cases, an imperfection in the original, such as a blemish or missing page, may be replicated in our edition. We do, however, repair the vast majority of imperfections successfully; any imperfections that remain are intentionally left to preserve the state of such historical works.

Forgotten Books is a registered trademark of FB &c Ltd.
Copyright © 2018 FB &c Ltd.
FB &c Ltd, Dalton House, 60 Windsor Avenue, London, SW19 2RR.
Company number 08720141. Registered in England and Wales.

For support please visit www.forgottenbooks.com

1 MONTH OF FREE READING

at

www.ForgottenBooks.com

By purchasing this book you are eligible for one month membership to ForgottenBooks.com, giving you unlimited access to our entire collection of over 1,000,000 titles via our web site and mobile apps.

To claim your free month visit:

www.forgottenbooks.com/free921655

* Offer is valid for 45 days from date of purchase. Terms and conditions apply.

English
Français
Deutsche
Italiano
Español
Português

www.forgottenbooks.com

Mythology Photography **Fiction** Fishing Christianity **Art** Cooking Essays Buddhism Freemasonry Medicine **Biology** Music **Ancient Egypt** Evolution Carpentry Physics Dance Geology **Mathematics** Fitness Shakespeare **Folklore** Yoga Marketing **Confidence** Immortality Biographies Poetry **Psychology** Witchcraft Electronics Chemistry History **Law** Accounting **Philosophy** Anthropology Alchemy Drama Quantum Mechanics Atheism Sexual Health **Ancient History** **Entrepreneurship** Languages Sport Paleontology Needlework Islam **Metaphysics** Investment Archaeology Parenting Statistics Criminology **Motivational**

The American Journal of Urology

GENITO-URINARY AND VENEREAL DISEASES

EDITED BY
WILLIAM J. ROBINSON, M.D.
OF NEW YORK

VOL. X

JANUARY-DECEMBER, 1914

THE UROLOGIC PUBLISHING ASSOCIATION
12 Mt. Morris Park West, New York

List of Contributors to Vol. X of The American Journal of Urology

Index to Principal Subjects

A

B

C

INDEX

R

S

T

U

INDEX

V

W

Y

THE AMERICAN JOURNAL OF UROLOGY

WILLIAM J. ROBINSON, M.D., EDITOR

VOL. X JANUARY, 1914. No. 1

DIAGNOSIS AND TREATMENT OF HEMIC INFECTION OF THE URINARY TRACT[1]

By PROFESSOR DR. THORKILD ROVSING, Copenhagen

I. THE DIAGNOSIS

HOW difficult it may be, and often is, to diagnosticate whether an infection of the urinary tract is of hemic or of other origin is best seen from this, that it has lasted so many years and cost so much labour to get corrected in the view, maintained by most of the authorities headed by Guyon, that, so to say, all urine infection was ascending, and entered from the urethra, and to get established the enormous frequency and importance of hemic infection.

No one has felt this more strongly than the author, who since 1889 has constantly fought for the recognition of the frequency of hemic infection and of its importance for treatment.

This does not so much concern the ordinary suppuration microbes staphylo- and strepto-cocci. Fairly early one recognized that pyonephrosis, occurring acutely during septicemia or pyemia, was of hemic origin. Far more does it concern the most frequent of all urine infections: *coli-nephritis*, *coli-pyelitis*, and *coli-bacteriuria*, and the most serious of all the infections of the urinary tract, *tuberculosis*.

Not till after I had procured, in my large work of 1897—*Clinical and Experimental Studies on the Infectious Diseases of the Urinary Organs*[2]—strong clinical and experimental evidences that coli-infection most frequently arises by way of the blood, did the correct conception begin to prevail among surgeons and urologists. But it is only a few years ago that, from the medical

[1] Read before the Urology Section of the XVIIth International Congress of Medicine.

[2] Published in German translation in 1898: *Klinische u. exp. Untersuch. über die infektiösen Krankheiten der Harnorgane,* Oscar Coblenz, Berlin.

(Lenhartz), pediatric, and obstetrical (Albech) side, one would still have maintained that coli-infection always, so to say, is of urethral origin, founding this opinion only on the fact that the disease is specially frequent with females, where the urethra is so short compared with that of the male.

As regards tuberculosis, I think every one now agrees that it is, as it were, always hemic and primary in the kidney. Pathological anatomy—Heiberg's work from 1891 in particular—has taught us this; absolutely in opposition to the clinical interpretation. This theory, which was to the effect that tuberculosis is always ascending and consequently inaccessible to surgical therapy, has, supported by Guyon's enormous authority, been extremely tenacious of life; and it is only since Guyon's pupils, Albarran first and foremost, at the beginning of this century came round to the correct conception that this, and therewith the only right treatment of tuberculosis of the kidney, became general.

These facts alone, that the greatest clinicians have for so long been able entirely to misjudge the hemic urine infections, make it obvious that the diagnosis whether a urine infection is hemic or not must involve serious difficulties. With our knowledge concerning the frequency of hemic infections and with our study of the aspects which they give rise to, we have dropped a number of these difficulties. Thus it is easy enough, now, when we have substantiated tubercle bacilli, pus, and albumen in the urine, to diagnose primary kidney tuberculosis; because now we are in possession of the fact established by operative autopsia that tuberculosis of the urinary tract, as a rule, is primary in the kidney. And it is often easy for us, after having found and described the typical aspect under which coli-nephritis most frequently begins, to diagnose this. Indeed, even where there has been no typically initial stage, or where this dates far back, or has been forgotten by the patient, we can diagnosticate with great certainty a present infection as hemic *in all cases where no instrument has ever been introduced in the bladder*, and *where the sphincter of this has hitherto always been healthy and capable of performing its functions.* Because no shadow of evidence has ever been shown to the effect that infection from without can enter the bladder so long as the function of the sphincter is uninjured. On the other hand, if Lenhartz and those who agree with him were right in thinking that the relative frequency of coli-infections with the female sex is simply due to the bacteria having an easy access to the bladder through the short urethra, all females would have coli-uria, while fortunately it is quite a small percentage in whom we do not find the urine absolutely sterile within the sphincter.

In cases, however, where instruments have been introduced without one's knowing the condition of the urine before the first introduction of these took place, it can be very difficult, or quite impossible, to diagnose whether the urine infection is of hemic or urethral origin. Whether albuminuria exists here or does not is by no means conclusive, because an ascending infection may cause nephritis, and the nephritic process, which generally is the beginning and cause of a hemic urine infection, may have passed away and left behind bacteriuria, pyelitis, or cystitis. It must be emphasized, however, that in cases where retention of the urine in the bladder does not exist, or has not existed, there are other momenta which might explain, or render probable, an ascending infection, and here the presence of albuminuria will speak in favour of the infection being hemic. This is particularly probable if the catheterization of the ureter shows that the urine of only the one kidney contains albumen and infection.

The most frequent of all hemic infection, coli-infection, is easy to diagnosticate when the *initial stage*—the primary nephritis—*occurs acutely and typically.* The patient then suddenly becomes violently ill with cold shivers, very high temperature (39–41°), pains across the loins or only in one of the kidney regions, and frequent, but generally painless, urination. The complaint very often begins with *strong hematuria,* which generally subsides quickly in the course of twenty-four hours or so, and is succeeded by *albuminuria* with diffusely turbid urine very rich in leucocytes and bacilli. *With coli-nephritis, on the other hand, one looks in vain for cylinders,* and the widespread superstition that the proving of cylinders is necessary for diagnosing nephritis is certainly the cause of so many of these cases being considered pure pyelitis. Sometimes the bleeding is so severe and the pains so considerable that the complaint is confused with renal stone colic. Not unfrequently such acute coli-nephritis starts from *acute appendicitis,* because the virulent microbes confined in the inflamed appendix enter into the circulation. If there is strong hematuria the severe appendicitis pains may give the aspect a deceptive similarity to kidney stone colic, and I have had several cases admitted for treatment under this diagnosis. The discovery of microbes in the urine does not contradict this, and the sensitiveness to pressure on McBurney's point fits in just as well with a stone in the ureter. The correct diagnosis, here, can only be given by the method of examination indicated by me: compression of colon descendens from below, upwards. If the indirect pressure produces pains in the right fossa iliaca, appendicitis is concerned; if not, a calculous or a retro-peritoneal inflammation.

In some cases the hematuria continues obstinately during weeks, even months, and can, in connexion with the patient's anemic, often sallow appearance, mislead one to the diagnosis of a malignant tumour. Even with a macroscopically pure hematuria, one ought, therefore, always to examine the urine microscopically, especially for microbes.

In other cases the hematuria is absent, and only after attacks of fever do albumen, pus, and bacteria occur in the hitherto normal urine.

While the acute febrile character of the disease in the great majority of cases—especially when a rational treatment is instituted—very quickly subsides, yet in certain cases it assumes a more perilous, fatal character *for the reason that the acute attacks recur time after time.* Sometimes one sees the attacks adopt the character of septicopyemia with confusion, delirium, and thrombo-phlebitis, often it puzzles one as to what these constantly renewed attacks are due: whether to renewed seed through the blood from the original focus from which the kidney was infected, or to a flare up of the infection at one time present.

In its typical form coli-nephritis is so characteristic in its symptomatic aspect, that from this alone one can make the diagnosis, but, superabundantly, we have the macro- and microscopic examination of the urine. This is acid, and diffusely turbid on account of the millions of bacilli which move about in it. The urine does not become clear when set aside, and on shaking it and holding it up to the light one sees with the naked eye shoals of bacteria being whirled round in the fluid. Microscopy and dispersed culture from the urine give the full diagnostic certainty.

Of other acutely arising hemic infections *staphylococcic and streptococcic nephritis* are the most frequent, and generally begin during acute infectious diseases such as *angina tonsillaris, osteomyelitis acuta,* &c.

With these infections the aspect of the complaint is generally much more acute and persevering than with coli-infections: high temperature often with violent fits of shivering, vomitings, and, on the whole, a very exhausted state of health in general. While patients with *coli-infection* generally recuperate quickly after each attack, patients with *strepto- or staphylo-coccic infections*, with *Proteus Hauser*, quickly assume the character of severe intoxication, and get a yellowish, sallow appearance.

Here, again, the decisive factor for the diagnosis of the nature of the infection is, naturally, *the examination of the urine.* The *sight and odour* of this are at once of great importance for the diagnosis. While coli-urine always, even when set aside, remains diffusely turbid throughout the whole column of fluid, with most other infections the urine quickly becomes clear when set aside, with a deposit of a larger or lesser sediment. Only by infection with *Proteus Hauser*, which like *B. coli* possesses a mighty power of propagation and lively self-motion, does the urine remain diffusely turbid; but to discriminate it from coli-infection we here find the urine ammoniacal with the typical, pungent ammonia smell, and of strong alkaline reaction, while the coli-urine has the typical insipid putrid odour, and reacts *acidly* on litmus paper. As with *Proteus Hauser*, all the pyogenetic forms of staphylococci and several forms of streptococci distinguish themselves by their ability to decompose the urea by forming ammonia, but as they are deficient in selfmotion, they sink to the bottom with the pus cells, the epithelium cells, and the crystals, while the urine above becomes clear. Besides the alkaline reaction and the ammoniacal odour, the *microscopical* examination of the sediment yields a fairly decisive contribution to the diagnosis of the nature of the infection: the discovery of the characteristic "*coffinlid*"*-shaped triple phosphate-crystals* tells us that a urea-decomposing microbe is concerned, and this is of great importance where such bacilli are in question, which, like *Proteus Hauser*, for example, deceptively resemble the coli-bacillus in the microscopical picture, or where we have a hybrid infection of coli-bacilli with urea-decomposing microbes.

As I proved some time ago by thorough investigations, the coli-bacillus by its numeric, enormous predominance can render it very difficult, or impossible, for us to find the less prolific microbes which perhaps are the real, or at least the most essential, cause of the disease. In such cases the ammoniacal condition of the urine may become the only sign which betrays to us that other and more active bacteria than *B. coli* are present.

Another peculiarity with the hemic infections of the urinary tract produced by ammoniogenetic bacteria is that we often find *cylinders*, and always find numerous epithelium cells in contradistinction to what we discover with coli-nephritis. The cause of this is the toxical and corroding effect of the ammonia on the kidney parenchyma, and on the epithelium cells everywhere in the mucous membranes of the urinary tract.

With these hemic infections of the urinary tract, therefore, we almost constantly see pyelitis and cystitis accompanying the nephritis, while these are very rare with coli-infection, that is if stone formation or retention (floating kidney, pyelitis during pregnancy, &c.) do not favour the development of inflammation.

For the diagnosis, moreover, it is of interest to know that the heterogeneous infection also stipulates for great distinction as regards the complication with *stone formation* in these complaints.

In a great number of cases the hemic infection of the urinary tract arises as a complication to, and on the basis of, primary nephrolithiasis, because the stones produce that solutio continui, that trauma which becomes decisive for the entrance of the infection and for its pathogenetic activity. If once the infection has arisen, the stone maintains the inflammation, partly by hindering the flow of the urine and causing retention, and partly by irritating the mucous membrane; but, vice versa, the infection also influences the stone disease, and this influence varies greatly according to the nature of the infection.

While all urea-decomposing microbes involve a quick growth of the stone by constantly depositing triple phosphate, most of the other microbes appear to be entirely without influence on the stones. Only one, but, on the other hand, the one that occurs most frequently—bacterium coli—has an *entirely opposite determining effect* on the concrements. This corresponds with bacterium coli being a *saprophyte* which consumes the organic stroma which binds together the crystalline elements of the stone, whereby these fall into gravel. But certain forms of *B. coli* have, besides, the peculiarity that they *devour uric acid.* A rapid waste of the stone then takes place, which generally is replaced by myriads of bacilli, leucocytes, and fibrin, which together with the remains of the organic stroma may then form most peculiar pseudomembranous formations, which resemble fruit peel, and most frequently remind one of boiled olive-skins.

These, or bits of these, pass with the urine from time to time under pains resembling colic. When one knows these formations one at once recognizes that a coli-infection on a calculous basis is in question, and for doctors who do not know this circumstance they often give rise to a faulty diagnosis. Sometimes they are interpreted as necrotic tumour masses, sometimes as displaced necrotic mucous membrane, and sometimes as mysterious formations which by some doctors—Morawitz and Adrian [3]—are termed albumin-stones (Eiweisssteine).

As early as 1897 I described a series of such cases under the title "pseudo-membranous pyelitis," [4] and later I have observed a number of cases with this interesting aspect.

The *differential diagnosis* between the *tuberculous pyuria* and the *pyuria* caused by *other microbes* is of great importance, because the therapy will, as a rule, be diametrically opposed in the first case and the last: with tuberculosis the diseased kidney ought to be removed as quickly as possible, while the treatment of the other infections is generally conservative.

With uncomplicated tuberculous infection the diagnosis is generally easy enough. Under the microscope the urine caught sterile from the bladder shows pus, and with the ordinary colour methods no bacteria; just as culture in the usual nutritive mediums gives a negative result. We know, therefore, with such great certainty that tuberculosis is in question that, even in those cases—10 per cent.—where in spite of all pains and the application of the best methods one does not succeed in proving tubercle bacilli, one ought to set to work operatively.

The diagnosis, however, becomes much more difficult where tuberculosis is complicated with infection of another kind, most frequently coli-infection, more rarely other microbes, whether by hemic infection or by catheterization performed at an earlier period.

If, here, one does not succeed in proving tubercle bacilli, or if one succeeds in proving only doubtful or faintly-coloured or stunted tubercle bacilli, the explorative production of the diseased kidney may become necessary for the diagnosis.

In the majority of cases palpation and inspection of the

[3] Morawitz u. Adrian, 'Zur Kenntniss der sogenannten Eiweisssteine der Niere, *Mitteil. a. d. Grenzgebiete d. Med. u. Chir.*, Bd. xvii, p. 579.

[4] *Hospitalstidende* and *Monatsberichte der Harn- u. Sexual-Apparate*, p. 1, 1897, and in my book, *Klin. u. experiment. Studien über die infektiösen Krankheiten der Harnorgane*, Coblenz, Berlin, 1898.

released and drawn forth kidney will give the diagnosis. In serious cases we find the kidney enlarged and the seat of abscesses or caves, but even in cases of very restricted tuberculosis, where the size and shape of the kidney are entirely unchanged, one will generally find small miliary bumps protruding from the surface of the kidney corresponding with a portion affected by tuberculosis, sometimes visible, but best perceptible to an expert finger.

It is well worth drawing attention, however, to the fact that, to the less experienced, the hemic coli-infection may present an aspect which deceptively resembles the miliary seed of tuberculosis; because the corticalis is often sown throughout with small abscesses which, like yellowy-whitish, often slightly projecting points, have a striking similarity to miliary tubercles. They differ from the miliary tubercles, however, partly by being surrounded by a hyperemic zone, partly by that part of them often being perforated at the tip, whereby a small crater-shaped decay appears. In cases of doubt, excision of a small piece of kidney tissue for microscopical examination will surely and quickly lead to the diagnosis, inasmuch as the microscope, in a case of coli-abscess, shows necrosis and pus containing coli-bacilli, while with tuberculosis it shows typical infiltration of the tissues with tubercle formation.

I need only just mention that cystoscopy and catheterization of the ureter naturally are of the greatest importance to the local diagnosis: if the urine caught from the ureters is normal and sterile, while the urine from the bladder is infected, there is no question whatsoever of hemic infection, and often in this way one can get the question of *hemic* or *non-hemic infection* solved. If hemic the catheterization of the ureter gives us the most important information as to whether both kidneys or only one is infected.

Röntgen examination of the kidneys and ureters is very important, in order to establish whether complication with stone-formation is present or not, which must greatly influence the therapy which has to be instituted.

II. THE TREATMENT

While a hemic kidney tuberculosis, provided it is unilateral, always indicates nephrectomy, in my opinion operative treatment is very rarely indicated with other uncomplicated hemic infections.

In some very few cases of unilateral *staphylococcic* and

streptococcic nephritis I have been obliged to perform resection or extirpation of the kidney in order to save the life of the patient. In two cases it concerned a *diffuse staphylococcic nephritis*, which involved, in addition to high fever and symptoms of intoxication, such violent and obstinate *hematuria* that nephrectomy appeared to me the only possible salvation, and it is my conviction that this encroachment really saved the patients from otherwise certain death. In a third case, with a left-sided *streptococcic nephritis* which had arisen in a twelve-year-old boy after *angina*, and had continued with pyuria and perilous attacks of fever, I found at the operation the upper third of the kidney sown throughout with *streptococcical* infarcts, while the rest of the kidney appeared healthy. By resection I removed the upper third of the kidney and the patient has been completely well during the twelve years which have since elapsed. In a series of cases I have opened *paranephritic abscesses* which were due to *hemic staphylococcic infection* in the corticalis of the kidney.

On the other hand, I have never found operative treatment necessary with uncomplicated *hemic coli-infection*, no matter how violent the initial nephritis may have been.

It is quite a different matter, however, when the infection is complicated with affections which favour the maintenance of the infection. Thus, *nephropyelitis calculosa* can be cured only when the stone is removed, and *pyelonephritis* with stable or intermittent hydronephrosis not until the passage through the ureter has been re-established.

If the stable hydronephrosis is due to a stone in the ureter, we must remove this by ureterotomy; if due to an acquired stricture, this must be dilated or removed; if due to congenital valvular formation at the entrance of the ureter into the basin of the kidney, Fenger's plastic operation is often able to remove the stagnation; if the valvular formation is situated in the lower end of the ureter a *ureteroneostomy* must be attempted. If a re-establishment of the ureter passage is impracticable owing to *multiple contractions* or total closing, then the infected hydronephrosis sack should be extirpated at once, "in toto"; whereas a mere opening and drainage of the sack is absolutely unadvisable, as the big relaxed sack obdurately retains the infection, while the *secondary performance* of extirpation becomes even more difficult on account of adherence to the surrounding parts: the peritoneum in particular.

As regards the intermittent hydronephrosis, floating kidney is most frequently the cause, and nothing is then so effective in preventing the constantly returning attacks of pyelitis as a *well-performed nephropexy.*

When faced with *pyelitis* during *pregnancy,* we know well that if we can weather the storm until the confinement takes place, then the retention, and with it the pyelitis, will be removed at one blow.

In most cases all goes well, as one limits oneself to the giving of medicamina which act as a disinfectant on the urine, and among these *salol* is in my experience absolutely the best. But if the condition becomes threatening, with high fever, cold shivers, and general indisposition, one must necessarily procure an outlet for the infected urine stagnating in the pelvis. Then one should first try catheterization of the ureter, with drainage of the pelvis, and a subsequent enema of ½ to 1 per cent. solution of nitrate of silver. Such a treatment often has a lasting effect, and by repeating it from time to time one can manage to pull the patient through until the confinement. If, however, one does not succeed by these methods in averting the perilous condition, one must adopt radical measures and face the difficult choice between *artificial delivery* and *nephro- or pyelo-tomy.* If the pregnancy is so far advanced that one can expect a viable child, one should as a rule choose artificial delivery, and only where the condition is so threatening that immediate outlet is necessary would one prefer *pyelotomy* through a lumbar incision. In earlier stages of the pregnancy it may often be difficult to choose between this operation and artificial delivery, and to a great extent the choice will depend on the importance of preserving the fetus.

With *uncomplicated coli-infections,* or in cases where the complication has been removed, operative treatment is not indicated; partly because, as a rule, nothing can be gained by operating against the little miliary abscesses which are often scattered over the whole corticalis of the kidney, and partly because, even in very serious hemic coli-nephritis, one can obtain much more effect by a rational internal treatment.

This treatment presents two problems:

1. *To avert the perilous condition and cure the nephritis,* which in the majority of cases one succeeds in doing by rinsing out the kidneys from within with big doses of water—distilled preferred—and salol 1 gr. three to four times a day.

2. The second problem is then *to remove bacterium coli from the urine,* and this problem is stated by many to be hopelessly insolvable. This, however, is unwarranted, but to procure a complete cure of the bacteriuria it is certainly necessary to apply my method of 1897. This consists in the application of the abovementioned treatment with distilled water and salol, *and putting the patient to bed with catheter à demeure,* through which the urine streams steadily and freely into a glass. The fact is, that the time betwen the two urinations is quite sufficient to allow the coli-bacilli in the bladder to multiply enormously, and thence to reinfect the upper urinary tract. *Only if one can establish a constantly flowing stream can one succeed in getting quit of the coli-bacilli.* By bacteriological examination of fresh samples of urine, one ascertains if one's object is attained, and if the result is favourable one removes the catheter after injecting immediately previously 50 c.c. of 1 per cent. solution of nitrate of silver, in order to kill the few microbes which possibly may conceal themselves in the folds of the mucous membrane of the bladder, especially in that place where the catheter is fixed. Where *women* are concerned I always use *Pezzer's* catheter, No. 22 or 23, which is most practicable because so easy to put into place, and to remove; moreover it is fixed *automatically.* Where *men* are concerned I use *Mercier's* formalin-sterilized rubber catheter, which is fixed by thread and sticking-plaster. The formalin sterilization hardens the catheter, so that this is able to lie à demeure for three to four weeks without being changed, while other catheters can remain only a few days. I then make the patient drink 3–4 litres of distilled water in the 24 hours, and take 1–4 grm. of salol. By this treatment I have succeeded with 50 per cent. of my cases in making the patient perfectly free from bacteria, and I am sure that a much greater percentage of cases could be so if all patients could and would devote sufficient time to this treatment; the difficulty is, however, to keep many of these patients confined to bed for so long a period, partly from economical reasons, and partly because they feel so exceedingly well in other respects.

Only in those cases where either one does not succeed in curing the nephritis, whereupon this becomes chronic, or where the kidneys are constantly reinfected from some hidden source of infection in the organism, it is impossible to obtain recovery on these lines. It is not easy to judge at the very beginning which cases will prove capable of resisting the water and salol cure; most often, I suppose, the violent nephritis which begins in perilous cases, but not always so. Sometimes one does see cases with insidious beginnings become persistently chronic, and, vice versa, one sees the most threatening cases completely cured by the water cure within a very short period.

Thus, there are in my material three cases where the patient was so ill that I considered an operation necessary, but by the operation I found that the kidney from end to end was infested with abscesses the size of a pin's head, so that all help by operation, with the excepting of *nephrectomy,* was excluded.

After having excised a small piece of tissue containing abscesses for microscopic examination the kidney was replaced, and an energetic water and salol cure with catheter à demeure established. After a few days the fever symptoms disappeared, and in the course of a fortnight the strongly pus-containing urine became perfectly clear, while in the course of a month the urine was free from bacteria. In one of these cases nephropexy was performed five weeks afterwards, and the appearance of the kidney was then found to be quite normal; only here and there on the surface were found small retractions: the remains of the abscesses. But of course the infection is not always benign. In some cases the disease flares up again acutely, just when one thinks the illness is overcome. In other cases the pyuria and the albuminuria become chronic, with indolent course, which is now and again interrupted by febrile periods. In these cases the salol and water treatment, though it cannot cure, is not quite impotent, as it can lessen the intoxication and soothe the acute cases. In a great number of these obstinately relapsing cases I have the impression that it does not concern the flaring up of the infection which the kidney has previously contracted, but constant new hemic infections from an *occult focus,* whether a wound in the intestine, a cholecystitis, appendicitis, or something to that effect.

With these cases especially, but on the whole with cases which—inaccessible to operative treatment—defy the ordinary internal treatment, we have in Wright's vaccination treatment a remedy which according to my experience is of great value.

At the German Urological Congress in Berlin in April 1909 I reported twelve cases of coli-infection treated with vaccination after Wright's method, with the improvement, however, that I did not employ "stock" vaccine, but always *cultures of the bacteria found with the particular patient in question.*

Especially in six very serious cases, where all other treatment had proved unavailing, the result was so surprising and encouraging that I felt myself bound to continue the experiments, and even at the International Medical Congress at Buda-Pest in the autumn of 1909 I had at my disposal 23 cases, which were submitted to the urologic section by my assistant, Dr. Ove Wulff, to whom I had handed over the question for thorough experimental and clinical study.

In 1911, in his book, *Studier over Fagocytose, Opsonin og Vaccine-behandling ved Urinvejsinfektioner,* by which he qualified himself as private docent at the university of Copenhagen, Dr. Ove Wulff has, moreover, reported his continued experimental and clinical investigations. With regard to the experimental investigations which have been performed at the Danish Institute for Serum Therapy I shall altogether refer to Dr. Wulff's publications. I wish only to emphasize one point which, in my opinion, seems to be of particular importance to the clinical applicability of the method. Dr. Wulff arrives at the result that the determining of the opsonic index previous to the vaccination treatment does not have that importance which Wright and Bulloch have attached to it. Partly the opsonic index can only be determined with about 20 per cent. of mistakes, and partly the diagnostic value as regards the condition of the patient and the danger of the treatment can only be extremely inferior. For this reason I think that it is not necessary to determine the opsonic index before initiating the vaccination treatment, provided only that one observes the necessary caution with regard to the commencing dose.

The effect of the treatment starting from the theory, should be, for one, an active immunity of the organism against the microbe in question, while it can hardly be expected to have any direct influence on the microbe proper. The clinical results are conformable to this, inasmuch as these consist in *decrease or cessation of the inflammation, the pus secretion, the albuminuria and of the general symptoms, whereas the microbes do not disappear from the urine as a rule.* In any case with bacteria with self-motion, such as the coli-bacilli, a bacteriuria generally remains, while pus and albumen disappear. The vaccination treatment, therefore, ought always to be combined with, or succeeded by, my usual antibacterial treatment: the administering of salol and large quantities of distilled water during a permanent drainage of the bladder, whereby we obtain a permanent rinsing from within, outwards, with antiseptic fluid. In my experience urotropine acts extremely whimsically and uncertainly in the urinary tract, and often produces an irritation of this which favours a flaring up of the inflammation.

It may, then, appear difficult to judge whether it is the vaccination or the other treatment which is acting. It must be remembered, however, that in practically all cases I have first, and for long in vain, employed the usual treatment before the vaccination therapy was adopted.

But, furthermore, Dr. Wulff has, for safety's sake, drawn a comparative statistical parallel with an equal series of cases from the time before the vaccination treatment; therefore, only of those treated according to the old method.

He found, of 38 *vaccinated*—

Before treatment.		*After treatment.*	
albumen	with 79 per cent.	albumen	with 16 per cent.
pus	with 73 per cent.	pus	with 24 per cent.
bacilli	with 100 per cent.	bacilli	with 76 per cent.

Of 40 *non-vaccinated*—

Before treatment.		*After treatment.*	
albumen	with 73 per cent.	albumen	with 50 per cent.
pus	with 100 per cent.	pus	with 70 per cent.
bacilli	with 100 per cent.	bacilli	with 75 per cent.

By comparing these figures one will see that, while albumen and pus diminish in a much greater percentage after the vaccination treatment, the quantity of bacilli is affected quite similarly in both series.

The importance of the vaccine therapy defines itself far more strikingly when one considers the *particularly serious cases* where the disease occurs in attacks, or permanently with grave suffering of the general state of health, with high temperature, shivering fits, indeed even with conditions resembling septicopyemia, which seem greatly threatening to the life of the patient. In a series of such cases—twenty altogether—as "ultimum refugium," the vaccination has undoubtedly cured the patients of the disease, which was incurable in any other way.

In the majority of these cases *coli-infections of a cryptogenetic nature* have been in question; in some of these it concerned acutely arisen violent bilateral nephritis, with severe hematuria and *albuminuria*, where the vaccine treatment seems to me in the most evident manner to have involved the decisive turn in the course of the disease.

In other cases—and these seem perhaps even more convincing—it concerned patients who during a series of years had borne nephritis and urine infection, and where, with certain intervals, acute, more or less violent attacks of fever, shivering fits, increased albuminuria and pyuria had lowered the condition of the patients more and more.

In some few cases it was thus that between the attacks the urine became completely normal, even free of bacteria, but the infection invariably reappeared until the vaccine treatment put an end to the disease.

But I have equally fine results in cases where the infection was due to *Proteus Hauser, staphylococci, or streptococci.*

A young lady, 22 years of age, who, twelve months previously, in accession to appendectomy, had contracted bilateral staphylococcic nephritis which had defied all treatment, was cured completely by only three weeks' vaccination treatment, and was discharged with completely normal urine free of albumen and bacteria, and has since then been completely well for eighteen months.

In June 1911, a man, 46 years of age, who, after having undergone treatment in vain in his own home during a month or so, was admitted with very serious *streptococcic nephritis,* with severe albuminuria and high jumping temperature, as high as 41°, which appeared in attacks with cold shivers and pains across the loins. *Complete recovery* after vaccination with *autogenetic streptococcic culture.*

Only in a very few cases has the treatment been quite *without effect* or only been attended with slight temporary improvement, without my having been able to find the reason thereof. Probably this has lain in the nature of the infection.

Serious drawbacks, as effects of the treatment, I have only seen in one case since the early time when we had not sufficient experience in the dosing. With this patient there was a rise in temperature and indisposition after each injection, and as, with the fourth injection, we even went up to 1,000 millions, this patient got convulsions, became confused, restless, and generally exhausted, a condition which, however, quickly passed away.

Otherwise I have not seen any secondary effects beyond the purely local reaction, with redness and soreness on the place of injection, which was observed in about 10 per cent. of the cases, but always passed away again spontaneously and quickly.

Our mode of procedure is as follows: from the purely cultivated bacteria of the patient's urine two emulsions of the destroyed culture are prepared, which contain 100–500 millions of microbes per c.c. respectively. Every second or third day was injected subcutaneously—

With adults,	25	millions once;
	50	millions once;
	100	millions three or four times running;
	250	millions two or three times;
and finally,	500	millions until the completion of the cure.

In some serious cases we have increased the dose up to 1,000 millions, but as a rule the dose ought not to rise higher than 500 millions.

Where *children* are concerned we begin with 10 millions and raise the quantity more cautiously on the whole.

I have no doubt, therefore, that Wright's vaccine treatment is a *most valuable augmentation of our expedients for contending with the hemic infections* of the urinary tract, a remedy which in most of these cases where all other expedients fail leads to recovery or very considerable improvement.

For The American Journal of Urology

POST-OPERATIVE HEMORRHAGE—AN UNUSUAL COMPLICATION OF PROSTATECTOMY

By Emory Lanphear, M.D., Ph.D., LL.D., St. Louis, Mo.

Professor of Surgery in the American Polyclinic.

HENRY W., age 66, patient of Dr. G. C. Eggers, of Clayton, Mo., was admitted to the Deaconess' Hospital Nov. 1, 1913, suffering seriously from urinary retention. He always has had excellent health except malarial fever 25 years ago. For about one year he has had some irritation of the bladder, with more or less difficulty in starting the stream of urine; past 2 weeks retention has been bad. Two days ago retention became complete; a doctor at Overland Park attempted catheterization with metal instrument but succeeded in securing nothing but a small quantity of blood, evidently from a "false passage" near prostate.

On admission to hospital his bladder was distended to the umbilicus, there was constant dribbling of urine—paralysis of overdistention, and general condition critical from uremic poisoning.

With great difficulty he was anesthetised but finally yielded sufficiently to permit enucleation of both lobes of the prostate thru a perineal incision. After removal of the unusually large prostate the bladder was explored for possible stone, with negative result. A strand of gauze was introduced into the bladder thru the urethra, and the wound packt tightly with gauze to check oozing. Before this was done a careful examination was made, as usual, to see if any vessels were bleeding, but nothing except minor oozing was found.

During the night following operation the patient was somewhat restless and may have disturbed the packing, tho there was no external evidence of hemorrhage and urine came away abundantly thru the gauze. Next day (24 hours after operation) the house surgeon reported patient to be suffering much discomfort in the bladder and that it seemed to be greatly distended, apparently with urine. Presuming that the urethra had become clogged with a blood-clot I ordered him to gently pull on the pack and make pressure over the paralyzed bladder; with the telephonic report that this had given relief and that the dressing was repeatedly saturated with slightly bloody urine.

Next day—48 hours after operation—the bladder was found distended to its limit, with absolute flatness on percussion to the umbilicus, altho the perineal dressings were saturated with urine of slightly red color. Suspecting what had occurred I removed the pack and found that the piece of gauze, which had been put into the bladder thru the remnant of prostatic urethra, had been forced out of the bladder and hemorrhage had occurred—into the bladder instead of thru the external wound; the bladder was filled with what appeared to be one enormous blood-clot around the back of which the urine was flowing into the gauze-pack. With great difficulty this clot was broken up, and then washt out with hot, boric-acid solution. Then the vesical drain was reestablisht by a gauze wick and the perineal wound packt tightly enough to control the oozing which was still persisting.

Strange to say the patient, who was fortunately of the full-blooded type, did not manifest any perceptible sign of this very large loss of blood—the pulse was of good volume, thirst was not markt, and there was no sign of hemorrhage at the perineal opening; yet he must have lost nearly two liters of blood during the 48 hours elapsing between operation and evacuation of the bladder.

He has made an excellent recovery.

This is only the second case of hemorrhage I have ever had in all the prostatectomies I have made. The other case was as follows:

Adolf K.— of Washington, Mo., patient of Dr. O. L. Muench, was admitted to St. Anthony's Hospital, July 14, 1908. He was 75 years of age, always well until 1904 when he began to have trouble with his bladder from enlarged prostate. For two years he had used the catheter which had induced a cystitis—very bad of late. After four days' treatment for the cystitis he was operated upon through the perineum—an extremely large fibroid prostate being removed. There was no hemorrhage at the time of the operation, so no ligatures were applied (in not more than one case in ten is it necessary to tie any vessel in performing perineal prostatectomy; the gauze pack controls all oozing). A large one-piece gauze pack was inserted into the wound and covered by a gauze pad sustained by a T-bandage. Eight hours after operation the pad was well soaked with blood and urine and in every other way patient was doing well. Some time during the night the patient pulled the gauze pack from the wound and in the morning was found dead from hemorrhage. If the gauze pack had been allowed to remain 72 hours, as is my custom in such cases, this patient without doubt would not have died as a result of the operative procedure.

SEXUAL IMPOTENCY IN THE MALE

By Victor Blum, M.D.

Assistant in Prof. von Frisch's Urological Department of the Vienna General Polyclinic

AUTHORIZED TRANSLATION. EDITED WITH NOTES AND ADDITIONS BY DR. W. J. ROBINSON

[Continued from the December Issue]

CHAPTER XXV

DEFINITION

We come now to a symptom-complex, which has attained, through the pioneer work of English and German investigators (Beard, Casper, Milton, Löwenfeld, Fürbringer, von Krafft-Ebing and others), the dignity of a disease sui generis: namely, the symptom-complex called Sexual Neurasthenia.

This represents partly the cause, partly the effect of the previously described functional disorders of the male sexual organs, abnormal losses of semen and impotence; but sexual neurasthenia also forms a combination of all those functional symptoms, so that it seems appropriate to close our studies of these individual symptoms of disease with a discussion of the sexual neurosis.

As subdivisions of general neurasthenia ("nervous exhaustion" of Beard), which is the most important neurosis in everyday practice, the sexual neurasthenic symptoms possess the greatest interest and deserve the most thorough and scientific appreciation. Not only do we find sexual injuries in almost all cases of general neurasthenia as contributory causes in the etiology of the affection, but also the signs of sexual irritation or exhaustion are hardly ever missing in the symptomatology of these cases.

The fundamental principle of Freud: "A neurosis is impossible in a normal sexual life," has indeed been combatted in this unqualified form by most investigators, and finally has been substantially modified and moderated by Freud himself.

But without doubt Freud deserves the credit of having pointed out the sifinificance of the sexual life in the etiology of the neuroses, and of having discovered the pathogenetic rôle of functional disorders of the male sexual organs for a large percentage of the cases of general neurasthenia.

The type of disease which we shall here consider, is characterized by a symptom-complex, which affects chiefly the male sexual functions. Alterations of the other nervous functions are to be observed only in the far-advanced stages of the disease.

ETIOLOGY OF SEXUAL NEURASTHENIA

Among the causes of sexual neurasthenia the different forms of sexual abuse take the first rank. Hence we shall devote a separate paragraph to the subject at the close of this chapter.

Masturbation, coitus interruptus, abortive excitements, forced abstinence, and venereal excesses may lead sooner or later to the development of sexual neurasthenia.

Just as an immoderate demand upon any other function of the human organism may produce those severe phenomena of deficiency, which we denote as general neurasthenic symptoms, so over-exertion in the sexual sphere may produce functional disturbances, which manifest themselves both locally in the genital organs and also by reaction upon the whole organism.

Of course one encounters great difficulties in any individual case in judging the pathogenic effect of the excessive demands made upon the sexual organs, since a normal standard does not exist for these functions, and accordingly a sexual injury may not cause any neurasthenic symptoms in one individual, which produces the severest derangements in another.

So it happens that men, who for a long time have indulged in the "vice" of masturbation, or have practiced interrupted coitus for many years, may suffer no disturbance of the general health, if they return in season to normal sexual activity.

Still other factors besides the above-noted sexual injuries produce an especial disposition to this nervous disease.

As in general neurasthenia, heredity doubtless plays a very important part in sexual neurasthenia.

Heredity was accepted by Charcot and his pupils as the true and certain cause of all neurotic diseases. The careful study of exact clinical histories, however, led to the now generally accepted view, that heredity represents the disposition to neurotic diseases, the well-prepared soil, in which on the addition of specific injuries (viz., sexual abuse) the seed of sexual neurasthenia germinates according to definite laws.

The inherited nervous predisposition of nervous and mental sufferers is ascertained from the direct and indirect ancestry of the individual. The reason why the same injury may produce a different impression upon different individuals lies in this inborn disposition. Especially, sexual noxæ can produce a severe sexual neurasthenia in the hereditarily disposed, while the same sexual abuse can remain without effect in persons of families with healthy nervous systems.

A congenital neurotic disposition often shows itself very early. The inherited tendency appears especially early among city children, corresponding to the extreme frequency of neurasthenia among city people; Beard indeed considers neurasthenia to be entirely an effect of civilization. The disproportionate demands made upon the physical and the mental development of children results only too often in a one-sided education and a " nervousness " of the children, which we can recognize by a very characteristic appearance and an abundance of general nervous symptoms (excitation, capriciousness, exaltation). But also local symptoms, for example nocturnal enuresis, nervous polyuria, premature appearance of conscious sexual excitement are not rarely to be found in young children.

Here we can often not resist the impression, that the premature awakening of the sexual feelings is one of the chief causes of youthful masturbation, so that in such cases the inborn nervous predisposition becomes the cause of the masturbation, which in its turn can considerably foster the neurasthenia. So the chain is completed, which unites the hereditary taint with the injury resulting from sexual abuse and of which the last link is sexual neurasthenia.

To be sure, a whole series of other injuries are added in the individual's life, which determine the time of the outbreak and the severity of the symptoms of the sexual neurosis and often also their localization.

There are psychic and somatic factors, which figure as accessory causes of neurasthenia. Such are all excitements of long duration, anxieties, examination worries, mental over-exertion, sudden grief, anxiety and fear, immoderate and unaccustomed bodily exertions, exhausted states after febrile diseases, injuries accompanied by great emotion (traumatic neurosis), intoxications (alcohol, tobacco), and finally exhausting diseases, syphilis, tuberculosis, etc.

The rôle of gonorrhea in the etiology of sexual neurasthenia will be considered separately.

All these injurious influences in the life of physical and mental workers are well adapted to produce conditions of nervous exhaustion, and to act as etiologic factors of general neurasthenia; only the operation of the " specific causes " is still needed to produce the clinical picture of sexual neurasthenia.

These specific causes lie in the sexual life of the individual concerned (Freud), " and are disorders in the present sexual life, or important events of this nature in the past."

"Masturbation and frequent nocturnal pollutions play the principal rôle in the etiology of general neurasthenia, which is characterized by the following symptoms: lassitude, disinclination, dyspepsia, constipation, spinal irritation, impotence, etc." We must not, however, disregard the fact that masturbation and spontaneous pollutions have to be considered already as SYMPTOMS OF GENERAL NEURASTHENIA in perhaps the majority of cases.

Freud has endeavored to separate the so-called " anxiety neurosis " (Angstneurose) as a completely independent symptom-complex from general neurasthenia. Its manifestation is characterized by the following symptoms: general irritability with auditory hyperesthesia and resulting sleeplessness, anxious apprehension, often taking the form of hypochondria and twinges of conscience, then the attacks of anxiety (phobias), agoraphobia, cardiac oppression, sweating outbreaks, trembling, diarrhea, dizziness, congestions, nocturnal fears, and paresthesiæ.

Freud regards the cause of this anxiety neurosis to be " sexual influences, which have in common the factor of restraint or of incomplete satisfaction, as *e. g.* interrupted coitus, abstinence with strong sexual desire, so-called abortive excitement and the like."

The gonorrheal conditions of the urethra and of neighboring glands deserve especial consideration in the etiology of sexual neurasthenia.

It is an only too common experience of every day practice that patients, who perhaps have shown the signs of general neurasthenia more or less markedly for some time, develop a typical sexual neurasthenia in connection with an acute attack of gonorrhea or the course of a chronic one.

Affections of the prostate and posterior urethra are of especial importance here, because for various reasons, they cause an especial nervous irritation in the patient.

To contract gonorrhea has of itself usually an extremely depressing effect upon impressionable, nervous persons; and if the course of the disease drags at all, the hypochondriac ideas of such patients grow from day to day. Each new complication becomes the source of the most serious fears. Such patients, whose whole imagination is concentrated upon their sexual sphere, get into a state of the most intense nervous excitement on account of their gonorrhea. Not a day passes, in which the patient does not believe he can discover a new symptom of some complication. The widespread opinion of the laity that gonorrhea is an incurable disease is embedded in the consciousness of these persons, and drives them sometimes to the rashest acts. There arises a permanent nervous excitability and depression.

The outbreak of the neurosis is favored by still other causes. The sexual abstinence of long duration, commanded by the physician, combined with the often much increased libido results in an over-stimulated state, which from lack of natural satisfaction may incite the patient to masturbation. Nocturnal pollutions then result, which produce renewed weakening and depression of the patient.

When the nervous system of such patients, who have mostly an hereditary neuropathic taint, has suffered from all these conditions, then a new factor is added during a chronic course of a posterior urethritis: namely, the PERMANENT IRRITATION OF THE SPINAL GENITAL CENTERS (Peyer) which proceeds from the prostatic urethra centripetally to the spinal cord. Insuperable impulses to sexual acts, and faute de mieux, to excessive masturbation, make their appearance.

The states of nervous irritation which we find in gonorrhea of the posterior urethra as well as in every case of chronic prostatitis, are also frequently found, when the posterior urethra is the seat of a congestive hyperemia and swelling of the mucosa, as is found in masturbators and persons who give themselves up habitually to other sexual abuses. The phenomena of spinal irritation and of nervous irritable impotence can develop on the basis of this permanent irritation proceeding from the prostatic urethra.

In what manner we must conceive the relationship between sexual neurasthenia and the different kinds of sexual abuse, will be considered in another place.

CHAPTER XXVI

SYMPTOMATOLOGY OF SEXUAL NEURASTHENIA

The polymorphism of the clinical pictures, which the sexual neurasthenics present to us, makes it appear a priori difficult to analyze the often very complicated cases and to reduce the symptoms to the basic types. It seems justified, however, to attempt a schematic presentation of the patients' various complaints and the symptoms and signs discovered in them, in short to draw a typical picture of sexual neurasthenia, inasmuch as a series of characteristic features can be deduced from all clinical histories. There are grouped, however, about these few typical symptoms various manifestations of disease, modified in each particular case, which may often so mask the main affection, that it requires an especially careful analysis of the symptoms, in order to avoid the often natural mistake of interpreting the case as a sexual or nervous disease of organic origin.

There is a famous case of sexual neurasthenia reported by Beard, in which the following diagnoses were made by the various physicians, whom the patient visited: oxaluria, phosphaturia, spermatorrhea, impotence, cerebral anemia, cerebral hyperemia, insufficiency of the ocular muscles, asthenopia, astigmatism, hypermetropia, dyspepsia, Bright's disease, enlargement of the liver, spinal irritation, spondylitis, neuralgia of the coccyx, hemorrhoids, cystitis, irritable prostrate, prostatorrhea, urethral stricture, hyperesthesia of the urethra, syphilis, malaria, exudative pleuritis, hysteria, hypochondria, cerebral congestion, emotional depression, general anemia, nervous exhaustion, tabes dorsalis, progressive paralysis, hallucinations, gout, rheumatism, progressive muscular atrophy, epilepsy, melancholy, and monomania.

It might here be *à propos* to precede a description of the separate symptoms with a typical clinical history, which a medical friend, who is a very good observer of his own trouble, has put at our disposal.

The man in question, a physician 37 years of age, consulted us for impotence and various other genital disturbances, which he describes as follows: (It should be stated at the outset that the man is of remarkably strong physique.) He is now much emaciated, has sunken cheeks, a pale yellow complexion, is prematurely gray, has dark rings about the eyes and deep wrinkles in his face. He gives the impression of a man of forty who has been brought low by disease. He comes of a nervous family, and was always weakly as a child; his intelligence awoke early, but also his sexual instinct. He began to masturbate at the age of 13, without having been seduced to the practice, at first alone, later in the company of other like-minded school comrades. During the trying time of his high-school (Gymnasium) examinations he suffered frequent nocturnal pollutions, which affected him severely. In the vacation after the final examinations he attempted coitus repeatedly, but always suffered from precipitate ejaculation though the erections were good. After this he contented himself, because of fear of infection, with letting himself be masturbated by obliging women, or with indulgence in solitary vice.

Pollutions occurred regularly under strong mental exertion

(such as cramming for examinations) and these were accompanied by dreams, which at the best presented acts of masturbation, but often enough represented merely indecent situations. He suffered also at such times from diurnal pollutions with conceptions of a sexual nature. Severe strangury followed each seminal emission, which was also followed exceptionally by nocturnal enuresis. Dyspeptic troubles began to distress him at about the age of 27; he complained of loss of appetite and constipation, alternating with diarrhea, and gastralgia after sexual acts. This resulted again in marked emaciation and bad appearance. Periods of long sexual abstinence cause depression of spirits: he becomes capricious, restless, quite incapable of work, unsettled, and he chases about town until he finds a woman, who performs manual masturbation for him. A stay in a hydropathic institute and later in the mountains brings decided improvement, and the success of a Weir-Mitchell rest-cure enabled him for about three-quarters of a year to support a liaison with a woman to the satisfaction of both. After breaking off this relation, renewed masturbation. He relapsed quickly into the old condition. Atonic pollutions by day and night. Indifferent dreams attending the pollutions. Complete loss of the erectile power on attempts at coitus, emaciation, disinclination to work, complete prostration; he can read for scarcely ten minutes; his eyes get so tired that the letters dance before them. He sleeps well, but complains of a feeling of extreme exhaustion in the morning after arising. After each pollution he suffers violent pains in the testicles and an itching sensation in the glans penis during the entire day. He suffers further from want of appetite, eructation, gastric cramps, and obstinate constipation.

Recently attacks of exhibition-mania, which cannot always be suppressed in spite of the most careful watching. Torturing strangury and spermatorrhea with micturition.

I have given this clinical history first, because it gives, quite free from confusing accessory symptoms of other local and nervous diseases, a typical example of sexual neurasthenia, in which one can also study the characteristic phase of development of this disease with perfect clearness.

According to Krafft-Ebing we can distinguish three stages of sexual neurasthenia as regards symptoms and pathogenesis. At first the affection manifests itself only as a local genital neurosis, which appears in functional, irritative disorders in the urinary and sexual organs. The next stage shows a characteristic neurosis of the lumbar cord, in which the patient complains not only of local troubles in the urinary and sexual organs, but also of irritative symptoms, which can be referred to the whole lumbar region of the spinal cord.

The symptoms in the third stage result from an extension of the neurosis of the lumbar cord to a general neurasthenia.

In this stage the cases really coincide with general neurasthenia, and it is often very difficult, by a careful history and analysis of the phenomena, to discover the sexual origin of the neurosis.

We shall also adhere to this division of Krafft-Ebing's in our description, since a gradual development of the three stages may be noticed even in the severest cases.

We may also observe by way of introduction that a division into phenomena of irritation and of exhaustion may be observed in almost all symptoms, the functional disorder manifesting itself first as an irritative condition and later, if the injury continues, as a state of exhaustion.

In most cases we can follow this sequence in each chief individual symptom of the sexual neurasthenia; in the disorders of sensibility, in secretion, and in the motor functions.

The local symptoms of the genital organs occurring in sexual neurasthenia often form the sole complaint of patients in the initial stage of the neurosis—which Krafft-Ebing for this reason denotes as the phase of "genital local-neurosis."

In this stage we find exclusively irritative conditions of the sensory, secretory, and motor functions of the urogenital organs.

One of the commonest early symptoms of the neurosis, which perhaps in some cases reaches back into earliest childhood and is the cause of sexual injuries in childhood (masturbation), is the irritation of the CUTANEOUS SENSIBILITY OF THE GENITAL ORGANS.

Marked hyperesthesiæ and later paresthesiæ frequently introduce the affection. The extreme sensitiveness of the skin of the penis and scrotum and especially of the glans penis produce a continual irritation, and concentrate the patient's attention unceasingly on his sexual organs.

One often encounters, to be sure, great difficulty in deciding, whether anatomical changes of the skin do not lie at the basis of this hyperesthesia, or whether it is to be explained as a purely nervous symptom.

Such a hypersensitiveness of the skin is often due to a phimosis, a collection of smegma in the sulcus coronarius, or a balanoposthitis. In the majority of cases, however, not one of all these pathologic states is to be discovered, and yet the patients complain of an intolerable pain at the end of the glans, which may come spontaneously or be produced by touching the organ and by friction against the clothing. A similar hyperesthesia often exists also in the scrotal skin; such patients seek to avoid this burdensome state by always wearing a suspensory padded with cotton. The painful sensations may also appear in the form of neuralgia, of lightning-like pains, which shoot from the anus to the tip of the penis or the scrotum.

The hyperesthesia extends often to the mucous membrane of the urethra and bladder, and here produces the well-known forms of dysuria. The patients feel the expansion of the bladder by the accumulated urine as a painful pressure in the cystic region and a painful need of passing water; but micturition occurs only with sharp pains. At first the urine feels very hot, later a disagreeable burning and feeling of heat comes in the whole penis and the anal region.

The morbidly increased sensibility, the irritation of the sensory nerve-endings, show itself further in an extreme sensitiveness of the testicles and the prostate, which we designate as prostatodynia and orchidodynia. The testicle becomes when touched, and also after long walks or much standing, the source of severe pressing and wrenching pains, which from time to time, especially after long sexual abstinence, are interrupted by torturing neuralgia, "irritable testis." This neurotic hyperesthesia of the testicles is probably also the usual cause of the popularly known "fiancé's testicle pains."

As in the testicles, so also in the prostate we observe a

series of painful sensations, which may occur spontaneously (as prostatic neuralgia), or provoked by defecation, micturition, and forced movements.

Seminal emission becomes a real pain to these patients. The hyperesthesia of the genital organs makes itself felt in the most unpleasant fashion in involuntary pollutions, the great frequency of which is a very constant symptom of the first stage of the disease, as well as in coitus.

We hear the complaint very regularly, that the patients are awakened at night out of sleep at the moment of ejaculation by a burning pain in the whole urethra and the anal region and by excruciating, stabbing pains in the prostate. A series of the most unpleasant painful sensations likewise appears in coitus in place of the orgasm and feeling of satisfaction, especially in the genital glands, and rob such sufferers of all pleasure in the practice of their sexual functions. This is a contributory cause for the severe emotional depression, from which our neurasthenics suffer even in the first stage of the disease, and which is in turn a source of the rapid advance of the general neurasthenia.

If we test the sensitiveness of the urethra by means of introducing a sound, we find there are two principal sites of this increased sensibility: first, the orifice, second the prostatic portion of the posterior urethra. Now we know from many endoscopic investigations (Grünfeld, Ultzmann), that in many cases this hyperesthesia of the posterior urethra has as an anatomical basis a swelling of its mucosa, partly congestive, partly inflammatory in nature. There are also congestive and chronic inflammatory processes in the prostatic parenchyma, which we can often regard as the cause of the prostatic pain.

As a rule manifold paresthesiæ appear simultaneously with the hyperesthesiæ of the skin and mucous membrane. A constant itching of the glans penis, the scrotal skin, the perineal skin and about the anus pursues the patient unceasingly, often even in sleep. Under the false diagnosis of a scrotal eczema all sorts of salves and applications are tried in vain; the patient's attention is continually absorbed by the genital organs because of the permanent itching, and he goes from one skin-specialist to another. Another, perhaps still more distressing form of paresthesia is the continual feeling of moisture at the external urethral orifice, the "feeling of the hanging drop," as it might properly be called. The patient cannot be dissuaded from his idea, that he suffers from a chronic discharge, a chronic gonorrhea, although he convinces himself a hundred times a day that there is no physical basis for the feeling of a drop of liquid. These patients are particularly frightened, when under sexual excitement they feel the escape of some drops of a watery fluid (urethrorrhea ex libidine). The thought that they suffer from an incurable seminal flow now establishes itself immovably in their hypochondriac consciousness.

A peculiar alteration of the sense of temperature ("Cryesthesia") or increased sensitiveness to cold, must be regarded as another paresthesia. We hear not rarely that the patients have a continual feeling of cold in the penis and scrotum, that even in coitus they do not feel the warmth of the female genitals. This cold feeling often occurs only in particular places of the genitals, *e. g.*, on the glans or the scrotum; often, however, the patients feel most unpleasantly cold over the whole surface of the body and shiver; and this sensation does not leave them even in the hot bath or on exercising on a hot day. As Milton declares, this feeling of cold often occurs in just those neurasthenics, whose general bodily constitution is quite satisfactory. Among 150 persons, who had suffered from spermatorrhea, Dicenta observed this feeling of cold in the genitals five times, and the "loss of internal heat" nine times.

Cold paresthesiae combined with hyperesthesia of the urethral mucosa is the reason why many patients feel the outflow as a decidedly cold sensation. They interpret this as a bad symptom, say that the loss of bodily heat is a sign of beginning impotence, of the "slow destruction of the vital forces," as one such hypochondriac complained to me.

These paresthesiae usually extend over the whole region of distribution of the pudic nerve. Hence it happens, that the annoying irritation is felt not only in the penis and scrotum, but frequently also in the perineal skin and the anus.

In some cases the itching is confined solely to the skin in the neighborhood of the anus, and torments the patients in the most unpleasant manner by day and night. Often in such cases hemorrhoids or hyperesthesia is discovered on palpating the prostate, a chronic prostatitis or an anal eczema are diagnosed. The paresthesiae remarkably resemble the symptoms of chronic prostatitis or irritative swelling and congestion of the prostate, which we see so often in masturbators, and the differential diagnosis is made possible only by examination of the secretion expressed from the prostate.

There is indeed a great difference between these two diseases as regards prognosis. The post-gonorrheal neurasthenia, which often develops in the course of a chronic prostatitis, almost never leads to the severe forms of the neurosis, which we shall consider later, and has always a comparatively good prognosis; while the masturbatory neurosis with its paresthesiae of the perineum and the hyperesthesia of the prostate is only an individual symptom of general neurasthenia, and without treatment and without return to normal sexual relations, goes on without fail to the severer degrees of the neurosis.

A patient observed by us for a long time had a tormenting paresthesia of the rectum as the chief symptom of his urosexual neurasthenia, and an extremely annoying itching about the anus. He inflicted severe abrasions upon himself in this region by his unceasing scratching day and night. Only the local treatment of his urethral hyperesthesia by cool sounds made this unpleasant symptom disappear.

Hyperidrosis of the genitals is a similar symptom, which is extremely unpleasant to the patients. This is usally an actually increased secretion of sweat on the scrotum, the intercrural folds, and the fold of the anus; but sometimes the normal secretion of sweat is felt as an *annoying evaporation* because of the abnormal sensations of cold in the genitals. Not merely the perspiration itself burdens the patients to so great an extent, but also the odor of the sweat which in extreme cases may so control the patient's imagination that he considers himself quite unfit for society merely on account of this more or less fancied odor.

This local hyperidrosis is fundamentally different from those cases, where an increased secretion of sweat on the entire body forms a prominent symptom of the neurosis. We observe occasionally in the severe degrees of sexual neurasthenia, perhaps as a partial phenomenon of a neurosis of the sympathetic, a universal or one-sided hyperidrosis, which together with other symptoms—tachycardia, tremor, anemia, etc.—reminds one of the "formes frustes" (abortive forms) of Basedow's disease.

Let us here mention in addition the other extreme of disorders of sensibility, which is, however, observed only in far advanced stages of the affection; namely, anesthesia of the genitalia.

Besides the disorders of sensibility in the skin of the genitals, it occurs not rarely, as a result of organic lesions of the spinal cord,—tabes, multiple sclerosis, and syringomyelia,—that patients complain of a diminished sensibility and especially of a diminution or disappearance of the sensibility of the glans penis. His anesthesia may be a cause of imaginary and of true atonic impotence.

Such cases of cutaneous anesthesia of the external genitals have indeed been observed only exceptionally in paralytic impotence, that is in the severest forms of sexual neurasthenia. The subnormal sensitiveness of the skin often gives occasion for peculiar masturbating manipulations of the urethra, the tactile sensibility of which usually survives that of the skin of the external genitalia.

[The diminished sensibility or complete anesthesia of the urethral mucous membrane in some patients of this category is quite remarkable. Inserting sounds which put the urethra to its highest stretch, instillation of strong solutions of silver nitrate, etc., elicit no pain. In their frenzied masturbatory acts they will insert rough objects, such as rusty nails, corkscrews, etc., into the urethra, and though the manipulations may cause severe hemorrhage, pain is not complained of. W. J. R.]

The first stage of the sexual neurosis includes besides the above-mentioned disorders of sensibility also symptoms of the motor, secretory and vasomotor functions of the genitals, and we must distinguish here also between the phenomena of stimulation and paralysis or exhaustion.

The vasomotor derangements manifest themselves in the already mentioned phenomena of congestive, active hyperemia of the posterior urethra and the prostate, in the local hyperidrosis, and in other phenomena, which we will now consider.

Many patients surprise us with the complaint, that their penis has become smaller, that it is shrunken, and that especially when they intend coitus, the organ, to their horror, becomes small and shrunken instead of becoming erected.

And it is actually a fact of every day experience, that when they undress, such patients, partly from psychic action (shame), partly as a result of the cold outer temperature, show a small, shrunken, cyanotic or livid penis, which feels to the touch like a firm, hard body.

Its consistency is increased by a tonic contraction of the smooth muscles of the blood-vessels in the corpora cavernosa. The vaso-constriction is shown also in the venous stasis, the purplish color of the skin. We can correctly designate this condition as one of " nervous penis."

The paralytic state of the vasomotor functions is shown in the loss of tone of the vaso-constrictors, which we can recognize, for example, in many cases of paralytic impotence by the relaxed condition of the organ. In such patients all the external genitalia are surprisingly withered; the penis and the scrotum are relaxed, the testes feel soft and flabby, and the tactile sensibility is diminished.

To be Continued

DISTILLED WATER VERSUS SALVARSAN IN THE TREATMENT OF SYPHILIS [1]

By G. Arbour Stephens, M. D., B. S., B. Sc., Lond.,

Honorary Physician, Royal Cambrian Institution for the Deaf; Appointed Surgeon Under the Factory Act.

THE simple treatment for syphilis herein recommended consists of the hypodermic injection of 6 to 10 c.cm. of distilled water every three days for two to four weeks.

I was induced to give this treatment a trial as the result of some research work I had done on surface tension, the results of which I published some fifteen months ago. I had previously published in the *Practitioner* an article on the Part Played by Colloids in Physiology and Pathology, in which I drew attention to the value of a consideration of surface tension. An experiment that I carried out to show the effect of the calcium salts on surface tension is rather interesting:

" When pure hydrogen peroxide is added to pure mercury in a clean test tube, catalytic action occurs and oxygen is given off, the mercury remaining unaltered. This reaction is due to an extremely fine film that forms on the surface of the mercury, but, on account of the tension, breaks almost as soon as formed, the making and breaking being rhythmic. On adding a small quantity of a 10 per cent solution of pure calcium chloride to the mercury, shaking well and draining it off, the mercury itself behaved peculiarly, its surface tension having been modified to such an extent that it could be induced to take up all sorts of shapes instead of the usual globular one. When the hydrogen peroxide was added the mercury was immediately changed into a grey colour and was then broken up into minute grey masses, many of which passed, as in the colloidal form, through filter paper; meanwhile the ebullition of oxygen was exceedingly great, and the heat generated sufficient to make the test tube very hot."

This experiment has been given at such length in order to show the marked effect of a slight alteration of surface tension.

The value of mercury in the colloidal form as an antiseptic is due to its possessing the powers of both classes of antiseptics — namely, the power of the heavy metals to combine with protein matter, and the power of chloroform, toluol, and the like to in-

[1] Dr. Stephens' paper in the British Medical Journal presents such a novel point of view that I believe it deserves to be presented to our readers. I refrain, however, from any comment.—W. J. R.

terfere with the surface tension of all living cells. It seemed to me, therefore, that it would be of interest to find out the surface tension of individual substances, and with that object I instituted some experiments.

In some of the experiments it was found that colloid mercury as well as mercury perchloride and carbolic acid have a tendency to reduce the surface tension existing between mercury and potassium chloride, and the fall is not complete at once, but is progressive. This fact is important, for with such a varying surface tension around a living cell the latter finds it very difficult to accommodate itself to its surroundings; in fact it fails, and its life ends.

The water soluble contents of coal-tar pitch, which no doubt are responsible for pitchworkers' cancer, have surface tensions that tend to drop considerably, whereas the soluble contents of blast furnace pitch have not this tendency, at least not to the same extent.

In the *Dublin Journal of Medical Science* for June, 1911, I gave the results of some experiments in which boiled yeast had been added to living yeast in a suitable growing medium, and I there showed that the effect of this addition was to stimulate the living yeast to marked activity, to a rapid life, and consequently to an early death. My experiments on the surface tension of boiled and unboiled yeast showed that whereas the surface tension of the latter was 70.62 dynes per centimetre, the surface tension of boiled yeast solution fell in twenty-four minutes from 70.96 dynes per centimetre, to 66.31, and in five hours to 61.02 dynes per centimetre.

I have previously shown that fertilizing with boiled bacteria stimulates the living ones to rapid growth and an early death. Boiled bacteria being vaccines, we can conclude that vaccines lower the surface tension, and by so doing produce their good results.

This lowering of surface tension is associated with a more rapid production of catalytic products in the cells, but the injection of vaccines is associated with the production of antibodies; therefore it seems but right to infer that the production of antibodies is closely associated with a lowering of the surface tension.

The addition of distilled water to blood corpuscles so affects the osmotic pressure as to cause a passage of water into the cell, which gets larger and eventually scatters its contents. In disease the rapid catalytic changes and the rapid production of antibodies are inter-dependent, and if one can induce these marked catalytic changes with or without a vaccine, one stands the chance of setting free a number of very useful and remedial antibodies.

In such a chronic disease as cancer it seemed to me that the process was allowed to continue owing to the absence of sufficient antibodies, or at least a sufficient number to act together at the same time, and if one could set free any catalytic antibodies in sufficient numbers one might get a good result.

Knowing of no vaccine to induce this antibody effect, it occurred to me that the injection of distilled water might so affect the surface tension as to bring about the osmotic effects, and with this object I determined to try the effect at the first opportunity, which I owe to Dr. Lloyd Edwards, Medical Officer of the Swansea Union, and to whom I desire to express my thanks.

Case I.

A man (in the infirmary), aged 62, who was suffering from immensely enlarged glands of the neck, secondary to an epithelioma of the lip. The glands were suppurating profusely, and the smell was so bad that the room had to be fumigated continuously. I injected 8 c. cm. of distilled water into the skin of the back, having previously rubbed it with alcohol to remove the grease (for the introduction of grease has a marked effect on surface tension). I did this every other day, and after the third injection the smell had disappeared almost entirely and the fumigation was discontinued. The surface of the sore seemed to be much cleaner, and the suppuration became more profuse, but otherwise the disease was not checked.

Case II.

A man who had previously been operated on for epithelioma of the lower jaw by Mr. Bilton Pollard, and soon after for clearing out the glands of the neck. This latter was an extensive operation, but the wound eventually healed up well and firmly. Within three weeks of his discharge from University College Hospital there was a return of the growth, and I thought that if injections of distilled water were started early enough one might be able to do some good. At this time the wounds were quite sound and firm, but after three injections, to my great surprise an abscess headed and burst about the middle of the scar. I continued the injections in the hope that this marked activity presaged a favourable catalytic change in the cells, but the growth increased rapidly and the suppuration came to a head in two other openings. Closely following the suppuration appeared a mass of granulation tissue arising out of the part where the wound had quite healed, which spread rapidly. During all this time the pus was inoffensive, and the nursing of the patient was never objectionable to the least extent."

The marked effect produced by the injections of distilled water made me feel certain that in any similar disease of less malignancy their effect ought to be still better, so with that object I undertook, with Dr. Lloyd Edward's permission, the treatment of the syphilitic patients under his charge. Both he and his assistant, Dr. Dunbar, were rather inclined to treat my mission as somewhat harebrained, but at the end of a week's treatment of my first patient I was able to prove to their satisfaction that the effect was excellent. The Wassermann reaction is, in my opinion, nothing but a very round-about way of determining the surface tension at which haemolysis occurs, and if this view is correct, the time ought not to be far distant when a simpler and more scientific method is introduced, and one that is not open to so many pitfalls.

It is easily understandable from the point of view of surface tension that in several diseases the haemolytic point may be the same although the antibodies may be different.

Case I.

An alcoholic prostitute, aged 26, had been in the infirmary since June, 1912, suffering from ulcers on the face and a large ulcer on the left shin. She was first admitted in August, 1910, having been infected a few months previously.

The area covered by the inflammation and ulcers was wing-shaped, covering both cheeks, upper lip, and a good part of the nose, and over the whole of this area there was considerable thickening. The ulcer on the leg looked indolent and unhealthy. She had not menstruated for two years.

I started treatment on October 25th, and continued it every other day until November 4th, but discontinued it on November 6th, *as she had started to menstruate.* I restarted treatment on November 8th, and continued it every third day till November 23rd, when the ulcer on the leg had healed. By November 9th, the ulceration on the face had cleared, although there was still some thickness, as well as dilated venules to be seen.

Her general health improved greatly, and she looked better and felt in better spirits than she had done for a long time.

The readiness with which the edges of the ulcer took on a healthy appearance was extraordinary, especially as she had ceased to respond to the ordinary methods of syphilitic treatment.

After each injection there was a marked reaction, the face becoming very flushed, and the temperature rising in a short time afterwards as indicated by the two-hourly chart. The four-hourly chart shows it still better.

Her general improvement was a matter of comment by all the others in the ward, and both Dr. Edwards and Dr. Dunbar were surprised.

Case II.

T. A., aged 35, had been in the navy, but after leaving was employed at some works in the neighbourhood, where he received a blow on the arm, as the result of which there was a thickness which persisted longer than the usual bruise. With a history of syphilis, I naturally concluded that this was a syphilitic thickening of the periosteum, and gave him the injections of distilled water every other day. At the end of the fortnight the swelling and pain had disappeared, and he returned to work.

Case III.

T. J., aged 46, was admitted to the infirmary on March 6th, suffering from multiple ulcers of the left leg and foot. There was the brownish scar on the right shin, which confirmed the diagnosis of syphilis. The ulcers on the left leg and foot would nearly heal and then again break down, but never assumed a healthy appearance. I started injecting distilled water on October 31st, and continued the treatment every other day until November 16th, when I did it every third day. By the end of the first week the edges of the ulcers had taken on a very healthy appearance, and the pain from which the man suffered had practically disappeared.

There were ten ulcers altogether, and by November 23rd seven of them had healed over, and the two largest were two-thirds covered with new tissue. The man appeared healthier, and some colour had returned to his face. He said he felt much better, and looked forward to the time for each injection.

A reference to his temperature chart shows that there was

a reaction after each injection, but the temperature did not rise nearly so high as in Case 1.

Case iv.

B. T., aged 24, had a hard chancre ½ in. in diameter on the dorsum penis, which appeared a fortnight before I saw him.

I started injecting him with distilled water on November 2nd, and injected him every third day, and by the 14th it had practically disappeared, as well as the enlargement of the glands in the groin. His general health improved rapidly, and he looked much better after a fortnight's treatment.

Case v.

M. S., aged 20, single, was admitted in November, 1911, as she was pregnant and infected with syphilis. After confinement and some treatment she was discharged, to be readmitted on November 11th, 1912, suffering from tertiary ulcers in different parts of the body. There was a small sore on the right ear and one on the right eye, whilst one seemed to be forming on the forehead.

Treatment was started on November 12th, and by November 19th there was considerable improvement, the ear and eye being practically well, and the swelling on the forehead had subsided.

All the other ulcers had taken on a healthy appearance, so that by November 25th they were all covered over.

Her general health improved greatly, she seemed brighter, looked healthier, and had colour in her cheeks, whilst the appetite improved. She much appreciated the treatment, although she cried on the first occasion.

The temperature reactions in this case were very marked, as in Case 1, rising a few hours after each injection to 100° F.

Case vi.

W. E., aged 26, admitted October 10th for sores on the right leg. Was infected with syphilis in the army.

Treatment was started on November 10th, and, after injections every third day, the gummata on thigh and leg were all covered over by healthy tissue on November 25th. A sore inside the right cheek also subsided, whilst his general appearance became more healthy.

SPECIAL ABSTRACT

INTRASPINAL INJECTIONS OF MERCURY IN GENERAL PARESIS

By Dr. Page. *Bulletin de la Société de Medicine de Paris*, 1913, p. 608.

Whereas the mercurial and arsenical treatment of the ordinary manifestations of syphilis gives prompt results, it has no such effect on general paresis. In fact many authors regard it as dangerous in the latter condition; at any rate it is conceded that even the most intensive specific treatment will not prevent the occurrence of a meningo-encephalitis.

The intravenous injection of salvarsan, also, is no more effective in destroying the spirochetae in the nervous system than are the older methods, even if there is no actual impermeability of the meninges, as Westphal suggested.

Page has hit upon the idea of introducing the medicament directly into the spinal canal. He uses the following preparation:

℞

Succinimide of mercury	0.02
Sodium sulphate	0.70
Sodium phosphate	0.30
Distilled water	100.00

This particular combination of salts is but slightly irritating. The author does an ordinary lumbar puncture and removes ten to twelve cubic centimeters of cerebro-spinal fluid which he saves for subsequent examination. He then introduces with a syringe, through the lumbar puncture needle, ten cubic centimeters of his preparation. This operation is repeated every week.

This method of treatment has practically no untoward effects. There is no pain; occasionally there is a feeling of warmth up and down the back. The night of the injection the pulse may become rapid and there may be headache. Very rarely is there any elevation of temperature or vomiting. The patient should remain in bed the rest of the day, on full diet.

The general effects of this treatment are: improvement in speech and writing, diminution of physical and mental fatigue, restoration of attention and memory, disappearance of tremors, and in one case diminution of pupillary irregularity and of Argyll-Robertson sign. Although remissions do occur in general paresis the fact that such improvement occurs immediately after treatment, that it appears to be lasting, that the Wassermann becomes negative and that the lymphocytosis decreases argues for a specific effect of the treatment instituted. Locally, there is at first an increase in the polynuclears and mast cells, followed by a diminution in the polynuclears, the lymphocytes and the albumen reaction, and finally by a disappearance of the mast cells. In one of the two cases treated in this manner the Wassermann in the cerebrospinal fluid became negative.

Now that, thanks to the researches of Noguchi, spirochaetae have been demonstrated in the gray matter of paretics, the profession should feel encouraged in adopting a method of treatment which attacks the spirochaetae in situ. Since nervous tissue does not regenerate, at least to any marked extent, it is essential to start such treatment early and we can best obtain evidence of beginning cerebral mischief by early and frequent examinations of the cerebrospinal fluid. Lumbar puncture should therefore be practiced systematically in all syphilitics suspected of having nervous system involvement.

The first case treated by the author was an undertaker, fifty-two years old. He was infected with lues fifteen years before, but had not been systematically cared for. His paretic symptoms were of four months' duration. His intelligence was disturbed and he was continually preoccupied with the state of his health. Argyll-Robertson pupils; slight tremor of lips; blood Wassermann positive. Examination of the spinal fluid showed increased amount of albumen, 27 lymphocytes and 2 polynuclears to the field, Wassermann faintly positive. Seven injections of 2 milligrams each of mercury succinimide were followed by a drop in the lymphocytes to 16 to the field, a negative Wassermann, and a striking improvement in the general condition. The mind became clear, the worries as to health vanished, as did the tremors, and the pupils became almost normal. Unfortunately the patient died soon from an intercurrent grippal pneumonia.

The second case was that of a lawyer ten years younger than the previous patient, who had a syphilis of seven years' standing and who had received systematic and thorough treatment. Nevertheless he became hypochondriacal, began to worry about his health, developed unequal pupils and showed characteristic paretic handwriting. Exploratory lumbar puncture showed 15 lymphocytes and 2 polynuclears to the field. Mercury was given by injection for one month, followed by four intravenous injections of salvarsan, but there was no change in the physical or mental condition of the patient. Eleven intraspinal injections of mercury were then instituted. After the first four there was a slight increase in the mononuclear and polynuclear cell count. The third was followed by slight fever and bilious vomiting, following the fifth injection there was a progressive diminution in the number of cells and in the intensity of the albumen reaction. After the eleventh injection the patient was able to assume the ordinary affairs of life. He hunted, went to business and wrote a letter in which it was impossible to find any indication whatever of the disease.

FREQUENCY OF ERUPTIONS AFTER THE USE OF BALSAM OF COPAIBA.

Dr. W. Fischer (Clinic for Skin Diseases of Prof. Blaschko in Berlin) (*Deutsche Med. Wochenschrift,* 1913, No. 18) reports upon the frequency with which eruptions were observed in the clinic of Prof. Blaschko after the use of balsam of copaiba in gonorrhea. The direct cause of this observation was the request of the Central Bureau of the Berlin Benefit Institution for the sick to employ balsam of copaiba in place of the more expensive preparations of the oil of santal. The after-effects of balsam of copaiba had almost been forgotten since the preparations of the oil of santal have been used almost exclusively for the last 30 years. Prof. Blaschko and many other physicians therefore favored the more extensive use of balsam of copaiba. It was soon found, however, that in fully 10 per cent. of the cases eruptions, generally with itching, appeared. Not rarely, there were also small petechiae which finally remained as brownish spots. The development of these blood extravasations shows that the process is not an altogether indifferent one for it proves that balsam of copaiba will either damage the walls of the vessels or else will induce hemolysis.

The author concludes as follows:

"The question is whether these observations justify the further employment of preparations of balsam of copaiba or whether it is imperative to again resort to the oil of santal. The latter is also not free from slight after-effects, usually in the form of gastric disturbance and pain in the region of the kidneys. They are usually however so slight and infrequent that they need cause no alarm. With the most popular preparations, santyl and gonosan, they are still less frequent. According to my own experience, santyl is tolerated best of all. I have never seen eruptions after giving santyl or gonosan. If others confirm the very common idiosyncrasy of the skin toward balsam of copaiba it would be best to drop this preparation and again return to the preparations of the oil of santal."

REVIEW OF CURRENT UROLOGIC LITERATURE

REVUE CLINIQUE D'UROLOGIE

July, 1913

1. Pseudo-cystitis as a Result of Functional Insufficiency of the Bladder.

In the cases studied by Reynès there was at the beginning of the disease, no organic disease of the bladder and no general, e.g., nervous, disturbance. Owing to infrequent emptying of the bladder there resulted a chronic condition of retention and distention followed by the usual consequences. This condition was met with at all ages and in both sexes. For example, children of from 5 to 8 years, intensely absorbed with their games or their studies, neglect the natural calls to urination. At first there is a period of tolerance, next comes the stage of vesical irritation, and it is then that the bladder, always distended, and seldom completely emptied, reacts with symptoms of cystitis; dysuria, cloudy, even purulent urine, and dribbling from incontinence. The author has seen cases in which the children empty their bladder only once or twice in twenty-four hours.

Exactly the same conditions have been observed in domestics who, owing to numerous, pressing, household duties, have postponed urinating from the time they arise, sometimes as long as to mid-day. Workmen and business men also suffer from this condition. In old people the consequences of such perverted hygiene of the bladder lead them to fear that their trouble is due to enlargement of the prostate.

Not only the patients themselves, but physicians as well, have been misled by this condition and erroneous diagnoses of cystitis, calculus, paralysis of the sphincter, enlarged prostate and tumors, have been made in such cases. A careful and detailed inquiry into the patient's mode of life is all that is necessary to determine the true nature of the affection.

The treatment is simple. A physiologic reëducation of the bladder is all that is required for a rapid and complete cure.

6. Foreign Bodies of the Urethra.

Tanton proposes the following classification of foreign bodies of the urethra:

1. Endogenous foreign bodies. This includes all bodies originating in the urinary tract itself. This is further subdivided into:
   - A. Bodies originating in the upper urinary tract and lodging in the urethra secondarily.
   - B. Bodies originating in the urethra itself, autochthonous foreign bodies. All endogenous foreign bodies are calculi.
2. Exogenous foreign bodies:
   - A. Bodies entering any part of the urinary tract by perforating its walls. This group is further subdivided into:
     - (a) Bodies foreign to the organism. These may be:
       - (*a*) Inanimate, such as needles or pins (pointed objects in general) which are accidentally swallowed and ultimately perforate the recto- or vagino-urethral septum and thus pass into the urethra.
       - (*b*) Animate, such as intestinal parasites, especially the teniæ. These pass into the urethra through recto-vesical fistulæ.
     - (b) Foreign bodies belonging to the organism. These are almost always sequestra of bones of the pelvis resulting from tuberculosis or osteomyelitis. Some of the cases reported under this head are very interesting.
   - B. Foreign bodies arriving in the urethra by the natural passages. These fall into two groups:
     - (a) Surgical foreign bodies, such as pieces of catheter, etc.
     - (b) Foreign bodies "of venery and of unconsciousness." These, as is well known, are of the most varied nature.

Localization.—The seat of the foreign body depends on its form. Irregular or pointed objects (pins, needles) become fixed in the mucosa and are usually found in the penile urethra. Rounded objects generally occupy one of the normal dilatations of the canal, such as the cul-de-sac of the bulb and become set there. Cylindrical bodies (pencils, pens) frequently sit astride the vesical neck, one-half in the bladder, the other in the prostatic urethra; they are then known as urethro-vesical foreign bodies. In women the only foreign bodies which occur in the urethra are pointed ones which perforate the mucosa; the others fall into the bladder as soon as they leave the hand. In general, all objects—except rounded ones which are expelled—show a marked tendency to travel inward toward the bladder. This results from erections or from traction on the penis by the patient in an effort to remove the offending body, the point of the pin, for example, which is anterior, becoming fixed when the organ is in a state of erection or traction, and then the whole body being forced backward when the penis becomes flaccid again.

Course.—Small round bodies may be spontaneously expelled during urination. Others may fall back into the bladder. Irregular bodies generally remain in the urethra and give rise to symptoms. The foreign bodies may remain in place for many years. Perhaps the most remarkable case is that in which a hairpin was removed from the penile urethra ten years after its introduction, it having caused no disturbance of micturition, of erection, or of coitus during this period. During their sojourn in the canal both the bodies themselves and the urethral walls undergo changes. Thus the foreign substance often becomes coated with phosphatic salts on the one hand, and the urethra dilates behind the body, on the other. Inflammation occurs and there is a discharge and perhaps a periurethritis. In the latter case a periurethral abscess occurs if the process is circumscribed, otherwise it is diffuse and there may be urinary infiltration. Actual strictures may occur and in some cases the entire urethral mucosa may be destroyed, necessitating a permanent perineal urethrostomy.

Symptomatology and Diagnosis.—The patients rarely present themselves for treatment until active symptoms occur. These are usually urethrorrhagia, acute localized, or dull, radiating, pain, frequency, vesical tenesmus and incontinence, especially diurnal, when the body is urethrovesical in situation.

The diagnosis is made on the history, when obtainable, by palpatiou of the canal when the object is in the anterior urethra, by rectal palpation when the object is in the posterior urethra, by sounding with the bougie à boule [and by endoscopy—Ed.].

Treatment.—Every foreign body should be removed as soon and as simply as possible, either by the natural passages or after surgical intervention (incision). The method of choice is by the Collin forceps through the Valentine-Luys endoscope. With pointed object it may be necessary to perform "version." In some cases (stones) it may be best first to push the object into the bladder and then to remove it with a lithotrite through a cystoscope. It is not wise to prolong such attempts as these, but to resort early to incision. This procedure, depending upon the location of the foreign body, will be either an external urethrotomy or a suprapubic vesical section. External urethrotomy is indicated whenever a foreign body is much encrusted and is embedded in the mucosa, whenever attempts at extraction through the natural passages have failed, and whenever the foreign body is located behind one or more strictures. Suprapubic cystotomy may be indicated when the foreign body is located in the prostatic or membranous urethra.

In women external urethrotomy may be indicated when forceps extraction fails because of the size or adherence of the foreign body. The incision may either be sub-symphyseal, or through the vagina. The latter is the method of choice. A fistula may be avoided by employing the technic advocated by Rochet.

JOURNAL D'UROLOGIE

Vol IV, No. 3, Sept. 1913.

1. Use of Radium in the Treatment of Cancer of the Prostate.

Radium has a definite action upon cancer of the prostate. The drug may be introduced into the gland, either

1. By operation, incising through the usual routes, perineal or vesical, or

2. Without operation, by the natural passages, rectum or urethra, which give ready access to the tumor.

This method of treatment is capable of so reducing a prostate originally inoperable, that a prostatectomy can be done without danger. In other cases it may bring about the cessation of hematuria and sometimes even the disappearance of the entire tumor and of some of the involved glands.

3. Nephrostomy as a Means of Permanent or Temporary Diversion of the Entire Urinary Current.

Nephrostomy is the best means of achieving the above result, for all other remedies such as implantation of the ureter into the vagina, into the urethra, or into the intestine end fatally, sooner or later, owing to pyelonephritis.

Ureterostomy alone is at all comparable to nephrostomy but it can be preferred only on the ground of its being less dangerous than the latter. On the other hand ureterostomy has the following disadvantages: 1. Drainage of the kidney is less certain. 2. There is a possibility of renal retention from an ascending ureteritis or from a kink of the ureter. 3. It is impossible to reëstablish the normal course of the urine into the healed bladder or into a new-formed bladder cavity.

The objections that can be raised against nephrostomy are first, that it hits the kidney directly and therefore exposes that organ to occasional attacks of nephritis or hemorrhage (which are rare), and, secondly, that it creates a fistula necessitating the wearing of an apparatus. This latter objection holds just as well for ureterostomy as it does for nephrostomy, but as a matter of fact the fistula is no very great inconvenience. With a good apparatus, and there are many such on the market, the patients lead a perfectly normal life. They do not exhale that urinous odor of which so much has been made. In this connection the author cites the histories of two patients. Both were men of the world who led very active lives, they travelled, hunted, went into society without any incommodation.

Disregarding the disadvantages of the fistula, nephrostomy presents the following advantages: 1. It permits of ready access to the renal lesions which necessitate the operation in the first place. 2. It allows of an ultimate reëstablishment of the urinary current, if this is desired. 3. Most important of all, it permits of such excellent drainage that the development of pyonephroses and the reproduction of calculi are out of the question.

4. Uretero-vaginal Fistula Cured by Permanent Ureteral Catheterization.

Boeckel reports the case of a woman of 45 on whom he performed a total abdominal hysterectomy for epithelioma of the cervix. He drained both through the abdominal wound and through the vagina. Recovery was uneventful until the 18th day when the patient complained of passing her urine per vaginam and of being constantly wet. An injection of methylene blue into the bladder failed to come through the vagina. The cystoscope showed no abnormal orifices in the bladder. There was therefore no vesico-vaginal fistula.

During cystoscopy, however, it was observed that no urine came out of the left ureteral orifice and on catheterization of that side an obstruction was met with at 5 cm. from the meatus. It appeared clear therefore that the wetting was due to the presence of a left uretero-vaginal fistula resulting probably from a ligation of the ureter during the operation with subsequent necrosis.

After several unsuccessful attempts, a fine catheter (No. 12 of the Pasteau scale) was passed by the obstruction into the kidney pelvis. Larger and larger catheters (up to No. 16) were passed and the tract irrigated with silver nitrate. The 16 catheter was allowed to remain in situ (with but one withdrawal) for about 10 days when it was permanently removed. The urine cleared up and there was no more leakage. The patient was well a year and a half after operation. She still admitted a No. 16 catheter.

5. Nephrectomy without Drainage for Renal Tuberculosis.

The patient was sent into the hospital with a diagnosis of appendicitis. Vaginal examination, however, revealed tenderness and a thickened cord in the right cul-de-sac which proved to be ureter. As the urine was purulent and contained tubercle bacilli the diagnosis of renal tuberculosis was made. Separation of the urines of the two sides with the Luys segregator was not successful owing to a marked bullous edema of the bas-fond which allowed of the mixture of the two urines through depressions between bullæ below the instrument.

It was only after catheterization of the left ureter was accomplished that a nephrectomy of the right side was decided upon. The wound was closed without drainage and healed by primary union.

Cystoscopy, done six months later, showed an absolute cure of the vesical lesions. All the subjective symptoms (pollakiuria, colic, etc.) had disappeared also.

7. Value of Our Anti-gonorrheal Armamentarium.

According to Janet we treat gonorrhea either by letting it alone, by balsamics, by antiseptics (local), by mechanical means, by caustics and operations, or by serotherapy. The first two methods are dismissed by the author as being pusillanimous. The last named method is of value only in the complications of gonorrhea. The others, with one exception, have only occasional indications; they are generally harmful. The exception is the method of treatment by local antiseptics, which remains our safest remedy. But by this means we do not actually destroy all the gonococci in the tissues, for those that are deeply located cannot possibly be affected by any external medicament. We simply destroy the superficial organisms and thus prevent reinfection at the same time, allowing the protective powers of the body a full opportunity to overcome the deeper-seated infection.

8. Clinical and Therapeutic Note on Bacillary Cystitis.

Bacillary cystitis is secondary to kidney involvement. Curative treatment would therefore necessitate nephrectomy and it follows that vesical treatment can only be palliative. It is a common custom to make medicated instillations into the naturally emptied (not catheterized) bladder. The author has found that of cases treated in this manner, apparently under the same conditions, some would show marked improvement whereas others would not respond to treatment. He attributes this discrepancy to the fact that in the latter cases the bladder was not completely emptied and that a much greater dilation of the medicament was used than was intended. He made a series of investigations in this direction and found that in more than 60 per cent. of naturally evacuated bladders he could withdraw with the catheter from ten to forty cubic centimeters of residual urine.

JOURNAL D'UROLOGIE

Vol. IV, No. 4, Oct., 1913

1. **Post-operative Treatment of Suprapubic Prostatectomy.**

Marion sets forth very clearly, step by step, his management of the patient after the operation. He takes up, in order, the local treatment, the general treatment, and the avoidance of complications.

Local treatment varies according to the four stages of recovery. During the stage of hemostasis which lasts 3 days, the gauze tamponade is still in place in the prostatic bed and the entire drainage is through the large (modified) Freyer tube introduced into the bladder through the hypogastric wound. If the drainage fluid is too bloody some ergotine may be injected. The dressing should not be changed unless absolutely necessary. During this period the patient may complain bitterly of tenesmus and of desire to urinate. Morphine and belladonna suppositories will usually suffice to control this pain until it ceases spontaneously on removal of the packings.

The stage of contraction of the hypogastric wound begins with the withdrawal of the packings and the large tube on the fourth day. A special elbow drainage tube with an irrigating attachment is then inserted and replaced by progressively smaller tubes every third or fourth day. The patient should be kept clean, the dressings being changed whenever they are soiled. The drainage stops being bloody on about the seventh day.

The stage of closing of the hypogastric wound begins on the twelfth day when hypogastric drainage is discontinued and a permanent catheter inserted into the bladder through the urethra. The abdominal dressings should be dressed as often as necessary. When the hypogastric wound is entirely closed the permanent catheter should be left in place 48 hours longer and then removed definitively. This stage is reached, on an average, 21 days after operation.

The last stage comprises the restoration of the bladder to normal. The urine may be cloudy and there may be burning on passing water but these symptoms usually clear up in three weeks to two months under appropriate medication. The best remedies are urotropine and nitrate of silver instillations.

As regards general treatment, it may be necessary to stimulate actively for the first 24 hours. After that sedatives are more likely to be in order; for example, suppositories of belladonna and morphine, and pantopon, 1 to 2 centigrams. The digestive tract needs looking after. On the second day milk and vichy may be given. The bowels should be moved on the third day and from then on the diet may be built up more substantially, except that nitrogenous foods should be restricted. The bowels should be kept loose to prevent hemorrhage from straining. The urinary system of course requires special watching. Proper diet, the forcing of fluids, and the administration of diuretics and urinary antiseptics, are the factors which prevent trouble from this source. Patients should not be allowed to leave the bed until the bladder wound is closed, otherwise they increase the chances of a phlebitis setting in.

As regards complications, secondary hemorrhages are very rare if the packing is not disturbed until the fourth day. Infection of the abdominal wall can often be prevented by putting a piece of gauze packing soaked in peroxide between the tube and the lips of the wound during the time the bladder is irrigated. Sometimes the permanent catheter functionates poorly; when this is the case a Lebreton sound will usually afford better drainage or else a small catheter may be introduced temporarily into the bladder through the abdominal wound. Delayed cicatrization or fistulization (failure of the abdominal wound to close after 35 days) is overcome by stripping the bladder from the abdominal wall, sewing the former together tight but leaving the latter slightly open, and introducing a permanent urethral catheter. Stricture of the urethra is treated by dilation or by urethrotomy. So much for the local complications.

Serious general complications are as follows: (1) Fever. This is generally due either to insufficient drainage of the prostatic bed or to the presence of the urethral sound. Treatment is self-evident. (2) Nephritis is controlled by a low nitrogen and salt diet, forcing fluids, and elimination. (3) Pyelo-nephritis should be treated by a milk diet, diuretic drinks and urinary antiseptics. (4) Urinary infection is readily overcome by continuous bladder irrigations. (5) Phlebitis may assume three types: (a) A mild form characterized by pain in the lower extremity, edema, and a slight elevation of temperature. (b) A more serious form is that in which the local manifestations are slight but the general reaction is severe. This type is an infective phlebitis and much mischief may result from the spreading of small microbic emboli through the circulation. (c) The most serious and insidious form is that in which there is a phlebitis of the deep periprostatic veins. It is in these cases that those large emboli are shot off which prove fatal. The treatment consists in confining the patient to bed, in immobilizing the affected part and in stimulation where necessary.

2. Wounds of the Bladder by Impalement.

In order for a condition of impalement to exist three features are required: (1) The wound should be caused by an object in the form of a pale or stake. (2) The point of entrance must be the perineum. (3) The pale must penetrate the pelvis through the inferior orifice of the pelvic girdle. It is immaterial whether the body falls upon an immobile pale or whether the pale is forced into the immobile body. A study of the etiology of this injury has shown:

(1) When the injury is produced by a blunt pale, but when the fall is not from a very great height, the foreign body will penetrate by the natural orifices and will affect, in men, the rectum and bladder, and in women, the vagina and bladder.

(2) When the injury is produced by a blunt pale, but the fall is great, the pale will penetrate at the point of application wherever this may be, and will determine severe injuries.

(3) When the injury is produced by a pointed pale the penetration will occur at the point of contact no matter how high the fall. Such injuries usually penetrate very deeply.

The first symptom to be complained of is pain. This may or may not be associated with general symptoms depending upon involvement of the peritoneum and viscera other than the bladder. Hemorrhage is always present and in some cases may endanger life directly. One of the most important symptoms is escape of urine through the wound, either immediately or after the lapse of a few days. On the other hand both anuria and retention of urine have been known to occur but it is important to bear in mind that escape of urine into the peritoneum may simulate either of these conditions. When the anus is torn the escaping urine may be mixed with fecal material and in recto-vesical empalings both gas and feces may escape through the urethra.

The diagnosis is made by examining the wound of entrance, by examining the foreign body if possible, by rectal palpation (important), by catheterization, cystoscopy and injection of air into the bladder, and by proctoscopy. Clinically it is important to distinguish intraperitoneal from extraperitoneal injuries.

3. Nephrostomy as a Means of Deviation of the Urinary Current (concluded).

Pakowski concludes his study of the subject as follows:

1. Of all the methods of high deviation of the urinary current, nephrostomy offers the maximum security as regards the conservation of the kidneys. The mortality is about 4½%.

2. The other methods of deviation are: implantation of the ureters into the skin, the urethra, the vagina or the intestine. All these have a much higher mortality than nephrostomy and subject the patient to the danger of pyelonephritis. Ureterostomy alone gives results comparable to those of nephrostomy but kidney drainage is much less certain and it is impossible to reestablish the urinary current into a new-formed bladder. On the other hand nephrostomy offers the possibility of attacking the renal lesions and by thorough drainage, preventing ascending infection, as well as offering a chance for the ultimate reestablishment of the urinary current. Pyelostomy alone would seem, theoretically, to be a superior procedure, as it drains the pelvis just as well without necessitating traumatism to the renal parenchyma.

3. Nephrostomy is indicated in the following conditions: (a) In acquired disease of the bladder (tumor, tuberculosis, etc.). The drainage may be temporary or permanent. (b) In congenital affections of the bladder (exstrophy, absence of vesical sphincter). In such cases this procedure would be the first step toward the establishment of a new bladder. (c) In disease of the pelvic organs invading the bladder or compressing the ureters (cancer of the uterus or prostate). (d) In traumatic lesions of the bladder or ureters, especially in persistent vesico-vaginal fistulae. The deviation is maintained only long enough for the lesions to be repaired. (e) In certain cases of renal lithiasis nephrostomy is the only means of preventing the continuous formation of calculi.

The paper is followed by a bibliography of over three hundred references.

4. **Unsuccessful Treatment of Renal Tuberculosis, Nephrectomy.**

The patient, a woman of 20, complained in 1910 of right renal pain and slight pyuria (40 leucocytes to the field of centrifuged urine). The right kidney was ptosed, but normal in size and not tender. Cystoscopically there was a raspberry-like proliferation of the mucosa about the right ureter opening; below the left ureter orifice, which was normal, there was a slight erythema with one or two small ulcerations. The right ureter could be catheterized for only 2 or 3 cm., the left was unobstructed. The right kidney urine showed slight evidences of suppuration, the left being clear. The following April (1911), the patient's condition remaining about stationary in the interval, injections of Maragliano's bacteriolysin were commenced. Every week 3 injections of 1 c.c. each were given for 3½ months (42 in all). The next July there was much less pus and albumen in the urine but there were a fair number of red blood cells, the latter being probably due to a congestion of the kidney caused by the bacteriolysin. A guinea pig was again injected with the urine with negative results. (An injection made the previous year proved positive.) The local and general condition showed much improvement so that the following October the case was presented before the French Urologic Congress as one of improvement under specific treatment.

This spring, however, the pains returned, the right kidney seemed larger and irregular, the urine was very purulent, and the cystoscope showed that the bladder condition had spread. Division of the urines proved that the left kidney was still intact. Nephrectomy of the right side was therefore proposed and successfully carried out.

Gauthier concludes that Albarran's advice as to renal tuberculosis still holds good: "Early diagnosis, early nephrectomy."

5. **Urethroceles in Man.**

Urethroceles are permanent and real cavities, lined with mucous membrane, and formed by the dilated urethra or by an open pouch of the canal. The cavity must be large enough to retain a part of the urine of a micturition. Pathologically urethroceles may be divided into those of the anterior urethra which are much the most frequent, those of the posterior urethra, and total urethroceles formed by extension of the first-named variety. In general urethroceles are located on the inferior wall of the canal, which is the weakest and least supported. According to their etiology urethroceles are divided into two distinct groups: Secondary urethroceles, which result from some pathologic lesion of the urethra, and primary urethroceles which appear without apparent cause either at birth (congenital), or in adult life (primary acquired urethroceles).

Secondary urethroceles result either from calculi, from strictures, which may be gonorrheal, traumatic, or congenital, or from traumatism. The latter may be external or internal (false passage). Finally, secondary urethroceles have been known to follow operations or chronic urinary abscesses when the walls become epithelialized.

As regards primary urethroceles, it seems pretty clear that those existing from birth (congenital) arise from a weakness of the urethral walls due to a defective calibration of the urethra. The primary acquired urethroceles, on the other hand, seem, according to the authors, to arise in most part from a blennorrhagic urethritis. The intermediary stage appears to be the follicular cyst, and when this has the right location, etc., it may enlarge, become epithelialized, and form a true urethrocele.

Symptoms—Characteristic of this condition is a tumefaction on the under side of the penis or in the perineum, which enlarges during micturition. Post-mictional incontinence is another important evidence of this condition. Pain is rare unless some complication supervenes; the same holds true of cloudy urine. Ejaculation is often difficult, the semen remaining in the cavity until the penis becomes flaccid. Sterility may result.

Physical examination, especially during micturition, reveals a characteristic fluctuating tumor on the ventral surface of the penis which can be transilluminated like a hydrocele. The diagnosis is further established by exploration with a sound, by urethroscopy, and by radiography after injection with a suitable opaque material.

Course—The tendency of the urethrocele is always to increase in size. Infection may occur at any time and fistulae may result from the breaking open of abscesses. Although the condition is not usually a serious one, a fatal issue may result from an ascending infection.

Treatment varies according to whether the urethrocele is or is not accompanied by urethral obstruction. Of course, if there is a stricture or stone, the indication is to remove these contributing factors. The only real cure, however, can be effected by excision of the urethrocele itself. The technic is described by the authors. They point out the danger of secondary fistulæ resulting from the use of a permanent catheter after the operation. The best means of deviating the urinary current, they say, is a suprapubic cystotomy.

6. Technique of Lavage without Urethral Catheter.

A. Lavage of the Anterior Urethra.—The patient lies on his back. The bottom of the irrigating vessel is raised one meter from the table. With two fingers of the right hand the operator grasps the rubber tube just outside the special canula (devised by Janet) and thus controls the latter. The pinch-cock being opened, a little fluid is allowed to escape but a bubble of air is caught in the canula to serve as an index. To lavage the anterior urethra the canula is successively introduced into and pulled out a bit from between the lips of the meatus, the flow being established in the former position and cut off in the latter, thus allowing for drainage of the canal. From time to time this procedure is discontinued and the fluid in the bulb massaged out through the perineum by the free fingers of the right hand. One must make sure that the fluid penetrates all the way to the bulb by noting whether there is a free return when the canula is withdrawn. If not, the pressure may be increased by slightly raising the irrigating stand. A tight prepuce or a pinhole meatus must be overcome in the usual manner.

B. Lavage of the Anterior and Posterior Urethrae.—Great care and gentleness must be exercised in this procedure. A liter of fluid is to be divided equally between the two parts of the urethra. The irrigating can is placed at precisely 1 m. above the bed level. The fluid must have a temperature of 38 to 39° (100–102F.). The anterior urethra is first lavaged; the posterior portion is then attacked by obturating the meatus with the canula and, at the moment when the sphincter is naturally relaxed, allowing the fluid to run into the bladder. Three procedures are available to achieve this end:

1. The meatus is incompletely obturated, thus allowing a small stream of fluid to escape alongside the canula. This affords a safety-valve arrangement when the pressure is increased.

2. The fluid is allowed to run in jets by opening and closing the fingers over the rubber tube.

3. Continued lavage is obtained by allowing the fluid to run directly against the sphincter, the meatus being closed all the time.

If these methods are unsuccessful novocainization of the canal may be tried. If repeated attempts fail, the height of the irrigator may be carefully varied, never increasing it above 1.3 m. above the bed level, and always stopping when the patient complains of pain. The pressure should never be increased above 1 m. in acute cases of gonorrhea. When all such methods fail, lavage may be carried out with a fine, well lubricated No. 13 Nelaton catheter.

C. Lavage of the Female Urethra.—This is very simple. A soft end canula is used and the meatus obturated in the usual manner, the patient being told to strain in the meantime as if passing her water.

Nephrolithotomy.

While the operative results of lithotomy have been very satisfactory at the hands of most renal surgeons, and it has been the operation of choice for renal calculi for the past twenty years, M. Krotoszyner, San Francisco (*J. A. M. A.*, November 8), sees in it some dangers which, he thinks, ought to lessen its popularity. The most important of these is postoperative hemorrhage, which lends to it an almost ominous aspect. Perirenal infection and the still graver septic nephritis are risks incurred in nephrolithotomy. An infected stone-kidney and fistula of shorter or longer duration is the rule, and in many cases relieved only by a secondary nephrectomy. Cases are reported of these complications and Krotoszyner thinks they are a serious drawback to the operation. Posterior pyelotomy for aseptic and moderately infected cases, and for the majority, nephrectomy, are advocated by him as the safest and best. He concludes as follows: "1. Nephrolithotomy is connected with serious immediate and remote untoward results. 2. It should be, wherever feasible, replaced by posterior pyelotomy. 3. Nephrectomy is the simplest, quickest and safest curative method for pyonephrotic stone-kidney, provided the function of the other kidney is satisfactory.

Implantation of Ureters.

Two cases of implantation of ureters into the colon by the oblique method, somewhat modified by allowing the ureter to dangle its free portion in the lumen of the bowel, are reported by Carl Beck (*J. A. M. A.*, November 8). He also gives a method of procedure and describes the methods of its performance. One of his patients survived the operation eighteen months without indication of disease of the kidneys until just before his death, which was due to tuberculosis of both lungs and kidneys, the former predominating as far as the symptoms were concerned, though the kidneys were found very badly disorganized. In the second case three operations were performed, the first for calculus, the second one for prostatectomy and in the third the ureters were transplanted, the right one into the appendix, the other more directly into the colon. The patient recovered promptly from the operation and was greatly improved. Beck closes his paper with the following conclusions: "I consider this process of temporary transplantation analogous to temporary gastroenterostomy for an ulcer of the stomach or duodenum. Though only the short period of a few months has elapsed since the implantation in the second case, I am inclined to believe that this patient also will, in course of time, develop pyelitis; but his bladder may have a chance to recover and become a healthy viscus, and a reimplantation of the ureters may be made into the bladder, if he does not prefer the present tolerable condition. In cases of tuberculosis, a permanent implantation made into the bowel is only palliative, but the method of free end implantation of the ureter or the implantation into the appendix insures a longer period of freedom from pyelitis than any other. I think it is even possible to implant both ureters into the appendix." The article is illustrated.

THE AMERICAN JOURNAL OF UROLOGY

WILLIAM J. ROBINSON, M.D., EDITOR

VOL. X FEBRUARY, 1914. No. 2

EROSIVE AND GANGRENOUS BALANITIS. THE FOURTH VENEREAL DISEASE. A FURTHER REPORT.

By B. C. CORBUS, M.D., Chicago, Ill.

IN May, 1909, Dr. Frederick G. Harris and I reported our observations on a specific form of balanitis, due to a symbiosis of a spirochete and a vibrio. This was the first time in this country that attention was drawn to this specific form of balanitis, although abroad Scherber and Müller [2] had classified this form of infection and proved conclusively that balanitis gangrenosa was identical with the "balano-posthite erosive circinee" of Bataille and Berdal,[3] only representing different degrees of severity.

Notwithstanding the fact that reports have come from McDonagh [4] in London, Scherber [5] in Finger's Clinic in Wein, Dind [6] in Switzerland, Romeo [7] in Italy, and Kallionzes [8] in Greece, since Scherber's and Müller's [9] publication in 1904, an extended search of the American literature and text-books still shows a lack of appreciation of the virulency of these organisms.

Scherber's [10] second and extensive communication, published in 1910, on the different forms of balanitis describes the condition in detail.

Definition. Erosive or gangrenous balanitis is a specific infectious venereal disease, caused by a symbiosis of a vibrio and a spirochete, with local and constitutional symptoms varying with the severity of the infection.

Occurrence. In private practice in this country the disease is uncommon, probably occurring once in two hundred cases. However, in the dispensary work where material comes from the lower walks of life, the infection is fairly common.

Scherber [11] reports eighty-one cases that occurred in Finger's Clinic in four years.

That more cases are not reported in this country, is, I believe, due to the lack of recognition and it is with this idea in view that I have had the accompanying pictures and photo-micrographs made.

Bacteriology. Abundant evidence is at hand to show that in noma and Vincent's angina the etiological factors are a spirochete and a vibrio. Rona [12] in 1905 says: "Noma begins without exception in gangrenous stomatitis. If the fusiform bacillus and spirochete found in the mouth are etiological factors in gangrenous stomatitis, since the organism is found in such abundance in noma, it must be due to the same cause."

In 1905, Weaver and Tunnicliff [13] described a fusiform bacillus which was isolated in pure cultures from cases of Vincent's angina and ulcero-membranous stomatitis. Later, Tunnicliff [14] described three strains of fusiform bacilli isolated in pure cultures from the normal mouth; these resembled the organisms she found in Vincent's angina and ulcero-membranous stomatitis.

In the first publication of this subject, by Harris and myself,[15] numerous authors were cited and abundant clinical proof was obtained to substantiate the pathogenicity of these organisms.

The accompanying photo-micrograph from Tunnicliff's [16] work shows typical vibrios and spirochetes cultured from a case of noma, and she believes the organisms to be one and the same, only representing different stages of development. Ellerman [17] takes exception to this, however, claiming the lack of motility of the cultured organism.

I have repeatedly examined the spirochetes found in Vincent's angina under the dark field illuminator. Here the organism is identical with that found in erosive and gangrenous balanitis, the motility being one of the characteristic and diagnostic features.

Since the conditions that favor the growth of these organisms, *i.e.*, heat, moisture, filth and absence of air, are more ideal in the genitalia than in the mouth, it is easy to conceive how an organism may leave its normal saprophytic domain and under proper anerobic conditions become pathogenic and produce extensive destruction.

Examination of vaginal secretions of one hundred normal women [18] showed bacteria and spirochetes similar to those found in smegma, but no spirochetes of balanitis.

In eleven cases of clinically evident vulvitis and vaginitis, vibrios and spirochetes were found.

Etiology. As shown by the micro-photograph that accompanies the pictures, the vibrio and spirochete are the predominating organisms found. We can easily argue, as did **Rona in 1905**, if the fusiform bacillus and spirochete found in the mouth are etiological factors in gangrenous stomatitis and gingivitis, since the organisms are found in such abundance in erosive and gangrenous balanitis it must be due to the same cause, especially since in the histories of all my cases unnatural sexual relations or a wetting of the labia was admitted.

A. Predisposing causes:
  (1) Long tight foreskin, excluding the air, always present in a more or less degree.
  (2) Wetting the labia or penis with saliva.
  (3) Unnatural sexual relations, due to alcohol.

B. Exciting causes:

The existing cause of this form of balanitis, as stated before, is a symbiosis of a vibrio and a spirochete. These two organisms are always found together. Both have been demonstrated in sections, in the blood vessels and in the inguinal glands.

The vibrio grows under anerobic conditions on serum agar. It occurs singly or in chains of two or more individuals. It is a slightly curved rod-shaped organism with pointed ends, measuring from 2 m. in length to 0.8 m. in width. It stains by the ordinary dyes and is Gram-positive, although the decolorization must be performed very carefully, as the organism gives up the gentian violet very readily. It is preferable to use 70 per cent. alcohol for this purpose.

The spirochete is Gram-negative, but stains with the ordinary dyes; with the Giemsa stain it takes a bluish red. These organisms are best seen with the dark ground illuminator. They average from 6 to 30 m. in length and about 0.2 m. in width. The windings are not acute and the ends of the organism terminate in the center of the spiral. The motion of the organisms is very rapid; they travel from place to place, resembling a small snake; they have a rotary motion, but this is not as pronounced as the backward and forward motion.

Scherber [19] does not believe in the pathogenicity of the fusiform bacillus after unsuccessful attempts at animal inoculation with cultures, and considers the spirochete responsible for the lesions.

A rapid and simple method of collecting the pus is by capillary attraction with small capillary pipettes. These may be pushed deep into the ulcers and a quantity of fresh discharge obtained. Either examine with the dark field illuminator or fix and dry and stain from two to three minutes with carbo-fuchsin. Examine without cover-glass with oil immersion. (This is the method that was used in the accompanying photo-micrograph.)

Pathology. The pathologic condition in the milder forms of balanitis erosiva circinata consists simply of a flaking off of the epithelium, leaving small superficial erosions. When the desquamation is more marked there are bright red ulcers, which are surrounded by a small white zone, the remains of the necrotic epithelium.

In the surrounding tissue there is an exudation of leucocytes and plasma. The organisms are found in the necrotic membrane. At times they can be demonstrated in the tissues and the blood vessels, as shown by Scherber and Müller.[20]

In the more severe grades of infection there is more venous stasis and more exudation, resulting in marked phimosis which predisposes to gangrene. As Scherber and Müller pointed out, the whole condition is one of degree only, but for clinical purposes we may distinguish two types: (1) balanitis erosiva circinata and (2) balanitis gangrenosa.

Symptoms. Balanitis erosiva circinata commences with the appearance of one or more small grayish-white patches in the preputial sac. At the time of the development of the erosion an offensive thin pus is produced, with a characteristic stinking odor and of the usual yellowish-white color; in the more severe cases it becomes grayish-white or grayish-brown.

Pus from lesions is innocuous (Berdal and Bataille [21]) and in its development the inoculation never becomes pustular, but necrosis of epithelium always represents the beginning and the future process is polycyclic.

Inoculation shows preference for sulcus coronarius, next on inside of prepuce and last on glans. In development all of glans penis is affected and under favorable anerobic conditions the whole fossa navicularis is affected. It must be borne in mind that more or less phimosis is an essential factor.

In the mild cases the foreskin may be easily retracted, but in the more severe forms marked phimosis develops; there is considerable itching and burning behind the glans; the act of urination is practically without pain. In contradistinction to the gangrenous form in this type of the disease, constitutional symptoms are slight or absent.

As the process follows no hard and fast lines there are certain deviations from the above picture. The process may be limited to the glans and the inner surface of the foreskin be unaffected. This may be extreme or mild, but is always present on the covered portions of the glans. The inflammatory condition may remain a purely erosive superficial process and may recover spontaneously.

Berdal says in simple cases healing takes place in four to five days. Scherber has seen spontaneous healing almost completed in 48 hours by simple washing and admission of air by retracting foreskin. He further states from observation, that the height of development usually occurs in 4 to 8 days after exposure to infection, and that he seldom saw cases of four weeks' incubation persist for three to four weeks.

In a number of cases the process does not remain superficial, but develops deep diphtheritic and gangrenous ulcers, which complicate the clinical picture in many ways. In some cases when one is able to retract the foreskin, one sees after removal of the pus, inside of the erosions small round ulcers varying in size from a pin-head to that of a pea. These ulcers are moderately deep and on the whole flat and surrounded by a red zone. They are covered by a closely adherent pseudo-membrane. In other cases the ulcers are more extensive and deeper, the average size being about that of a dime. These may become confluent and extend over the whole surface of the sulcus or the inner surface of the foreskin.

These balanitic ulcers are of a somewhat irregular outline and are surrounded by a small inflammatory, slightly elevated border. This border is clean-cut and the sides somewhat slanting; the base is uneven, with a firm yellowish-white or yellowish-brown membrane which is often edematous and swollen. When more edematous this false membrane appears as a sort of friable slime. Here and there may be hemorrhagic spots which sometimes give rise to hemorrhages from the base of the ulcer.

In the severe forms the constitutional symptoms are more marked. Scherber and Müller noticed in a majority of their cases chills and fever, and at the onset vomiting; the average temperature ranges from 100 to 101 degrees. There is marked edema, the external skin being red and edematous; the infiltration may extend to the root of the penis in some cases. The dorsal lymph cord is usually palpable and the inguinal glands are enlarged, but not painful. Unless the phimosis is complete there is no pain on urination; when, however, the urine is not able to pass freely and dilates the preputial sac there is considerable pain. The discharge is the most profuse in this type of disease. By gently irrigating the preputial sac with sterile water and wiping the external urethral orifice we can easily exclude a gonorrhea by having the patient urinate in two glasses.

In the majority of cases of balanitis gangrenosa there occurs a marked edema of the subcutaneous tissue of the penis, which extends to the root and causes a marked phimosis. If the ulcer is situated on the inner surface of the foreskin it shows externally as a dark, bluish-red area within the surrounding bright red inflammatory tissue. The congestion and abnormal pressure, due to edema, favor in a marked degree the progress of the disease. Soon the foreskin over the ulcer becomes black, and a complete necrosis of the part occurs. If the ulcer is situated on the glans, in a short time it may produce complete destruction of the same, or may even cause an extremely rapid gangrene of the organ which may extend even to the root of the penis, as may be seen by the fourth case reported in this paper. The ulcers in these cases are deep, the edges sharp and perpendicular, the base grayish-green or brownish; or it may show hemorrhagic areas or be changed into a black necrotic mass.

The discharge at this time is more offensive than in the erosive type; it has a grayish-yellow or yellowish-brown color and at times it may be slightly hemorrhagic, but always with the same characteristic odor. The inguinal glands are enlarged; there is a mild grade of sepsis present. General malaise is marked. There may be vomiting and the temperature may reach 104. The tenderness of the part is extreme.

Diagnosis. This disease is not so uncommon as one might suspect; unfortunately it is usually mistaken for chancroidal infection. The period of incubation may be the same in the two conditions; but with the characteristic thin yellowish-white offensive discharge, in which one finds vibrioform organisms and a spirochete, the diagnosis should not be difficult.

The ulcers of the two forms of infection may simulate each other very closely. In this form of balanitis when the infection is at all severe there is marked phimosis and considerably more inflammatory reaction. The enlarged inguinal glands are painless, while with a very insignificant chancroidal sore a suppurating bubo is often present.

Chancroidal ulcers are as a rule multiple, but they do not spread with as great rapidity as do the ulcerative forms of balanitis. Whereas the ulcers in both diseases have a clean-cut punched-out appearance, there is greater tendency to undermine the wall in a chancroidal infection.

On account of the indolent adenopathy that accompanies balanitis erosiva, it must be differentiated from syphilis. In syphilis the period of incubation is longer, although the two infections may occur simultaneously, as reported in one of Scherber's cases as well as in one of my own. When such a condition exists we may be compelled to defer our diagnosis of syphilis until the period of incubation for syphilis has elapsed; or in case of a mixed lesion the spirocheta pallida may easily be demonstrated by the dark ground illuminator and is so characteristic as to be easily differentiated from the spirochete of balanitis.

Herpes preputialis always occurs as groups of small insignificant vesicles in which local reaction is mild or entirely absent. This condition simulates somewhat the mild form of balanitis erosiva, but in herpes one fails to find the organisms characteristic of balanitis.

Treatment. As a prophylactic measure the practice of circumcision should be encouraged; it is absolutely impossible for balanitis to exist in an individual who has been circumcised.

In many cases in which the condition is mild and the foreskin can easily be retracted, all that is necessary is a thorough cleansing, but in the mild ulcerative forms in which there is the slightest evidence of phimosis a dorsal incision should be performed. As the organism of balanitis is anerobic, this incision serves a twofold purpose, that is, of admitting air and exposing the diseased parts for treatment.

The natural tendency is to burn all the sloughing ulcers in this disease, but such treatment subjects the patient to needless punishment. As has been said, the organisms of the disease are anerobic, and as hydrogen peroxid liberates oxygen when in contact with organic matter, it acts as a specific for this form of infection. The ordinary 2 per cent. solution is sufficient, but in severe cases of gangrenous balanitis, 25 per cent. may be procured and painted on the parts.

CASE I. Erosive type. Previously reported.

History. The patient, M. M. W., aged 40, married, denied all previous venereal history. After four days' incubation the patient noticed itching and burning around the glans penis. There were no constitutional symptoms. During the first week this continued as a mild balanitis. The patient was able to retract the foreskin. Treatment was neglected. At the end of the first week conditions suddenly became worse; the foreskin began to swell and the patient was unable to retract it. At this time he presented himself for examination.

Examination. The general muscular development was good; there were no scars or evidence of previous venereal disease. The penis was swollen and edematous; the edema extended about half way up the shaft of the penis, giving it a pear shape. The skin over the glans portion was red and slightly infected. There was complete phimosis. Exuding from the opening was a thin, yellowish-white pus, with a penetrating odor, in which was found a vibrio and spirochete. There was constant burning pain, which was increased on slightest pressure. There was no urinary pain. The dorsal lymph cord was easily palpable; the inguinal glands were enlarged but not tender. There was no fever.

Treatment. With a small hand syringe 2 per cent hydrogen peroxid was injected every hour into the preputial sac. By the second day the foreskin could be retracted, showing numerous small ulcers with sloughing bases with sharp borders, involving the sulcus and the covered portion of the glans. These healed rapidly under the above treatment.

CASE II. Erosive type, complicated by syphilitic infection.

History. C. E., male, age 19 years, single. No previous venereal disease. Gives history of many exposures, last exposure four days previous; unnatural relations. After six days of incubation, patient presented himself at my clinic at the Post Graduate Hospital.

Examination. Well-developed individual; general examination negative. Pulse and temperature normal. No glandular enlargement; profuse yellow discharge from the preputial opening.

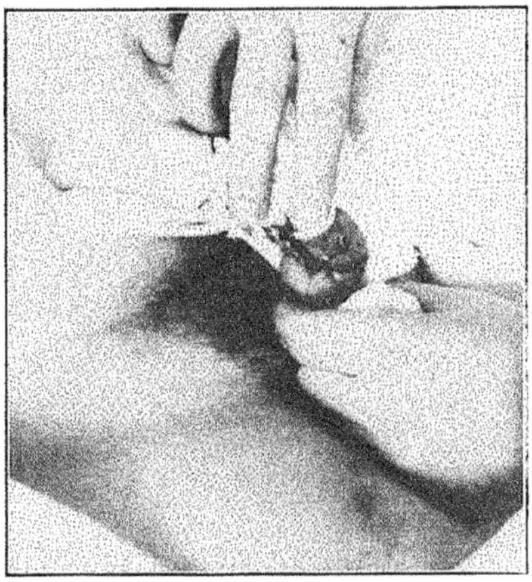

ase No. 3. Erosive Type, more advanced stage. Foreskin retracted after dorsal incision. Deep erosive ulcers with necrotic bases just back of the sulcus coronarius.

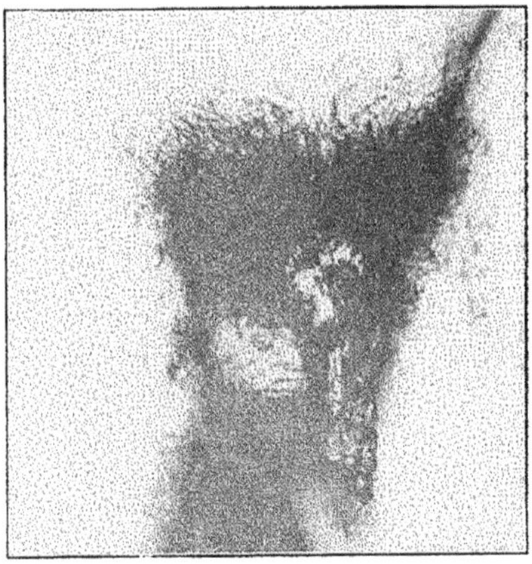

Case No. 4. Gangrenous Type, appearance 48 hours later.

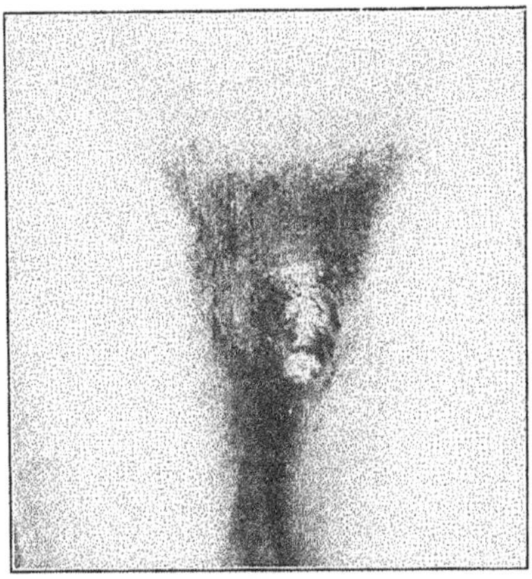

Case No. 4. Gangrenous Type, appearance upon examination.

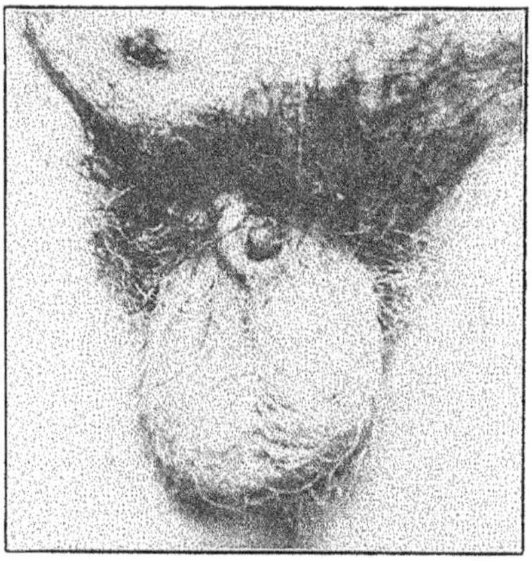

Case No. 4. Gangrenous Type, appearance five months after, showing small stump left.

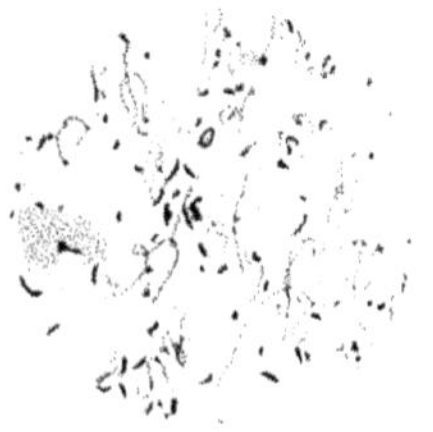

Etiological factors in erosive and gangrenous balanitis.

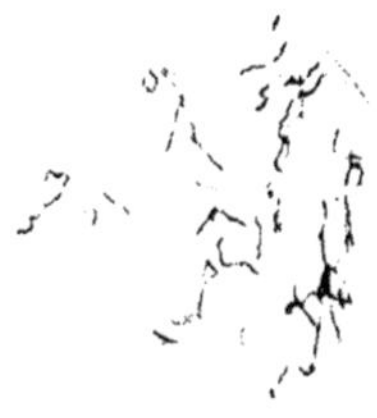

Vibrio and spirochæte. Culture from case of noma.
Slide from culture by Dr. Ruth Tunnicliff.

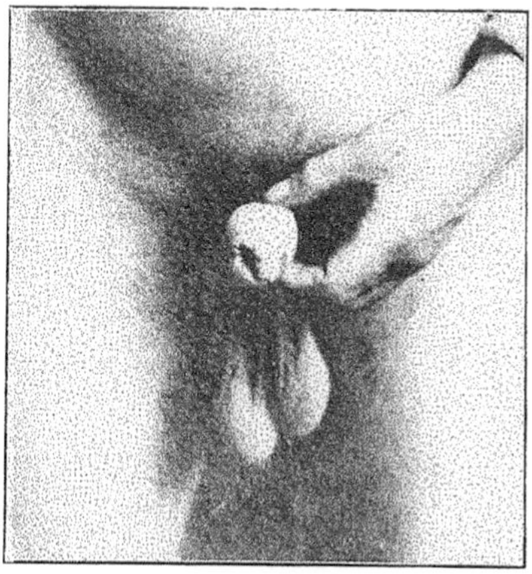

Case No. 1. Erosive Type. Balanitis erosiva. Foreskin not retracted. Ulcers seen on margin.

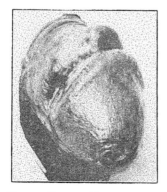

Case No. 2. Erosive Type, complicated by syphilitic infection. Foreskin retracted. Grayish purulent secretion in sulcus coronarius and few small erosions on glans penis.

Moderate amount of phimosis present. Foreskin was retracted with little difficulty, showing numerous typical superficial erosive ulcers, both in the sulcus coronarius and on glans penis. Complicating this, however, was a hard indurated erosive chancre, seen just back of the corona on the patient's left side. Sulcus filled with purulent discharge, as seen in picture.

Here by examination with the dark field illuminator it was possible to make a differential examination at once, for there were present both the spirochete pallida and the spirochete of erosive and gangrenous balanitis, also numerous vibrios. No other method could have given such prompt diagnostic technique.

Treatment. Two per cent. hydrogen peroxid and salvarsan, with prompt resolution of erosive condition.

CASE III. Erosive type, more advanced stage.

History. F. P. E., male, age 21 years, single; private patient. No history of any previous venereal disease; incubation six weeks, at which time unnatural relations were performed with the idea of avoiding exposure by the ordinary channels.

Examination. Large, corpulent individual; general examination negative. Pulse and temperature normal. Considerable phimosis present, penis slightly swollen. Extreme tenderness upon examination. Foreskin was not retractable. Patient stated that during month previous there was a little itching behind glans but that twenty-four hours previous to presenting himself for examination it suddenly began to swell and was extremely painful upon examination. Profuse stinking discharge. Dorsal lymph cord was palpable, slight painless inguinal adenopathy present.

Operation. Dorsal and ventral incisions were performed, showing both superficial and deep necrotic ulcers present at borders of glans and sulcus coronarius, as seen in the cut. Numerous vibrios and spirochetes obtained from necrotic ulcers.

Treatment. Two per cent. hydrogen peroxide, thorough cleaning with hand syringe every two hours. Prompt recovery; unable to obtain second photograph. There is no doubt that this case would have gone on to gangrene had not prompt treatment been instituted.

CASE IV. Erosive type.

History. P. O. S., male, age 26 years; history of previous gonorrhea. Unnatural relations were performed thirty-six hours previous.

Examination. Typical pear-shaped swelling of the penis, foreskin retracted. Whole of glans penis and sulcus coronarius covered with superficial ulcers, average size about the head of a pin; profuse purulent discharge, containing vibrios and spirochetes. Dorsal lymph cord palpable, no adenopathy.

This patient was so slovenly and careless, that after two days of marked improvement he discontinued treatment and had a recurrence, with a later cure.

Case V. Erosive type. Previously reported.

History. The patient, M. W. M., aged 26, denied syphilis; had had a supposed chancroidal infection two years previously. Two weeks before presenting himself the patient had intercourse. After three or four days there was a little itching beneath the prepuce. At the end of six days he presented himself for examination.

Examination. The temperature and pulse were normal. The general nutrition was good, and there were no signs of latent syphilis. There was a large indurated swelling of the penis. From the perputial orifice exuded a thin, yellowish-white, stinking discharge. This was examined for gonococci but none were present. There was phimosis, but not complete. With dilation, the little finger was gently passed between the foreskin and the glans. The whole covered portion of the glans and the inner leaf of the foreskin was covered with small ulcers, having necrotic sloughing bases. Those on the inner leaf extended to the border of the preputial fold; by gently pulling back the foreskin the whole could be plainly seen. The dorsal lymph cord could be plainly felt and the inguinal glands were enlarged but not tender. There were no constitutional symptoms.

Treatment. The patient was given a wash of hydrogen peroxid, full strength. As he did not return to the clinic, we presume that his condition was satisfactory.

Case VI. (No. 4 in picture.) Gangrenous type. Previously reported.

History. The patient, A. G. G., aged 43, denies all previous venereal history. He had had intercourse nine days previous; at this time, the patient said the prostitute lubricated her labia with saliva. The following day the glans portion began to swell; there were chilly sensations, no nausea or vomiting. Previous to this time the patient's glans penis was exposed between the preputial fold and the foreskin could be retracted. On account of the rapid phimosis that developed this could not be accomplished later. The local symptoms increased rapidly; by the third day gangrene had set in.

Examination. When the patient presented himself at the clinic he was well nourished; muscular development good. There was slight septic intoxication. The entire preputial covering for a distance of three inches was one black, necrotic mass. By gentle manipulation the necrotic mass could be drawn away and deep sloughing ulcers, with sharp borders, could be seen extending into the penis above the glans. There was considerable thin, slimy pus, with an odor of necrotic tissue present. Here we were able to find the organism in large numbers. The remaining portion of the penis was dark red and infiltrated, the edema extending to the root; the inguinal glands were enlarged. The patient's temperature was 102; malaise was marked.

Treatment. The patient was sent to the county hospital. Here the necrotic foreskin was cut away, and just above the glans portions, at the site of the inner preputial fold, could be seen two deep ulcers. The glans portion was necrotic. In forty-eight hours the entire glans portion, together with about one and a half inches of the shaft of the penis, sloughed off, leaving a short stump. The patient was treated with irrigations of potassium permanganate three times a day, but the organism had already invaded the deeper layers and gangrene was unavoidable.

In the summer of 1912, I was permitted to exhibit in my clinic, from Dr. Sullivan's service at the Post Graduate Hospital, an extensive case of gangrenous balanitis with destruction of one-half of the shaft of the penis. This had been previously treated with aseptic dressings and no organisms were found at the time I saw him.

At the present writing, on the service of Dr. Oliver Ormsby at the Cook Coutny Hospital there is a case of gangrenous balanitis.

Since reading Scherber's last publication, I am positively convinced that this same condition may produce distinct pathological lesions in the female. Only recently, I had under observation an individual with distinct erosions on the inner border of the labia minoris, with profuse foul-smelling acrid discharge. I was only able to find the vibrio, but prompt and permanent healing was effected by means of tampons applied daily of 2 per cent. hydrogen peroxide.

It must be borne in mind that erosive and gangrenous balanitis only represents different stages of development in the same infection and that prompt treatment may often save an unfortunate individual from the destruction of the whole part of the sexual organ.

BIBLIOGRAPHY

1. Journal A. M. A., May 8th. Vol. LII, page 1474–1477.
2. Arch. f. Dermat, u Syph. LXXVII, page 77.
3. Med. Moderne, 1891, Vol. II, page 340.
4. West London Med. Journal, London, 1911. Vol. XVI, page 131.
5. Handbuch der Geschlechts Krankeiten, 1910. Vol. 1, page 153.
6. Rev. Med. de la Suisse Rom. Geneve, 1911, page 592.
7. Gazz. d. osp., Milano, Oct. 4, 1910. N. 119, page 1257.
8. *Ibid.*, 1910. XV, pages 385–387.
9. Arch. f. Dormat. u. Syph. LXXVII, page 77.
10. Handbuch der Geschlechts Krankeiten, 1910. Vol. 1, page 153.
11. *Ibid.*
12. Arch. f. Dermat. u. Syph. LXXIV, page 171.
13. Journal Inf. Diseases, 1905, 2 page 446.
14. Journal Inf. Diseases, 1906, 3 page 148.
15. Journal A. M. A., May 8th, 1909. Vol. LII, pages 1474–1477.
16. Journal Inf. Diseases, 1911. Vol. 8, No. 3, pages 316–321.
17. Centralb. f. Bacteriol. XXXVIII, page 383.
18. Handbuch der Geschlechts Krankeiten, 1910. Vol. I, page 153.
19. *Ibid.*
20. Arch. f. Dermat, u Syph. LXXVII, page 77.
21. Med. Moderne, 1891. Vol. II, page 340.

EPIDIDYMOTOMY

THE RADICAL OPERATIVE TREATMENT OF EPIDIDYMITIS [1]

LAUREN S. ECKELS, M.D.

First Lieutenant Medical Corps, U. S. Army, Fort McKinley, Me.

NO operative procedure which has been recently suggested has given more gratifying results to both the surgeon and the patient than that for the relief and cure of acute epididymitis. The comparatively easily attained results are all that could be desired by the surgeon and are almost miraculous in the immediate relief they bring to the suffering patient. The relief is so immediate as to render the continuance of the internal administration of sedatives and opiates as well as the loathsome external applications entirely unnecessary. After the operation, the abatement of the fever takes place in twenty-four and not more than forty-eight hours, as a rule, and in from four to eight days the patient is able to resume his usual duties if not too violent. In view of these facts, and since I believe that this operation is devoid of risk to the patient's life, if accomplished with proper aseptic surgical surroundings, it seems to me that it should be the procedure of choice.

Epididymotomy (incision and opening of the epididymis) is an entirely rational procedure based on an accurate study of the pathology of the existing lesions. The catarrhal inflammation present causes the secretion of a varying quantity of serous fluid by the tubular glands of the epididymis, and frequently there is an exudation of some of this fluid into the tunica vaginalis, forming a hydrocele. The usual symptoms of the disease, swelling, tenderness, pain, dragging, etc., are proportionate to the amount of fluid secreted. Consequently, the liberation of the fluid from its sacs of restriction immediately relieves all symptoms.

It is customary for patients with epididymitis to appear for treatment some days after the onset of the symptoms, when pus and abscess formation will in all probability be present. If, however, the disease can be arrested in its first stages by the method under consideration, this pus and abscess formation can usually be avoided. Thus it argues that in an attack mild in character and seemingly amenable to medicinal treatment, the operative plan is more expedient, obviating as it does the possibility of future development of pus and abscess; but if the disease has progressed

[1] J. A. M. A.

to the point of pus, this pus is usually confined in the intertubular connective tissues, and the abscess formed is small. It is rare that the focus of the abscess is large except in old and neglected cases. Again, the judicious method of treatment is to open the abscess and liberate the pus.

The operation which I perform is one of comparative simplicity, being a modification of that suggested by Hagner of Washington, D. C. The time required for its accomplishment is short, rarely being more than from five to ten minutes. The preparation of the patient is the same as that for the administration of a general anesthetic, as local anesthesia is not advisable. The local sterilization of the scrotum may be accomplished in any satisfactory manner, but I have always used the simple method of applying a weak alcoholic iodin solution (from 2 to 3 per cent.) after the parts were properly shaved; always with the precaution of applying the iodin solution only after the skin is thoroughly dried.

The incision in the scrotum is made over the most prominent portion of the swelling. It varies usually from 2 to 4 inches, but should be of sufficient length to allow of the delivery of the testicle, which is wrapped in cloths moistened with warm sterile water or saline solution. A small incision is made in the tunica vaginalis which allows the fluid of the hydrocele to escape. Then the portion of the epididymis which is inflamed is punctured in numerous places with a blunt probe or grooved director. This relieves the tension by allowing the restricted fluid to escape. If pus is present, it will be seen escaping from the punctures, in which case an incision is made in the epididymis in its longitudinal axis to allow free drainage. A probe directed into the pus focus with the addition of mild pressure will free the focus of the greater parts of the pus. After thorough washing of the organ with warm normal saline solution, a short drain composed of a half-dozen strands of silkworm gut is inserted into the pus focus. The testicle is returned to the scrotum, which has previously been cleansed with warm normal saline solution, the subcutaneous tissues united by one or two sutures of small catgut, and the skin united by silkworm gut sutures, with the drain passing out at the lower angle of the wound. When the swelling is great, it may be necessary to observe certain precautions to prevent the silkworm gut sutures from tearing out of the inflamed friable tissues, in which case I make use of the button suture, which fulfils this requirement admirably.

After the operation, a simple gauze dressing is applied which

I change at the end of forty-eight hours, when I remove the drainage, if present. During this period a T bandage supports the scrotum. One other gauze dressing is usually all that is necessary and is removed on the fifth or sixth day following the operation when the silkworm gut sutures are removed. Most patients are fitted with suspensory bandages and allowed to be out of bed from the third to the fifth day and return to their usual duties from the fourth to the eighth day.

If no pus focus is discovered, the testicle is returned to the scrotum with no drainage, the convalescence being simpler and quicker,

The immediate results of this operation in acute cases are astonishing. The pain vanishes at once, the swelling disappears rapidly, and the tenderness subsides with the swelling. The patient is comfortable from the time he recovers from the anesthetic.

The remote results of the operation are just as remarkable when it is considered that relapses never occur. In a series of one hundred cases, in which I have operated in twenty-five, I know of no relapses. The most gratifying results occur in acute cases or in cases in which the tissues have not become permanently swollen and indurated. The pain is relieved instantly in all cases, but the less the induration, the more rapid and complete will be the return to normal in size and shape of the testicle, and the less apt there is to be occlusion of the vas deferens and the epididymis with the resulting sterility, especially if the attack be bilateral.

I am unable to state the influence of epididymotomy on sterility. But from the logical point of view it appears to me that a patient will have a far greater opportunity to recover without the occlusion of the vas deferens or epididymis if the continuity of the inflammation is aborted and the products of the inflammation are removed. I cannot understand how the operation itself would cause the obliteration of either the vas deferens or the epididymis. Any influence it has shortens the course of the disease and carries away the products of the inflammation. Doubtless it has the same beneficial effect on the retaining of a patulous canal as it has on the disease itself.

In conclusion, it is my belief that epididymotomy should be the treatment of choice in all cases of epididymitis, whether caused by traumatism or by infection with either the gonococcus or other organism. Every case from the mildest to the most severe should be operated on as:

1. The relief from pain is instantaneous.

2. Internal administration of sedatives and opiates and loathsome external applications are unnecessary.

3. The abatement of fever takes place in from twenty-four to forty-eight hours.

4. Pus and abscess formation is prevented.

5. Swelling, tenderness and other symptoms rapidly disappear.

6. There is no tendency to relapse.

7. It insures a minimum of time lost from usual activities.

8. There is probably a smaller percentage of sterility following the disease.

TRANSPLANTATION OF THE TESTICLE.

V. D. Lespinasse (*J. A. M. A.*, November 22), after briefly noticing the experimental work hitherto done, says that the size of the transplanted organ has a great deal to do with the success or failure of the operation. If the testicle is transplanted *in toto* it is almost certain to necrose, but if cut in thin slices and transplanted into a vascular bed it will grow and in frogs and chickens it will produce spermatozoa. In the higher animals this does not occur and the spermatogenic cells disappear in less than thirty days. The Sertoli cells and the Leydig cells, however, do not degenerate but seem to preserve their life and function. His own experimental results were confirmatory of these facts. Experimental transplantation with blood-vessel anastomosis is practically impossible though there is one human case on record where it was tried but atrophy followed. He reports a case of his own in which he transplanted slices of normal testicle into the scrotum and also into the rectus muscle with strikingly great improvement in sexual power and desire. "Transplantation of the testicle is a perfect operation in frogs and chickens; spermatogenesis and sexual characteristics are preserved. In guinea-pigs, rabbits and dogs the results are variable. Some experimenters report that there is no success at all; others assert that the interstitial cells remain and functionate. In the two human cases that have been tried to date, the one with the blood-vessel anastomosis was certainly a failure as far as spermatogenesis is concerned; but the interstitial cells may be and probably are present. In my own case the result clinically has been absolutely perfect. The man has regained his sexual powers completely, both as to desire and as to ability to perform. Furthermore, these powers have remained present for two years."

SEXUAL IMPOTENCY IN THE MALE

By Victor Blum, M.D.

Assistant in Prof. von Frisch's Urological Department of the Vienna General Polyclinic

AUTHORIZED TRANSLATION. EDITED WITH NOTES AND ADDITIONS BY DR. W. J. ROBINSON

[Continued from the January Issue]

CHAPTER XXIV—*Continued*

SYMPTOMATOLOGY OF SEXUAL NEURASTHENIA

The motor and secretory derangements, which occur in the stage of local urogenital neurosis, concern partly the genital functions and partly micturition.

We must consider first of all the disturbances of innervation in the cremaster muscle. Convulsive states of this muscle dominate during the early stages of the neurosis. One often hears the complaint from these patients that the testicles are in continual movement; they wander from the bottom of the scrotum into the inguinal canal and in so doing often cause most unpleasant sensations. In a far-advanced stage, on the contrary, in paralytic impotence for example, an atonic condition is found. The cremaster no longer reacts even to stronger tactile or electric stimuli.

Those anomalies of micturition, which are due to paresthesia, hyperesthesia, and dulness of the tactile sense of the urethra have already been considered.

The motor functions in micturition are often found affected even in the early stages of sexual neurasthenia. The symptoms from the urinary organs are often so striking, that we can rightly call the whole symptom-complex a "urosexual neurosis" or "urogenital neurasthenia."

The motor acts in micturition consists of the following phases:

The contractions of the detrusor muscle, set in action by the parietal tension of the full bladder, transmit to our consciousness the feeling that we need to pass urine. Then at the proper opportunity for urination the volitional impulse is conducted from the brain to the periphery, and micturition occurs in the following process: the sphincter of the bladder relaxes and opens, and by the simultaneous powerful contractions of the muscular walls of the bladder the urine is expelled in a stream. Powerful contractions of the bulbo-cavernosus and ischio-cavernosus muscles void the last drops of urine from the urethra. The ejaculation of the last drops of urine (" coup de piston ") at the end of the urination occurs in this way.

The sexual neurasthenic may suffer derangements in any of these phases of the act of micturition. They may be based upon the increased irritability of the peripheral nerve-endings; but the cause lies partly in changes in the spinal centers for micturition.

We have already referred to the affections of the genito-spinal center, its small capacity for meeting demands, and its easy exhaustibility. But the centers for the male genital and vesical functions are so closely associated, both in space and function, that as a rule any disturbance in the genital reflex-centers also produces a disturbance in the center for micturition.

The irritability of the periphery, which shows itself in the hyperesthesia of the mucous membrane, goes hand in hand with the irritation of the spinal centers for micturition, which become more easily excited than normal and more easily exhausted, just as do the genital-reflex-centers.

A slight filling of the bladder with urine now suffices to excite contractions of the bladder musculature, so that the need to pass urine comes much earlier than under normal conditions. The hypersensitiveness of the cystic mucous membrane to expansion is alone sufficient to excite such contractions. The well-known nervous pollakiuria results, which accompanies almost every case of sexual neurasthenia. The patients have to empty their bladder every hour, or indeed much oftener; this is at first, quite painless. There is no disturbance during the night, however, for the sleeping state diminishes the irritation coming from the hypersensitive mucous membrane of the bladder.

At first, we usually hear only one complaint from these patients, that they must urinate much too often during the day, " for the bladder is evidently too small." The expert physician, after hearing this complaint, which he finds has no anatomical basis, will at once inquire about the genital functions, and will usually satisfy himself that the urinary disturbance possesses only a secondary significance among the patient's troubles, that derangements of the sexual power, pollutions and the like play a much more important rôle. The patient often shrinks on account of embarrassment and false modesty from laying his sexual troubles before the physician. He wishes usually to conceal these conditions, because he is firmly convinced that he has brought these "states of weakness" upon himself by excessive coitus, masturbation, etc.

A reasonable hygiene, preferably "the hygiene of the marriage-bed," usually cures the genital disorders and with them the nervous pollakiuria.

In more advanced cases, the symptoms of dysuria and strangury are added to that of increased frequency of urination. The hyperesthesia and in many masturbators the hyperemia of the posterior urethra, its inflammatory swelling, produce the symptom of strangury., Whereas, formerly the patient had the need for passing urine only more frequently, which he could if necessary restrain for some time, he suffers now at each micturition a violent strangury, which he must satisfy at once. The emptying of the bladder is made difficult, however, by unseasonable contractions of the sphincter, and the patient passes a few drops of urine only with difficulty and very painful straining, and soon after the same tormenting tenesmus begins again (DYSURIA AND STRANGURY).

Later the dysuria no longer disappears at night, and the patient is continually tormented by the frequent need to urinate, which in conjunction with the annoying paresthesiae, the itching and burning in the urethra produce an intolerable condition. The intervals between the frequent urinations are now filled out by an unpleasant feeling in the bladder, by feelings of pressure and tension, heat and weight above the symphysis and in the groins.

The strangury often increases to true bladder-cramps, cystospasm, which may be distinguished by especial painfulness (irritable bladder).

If now a reflex cramp of the urinary sphincter occurs, the well-known symptom of nervous retention of urine results. Happily these severest forms of strangury are seen only exceptionally. Neurotic retention of urine is only rarely a complication of the urogenital neurosis.

The symptoms of pollakiuria and diurnal dysuria with undisturbed sleep is almost pathognomonic for "nervous bladder."

The spasm of the sphincter, which often occurs most untimely during micturition, produces the familiar hesitation or "stuttering of the bladder." The stream of urine is suddenly and repeatedly interrupted by energetic contractions of the sphincter, and the patient has to renew his attempts again and again to empty his bladder.

It may also frequently happen, that the patient loses the feeling of the emptied bladder, and imagines that he always retains a certain residue in his bladder. In uncomplicated cases the passing of the catheter shows us that this is not the case.

The hypochondriac ideas of the patient also obtain new encouragement from the symptom of dribbling of the urine after urination. A typical idea of these neurasthenics is the conviction that they have a urethral stricture, for they know from their popular treatises that dribbling of urine may be a sign of stricture.

As a matter of fact, however, it is only an affection of micturition, consisting in this, that the closing act of the process does not take place by a powerful ejaculation ("coup de piston"), but the urine, evidently because of deficient contraction of the muscles surrounding the urethra, drops slowly after the ending of the stream, and soils the patient's clothes.

This is the only form of "urine-dribbling," which we have observed in neurasthenics. We have never seen a true incontinence of urine—an enuresis. Eulenburg, however, also includes the latter symptom, enuresis, among the signs of sexual neurasthenia.

Finally, we have still one more symptom to consider, which we must include among the morbid changes of micturition;

namely, the peculiar feelings, with which the organism reacts in such patients after urination. Whereas, the healthy man has a feeling of relief, the sensation of an empty bladder after micturition, sexual neurasthenics have many feelings of discomfort after passing urine. Apart from the local pains, which often outlast urination a long time, many patients feel weakened and tired, complain of pains in the legs, sciatica, and the like.

Another symptom is the SLIGHT SHIVER at the close of micturition, which Ziemssen denoted "urethrismus" (urethral spasm), and which also occurs in healthy men after forced suppression of the desire to urinate. In our urosexual neurasthenics this slight shudder is aggravated to a true nervous chill. Ziemssen also noticed this peculiar symptom of urethral spasm during a prolonged preliminary stage of coitus, and assumes for its explanation a spasm in the prostatic urethra. These spasms form an analogue to the familiar symptom-complex of vaginismus.

[THE LITTLE SHUDDER

That little shudder or shiver, which I had thought I was the first one to discover, is a very unique characteristic symptom in sexual neurasthenics. It had been called to my attention by a very intelligent and observant patient. The little shiver would take place at the end of each urination; it would either be localized in a small portion, usually the center, of the spine, or it would take place throughout the entire spine. Occasionally the entire body would participate in the shiver, so that the knees would suddenly flex and the head would shake. Since I became familiar with this symptom, I have made it a point to inquire of each sexual neurasthenic as to its presence, and in the largest percentage of cases the answer would be in the affirmative. Patients who present this symptom do not have it constantly. It appears with some urinations; it is absent with others. In trying to solve this point—why patients experienced it at some urinations and not at others—I made a microscopic examination of a large number of specimens of urine, and I have discovered the following peculiar fact:

Whenever the patients experienced the shiver, the urine contained semen and spermatozoa; whenever the shiver was not experienced the urine was usually free from spermatozoa, and it is my opinion that the shiver occurs only when there is an ejaculation of semen, however slight that may be. It would perhaps be correct to state that the shiver or shudder is the accompaniment of a spasmodic contraction of the seminal vesicles, resulting in an ejaculation. As mentioned above, I pay great attention to this symptom, and its disappearance is a sign of positive improvement in a patient's condition. Its reappearance is an indication that the patient is "going back." Besides local urethral treatment, which is *always* necessary in sexual neurasthenics, massaging the back, vibrating it or painting it with counterirritant solutions has an unmistakably beneficial effect on this symptom. W. J. R.]

In order to avoid repetitions we will not describe here in detail the motor, secretory, and functional nervous disorders of the genital organs, which characterize the various stages of sexual neurasthenia. The reader is referred to the corresponding chapters—seminal losses, impotence, priapism.

We will only emphasize here again the fact that the genital disorders also may be referred to analogous alterations in the periphery and in the centers. The hyperesthesia of the genital organs leads to permanent irritations, which manifest themselves in frequent erections, pollutions, and diurnal ejaculations.

The centers for the sexual functions show a pathologically increased responsiveness to demands, and little endurance; they are further easily exhausted. Finger emphasized the fact that "the erection center is more easily excited, but also more easily exhausted; whereas the ejaculatory center is more difficult to excite, but also more difficult to exhaust, more resistant."

The particular forms of impotence, which result from alterations of the separate acts of normal coitus; namely, libido, erection, ejaculation and orgasm, have been considered independently in the chapter on impotence.

We recognize of course, that the disorders of the male sexual functions are as a rule the cardinal symptom of sexual neurasthenia; yet we must reject the idea that the alpha and omega of the neurosis consist of the individual forms of impotence, as is claimed for instance of Gyurkovechky in his work on impotence.

As we proceed in our description of the symptoms of the separate stages of sexual neurasthenia, we must glance again here at the original classification of Krafft-Ebing. The symptoms hitherto described concern exclusively the urinary and sexual organs, although, to be sure, in different degrees. They form the characteristic features of the first stage of the classification sexual neurasthenia proposed by Krafft-Ebing, that of local genital neurosis.

These symptoms indeed persist in the further phases of development of sexual neurasthenia; they merely fall in part into the background in the course of the disease as compared with other symptoms. A careful examination of the patient, however, always discloses the phenomena of a local genital neurosis even in the most complicated cases.

The second stage, that Krafft-Ebing assumes, the stage of neurosis of the lumbar portion of the spinal cord, only represents a higher degree of the stage that has just been described. The local symptoms are more sharply marked, the forms of impotence, which characterize this stage, correspond to severer anomalies of the genital functions. The picture of "irritable weakness of the genital centers" is complete.

Sexual desire is increased, diurnal pollutions occur, and ejaculation appears prematurely on attempts at coitus. The centers need a longer time for recovery than normal. Repetition of coitus is impossible until a long period of rest has been enjoyed. Derangements of the uropoietic system and of innervation proceeding from other regions of the lumbar cord, (in the plexus lumbalis, and sacro-coccygeus), are regularly associated with these disorders of the genital functions.

We also find derangements of sensibility, of motor and of secretory functions in the realm of those centers of innervation which are adjacent to the sexual centers. In this stage the patients complain of tormenting sacral pains, of pains in the rectum and anus, which radiate toward the kidneys, into the thighs and even to the feet. There is a continual feeling of cold in the feet and frequent paresthesiae (formication, tickling), and the patients are unable to walk or stand for any length of time. Especially after any sexual act, such as masturbation or pollution, they suffer such an alarming feeling of weakness in the legs that they are obliged to rest in bed for hours in order to recover. The pains may appear only in the region of the kidneys, and in this way by spinal irritation imitate the typical clinical picture of renal colic. The differential diagnosis in such cases between a nervous renal colic and a genuine renal colic due to calculus may sometimes be very difficult.

Also a marked COCCYGODYNIA can temporarily or permanently dominate the picture.

In this second stage of sexual neurasthenia the disorders of sensibility and motility of the urogenital organs are already extremely unpleasant. Violent neuralgia of the urethra and prostate, pain in the testes, painful cramps of the bladder (irritable bladder), and temporary dysuria and strangury characterize these disturbances of the urogenital organs.

The THIRD STAGE of sexual neurasthenia is characterized by the EXTENSION OF THE NEUROSIS OF THE LUMBAR PORTION of the spinal cord to GENERAL NEURASTHENIA.

We find here fully developed the whole symptom-complex, which was formerly called "spinal irritation." The irritative states are not now confined to the nervous regions supplied by the lumbar cord; on the contrary the whole spinal cord and the sympathetic nervous system take part in the development of the symptoms.

In this stage also we have to distinguish between first irritations and later paralytic phenomena in the sensory, motor, vasomotor, and secretory realms.

For the sake of clearness we will consider the symptoms in order as sensory and motor disorders, visceral derangements, and finally the influence of the sexual neurosis upon the patient's PSYCHE.

Among the sensory disorders in our patients appear spontaneous pains, which are located in the back, in the spine, and often only in particular parts of it. These painful sensations often radiate toward the shoulders, the hips, and the upper and lower extremities. The pains are described as "rheumatic" conditions and oppressive sensations, they often appear in a neuralgic form like lancinating pains (intercostal neuralgia). Also headaches, localized in the forehead and occiput, are often complained of, likewise migraine, and not rarely the feeling of a constricting band about the entire head.

The painful parts of the spinal column are also very sensitive to pressure, and there is often an extreme hyperesthesia of the skin. Thus with one of our patients the hypersensitiveness of the skin of the back, which caused any heavy article of clothing to be felt as an unbearable pain, formed his principal complaint and was the source of all the hypochondriac ideas imaginable.

The paresthesiae, which in the course of the local genital neurosis affected only the skin and mucous membrane of the genital organs, now extend over nearly the whole body surface. There may be attacks of general itching of the skin, formication, and a dull, pasty feeling in the lower limbs, rarely also in the fingers and upper arms. The special sensitiveness to cold, which in the first stage exists only in the sensations of cold in the penis and scrotum, extends to larger regions of the body; the skin of the back and the abdomen is especially sensitive to low temperature and is often the seat of abnormal, subjective sensations of cold.

The motor phenomena consist above all in great exhaustibility. In spite of a good night's sleep the patients feel so prostrated, flabby, and tired on arising next morning, that they would rather get back into bed. Walking or standing for any length of time becomes almost impossible for them. Even speaking, indeed, may seem hard to them. A characteristic symptom, which is often observed, is to be noted here; THE ABNORMAL EXHAUSTIBIILITY OF THE MUSCLES OF ACCOMMODATION OF THE EYE, which is the essential feature of asthenopia.

We observed one patient, who acquired a severe degree of neurasthenia as a result of masturbation and diurnal and nocturnal pollutions. He considered himself quite impotent, and did not dare to attempt coitus. Recently since 1906 almost every night one or two pollutions, often without erection. He complains that his vision becomes exhausted extremely easily, especially in the morning after arising. His eyes close involuntarily from exhaustion. He is unable to read or write. When he has read for a few minutes, the letters swim before his eyes. He also becomes tired very quickly in talking, so that he speaks through his nose, evidently from insufficiency of the palate and tongue muscles. His memory has failed, and he is greatly emaciated. In the physical examination an insufficiency of both external recti, a lessened sensibility to pain of the right half of the face, tremor of the hands, hyperidrosis, increased knee-jerks, and ankle clonus were noted.

The picture that the patient presented in this condition was quite similar to the classical picture of myasthenia gravis pseudoparalytica; yet the fatigue-reaction could not be demonstrated either actively or electrically. The patient was completely cured by appropriate psycho-therapy and local therapy of the urethra.

Besides this abnormal liability to fatigue and the loss of muscular tone we observe a neurasthenic tremor and an increased reflex excitability as motor disorders. The knee-jerks are much increased, and in many cases there is a suggested or clearly marked ankle-clonus.

Paralyses of the limbs, paraplegia, phenomena which are probably always present in the patient's imagination as a result of reading the conscienceless exaggerations in popular sexual literature, are perhaps never observed in uncomplicated cases of sexual neurosis. The scientific literature on this subject from the beginning of the previous century (Lallemand, Tissot, etc.) also speaks always of the possibility of tabes and other severe spinal diseases as a result of masturbation and venereal excesses. These exaggerated notions got into the literature dealing with sexual errors and sexual hygiene, which is always at the disposal of the laity. The fear of tabes as a result of sexual excesses in youth dominates the imaginations of our severe neurasthenics with surprising uniformity. These unfortunates see the symptoms of tabes in the dulness of the senses and paresthesiae, in the impotence and great fatigability, and above all in the asthenopia, and often all the physician's attempts at persuasion cannot convince them that they are mistaken. The patient obtains support for his fear of tabes ("Tabophobia") in the VISCERAL SYMPTOMS of sexual neurasthenia.

In connection with the latter we will also consider the vasomotor phenomena, since both depend partly upon disturbances in innervation of the cerebral centers (medulla oblongata) for respiration, the heart's action, the vagus nerve, etc., and also partly on disturbances in innervation of the sympathetic nervous system.

The abnormal excitability of the vasomotor nerves is shown in the tendency to uncalled for constrictions and dilatations of vessels.

The sudden blushing, often without any reason, makes the patient socially impossible, for he fears that by this annoying occurrence he will betray his carefully concealed sexual neurasthenia. Moreover, the feelings of congestion of the head, of the hot blood in the scalp and face make themselves most unpleasant. The patients complain often of cold feet and hands, and are inclined to chilblains. The symptoms of dermographia, which is a sign of abnormal vasomotor excitability, is almost always clearly marked.

The extremely common hyperidrosis is a perfect torment to the patients. The slightest excitement produces sweating of the face and body. We have also observed one-sided sweating in one such case. The vasomotor symptoms in connection with the phenomena of the circulatory organs to be considered later—tachycardia, cardiac palpitation, etc.—often imitate the clinical picture of Basedow's disease.

As we have already indicated, there are often considerable disturbances of the circulatory organs in severe cases of sexual neurasthenia.

Especially in the masturbatory neurosis the patients complain of attacks of cardiac palpitation; the pulse is very frequent, small, and not rarely one also finds real irregularity of the heart's action, an unequal and sometimes an intermittent pulse.

The affections of the heart's action are aggravated by each sexual or masturbatory act, and this can reach such a degree, that the patients fall into a condition of collapse after masturbation, which may sometimes assume very dangerous forms. We have also seen in a few cases attacks of pseudo-angina pectoris of sexual origin, which can imitate perfectly the clinical picture of true angina.

Severe disorders of the respiratory organs also develop: attacks of dyspnea and oppression cause severe states of anxiety in these patients. Deep inspiration is frequently very painful, and in such attacks they can breathe only with difficulty and with the help of the accessory muscles of respiration. We call these attacks "sexual asthma." In almost every case of severe sexual neurasthenia we find more or less serious derangements of the digestive organs.

It is usually indeed, the digestive troubles that induce the patient to consult a physician, and only by means of a careful consideration of each separate symptom, of the history and the course of the disease can one exclude an organic cause for the digestive disorder and diagnose a nervous affection. But on careful study of the cases one will be astonished to find how often the nervous digestive troubles owe their origin to sexual disorders.

The dyspeptic complaints manifest themselves in all parts of the gastro-intestinal canal.

Nervous dyspepsia is usually introduced by an unpleasant, pasty taste in the mouth and dryness of the tongue and throat. The appetite is not affected at first; one often sees on the contrary a marked increase of appetite and attacks of bulimia. Not until the advanced stages of the disease, when the nervous derangements of secretion and motility of the stomach and intestine have produced a general catarrhal condition of the mucous membranes, does the appetite suffer, and there exists a marked aversion to certain foods, such as meat and milk.

The lowered muscular tone is often seen in the function of the esophagus. Difficulties in swallowing occur during meals of some duration, and spastic states of the cardiac opening of the stomach prevent the smooth transmission of food into the stomach.

The stomach itself shows derangements in motility and in the secretion of the digestive juices. Tonic contractions of the pyloric sphincter, which are often very painful, produce stagnation of the gastric contents. The secretory activity of the glandular cells is often influenced in both extreme directions. At first there usually exists hypersecretion with hyperchlorhydria and heartburn. Vomiting of sour masses now occurs with convulsive contractions of the stomach. Complete achylia with its characteristic symptoms may also occur in the course of sexual neurasthenic dyspepsia. The patients have no appetite, have a marked revulsion against meat, while they often bear coarse and indigestible foods very well; they suffer from eructation of stale smelling gases, and occasionally vomit with extreme cardialgia.

The absence of chyle is accompanied typically by attacks of colic and diarrhea.

But the patients suffer oftener from obstinate constipation, due to the derangements of motility as well as to the secretory changes in the intestinal glands. The atony of the intestine produces an annoying flatulence and distension of the abdomen.

The natural result of these digestive disorders and the lack of nourishment following their loss of appetite, is that these patients suffer severely in their general health. They lose flesh, and acquire finally a characteristic, emaciated appearance. The complexion is sallow, the cheeks sunken, the eyes lie deep in their sockets with dark rings about them. The embarrassment, shyness, and anxious expression—symptoms, which are especially striking in the neurosis of masturbation—give the patient's appearance such a characteristic stamp, that one is often tempted to make the diagnosis of sexual neurasthenia due to masturbation at first sight.

Certain very characteristic disturbances of the urine belong to the secretory disorders of sexual neurasthenia. We see considerable alterations in the amount of urine produced under nervous influences. Everyday experience shows us that the neurasthenic gets a surprising POLYURIA under the nervous excitement produced by the medical consultation. Although he has passed his urine perhaps only an hour before, he produces a very large amount of a pale, watery urine of low specific gravity. There occurs a dilatation of the renal vessels, perhaps as a result of the instability of the vasomotors, and the parenchyma is incited to abundant and rapid production of urine.

PHOSPHATURIA is a second very common symptom of neurasthenia and according to some authors a typical physical sign of the neurosis. It occurs in two forms; either as *manifest* phosphaturia, in which the urine is opaque and clears up at once on adding acetic acid, or as latent phosphaturia, in which the urine is not clouded until boiled, when the precipitated phosphates make it opaque.

The patients usually attribute great significance to this symptom. The opaque urine frightens them, and based upon this and also upon the dysuria and pollakiuria of long duration, a diagnosis of cystitis is made by them and unfortunately also only too often by the superficial physician.

The excessive excretion of OXALIC ACID is also a frequent accompaniment of the neurosis. The urine laden with crystals of calcium oxalate causes a burning sensation when passed and pains AT THE CLOSE OF MICTURITION, as is also the case in phosphaturia.

We must not leave the symptoms of sexual neurasthenia without speaking of the important effects of the nervous symptoms upon the mental state of the patient. Indeed the mental changes in sexual neurasthenia are so important, that one can truly say, these psychic changes first give the characteristic stamp to the disease. And after a little experience and in uncomplicated cases one can assume the sexual etiology of the neurosis from one's judgment of the patient's mental state, with great probability.

These patients are nervous. Although we will not go so far as to say that every kind of nervousness is due to sexual injuries, still we must recognize that a certain form of nervousness—of which we shall next speak, is almost always an expression of sexual neurasthenia.

The patients react in a peculiar, abnormal fashion to slight impressions of an irritating or depressing kind upon their minds. They are pained or delighted quite out of proportion to the triviality of the occasion. But it is chiefly states of mental depression that dominate these sufferers! From the most trifling symptoms, quite unnoticed by normal people, they draw the most serious conclusions as to their state of health. They become hypochondriacs in this way, and indeed, as we shall later see, pseudo-hypochondriacs.

We are often enabled to observe the change of character right under our eyes, for example in such cases of sexual neurasthenia as develop in the course of or after a chronic gonorrhea (prostatitis). Patients, who have succeeded excellently in their profession because of strong character and marked abilities, begin to complain that they can no longer do justice to their work. We can usually assume some exaggeration in this statement, since the emotional depression of these patients makes all their symptoms appear much much serious than they actually are.

To the main features of the psychic condition, abnormal excitability, pessimism, and depression of spirits, are now added failure of memory and inability for mental work. This occurs chiefly because the observation of their physical state creates so much thought, worry, and anxiety that not enough time or peace of mind are left for their professioal or intellectual work.

The dulling of the mental faculties shows itself not only in the failing memory, but also in the actually diminished work done by the sensory organs.

We have already spoken of nervous asthenopia or insufficiency of accommodation. Disturbances of hearing also occur. At first there exists only a certain painful auditory hyperesthesia, which causes considerable sleeplessness. Subjective noises appear later—tinnitus aurium, hammering, knocking, etc., and finally actual diminution of the hearing power may ensue.

In other patients idiosyncrasies of smell dominate the mind. Somatic conditions, paresthesiae and dulness of the senses and visceral disorders intervene, and form a constant source of exaggerated complaints.

States of anxiety further belong to the characteristic signs of sexual neurasthenia. They are seen so regularly in cases of sexual neurosis and quite definite sexual injuries are so constantly discoverable in the previous history of patients who suffer from nervous anxiety, that Freud thinks himself justified in differentiating from general neurasthenia a symptom-complex, the anxiety neurosis ("angst-neurose"), which he considers to be invariably due to sexual injuries. Freud went indeed so far as to express the formula:—"anxiety is essentially sexual desire diverted from its proper application."

While the polymorphous symptoms of general neurasthenia may be reduced to certain basic types (fatigability, flatulence, constipation, paresthesia, sexual weakness), only such symptoms enter into the anxiety neurosis as stand in a definite relation to the central symptom—fear or anxiety—that is to converted libido.

The general anxiety, which forms the main feature of the mental state of these patients, may be accentuated even to "morbid doubt" (maladie de doute) in pronounced cases, which are close to the border of the psychoses.

The general anxiety may be projected on the outer world, and so give to the character the various traits of unsteadiness, indecision, weakness and lack of energy.

The egoistic manifestations of anxiety are still more characteristic; they are expressed in the various phobias; which are very characteristic of sexual neurasthenics.

The commonest of them is a morbid fear of disease, which we are accustomed to call hypochondria according to old custom. According to Barruco we have in general to distinguish a true hypochondria [and for which imagination there is no justification as he has *no* symptoms] in which the patient imagines a disease that he actually has not got, from a false hypochondria or preudo-hypochondria, in which the patient imagines that he has a disease on account of more or less marked symptoms, which he greatly exaggerates. We have to do with this pseudo-hypochrondia in our sexual neurasthenics. The manifold somatic symptoms are the source of the hypochrondriac ideas.

At the head stands the fear of tabes, which with remarkable constancy dominates the emotional life of our patients. As has been already mentioned, this fear comes from the popular "scientific" books, in which tabes is represented as the sure consequence of sexual errors.

It is perhaps unnecessary to point out, that although the two diseases have some symptoms in common, such as the visual disorders, the paresthesiae, the impotence, etc., no direct etiologic connection between the two exists.

The patients' fear of mental disease, paralysis, and insanity is similar. Here again the patients draw upon their actual symptoms—the failure of memory, the compulsory ideas, etc.—in order to establish their fear of the psychosis.

As a matter of fact sexual injuries may well occasionally figure as accessory causes, as the exciting agent of tabes and general paralysis, only, however, when other predisposing causes, especially syphilis, are present.

[Syphilis is so preëminently the cause of locomotor ataxia that to admit the possibility of any other cause seems to be unscientific. And while I am fully aware of the fact that Lallemand's and Tissot's claims often lacked the proper scientific foundation; while I know that those authors did not always subject their data to careful critical analysis, still I do not wish to be so dogmatic as to assert that tabes and general paralysis can *never* be the result of sexual abuse alone, without syphilis. I have now a patient who used to practice masturbation as many as 20 and 24 times a day. He has never had any sexual intercourse, nor any venereal disease. He has no tabes, but the symptoms he presents are very markedly tabetic. I have had quite a number of patients who for a considerable period of time had practiced intercourse 10 and 15 times a day. It is conceivable that such immoderate excesses, either in masturbation or in normal coitus, might lead to organic changes in the spinal cord. *Severe functional abuse may lead to organic anatomical alterations in any part of the body*, and it is my opinion that very severe and prolonged sexual abuse may lead both to tabes and to general paralysis.—W. J. R.]

Another very common phobia is agoraphobia and its related

phobias, "all of which are characterized by their relation to locomotion. A previous attack of vertigo is often the foundation of the phobia" (Freud).

Agoraphobia occurs on crossing great squares or broad streets. Similar states of anxiety occur, apparently in remembrance of an attack of fear suffered in a certain situation, in the theater, in parties, in the railway, etc. We call these phobias according to Jolly "situation anxiety."

It is Freud's merit to have discovered by means of anamnestic and psycho-analytic deductions the relations of all these phobias to sexual injuries: injuries due to deficient satisfaction—coitus interruptus—abortive excitements, etc.

Among the anxious states we must finally include the well-known attacks of anxiety which are often observed as accompanying phenomena of the attacks of tachycardia with oppression and feelings of impending death in our sexual neurasthenics. These are pseudo-anginous attacks.

We can not go further into all these psychic abnormalities, which are often quite strikingly developed among our patients, and which in many cases represent the transition to real psychoses, since they do not belong to the province of our functional symptoms, but rather to the psychiatric and psychologic textbooks.

It seemed to me, however, desirable to describe briefly the peculiarities in mind and character of our sexual neurasthenics, since the knowledge of these conditions must often be adduced in order to explain the somatic troubles.

The often extremely complicated picture of sexual neurasthenia, in which pains in the urinary and genital organs, paresthesiæ, strangury, etc., suggest the thought of organic diseases of these organs, will often turn out, after analysis of the psychic symptoms, to be a functional neurosis—sexual neurasthenia.

DEPARTMENT OF SEXUAL PSYCHOLOGY

NOTES ON THE PSYCHOLOGY OF SEX

III

By Douglas C. McMurtrie

SEXO-ESTHETIC INVERSION

THE most important recent contribution in the field of sexual psychology has been made by Havelock Ellis in his study [1] of sexo-esthetic inversion. Students of medical psychology have frequently encountered persons tending toward some of the habits of the opposite sex, who have yet exhibited no evidence of homosexual desires. As methods of dress constitute the most intimate habits associated with one sex or another, the anomaly referred to has found most frequent expression in this field. We encounter men with a passion for articles of female attire and for activities and attributes (non-sexual) of women. We also find women who ape the dress and manners of men. Yet the subjects in these cases have heterosexual attractions and can certainly not be classed as sexual inverts.

The field of dress has provided us with the most plentiful evidence regarding the tendency under discussion and Hirschfeld has dealt with the subject in an extensive book [2] on "cross-dressing," that is, men dressed as women and women dressed as men.

He emphasizes particularly the characteristics of dress, but also makes clear that in most cases there is no sexual inversion.

In the past these tendencies would have been unhesitatingly diagnosed as tributary to homosexuality but we know now that this is not the truth. Many of the subjects are completely and enthusiastically heterosexual in their physical attractions and desires.

What then causes this longing for the clothing of the opposite sex? It is a question difficult to answer, but Ellis has addressed himself successfully to the solution of the problem.

[1] Havelock Ellis. Sexo-aesthetic inversion. *Alienist and Neurologist,* St. Louis, 1913, xxxiv, 156–167; 249–279. Also: Sexo-esthetische Inversion, *Zeitschrift für Psychotherapie und medizinische Psychologie,* Stuttgart, 1913, v, 134–162. In the spelling of the word I have followed the most approved American usage and dropped the diphthong.

[2] Magnus Hirschfeld. *Die Transvestiten: Eine Untersuchung über den erotischen Verkleidungstrieb.* Leipzig, 1910.

"There are at least two types of such cases;. one, the most common kind, in which the inversion is mainly confined to the sphere of clothing; and another, less common but more complete, in which cross-dressing is regarded with comparative indifference but the subject so identifies himself with those of his physical and psychic traits which recall the opposite sex that he feels really to belong to that sex, although he has no delusion regarding his anatomical conformation." Ellis presents several case records showing the particuar channels which the tendency has taken in each instance.

The theory which Ellis advocates is then stated. "When we attempt to classify or to account for the cases here brought forward the task is scarcely easy. We may well assert that they illustrate that universal bisexuality which is now so widely accepted.

"But if we proceed to co-ordinate these views of sexo-esthetic inversion with ordinary sexual inversion, now commonly regarded as most easily explicable by this same organic bisexuality, we encounter difficulties. We may be inclined to regard esthetic inversion as a slighter degree of the same sexually intermediate state of which we find a more advanced stage in sexual inversion. But a little consideration shows that that is scarcely correct. In the narrow sphere of the sexual impulse itself esthetic inversion shows indeed but little if any approximation to the opposite sex. But in the wider non-sexual psychic sphere, on the other hand, it goes farther beyond all the most usual manifestations of sexual inversion. The two conditions are not strictly co-ordinate. They may rather be regarded as, so to speak, two unlike allotropic modifications of intermediate sexuality. Sexual inversion when it appears in esthetic inversion would appear to be merely a secondary result of the esthetically inverted psychic state. Esthetic inversion, when it appears in sexual inversion, is perhaps merely a secondary result of the sexually inverted psychic state.

"Thus, on a common basis, we seem to be presented with two organic conditions which are distinct, do not easily merge, and are even mutually repugnant. A large proportion, perhaps the majority, of sexual inverts have no strongly pronounced feminine traits, and even so far as they possess them not infrequently desire to slur over or disguise them. The majority of sexo-esthetic inverts on the other hand, indeed nearly all of them, are not only without any tendency to sexual inversion, but they feel a profound repugnance to that anomaly.

"Psychologically speaking, it seems to me that we must regard sexo-esthetic inversion as really a modification of normal heterosexuality. It is a modification in which certain of the normal constituents of the sexual impulse have fallen into the background, while other equally normal constituents have become unduly exaggerated. What are those two sets of constituents?"

In the discussion of these constituents is brought forward a most acute analysis of the love process. "In normal courtship it is necessary for the male to experience two impulses which are, on the surface, antagonistic. On the one hand, he must be forceful and combative; he must overcome and possess the desired object. On the other hand, he must be expectant and sympathetic; he must enter into the feelings of the beloved and even subject himself to her will. The lover must be both a resolute conquerer and a submissive slave. He must both oppose himself to his mistress's reticence, and identify himself with her desire. This twofold attitude is based on the biological conditions of courtship.

"In civilized human courtship there is a tendency for the first and aggressive component of the sexual impulse to be subordinated, and for the second and sympathetic component to be emphasized. This tendency was set forth some years ago by Colin Scott as the 'secondary law of courting' by which the female (who is already imaginatively attentive to the states of the excited male) develops a super-added activity, while the male develops a relatively passive and imaginative attention to the psychical and bodily states of the female. This 'imaginative radiation' and 'development of the representative powers' is favored, Colin Scott points out, by the restrictions imposed by civilization, and the larger mental capacity involved.

"The secondary component of the sexual impulse, the element of sympathy and identification, may be said to be connected, as Colin Scott seems to have recognized, with an esthetic attitude. It is worth while to insist on the connection for it may furnish a deeper reason than I have yet suggested for applying the name 'esthetic inversion' to a condition which, as the reader will by now have perceived, is to be regarded as an abnormal and perhaps pathological exaggeration of the secondary component of the normal heterosexual impulse.

"The philosophic students of esthetics have frequently shown a tendency to regard a subjective identication with the beautiful object as the clue to esthetic emotion. They hold that we imaginatively imitate the beauty we see, and sympathetically place ourselves in it.

"Here we may perceive a deeper reason than we have yet reached for describing the psychological anomaly which we are here concerned with as esthetic inversion." Ellis does not find any physiological conditions analogous to the psychic state.

URETHRAL MASTURBATION

There will be encountered frequently among men who, by reason of age or otherwise, have lost the power of erection, a habit of masturbation through the urethra. The sensation is produced by tickling the interior of the urethral passage near the head of the penis by means of various articles. In one case which came recently to the attention of a New York hospital, the man had used a pin with a round ball head, this head being inserted up the urethral orifice. In its manipulation, the grasp on the point end of the pin was lost and the article became lodged up the urethra. The point of the pin finally came out near the base of the glans and infection set in. It was this condition that necessitated the visit to the hospital for removal of the pin and treatment of the infection.

CRIMINOLOGY AND PROSTITUTION

In a recent authoritative study on criminology Gustav Aschaffenburg has devoted considerable attention to prostitution which he classifies among the social causes of crime. He summarizes [3] its history and development as follows. "Prostitution, that is, self-surrender for payment, originally instituted by priests for the honor of the divinity and the benefit of the temple, and later put into practical form by statesmen like Solon, has existed in all ages and will always continue to exist. The most ancient historical documents speak of it; but they also tell us—a fact that is important for legislation—that all conceivable means of repressing it had already been tried. In vain! With the weapons of religion and Christian love Louis XI of France, for instance, attempted to abolish it altogether and founded places of refuge for fallen women. On his return from Palestine he ordered it to be completely exterminated. The concealed prostitution that immediately began to flourish everywhere, however,

[3] Gustav Aschaffenburg. *Crime and its Repression.* English translation by Adalbert Albrecht. Boston, 1913.

compelled him, before a year had elapsed, to repeal the order and to assign certain streets to the use of prostitutes. The harshest measures (flogging, the pillory, and capital punishment) proved of no avail in repressing the evil, which continued to spread and thrive only in a more secret and dangerous form, and they were always given up after a time. Thus, in all countries, legislation has oscillated between extremes, turning from the method of herding prostitutes together in barracks to allowing them unlimited freedom, from occasional superintendence to the strict supervision of every individual. The tendency to respect the rights of the individual and to place them above those of society on the one hand, and, on the other, the moral fear of sanctioning the evil by legally allowing it, have always led to the repeal of regulative measures. This has been followed by such a spread of prostitution in its most dangerous, clandestine form, that it later became necessary to recognize and regulate it again. We may regret, but we must not ignore, the fact, that the tendency to immorality cannot be exterminated by laws. The man who had the most extensive knowledge of prostitution, Parent Duchatelet, said that, wherever people congregated, it was as unavoidable as sewers or cesspools. But, because it seems to be impossible to abolish this evil, it does not follow that it should be allowed to grow and spread in all directions. Its repression should be striven for as far as possible, and for that, it is essential, above all, that its dangerousness should be thoroughly understood."

Prostitution among females is often regarded as equivalent to criminality among males. There is much to support this view, notably some of the studies of degenerate stocks where most of the men turned to crime and most of the women to prostitution. In this connection Aschaffenburg renders a careful and deliberate opinion. "We cannot fail to recognize that prostitution does absorb a considerable percentage of criminally inclined women. Every prostitute lives without working, at the expense of society; she corresponds in a measure to the male beggar and the vagabond. In a period of three years Baumgarten found only 32, 30, and 41 convictions among 2400 prostitutes, and altogether only 21 cases of theft. He accounts for this by the prostitute's absolute lack of energy. Those few prostitutes who make a practice of robbing, he believes to be, first of all, thieves who have turned to prostitution because it affords easy opportunities of stealing from men. Ströhmberg contrasts the prostitutes of the passive, indolent type, with another group that consists of those who have some secondary occupation as well. But only in very rare cases is it honest work; generally it is thieving. Of the 462 prostitutes that Ströhmberg examined, 175 were thieves, of which 32 came from notorious families of thieves. His figures, which, though dealing with small groups, are, nevertheless, noteworthy because they are so reliable, show that prostitution is neither a contrast nor an equivalent to crime, but rather than the two are often united. It must, however, be admitted that a large percentage of prostitutes, in spite of their passiveness, would turn to crime if the possibility of living by prostitution did not exist.

"On the other hand, it cannot be denied that the necessity that sometimes makes a man a thief may as easily drive a woman to prostitution. The low pay received by certain classes of working women, especially waitresses, second-rate actresses, and dressmakers' assistants, makes it necessary for many a girl to supplement her wages in some way. But we must not forget that a large number are led to adopt these dangerous occupations, instead of becoming domestic servants, for instance, by their strong sexual impulses and their love of dress and an apparently comfortable life.

"Just the figures that Bebel, Blaschko, and others give in support of the view that it is poverty that drives women to prostitution seem to me to prove the contrary. It is true that working women, saleswomen, dressmakers, and, above all, former domestic servants, predominate, but they also form an unusually large part of the population. Behrend's proofs that 5.3% of all prostitutes live with their parents must make us suspicious. These better situated women belong to the not inconsiderable number who have not officially turned to prostitution, but they differ from the girls who are under police supervision only in the manner in which they carry on their occupation. Ströhmberg found poverty given as the cause of prostitution only in one case, and in that particular instance he ascertained that it was absolutely untrue.

"I would not, however, deny the significance of economic wretchedness. Girls that come from the very lowest proletarian classes, the daughters of drunkards and prostitutes for instance, never, of course, learn to look upon prostitution as anything degrading. Still graver in its consequences is the present custom that prevents prostitutes from being restricted to certain localities. They now live, as a rule, in workingmen's families. From their earliest childhood onward the children in the house see the practice of this occupation, and it is the outward brilliance that often impresses them, rather than the underlying misery; daily they see work, hunger, and scanty clothing in their own families in crass contrast to the life of idleness, theatres, concerts, balls, and luxury in dress that the prostitutes enjoy. These impressions remain and facilitate the first step towards vice. If, later, necessity or temptation, love of adventure, and envy of a friend's smarter clothes, confront a young girl, the force of habit and knowledge of the life have dulled her sensibilities in that direction to such an extent that resistance is possible only to an unusually strong character.

"This, it seems to me, is the course of development in most cases, and on it my opinion is founded. Undoubtedly our social conditions—miserable economic circumstances and the fact that prostitutes are not restricted to certain localities—are the cause of prostitution, but these factors are effective only when descent and training, and, above all, natural disposition, prepare the ground for them. And natural disposition or temperament is, indeed, of the most importance; not so much pronounced sexual instincts, for just among prostitutes they are often lacking, but general inferiority of the mind. 'In many cases prostitution is to be regarded solely as a symptom of a defective psychic condition,' says Bonhöffer, who, among 180 prostitutes, found that only one-third were without psychic anomalies. Just as the weak are the first victims of great epidemics, so, too, in the struggle for existence, it is the many defective natures that first sink into the morass of prostitution."

MENTALITY OF PROSTITUTES

More and more attention is being directed at the present time to the study of mentality among prostitutes. The early results seem to indicate that a high proportion of them are clearly mentally defective. In an analysis of one hundred consecutive admissions to the New York State Reformatory for Women at Bedford Hills, 28 girls were found to be mentally defective, below the moron grade, and considered in need of permanent custodial care. Eight had psychoses of one kind or another which would probably result in insanity. Three of these have already been transferred to an insane asylum. Further studies along these lines should show valuable results.

AN EARLY CASE OF FEMALE INVERSION

The first mention of sexual inversion in the female in the literature in English was reported[4] in 1881 by Julius Krueg. After giving a full report of a case of male inversion, he records circumstances regarding a young woman which, in his opinion, point to a similar condition. He describes the case as follows: "The patient was a maidservant, twenty-five years old. Little is known of her previous history, except that she changed her place with extraordinary frequency, until she obtained her present situation with four young ladies (orphan sisters), with whom she has been for three years. And now she vows she will throw herself into the Danube if she receives notice to leave. She says she cares nothing for men, and other circumstances confirm this, for she is such a well-favoured woman she would certainly have long since found a lover had she cared for one. She is, however, passionately devoted to her ladies, and will cry all day if she thinks one or other of them has looked black at her, going about moaning that Miss does not want her any more, etc. She is a tolerably big woman with strong but pretty features, not at all unwomanly in appearance, and, so far as can be judged, normally developed."

SEGREGATION AND PERSONAL PROPHYLAXIS

Feeling the inadequacy of education along the lines of fear toward the elimination of evil results of prostitution Christian[5] suggests that a "red light" district with police regulation and control, such as now exists in Europe, while not in every respect efficient or satisfactory, is certainly a step far in advance of our present condition with spasmodic raiding and "graft" for police protection. Even with regulation, however, the clandestine prostitute, the most dangerous of all, still remains. Personal prophylaxis soon after exposure to venereal disease should afford the public a certain degree of protection. The prompt and adequate provision for the treatment of infected persons he considers vitally important.

[4] Julius Krueg. Perverted sexual instincts. *Brain,* London, 1881–1882, iv, 368–376.

[5] Hilary M. Christian. The social evil from a rational viewpoint. *Pennsylvania Medical Journal,* xv, 788–791.

PROSTITUTION AND PERVERSION

In all the recent vice reports there have been allusions to the growing prevalence of perverted practices. Exactly what these are scientifically is not stated though it is presumed that *fellatio* and *cunnilingus* are referred to. If there is to be any intelligent effort to combat the spread of these practices it is important that the scientific data gathered regarding them be made available through some proper channel. It is natural that the prostitute, regarding sexual relations in a coldly business light should endeavor to present for approval as wide a variety of wares as possible. Furthermore such practices are usually charged at a higher rate, and are thus more profitable.

ONE ANALYSIS OF SEXUAL ETHICS

There are few persons in this country who have taken a more earnest interest in standards of sexual ethics than Richard C. Cabot of Boston. A short time ago Dr. Cabot spoke in New York before the Society of Sanitary and Moral Prophylaxis on the subject: "Are sanitary and moral prophylaxes natural allies?" and held that they were not. The conclusion reached was that the moral considerations were so paramount that sanitation could only be regarded as playing a minor or insignificant rôle. Dr. Cabot's address was a brilliant example of exposition but his main points were not fully comprehended by the majority of the audience and most of the discussion was not in the least germane to the questions proposed. Dr. Cabot's position is almost unique and, although it would not meet with general acceptation, it is entirely consistent and of great interest. It being impossible here to give a full synopsis of his argument, I hesitate to hazard a statement of his thesis. The idea was, however, that sanitation is largely a matter of information which can be conveyed by word of mouth or instruction; while morality is in no sense a matter of information but purely dependent on character. His contention was that improvement in sexual ethics will be effected only through building up the character of individuals.

A delightful series of essays by Dr. Cabot is now running in one of our leading literary monthlies. In "Some Allies of Love" he sets forth [6] one view of prostitution from the moral aspect.

[6] Richard C. Cabot. Some allies of love. *Atlantic Monthly*, Boston, 1913.

MARRIAGE OF PROSTITUTES

Freyer finds [7] that prostitutes in classic times occupied a position of marked preference to married women. The prostitute of today in many cases is inclined to marry, if she finds a husband who sees no drawbacks in her former profession. In Japan an honorable Japanese will marry a prostitute and make an ideal wife and mother of her.

ECONOMICS OF VENEREAL DISEASE

Willson has dealt [8] with the economic cost of the diseases incident to prostitution. He mentions general estimates ranging from 500,000 to 2,500,000 cases of syphilis constantly existing in the United States. Here are also a vast number of new infections each year. For every case of syphilis it may be estimated that there are several (from 4 to 10) cases of gonococcus disease. The economic cost of the treatment and possible cure of venereal disease and the expense of pelvic operations on women is tremendous. The treatment of chronic and acute eye disease, the support of blind asylums, the operation of the divorce courts and the maintenance of large numbers of the insane all represent items, part of the cost of which is chargeable to the effects of the social diseases. The great stream of incoming immigrants, none of them examined for venereal disease, constitutes, in Willson's opinion, another menace to national welfare. He believes the most effective weapon to combat prostitution and its sequelae is sex education of the younger generation.

[7] W. Freyer. Prostituierten—Ehen. *Sexual-Probleme,* Frankfurt a.M., 1912, viii, 293–300.

[8] Robert H. Willson. The economic relations of social disease. *Pennsylvania Medical Journal,* xv, 843–855.

REVIEW OF CURRENT UROLOGIC LITERATURE

ANNALES DES MALADIES VENERIENNES.

Vol. VIII, No. 9, September, 1913

1. The Antigen in the Wassermann Reaction.

The authors begin this communication by describing the cholesterin antigen of Desmoulière, its mode of employment, and the interpretation of the results with the colorimetric scale, all previously detailed in four papers published in the *Annales* and abstracted in this journal. (See especially Am. Jour. Urology, Vol. IX, No. 7, July, 1913.) The authors then go on to report their results with three different antigens, which they designate DP (a cholesterin base dissolved in an alcoholic maceration of powdered liver extracted with ether), C (a cholesterin-lecithin-soap base) and F (alcoholic extract of powdered heredo-syphilitic liver), respectively. They divided their cases into seven groups, as follows:

(1) Subjects free from syphilis, (2) Untreated or latent syphilis, (3) Primary syphilis, (4) Syphilis of less than one year's duration, (5) Syphilis lasting from one to three years, (6) Syphilis of more than three years' duration, (7) Hereditary syphilis.

Paris and Desmoulière concluded from their numerous examinations that their DP antigen gives a more sensitive Wassermann test than either of the other two antigens. To be specific:

1. In the one hundred fifty-four individuals who were free from syphilis the results were the same: all had negative Wassermanns with each of the three antigens.

2. In latent syphilis antigens F and C fail to demonstrate the presence of the disease in 20 per cent. of the patients in whom either antigen DP, clinical examination, or the therapeutic test justify the assumption that specific disease is present.

3. In half the cases of primary syphilis, whereas the results obtained with antigens F and C are at first doubtful or even negative, those given by antigen DP will permit the diagnosis of syphilis, eleven to thirteen, sometimes even as soon as eight, days after the appearance of the chancre.

4. In syphilitics of less than a year's standing the results are identical where the patients have not been treated. When the disease has been combated with salvarsan or with mercury, however, one-third of the patients treated with the former drug, and one-half of those treated with the latter would be considered cured with the F and C

antigens whereas with the DP preparation the Wassermann would remain positive.

5. Syphilitics of from one to three years' standing were too few in number for any definite conclusions to be drawn. It was observed, however, that antigens F and C gave only 54% positive results whereas antigen DP gave 74%, the difference between the two figures being represented by patients treated with salvarsan or with mercury.

6. For syphilitics of more than three years' standing the figures read: 60% positive with F and C antigens as against 75% positive with DP antigen. Most of the syphilitics examined had received specific treatment.

7. In late hereditary syphilis the difference is still more striking: 86% positive with DP antigen as against 41% positive with F and C antigen.

2. Salvarsan Does Not Sterilize Syphilis.

Lévy-Bing injected ten patients with salvarsan as soon as possible after the appearance of the initial lesion, viz., from three to fifteen days after infection. In all but one of these cases the Wassermann reaction was still negative and even in the exception it was negative with ordinary procedure but positive with the refined technique of Desmoulière.

The doses employed by the author were rather large, 0.4 to 0.6 grams of salvarsan and 0.4 to 0.75 grams of neosalvarsan. Many of the cases were started off with an initial dose of 0.6 grams of salvarsan. Salvarsan was used in eight of the cases, neosalvarsan in only two. The number of injections was never less than two (as in the case where secondary manifestations appeared before the third injection) and once it was as high as seven. The injections were repeated at the most at intervals of a week, in some cases oftener.

Nevertheless all the patients but three showed severe secondary manifestations. These symptoms appeared rather soon after the last injection: seven days in one case, three weeks in another, one month, one month and a half, two months, and five months in the others. The three patients, who up to the time of writing, did not present any actual manifestation of syphilis, have or have had positive seroreactions.

In the face of such evidence one is forced to admit that it is extraordinarily difficult, not to say impossible to *sterilize* syphilis even if one attacks the disease at its very onset when it still seems to be a local condition and when one employs large and repeated doses of salvarsan. Lest the objection is raised that this particular series of cases was in some way an unfavorable one, the author points out that the conditions were in effect as near ideal as it was possible to get them, treatment being begun in one case on the fourth day after the appearance of the chancre.

Cases of cure of the disease and of reinfection are doubtful, for the two criteria of cure at our disposal (absence of manifestations and negative Wassermann reaction) are still not entirely reliable and do not really prove that the syphilis has been sterilized. Syphilitic infection may long remain latent without disappearing entirely. Even a conceptional syphilis, which has never given any trouble, may manifest itself years afterward by a hemiplegia or some other severe tertiary lesion.

As for the negative Wassermann after 606, it may very readily become positive; besides, there are numerous cases in which syphilitic symptoms have made their appearance during a negative period.

In short, the author believes that salvarsan is not capable of sterilizing syphilis and that despite the most favorable experimental conditions he was not once able to realize the ideal of the *sterilisatio magna* claimed by Ehrlich.

3. Two Cases of Syphilitic Reinfection.

The first case is exceedingly well worked up by the author; he has even established the fact that the woman with whom the patient had intercourse was in a florid state of syphilis at the time of the act. The case under discussion was that of a man of 21 or 22 in good general condition, who during the course of a year and a half went through two complete cycles of primary and secondary syphilitic infection. Both infections were observed personally by the author.

In the first infection the constitutional symptoms assumed a relatively grave aspect: pustular syphilides, meningeal irritation (headaches). An intensive course of combined treatment was instituted: a single injection of 0.6 gram salvarsan and 17 injections of salicylate of mercury (0.1 gram each) in 110 days. There was no other treatment following this. The Wassermann was negative in June, 1912, and December, 1912, and even on May 2, 1913, despite the presence at that time of primary indurations of the second infection. The sequence of events at this stage was as follows: coitus at the beginning of April with a woman in the secondary stage, appearance of primary ulcerations on the 28th of April, 1913. May 2, Wassermann negative. May 20, Wassermann positive (four plus). Successive involvement of the lymphadenous system: inguinal glands, May 19; mastoid glands, May 24; left epitrochlear, May 30; and posterior cervicals, June 4. On the same day there developed a typical recent roscola involving the chest and abdomen. The peculiar features in this case are:

1. The proximity of the two syphilitic infections, evolving successively, and in the short space of a year and a few months.

2. A single course of combined specific treatment, short, but sufficiently intensive to overcome the first infection (negative Wassermann).

3. The different character of the secondary symptoms in the two infections. In the first case they were sufficiently severe to be called "syphilis secondo-tertiaire," and might have been regarded as a precocious tertiary or even a malignant syphilis. The secondary symptoms of the second infection were quite ordinary and benign.

The second case of reinfection is by no means so conclusive, as the author did not have the opportunity of personally observing the first infection. The latter was mild and disappeared after a moderate amount of treatment, whereas the second manifested from the beginning a most malignant character even though it did not attack any organs of vital importance and was cured rather easily by specific treatments.

ANNALES DES MALADIES VENERIENNES

Vol. VIII, No. 10, October, 1913

1. The Present-day Treatment of Syphilis.

The ideal treatment of syphilis, according to Neisser is the following:

1. Always begin with small doses (0.1 or 0.2 gm.) of salvarsan. Do not repeat the injection before eight to ten days have elapsed. Then give the same dose or a slightly larger one.

2. At the same time or even before, begin mercurial treatment.

3. If the first two intravenous injections of salvarsan (small doses) have not given rise to any untoward effects (as regards the nervous system or the gastro-intestinal tract), the dose may be increased to 0.4 to 0.6 gram for a man, or 0.3 to 0.5 gram for a woman.

4. The eliminative functions of the kidneys and intestines should be very carefully watched.

5. The very greatest care should be exercised with alcoholics, neurasthenics, and hepatics.

Unfortunately, the greatest obstacle to such procedure, in only too many cases, is the patient himself. The anxiety with which he begins treatment with 606 is only equaled by the carelessness with which he neglects to follow the most indispensable precautions—such as rest after the injection, restriction of food and drink on the evening before and the morning of the injection—after the treatment is well under way. There is an additional point to be considered, namely, the high price of the medicament. It is to be hoped that the cost will soon be diminished so that the most modest purse will be able to meet the expense.

Neisser also takes up Ehrlich's "418," or arsenophenylglycine, which he regards as a very valuable substitute for salvarsan, and which he recommends whenever the latter drug cannot, for any reason, be employed either intravenously or intramuscularly. Arsenophenylglycine when dissolved (with the same precautions as with salvarsan) in the proportion of 1 to 10 (i. e., 0.5 gm. to 5 c.c.) in a 1% solution of novocaine can be injected almost painlessly into the muscles of the buttock. The author has employed the drug in more than one hundred cases and can recommend as a safe dosage: 0.3 gram for the first injection, then four doses of 0.5 gram each, separated by weekly intervals. The total dose for an adult is thus 2.3 grams. Neisser has observed especially favorable results in intractable leucoplasias. Very large doses or cumulative action due to improper spacing of the injection may be followed by the same untoward results as are associated with salvarsan under the same circumstances.

2. Latest News from the London Congress.

Carle describes very graphically a meeting of the urologic section, held in Albert Hall, under the chairmanship of Dr. Malcolm Morris. The subjects for discussion were:

1. The compulsory declaration of syphilis by the physician.

2. The best measures to be taken by the public authorities for the diagnosis and treatment of this disease.

The author seriously questions the wisdom of selecting the first subject as a fit topic for debate, first, because the members were not sufficiently prepared and secondly, because all satisfactory discussion was impossible because of the enormous size of the hall. Professor Gaucher, with his accustomed energy, opposed the measure on the ground of professional secrecy in such matters and Dr. Carle explained how an innovation of this kind would be incompatible with French thought and feeling. The discussion was prolonged to such an extent that many members had already left the hall when the question was put to the house for a vote. It was decided in the affirmative but Dr. Carle feels that this was by no means the sense of the assemblage. Moreover, he points out that such questions should not be decided hastily by a single vote at the end of a session but that the ground should be gone over carefully beforehand, and that the results already obtained elsewhere (the reporting of syphilis is compulsory in the Scandinavian countries) should be published and familiar to all. Steps have already been taken toward this end, in connection with the next international congress to be held at Brussels.

3. A Case of Diffuse Cerebrospinal Syphilis.

The subject was a woman of 38 who had suffered previously from occasional headache, anemia, and fatigue without apparent cause. At one time she had an attack of edema of the extremities and of albuminuria. She was never pregnant; she never miscarried. Toward the end of last March she had an attack of slight headache which lasted two days and which was followed by poor vision and a paralysis of the right external rectus muscle. This was treated with intravenous injections of enesol.

From the end of April the patient began to complain of great difficulty with walking. On her admission to the hospital, May 8, her lower limbs were very weak, but there was no ataxia. The reflexes were diminished, but normal. There was steppage gait and the patient showed the utmost "weakness" on her feet. There was no difficulty with the sphincters. The right eye showed a marked convergent strabismus. The left pupil was smaller than the right and did not react to light. The pupils contracted together in convergence and in accommodation. The eye grounds were normal.

Combined treatment was begun on May 9; the patient received each day, 2 centigrams of benzoate of mercury by injection and 2 grams of potassium iodide. The Wassermann reaction was strongly positive. The next day movement of the lower extremities was almost absolutely impossible; The Achilles reflex was gone, the knee jerks were still present; there was bilateral Babinski. From then on improvement was steady (treatment being continued as above described) until the patient was discharged on July 25. At that time there was no difficulty with the patient's posture or gait. There was no more headache and no more fatigue. The Achilles and knee reflexes were completely abolished. There was no sensory disturbance. The paralysis of the right external rectus persisted unchanged.

There are several interesting points in connection with this case. (1) The unilateral Argyll pupil on the side opposite to that of the palsy. (2) The multiplicity of localizations in this case of syphilis of the central nervous system: paralysis of right external rectus, Argyll pupil on left side, flaccid paraplegia. (3) Perhaps most interesting of all is the mode of onset of the paraplegia. During the course of a walk, in which the patient noticed nothing abnormal, she attempted to cross the street and narrowly missed being run over by a carriage. She was not hurt but under the stress of emotion she collapsed and had to be carried to her home. From that moment on, she had increased difficulty with locomotion, until in less than two weeks she was suffering from a complete flaccid paraplegia. It appears, therefore, that in this particular case a latent specific lesion was brought to light by emotional stress alone.

ZEITSCHRIFT FÜR UROLOGIE

Vol. VII, No. 11, 1913

1. Renal Hemorrhages in Hemophiliacs. By Otto Mankiewicz. P. 865.
2. A Case of Misinterpretation of a Kidney Röntgenogram. By A. W. Wischnewsky. P. 879.
3. Arthigon in Anterior Urethritis. By Dr. Orlowski. P. 882.
4. Spina Bifida, Retentio Urinae, Hydro-ureteropyelonephrosis Bilateralis, Diverticulae Vesicae Urinariae. By M. A. Mucharinsky. P. 885.

1. Renal Hemorrhages in Hemophiliacs.

Mankiewicz reports two cases. The first was a traveling salesman, 31 years old, who had a renal hemorrhage in May, 1908, following a hot bath. He had previously had severe hemorrhages from an operation on cervical glands, and a tooth extraction. Examination at the time of the hematuria showed that the prostate, bladder and kidney regions were entirely normal. He was given gelatin internally, also ergot, castor oil and morphine. Later on 15 drops of adrenalin were administered, three times a day. The filtered urine was red (hemolysis). In less than ten days the urine was free from blood. The patient died a few months later from heart failure.

The second patient was a cutter, 25 years old. His hematuria began on Feb. 4, 1913. He had taken a steam bath 2 or 3 days before on account of pains in the left elbow (hemarthrosis). Both knees showed greater or lesser changes of arthritis deformans resulting from old hemorrhages. He was ordered rest in bed, gelatin by mouth, and about 2 drams of ergot t.i.d. On February 11, calcium chlorid was begun (about 7 grains, 4 times a day). The condition cleared up but on the 23d blood reappeared in the urine. Calcium was again given and styptol was begun. On March 1, 30g. of gelatin (Merck) were given subcutaneously. On March 5, 40c.c. of horse serum were administered subcutaneously. On the 13th a strict dry diet was commenced, and on the 15th, 15 c.c. of horse serum were given intravenously. For the next two weeks the patient passed blood clots occasionally; after that the condition cleared up entirely (except for an inflammation of the left knee) and when last seen, on August 8, he was well, having gained about 8 pounds.

The author summarizes similar cases reported in the literature and then takes up the various modes of treating this condition. Perhaps the most popular procedures are as follows:

1. Improvement of the general condition. [Avoidance of exposure—especially to changes in temperature—seems to play an important part in prophylaxis.—Ed.]

2. Injection of serum up to 40 c.c. at a time. Either human or horse serum (diphtheria anti-toxin answers the purpose) may be used.

3. Transfusion of blood directly into the veins. The author takes up in detail Soresi's and Elsberg's methods.

4. Administration of gelatin by mouth or subcutaneously. Cmunt has shown that 40c.c. of 10% gelatin given subcutaneously increase the viscosity of the blood 1.4%, whereas 2000c.c. of 3% gelatin given by mouth in ten days increase the viscosity of the blood 0.6%. Unfortunately the blood pressure is also increased. To be of any great value gelatin must be administered over long periods. It is not of much use in emergencies.

Calcium salts (chlorid or lactate) do not seem to be of much value.

One liter of milk a day will introduce more calcium into the system than the most intensive calcium treatment.

5. Restriction of fluids. A dry diet, as carried out for the first time in this condition in the author's second case, seems to be of distinct value. For fifteen days no fluids whatever were taken and the solid food was prepared as dry as possible. The coagulable substances seem to be increased in proportion to the blood volume, as a result of this treatment.

Mankiewicz recommends that in all cases of hemorrhage in general, but in hemophiliacs especially, dry diet be given in conjunction with gelatin over a long period. In this way the necessity of transfusion may be avoided, as was accomplished in the second of the author's cases.

2. A Case of Misinterpretation of a Kidney Röntgenogram.

The patient, a girl of 22, consulted the author for bleeding from the bladder. The patient had been treated for stone. Five years before she had had pain in the right lumbar region. At this time an abscess had formed at the crest of the right ileum and was opened. It was supposed to have been tuberculous in nature. An X-ray picture was taken and as a result the diagnosis of renal stone was made.

When the patient was examined by Wischnewsky she presented great tenderness in both renal regions, and a painful cystitis with attacks of tenesmus every quarter of an hour. The general condition was much run down although the heart and lungs were supposed to be normal. The temperature was for the most part normal, but occasionall rose to 100.4°.

Catheterization of the bladder gave at first urine, then a large quantity of pure pus mixed with blood. There was clearly a tuberculosis cystitis secondary to a similar process in both kidneys. At this point the author was enabled to examine the X-ray plate which had been made five years before. The affected kidney appeared in the form of a shadow like a bunch of grapes. There was no question of simple calculosis; it was clearly a case of fibrosis with calcareous changes due to tuberculosis.

The patient died 3 weeks later. A guinea pig inoculated with the bladder urine showed typical lesions of the viscera and peritoneum.

The author feels that had the case been properly diagnosed when the X-ray picture was taken the patient's life could have been saved by nephrectomy as the other side was probably not affected at that time.

3. **Arthigon in Anterior Urethritis.**

Orlowski distinguishes two types of recurrent anterior urethritis. The first, which is the more common, is characterized by the onset 2 or 3 days after the cessation of irrigations, of a heavy pus discharge accompanied by itching which results, pathologically, from an infection of the urethral adnexa: lacunae of Morgagni and glands of Littré.

In this type Arthigon treatment is of no avail. The second type, however, is very favorably influenced by Arthigon. In such cases the discharge reappears on the day after the irrigations are stopped, there is no itching, the first portion of the urine contains flakes. Anatomically there is no infection of the mucosa and since such individuals possess no accessory glands or lacunae the urethral wall is attacked only by isolated organisms which cannot penetrate, become parasitic, and supply a continuous discharge of pus from small abscess cavities. In such cases the author injects 2 to 2½ grams of Arthigon intramuscularly. Three injections usually suffice. They must be followed by a slight temperature rise and local irritation, otherwise they are of no avail.

Orlowski uses this serum treatment in still another class of cases, namely, in the acute exacerbations, resembling primary infections, of old gonorrheics. In such cases the author gives 8 injections, of ¼ to ½ to 1 gram twice a day, with good results.

4. Spina Bifida, Retentio Urinae, Hydro-ureteropyelonephrosis Bilateralis, Diverticulae Vesicae Urinariae.

The patient, a young man of 17, had been suffering from nocturnal incontinence since birth; during the day, he passed small quantities of urine every 15 to 30 minutes. In the region of the sacrum he presented a soft scar with a yielding center. This condition was due to an operation which he had had 9 years before for spina bifida.

The patient could void 60 c.c. of urine spontaneously, but 600 c.c. could be drawn off with the catheter. Cystoscopically, the vesical neck and a part of the trigone were swollen with bullous edena, the ligamentum interuretericum was thickened, the fundus was trabeculated. The ostia of the ureters were not visible but in their place, and elsewhere, rather large diverticula were present.

The quantity of urine was 3 liters in the 24 hrs., the specific gravity was 1006, but 0.3% albumen was present. There were a few leucocytes in the sediment. The left ureter could be readily catheterized through its dilated ostium. The right ureter could not be catheterized owing to a kink in its intramural portion. Collargol was injected into the bladder and up the left ureteral catheter. By this means it was shown that the bladder was very small, 4½ by 4½ cm., with two diverticula and the ureters very much dilated, being about 1 cm. across at their vesical insertion, 2 cm. at the linea innominata, and 2½ cm. at their renal end.

Mucharinsky compares his case with others reported in the literature. He believes that the abnormalities he presents are of central origin and depend upon the existence of the spina bifida. In fact the trabeculae, the diverticula, the dilatation of the kidney pelves and ureters, all depend upon the poor development of the bladder and the predominance of the sphincters over the detrusors. There was no real incontinence but merely a paradoxical incontinence from retention with overfilling. By conservative treatment—such as systematic catheterization of the bladder—these conditions were much improved. Radical operation with construction of a new bladder would be very dangerous because of the almost certain ascending infection which would follow. In case operative interference was indicated it would be necessary to perform a uni- or bilateral nephrostomy, to free the ureters from adhesions, and to do a plastic on the kidney pelvis to avoid pyelonephrosis and the further stretching and destruction of kidney tissue.

MISCELLANEOUS

Salvarsan.

H. E. Robertson, Minneapolis (*J. A. M. A.*), has carried out studies of the effects of salvarsan on the muscles of animals compared with that on the muscles of man, and also of the effects of neosalvarsan, and of both of these drugs compared with those of deep injections of the ordinary mercurial preparations still used in the treatment of syphilis. Dogs were used in all the animal experiments and the results are given in tabulated form. The facts developed are reported as follows: "1. The lesion in these cases consists of hemorrhage and necrosis with edema which develops almost immediately following the injection. Leukocytes early invade the tissue and tend to form a zone around the necrotic area. 2. Salvarsan invariably leaves a deposit of insoluble yellow pigment which acts in every respect as a comparatively inert foreign body. 3. There is no appreciable difference between the severity of the lesions which appear after the intramuscular injections of either salvarsan or neosalvarsan. If anything, neosalvarsan tends to give a slightly more diffuse zone of destructive inflammation. Reparative processes begin in about a week, but the absorption of the necrotic material proceeds very slowly and usually is not completed until a period of at least two months has elapsed. 4. Variations of the amount of the drug injected from one-half to twice the amount advised does not appreciably affect the extent of the lesion. 5. No changes in the general health of the animal could be observed, and there was no evidence of any marked tenderness at the site of the injections and no apparent limitation of motion unless abscesses developed." A second series of experiments was made with the ordinary mercurial preparations with similar results though not quite so severe. Two cases of necropsy of human beings showing the necrosis produced by the intramuscular injections of salvarsan are also reported. They conclude that the use of such preparations in this manner is in the majority of cases an unjustifiable procedure. The article is illustrated.

Genital Tuberculosis in Children.

Including under this head the localization of tuberculosis in the prostate, seminal vesicles, epididymis, or testicles, Oliver Lyons,

Denver (*J. A. M. A.*, December 6), says such cases occur and have no restriction as to months or years of life. Their frequency, however, is disputed, and he does not agree with those who claim that they are as common in children as in older persons. He believes that primary tuberculosis may occur in the male generative organs but is rare compared with secondary infection. Primary tuberculosis in the seminal vesicles and prostate is according to his experience a rare occurrence. Predisposition may be a factor in its occurrence and Lyons puts more faith in this view than do some authorities. The frequent localization of the tuberculous lesions in parts of the body not readily exposed to external infection must, he says, be regarded as congenital. The entrance of the tubercle bacilli through the urethra must be very rare and the history of tuberculosis in childhood is generally against any exclusive port of entry. The onset may be sudden or gradual and when confined to the genital organs may give rise to no symptoms calling attention to it. A discoloration or swelling is perhaps the first symptom as in cases reported. Acute tuberculosis of the epididymis or testes is rare and begins suddenly with acute symptoms. It has probably been preceded in some cases by preëxisting tuberculous nodules that were unnoticed. In the differential diagnosis, congenital syphilitic orchitis is the most common and the most difficult disease to exclude. The chief aids are the other signs of congenital syphilis and the therapeutic test. Sarcoma is the next most frequent disease but can usually be recognized; clinically the treatment would be the same. Hydrocele usually presents no difficulties but should be remembered as often a symptom of tuberculosis. Benign tumors are so rare they need little consideration. The prognosis of primary tuberculosis of the genitals in children is usually favorable and it is important to know that tuberculosis of these organs remains almost always the only tuberculous focus in the body, differing in this respect from that in adults. Operation therefore may produce permanent cure though this is not certain. It should always be advised.

Bladder Suture Four Years After Operation.

Judd describes the appearance of the bladder four years after operation (*J. A. M. A.*, December 6). There were no adhesions along the suture line. Careful search revealed no trace of the continuous silk suture which was used.

Case of Foreign Body in the Rectum.

Conlin reports (*J. A. M. A.*, December 6) a case of foreign body in the rectum with operation and an uneventful recovery. The foreign body was a cup measuring 3¼ inches by 3½ inches and about ¼ inch thick.

A CASE OF PELVIC KIDNEY

Dr. G. J. Thomas reports from the Mayo Clinic (*Annals of Surg.*) a case of pelvic kidney diagnosed before operation. The patient was a married woman, aged thirty-two. The vagina was about one inch in length, and no uterus was discoverable on palpation. She had never menstruated but had distress and pain over the region of the ovaries every two months. A rounded mass about the size of an orange high in the left inguinal fossa, tender to touch. For about a year she had been suffering from attacks of frequent urination, which lasted about a week and then disappeared. Complains of a low abdominal pain, alternating from one side to the other, cannot lie on her left side, and has been confined to bed for two or three days at a time with marked soreness in the left pelvis. Cystoscopy showed the urethra and bladder to be normal. It was difficult to pass the left ureteral catheter more than 2¼ inches from the bladder. The right side appeared to be normal. Amount and character of the urine from the left side compared favorably with that from the right side. A double injection of colloidal silver by the gravity method was made and a radiogram taken, which shows the pelvis of a hydronephrotic kidney lying well down in the left bony pelvis. The ureter was 3½ to 4½ inches in length. The pelvis of the kidney was upward and inward from the cortex, and the ureter's course upward and outward then downward and inward. The patient was operated by W. J. Mayo, and the position of the kidney was found as above. The blood supply to this kidney came from two or three renal arteries from the left common iliac about one-half inch below the division. The renal vein entered the vena cava just at the bifurcation and was closely adherent to the kidney-mass. All of the left external iliac vein could not be found. It may have become fused with the internal or it may have been very small, due to the pressure of the adherent kidney.

BOOK REVIEW

Our Nation's Health Endangered by Poisonous Infection Thru the Social Malady: The Protective Work of the Municipal Clinic of San Francisco and Its Fight for Existence. By Dr. Julius Rosenstirn, Chief of Staff and Attending Surgeon, Mt. Zion Hospital; Chairman Advisory Committee Municipal Clinic of San Francisco. Baker & Taylor Co., 33 East 17th St., New York, 25 cents.

All those who are interested in fighting venereal disease and who are not blinded by bias and prejudice will do well to read Dr. Rosenstirn's pamphlet. There is so much hysterical gush poured out on the subject of prostitution that it is a pleasure to read occasionally some common sense utterances.

THE AMERICAN JOURNAL OF UROLOGY
WILLIAM J. ROBINSON, M.D., EDITOR

VOL. X MARCH, 1914. No. 3

PYELITIS FOLLICULARIS

By HERMAN L. KRETSCHMER, M.D., Chicago, Ill.

THE terms pyelitis follicularis and pyelitis granulosa have evidently been used for describing the same pathological condition. Paschkis says that we should differentiate between the cases of pyelitic granulosa reported by von Frisch with their concomitant bleeding, and pyelitis follicularis, which is often seen as a co-existing condition in various pathological lesions, as for example, hydronephrosis or nephrolithiasis. According to this more or less arbitrary classification, the following case should be reported as one of pyelitis follicularis, because of the absence of profuse hematuria:

Mrs. S., aged 36, referred by Dr. George Parker, Peoria, Ill., Aug. 19, 1912. She dates her present illness back ten years. In February, 1902, albumin was found in the urine. This occurred before her first confinement, and she was kept in bed for six or eight weeks prior to delivery. At this time her feet were badly swollen. During her second pregnancy she had no albumin. Following the second confinement she again had swollen feet. After this she was under observation for a long time, but the albumin never disappeared.

Two years ago she went to the hospital and was operated on for a perineal laceration. During her convalescence a high fever developed, which was called malaria, for which she was treated for over two months, without being free from fever. At this time the consulting physicians found pus in her urine, and the pus has been present ever since. The administration of large doses of urotropin seems to control the fever, and the amount of pus becomes less, but the urine is never completely free from pus.

She has attacks of fever which come on without any regularity, and are accompanied by very severe chills. The temperature after the last attack was 103 F., eight hours after the chill.

For many years she has had a backache. No matter where the pain in the back begins, or where it is most severe, it always winds up on the left side. There have never been any urinary symptoms, nor has she ever noted blood in the urine. Physical examination was negative. X-ray examination was negative. Blood-pressure was 112.

Cystoscopic Examination. The bladder was negative, except for the presence of a slight edema of the trigone. Double ureteral catheterization. No obstruction to catheters.

Urinary Examination.

RIGHT	LEFT
Turbid	Clear
Neutral	Acid
Urea 0.4%	Urea, 0.3%
Albumin, + + +	Albumin, + +
Sugar	Sugar, 0
Pus present	No pus
Casts, 0	Casts, 0
Blood, 0	Blood, 0

Phenolsulphonephthalein Test.

	RIGHT	LEFT
Time of appearance	7 minutes	4 minutes
Amount of elimination	2 per cent	15 per cent

Bladder leakage, 22 per cent
Total phthalein output, 39 per cent

On Sept. 12, 1912, the patient was operated on in her home town. Right-sided nephrectomy was done. A very small pus kidney was removed. Recovery was uneventful. Five weeks after the day she was operated on she had a severe chill, and a temperature of 101.5 F. The chill lasted for fifteen minutes, but she was cold for about one and a half hours. The temperature after this attack remained high for three days, whereas prior to her operation the temperature returned to normal after the chill.

A specimen of urine examined by her physician showed the presence of a large amount of pus and bacteria. A second cystoscopic examination, Nov. 7, 1912, showed a slight difference in the appearance of the ureteral orifices, the right being a little larger than the left. Some edema of the base of the bladder was present.

Double Ureteral Catheterization.

RIGHT	LEFT	
No urine	Clear	Bacteria, many
	Albumin, +	No pus
	Casts, 2	

Phenolsulphonephthalein Test.

Time of appearance, 4 minutes
Total output in 30 minutes, 41 per cent

Shadowgraph catheters were passed into both ureters and an X-ray was taken. The right catheter did not move with respiration, and the upper three inches of the catheter are very plainly visible, so that the eye of the catheter and even the fabric of which the catheter is made are distinctly seen on the X-ray plate. From this it is evident that the catheter lies very close to the X-ray plate and hence must lie in a cavity close to the back.

Examination of the Kidney. The specimen is two inches long, and one inch wide and weighs 15 grams. The parenchyma of the kidney has been reduced to a mere shell, being replaced by large sacculations. The pelvis is apparently very much thickened and feels hard. The mucous membrane is thrown up into folds. Situated within the mucous membrane and projecting well above its surface were seen many small nodules, the largest being about the size of a millet seed.

Microscopic Examination. Upon histological examination the nodules were seen to be composed of a light center area, which is surrounded by a darker zone of small lymphocytes very closely crowded together. The center consists of lymphocytes which do not stain as deeply as do the cells at the periphery. The nodules as well as the surrounding areas are very vascular. The smaller nodules are covered by the mucosa of the ureter. The larger nodules project well above the surface of the mucosa and are only partially covered by it. No ulceration of the follicles was seen. The picture is one of a lymph follicle with a germinal center. (Fig. 1.) Some of the nodules show the presence of two germinal centers. By far the larger numbers of nodules project above the surface of the ureteral mucosa.

Up to the present time most of the work on this subject has been done by the pathologists and the results of their work will be taken up later in this paper. Recently this subject has received more attention from the clinicians, and for this reason it might be well to consider the reported cases in detail. In the literature at my command I have been able to find records of only the following seven cases.

Solieri and Zanellini [1] report a case occurring in a patient aged 42, who was suffering with attacks of profuse hematuria, associated with frequency of micturition and pain at the external urethral orifice. The hematuria rapidly became worse, the hemoglobin going down to 35 per cent. Suprapubic cystotomy showed the blood coming from the left ureteral orifice. Left-sided nephrectomy was done. The pelvis of the kidney was studded with small excrescences like grains of sand. Microscopically they found lymph follicles made of a connective tissue reticulum with a tendency to capsule formation, being identical in structure to Peyer's patches of the intestine. The follicles for the most part were large and round. Blood-vessels were abundant in and around the follicles. In some areas the follicles were ulcerated and opened into the lumen of the pelvis.

The case reported by Taddei [2] occurred in a woman, aged 23. The first attack of hematuria was painless, of four weeks' duration and the hematuria ceased with drug treatment. One year later a second attack of hematuria occurred. Cystoscopy showed that the blood came from the right ureter. Nephrectomy. The pelvis showed the presence of miliary nodules. The cells which constitute the follicles have the characteristics of lymph cells. The most superficial lymphatic follicles raise up the epithelium of the pelvis, protected everywhere by its characteristic cellular plan. The lymphatic subepithelial follicles are found to diminish as we recede from the ureteral orifice of the pelvis.

Loewenhardt's [3] case concerned a woman, aged 33, whose only complaint was hematuria. The origin of the hematuria was proved to be from the right kidney by a cystoscopic examination. Nephrectomy. Six months after the nephrectomy she had another milder attack of hematuria. A cystoscopic examination at this time showed a nodular appearance of the mucous membrane in the region of the trigone. The mucous membrane of the pelvis appeared hypertrophic and nodular. Microscopically,

[1] Solieri and Zanellini: Clinica Chirurgica, 1905, xiii, No. 96.

[2] Taddei: Ann. d. mal. d. org. gen.-urin., 1907, No. 55.

[3] Loewenhardt: Arch. f. Dermat. und Syph., lxxxiv.

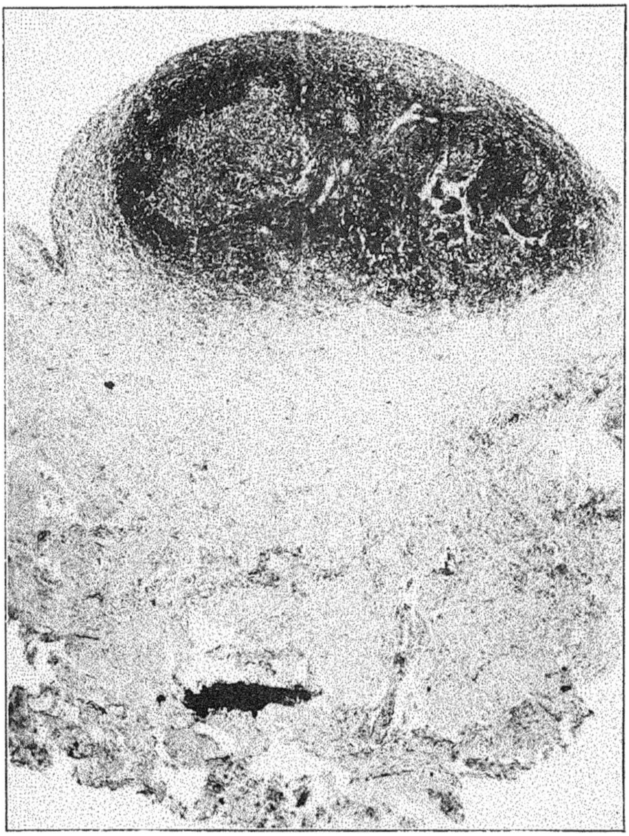

Fig. 1.

Microphotograph of section through lymph follicle.

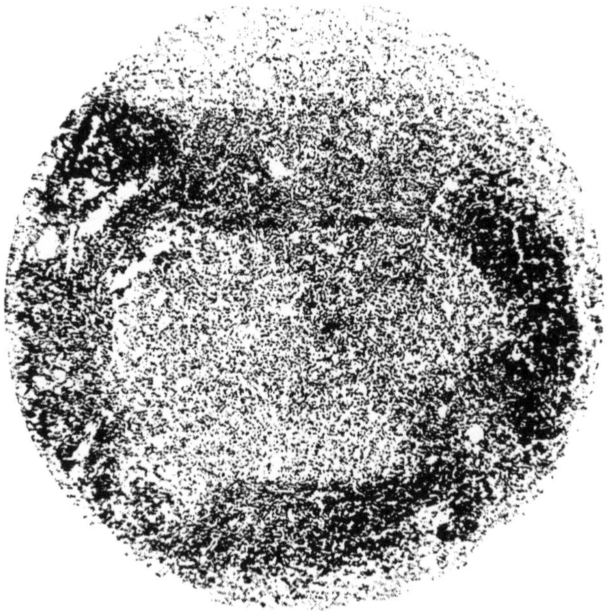

Fig. 2.
Microphotograph showing a part of
Fig. 1 under higher power.

there were seen rounded subepithelial masses of round cells, resembling lymph follicles. He also noted an extraordinarily rich vascularization.

Von Frisch [4] had the good fortune to be in a position to report three cases. In all three cases there was a profuse intermittent hematuria and a pyelitis granulosa. The kidney pelvis was studded with grey or reddish-grey nodules, the size of millet seeds, which protruded above the surface of the mucous membrane. The mucous membrane of the pelvis showed a diffuse round cell infiltration. Near the surface of the mucous membrane the mononuclear cells are grouped, forming lymph-follicle-like structures, which resemble the solitary follicles in the large intestine. He also found the presence of germinal centers. The blood-vessels were markedly dilated in the neighborhood of the follicles, being well filled with red blood-cells.

Paschkis' [5] article contains an illustration from a case of pyelitis follicularis showing germinal centers, but no clinical history is given.

Associated Lesions. Taddei's case had associated inflammatory changes in the kidney. Loewenhardt's case, a subacute pyelopapillitis and an interstitial nephritis. In von Frisch's first case, the pathological process was limited to the pelvis and papille; in the second case, pyelonephritis, and in the third case a severe degeneration of the entire kidney.

In the above-reported case there were two gross kidney lesions; first, the small size of the kidney, and second, the almost complete destruction of the kidney by a pyelonephritic process.

The kidney was free from associated lesions in von Frisch's case and in the case reported by Solieri and Zanellini. In two cases, von Frisch's third and in my own case, B. coli communis were found.

Pathogenesis. Various theories have been advanced by different authors as possible explanations for this rather rare condition. Solieri and Zanellini, who probably were the first clinicians to report a case, advanced a theory which they based on embryology. Their conclusions exclude lymphosarcoma, leukemia and pseudo-leukemia, because the follicles described have characteristics identical with normal lymphatic follicles, with characteristic reticulum and medullary texture. They cannot be com-

[4] Von Frisch: Verhandl. d. Deutsch. Gesellsch. f. Urol., 1911.
[5] Paschkis: Folia Urologica, 1912, vii.

pared to ordinary granuloma. "We cannot speak of an infectious process unless we wish to admit the existence of special micro-organisms not revealed by ordinary stains, not transportable and non-inoculable, and which are capable of inducing new formations with the attributes of normal lymph follicles. Owing to these considerations and because the renal pelvis has diverged from the kidney, derived from the allantois, which is of intestinal origin, we are inclined for want of another opinion to admit an aberration of these same embryonic germs which under the ordinary circumstances give follicles of Peyer."

Taddei does not agree with Solieri and Zanellini for two reasons: "In the first place, there is no need to say that this quantity of lymphoid tissue in the submucosa of the kidney pelvis is absolutely abnormal.

"In the second place, all embryologists are not in accord as to the derivation of the renal pelvis from the allantois."

This brings us to the question as to whether lymphoid tissue is a normal constituent of the renal pelvis. There still remain some differences of opinion among the various writers on this topic.

Chiari [6] published the results of his examinations, in which he reports that in the mucous membrane of the urinary apparatus in man, under pathological conditions, there frequently occur collections of lymphatic tissue. He lays stress on the pathological significance of this, because as a result of many repeated examinations in which the mucous membrane was normal, he was never able to find lymphatic tissue present. The pathological conditions which may play a rôle in this formation are inflammatory in nature, especially catarrhal conditions, during the presence of which the follicles gradually develop, may persist for a long time and gradually completely disappear by resorption.

Prezowski [7] comes to some rather startling conclusions in his report of three cases coming to autopsy. He has seen a total of fifty-eight cases of this rather rare condition, a number which far surpasses the report of any one else. It must be borne in mind, however, that his report is based on his findings in the post-mortem room. In regard to his conclusions, he states, first, as these follicles are absent in the mucous membrane of the urinary tract of the new-born, they must therefore be looked on as the

[6] Chiari: Med. Jahrb., 1881, page 9.
[7] Prezowski: Virchow's Archiv., Vol. 116.

result of later development; second, inasmuch as they are often completely absent in adults and in old age, they cannot be considered as normal constituents of the body; third, the nodules vary in one case in size and number and in what appears to be development, so that one cannot help but think that they may develop at any period of life; fourth, the presence in some of the nodules of fatty changes, as well as the presence of ulceration in consequence of suppuration in the nodules, demonstrates that the nodules can disappear at any time. Further, that they are more numerous in a mucous membrane showing inflammatory changes is suggestive that the catarrhal mucous membrane conditions are most favorable for their development. Upon all of this evidence, he thinks that these nodules resembling lymphoid follicles are in the large majority of cases, if not in all, pathological in their origin.

Stoerck [8] says that he examined a large number of bladders in infants, from a large series and from various parts of the bladders, for the presence of follicles, with the same negative results as were obtained by other authors. There are, however, many other authors who look on these follicles as constituents of the normal mucous membrane. Thus, for example, Weichselbaum, who examined the bladders of five young men, aged from 20 to 23, who had either committed suicide or were hanged, found lymphoid tissue in all five and comes to the following conclusions as a result of his examinations: He believes that one is justified in asserting that under normal conditions lymphoid tissue may occur in the human bladder, though whether or not they must always be present can hardly be determined definitely from the examination of five cases. He believes that these lymphoid follicles may be present normally but very sparingly, but not until they become swollen and enlarged by pathological changes do they become visible microscopically.

Also in the text-books on histology, we find equally rather unsettled views regarding the histology. Stöhr's, Gray's, and Quain's Anatomies do not mention the presence of lymphoid nodules in describing the normal histology of the kidney pelvis and the ureter. Piersol, quoting Toldt, says that occasional aggregations of lymphoid cells occur, which in the vicinity of the calices sometimes form distinct minute nodules within the mucosa. Ferguson, Bailey, Szymanowicz and MacCallum describe the for-

[8] Stoerck: Ziegler's Beitrage, Vol. 26.

mation or the occasional presence of small collections of lymphocytes which sometimes form solitary follicles. They do not regard them as of constant occurrence. Regarding the statement of Chiari that these follicles may persist for a long time and gradually completely disappear by resorption, I should like to mention a case previously reported,[9] in which I had the opportunity of seeing this phenomenon occur. The follicles were present in the bladder during the time of the patient's illness and were seen with the cystoscope. Some of the nodules were removed and examined microscopically, so that the nature of the nodules seen with the cystoscope was proved microscopically. About four or five months after the patient left the hospital and when he was free from all symptoms, he was again cystoscoped and at this time the nodules had disappeared. Whether a similar occurrence might take place in the pelvis or kidney, I will not attempt to say.

In regard to the diagnosis, this probably can never be made except at the time of operation. In those cases presenting the clinical symptoms of profuse hemorrhages, it might be well in going over the possibilities to consider the presence of pyelitis granularis or follicularis. Further than that I do not think we can venture.

In regard to treatment, I think the treatment will depend on the conditions found at operation. If the kidney is perfectly normal, as occurred in one of von Frisch's cases, and in the case of Solieri and Zanellini, I think measures other than nephrectomy should be instituted, unless, of course, there be danger due to loss of blood on the part of the patient. It might be well to consider the use of pelvic lavage; in those cases in which bacillus coli communis infection is present, to employ vaccines. There are only two cases on record in which the colon bacillus was found, one of von Frisch's cases and in the case just reported.

[9] Kretschmer: Surg. Gynec. and Obst., Nov., 1908, page 510.

SUDDEN DEATH FOLLOWING PYELOGRAPHY

By E. O. Smith, M.D., Cincinnati, O.

ON January 14th I was asked to make a cystoscopic examination of Mrs. M. at the Cincinnati General Hospital, on account of a mass in the right side of the abdomen. The patient, aged 64 years, appearing much older, was thin, poorly nourished, but was able to walk into the cystoscopic room without assistance. The bladder was found to be normal and both ureters were catheterized without difficulty. The same amount of urine came from each kidney over the same period of time. There was neither pus nor blood in either specimen. It was decided to photograph the pelvis of the right kidney, which was done two days later. Twenty cubic centimeters of 10% collargol preparation was injected through a ureteral catheter with a small hand syringe. But little force was used, and further injection stopped as soon as the patient complained of pain.

The accompanying radiograph was taken by Dr. Sidney Lange. From the beginning of the introduction of the cystoscope until it was removed after the radiograph exposure was not more than six or eight minutes. Before removing the catheter, collargol was seen coming from the ureter. The patient was placed on a carriage to be returned to the ward. I left the room but was quickly recalled by the orderly stating that the patient was not "doing very well." When I returned she was dead. This was not more than five minutes after I had removed the cystoscope. This death was so unexpected that a post mortem examination was made by Dr. C. F. Hegner to determine the cause of death.

Autopsy Report of S. M., Jan. 16, '13· Dr. Hegner.

Body that of a poorly developed and poorly nourished adult white female, apparently seventy years of age.

There is a moderate lordosis of the dorsal spine, and a lateral contraction of the thorax. The eyes are somewhat puffy, and the legs are slightly edematous to the knees. The abdomen is rather prominent, and the bowels moderately distended with flatus. A tumor can be felt on the right side of the abdomen extending from the right costal arch to the pan of the ilium.

On opening the chest, both lungs were found firmly adherent

to the chest wall, over an area corresponding to their upper lobes. Both lungs were markedly emphysematous. Large fibrous tuberculous nodules were noted in the apices of the upper lobes of both lungs. The bronchi showed a moderate bronchitis and bronchiectasis and contained a considerable amount of mucopurulent material.

The heart was very greatly enlarged, the myocardium firm and of good color. The coronary vessels were sclerosed. The aortic ring was completely ossified. The aortic leaflets were very stiff and one was so contracted as to make closure of the valve impossible. The mitral leaflets were thickened and fibrous. The pulmonary valves and tricuspid valves showed no gross lesion. The aorta was markedly atheromatous.

The abdomen: Bowels were distended with flatus, the transverse colon and the duodenum were adherent to the greatly distended gall-bladder. The gall-bladder was the size of a man's fist, very tense and filled with creamy pus, which contained twenty-five gall-stones. The liver extended one and one-half inches below the costal arch. It showed a pronounced cardiac cirrhosis. Beneath the liver and behind the gall-bladder was a secondary abscess. This abscess was well walled off and communicated through a small opening with the gall-bladder.

The mesenteric lymph glands were somewhat enlarged, especially those in relation with the hepatic flexure of the colon and that part of the small intestine adherent to the gall-bladder. There was no evidence of malignancy.

The intestines with the exception of the before mentioned adhesions showed no gross lesion. The spleen was small and fibrous.

Kidneys: The right was firm and moderately contracted. The pelvis was comparatively large. On section a considerable quantity of dark fluid (collargol solution) escaped and stained the section. On close examination of the surface of this section as well as of one made at right-angles to it, one could see striations of similar dark color extending with the uriniferous tubules to the cortex near the capsule. The glomeruli were very prominent. The renal vessels were sclerosed. The cortex of the kidney was irregularly contracted and the capsule was irregularly adherent. The ureter of the right kidney contained a few drops of the same dark fluid. The bladder contained about one and one-half ounces of the same.

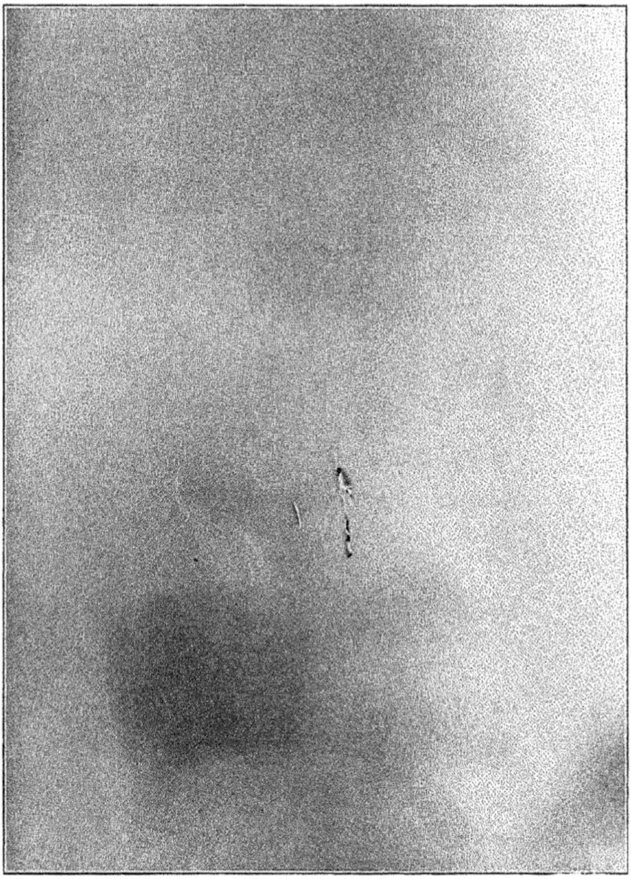

Radiograph of kidney pelvis. 10% collargol. 20 c.c. used.

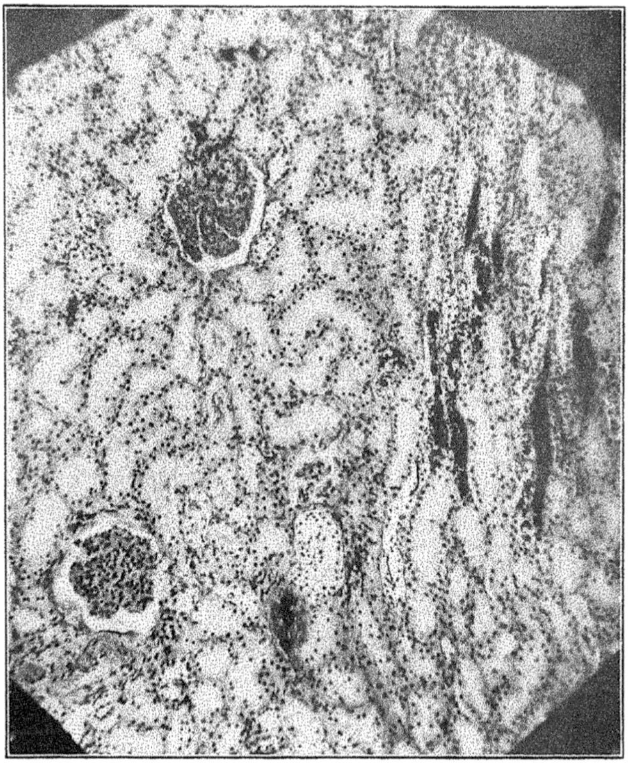

Showing collargol in the tubules, outside the tubules, and in a few cells.

The left kidney showed much the same lesions with the exception of the dark fluid and the staining therewith.

The kidneys were demonstrated before the Clinical Society of the Cincinnati Hospital, and sent to the laboratory for microscopical examination.

Summary: Emphysema, Bronchitis, Bronchiectasis, Aortic Stenosis, Aortic Insufficiency, Arterio-sclerosis. Empyema of the Gall-bladder with secondary abscess, Cholelithiasis. Cirrhosis of the liver (cardiac), Acute and Chronic Interstitial Nephritis (arterio-sclerotic type).

Dr. Paul G. Woolley, Pathologist.
No. 272, Ward N, S. M., Jan. 17, '13·

Report: Both kidneys show an acute interstitial nephritis, superimposed upon a subchronic diffuse (interstitial-arterio-sclerotic) process. Right kidney contained a (nitric ac. or H. C.) soluble black pigment in the tubules.

A very small amount of pigment was also present in occasional tubules and in a few cells.

Photo-micrograph. This was a patient who, although able to be about the ward, had so many pathological lesions that it required but little to turn the tide. The mere handling and manipulations necessary to make the pyelograph, plus the shock of the collargol in the kidney, were sufficient to break the slender thread that held life in her body. We have learned the lesson that it is wise to take into consideration the patient with his weaknesses other than those that may be of urological interest, and that there is some positive shock attending pyelographic examinations. We have further learned that it is possible to force some silver preparation into and beyond the uriniferous tubules into the kidney substance, and when this does happen it evidently produces shock. After having studied this specimen, and having observed the general invasion of the kidney by the collargol, I think we are in position to *explain* the causes of the shock and elevation of temperature that sometimes follow this examination. Just how much damage, either temporary or permanent, has been done to kidneys in this way will never be known. I am convinced that no preparation should be *forcibly* injected into the pelvis, but that it should be introduced only by the force of gravity.

MASTURBATION

By Victor Blum, M.D.

Assistant in Prof. von Frisch's Urological Department of the Vienna General Polyclinic

AUTHORIZED TRANSLATION. EDITED WITH NOTES AND ADDITIONS BY DR. W. J. ROBINSON

IN a consideration of the functional disorders of the male sexual organs masturbation deserves proper recognition.

The chief reason for this lies in the circumstance that we meet sexual abuse and especially masturbation in the etiology of most other functional genital symptoms, hence we must discuss this " disease " as a most important pathogenetic factor in the etiology of the genital neuroses. Moreover masturbation represents an important functional disorder, which shows such characteristic features in its manifestations and its clinical results that we can treat this disease here as an independent group of symptoms. We may also devote a separate chapter to masturbation for this reason, that this disease has an etiology and a symptomatology of its own, and because the results of masturbation occupy to a certain degree a unique position in the symptom-complex of sexual neurasthenia.

The word masturbation (from *manus*, hand, and *stuprare*, to debauch) has many snyonyms in colloquial and medical language; namely, onanism, self-abuse, self-pollution, the sins of youth, the solitary vice, etc.

Very few of the definitions which have been made of masturbation are satisfactory. The latest, by Fürbringer, is as follows: " The artificial excitation of the outer genitalia performed of one's own accord and by one's own manipulations without the participation of the other sex and continued until ejaculation, or in women and children to the climax of excitement "; but this does not include all forms of masturbation, since neither " one's own manipulations " nor " absence of the other sex " is necessary to the idea of onanism.

The definition of Pouillet's (" L'onanisme chez la femme,"

Paris, 1877) seems to me the most precise: "Onanism is an act contrary to nature performed with the help of a living organ (hand or tongue) or any instrument (such as a pencil-case or an artificial penis) with the object of exciting the venereal orgasm; whether performed alone or with other persons."

One important form of masturbation, however, is not included even in this definition; namely, imaginative, mental masturbation, which we shall soon see plays a very significant part in the masturbatory neurosis.

I define masturbation as follows: "Any intentional manipulation, brought about by psychic or unnatural means, or tolerated from others, which has the object of producing sexual voluptuous feelings without conjunction of the opposite sexual organs."

We can then distinguish between active and passive masturbation. To the objection that also homosexual acts, pederasty, etc., fall within this definition of onanism I reply that most homosexual acts must really be considered as onanistic, and that "amor lesbicus" (Lesbian love) is also included in all the works on our subject among the forms of female masturbation.

Following our definition we shall consider in this chapter in order, manual masturbation, active and passive (mutual), imaginative, psychic, and instrumental masturbation.

Masturbation is one of the most widespread epidemics which exist; indeed, one may say it is *the* most widespread (Rohleder). We are not justified in calling it *vice.* The conception of vice and sin supposes the knowledge in the person concerned that the action in question is forbidden. But as a matter of fact the practice begins as a rule at an age when the individual can take no account of the impropriety of the act.

Masturbation occurs at all ages of life, in all countries, at all times, and spares neither the upper nor the lower classes of society.

We meet this kind of sexual abuse extremely often in the history of most functional disorders of the male genital organs (impotence, chronic nocturnal priapism, morbid seminal losses, etc).

It is indeed doubtless true that masturbation in many cases, even when practiced in relative excess, *does not necessarily lead to any nervous symptoms;* and many authors felt obliged to draw the conclusion from this fact that the continually emphasized injurious effects of masturbation are exaggerations.

The severest results of masturbation that we are familiar with—severe sexual neurasthenia, impotence, and spermatorrhea—are partly attributed by these authors to other causes, such as overexertion in professional work, excesses in the natural satisfaction of the sexual need, dreams, etc. In part also they assign to masturbation only the significance of a secondary cause, and see the primary cause of these severe disturbances in general neurasthenia and in other severe derangements of the nervous economy.

We take quite a different standpoint in this question. We admit at once that masturbation does not necessarily have a pathogenic effect in all cases.

But *excessive* masturbation is probably never tolerated without injurious effect. When we hear, for instance, from Lallemand (Les Pertes Seminales) that one of his patients was accustomed to masturbate from his eleventh to his fifty-third year and estimated his excesses even in the last five years at about ten every day (!), we cannot be surprised that such an excessive masturbation must have an absolutely pathogenic effect.

But if we disregard such excessive masturbation, we must recognize that *severe* results can occur in other cases of *moderate* masturbation *only* when another cause coöperates beside the onanism; and we must regard a special nervous predisposition as such a cause. But there is here a suspicious concatenation, for we know on the one hand that an hereditary nervous constitution may cause an early beginning of masturbation, and that on the other hand this precocious masturbation must be the origin of the severe nervous phenomena occurring later.

The reasons for the great injuriousness of masturbation are manifold:

There is at the outset a great error in the oft-repeated

supposition that, in a mechanical respect and with regard to the end-result as well as to the processes in the nervous system, the act of masturbation should be considered as hardly differing in nature from coitus.

The masturbatory act supposes a much greater activity of the imagination; the immediate erotic impressions and sensations, which come spontaneously in coitus, must be replaced in masturbation by increased mechanical stimuli and by excessive demands upon the erotic conceptions. All these powerful accessories to sexual activity, which we receive in normal cohabitation from visual impressions, tactile sensations, kissing, sensations of smell (perfume) and of hearing, all these immediate perceptions must be replaced with the manual masturbator by the power of the imagination—truly an excess of mental effort, a waste of valuable nervous substance!

In coitus a gradual increase of the libido and the stimulus, up to the discharge of ejaculation, necessarily results from the normal course of sexual congress; whereas in masturbation disturbances in the normal sequence of the reflexes interfere, disturbances which arise from the wish for a quick ending of the sexual act.

The masturbator aims in the first place at the quickest possible conclusion of his sexual manipulation. When erection has once taken place, he will hasten the arrival of ejaculation by increasing the mechanical friction, and as soon as the former has arrived not enough time is given to the congested sexual organs, as must be the case in coitus, gradually *by means of depletion of the hyperemic organs* to pass over temporarily into a state of rest.

To this are added all kinds of disturbing psychic processes: The masturbator must secure absolute secrecy for his "sin," and for this purpose the most out-of-the-way places are sought, where his desire is indulged, usually in a standing position in the greatest haste. As soon as the ejaculation has come, a sense of bitter disillusion ensues; the victim regrets the vice, makes the worst possible self-reproaches, and declares this is the very last time.

The individual act of masturbation is thus in course and

effect wholly different from normal cohabitation. The mechanical manual friction of course does not correspond to the specific sensations received from the vagina, the reflexes are voluntarily influenced, and in place of the satisfaction and general relaxation with voluptuous feelings, which come at the close of normal coitus, there appear quite opposite sensations.

The abnormalities in the course of the individual onanistic act also furnish explanations for the different pathologic effects of masturbation.

One of the earliest is ejaculatio præcox, which also figures in masturbation as to the voluntary ending of the sexual act; on attempts at coitus the lessened resisting capacity of the ejaculatory center becomes evident. The disorder of the erectile power, a very annoying result of previous masturbation, finds its explanation in the fact that the masturbator in the course of time has accustomed himself to masturbate also without complete erection; at bottom he cares only for the outcome, the seminal ejaculation.

The absence of orgasm, which so depresses reformed masturbators, when they take up regular sexual activity again, seems to us quite natural and easily explained by the strong feelings of disgust which had followed each separate act of masturbation formerly.

The impotence in many cases of masturbatory neurosis is characterized by the absence of libido. This derangement of the male genital functions will also become quite intelligible to us when we consider the characteristic circumstances accompanying masturbation.

After what has been said we must admit that there is a great and important distinction in the nature of the masturbatory act from that of normal coitus.

There are still other factors which weigh down the scales against masturbation in favor of normal coitus, even when practiced to excess.

A most important factor is that masturbation is often begun extremely early. According to authenticated reports by various authors one meets this "vice" occasionally even in infancy. One observation of Hirschsprung's (Hosp. Tid. 1885) concerns a child of four or five months. According to the reports of Hirschsprung, Kraft, Rohleder, Vogel and Bloch children from one to three years of age were repeatedly caught masturbating.

It is at once intelligible that this tender age, when the young brain is still developing rapidly, masturbation must have a decidedly injurious effect upon the whole nervous system. And the histories of these children regularly show convulsions and other severe nervous disturbances in immediate sequence to the attack of masturbation or later.

Such early sexual injuries in childhood make ineffaceable impressions upon the mind and nervous system in later life. We frequently succeed, in studies in psychoanalysis in neurotic diseases of adults, in discovering sexual traumata in childhood of the nature of masturbation and similar acts as the cause of the neurosis.

A further circumstance, which tends to make masturbation especially injurious, is that the temptation is unusually strong to excessive indulgence of the sexual impulse.

The often limited opportunities for practicing coitus, on account of various external reasons, constitute a leading factor in preventing excesses in true venery. The latter require time and preparation, money and an understanding with the other party; whereas all these considerations do not come in question in the masturbatory satisfaction of sexual desire. Every momentary libidinous impulse can be indulged in at once.

The great danger of venereal diseases enters in as an important preventive factor against venereal excesses. This often exaggerated fear of infection and also the fear of impregnation may form an incentive to self-abuse.

Experience teaches that masturbation has an extremely weakening effect upon the human will; to break off the vice an expenditure of energy is required, which the patient can no longer command, and so he remains a slave to his lonely enjoyments and sinks deeper and deeper into the slough of masturbation and its injurious consequences, with each act.

We have already indicated how differently masturbation

and natural coitus affect the morality, the ethics, and the esthetic feeling of man.

The sexual sphere of the masturbator claims his whole mental life; ideas, which are felt as completely indifferent by the normal man, awake libidinous sensations. Hardly any energy is left for the development of the mental faculties; hence masturbators fall behind in school; and gradually the destructive nature of their vice reaches their consciousness. They cannot muster enough energy of will to consult a reliable physician or adviser; they live in continual anxiety of being discovered and in the fear that people can read in their face what passions they indulge; so they become insincere and shy, are always depressed, and completely lose their self-confidence.

Natural coïtus has exactly the opposite effect upon the human psyche. It elevates the self-consciousness, the feeling of well-being, the joy in work, and the creative energy.

"Nothing is more calculated to cloud the source of noble, ideal sentiments, which evolve of themselves from normally developing sexual feelings, and under some circumstances to dry it up entirely, than masturbation practiced at an early age. It strips scent and beauty from the bud, which should unfold to a perfect flower, and leaves behind only the coarse-minded, animal instinct for sexual satisfaction. If such a ruined individual arrives at the procreative age, he lacks the esthetic, ideal, pure, and ingenuous attraction, which attracts to the other sex. The glow of the sensual perceptions is quenched, and the inclination to the other sex is considerably weakened. This defect influences the morality, ethics, character, imagination, mood, feelings and impulses of the youthful masturbator, whether male or female, unfavorably, and in some cases extinguishes the desire for the other sex entirely, and causes masturbation to be preferred to any natural sexual intercourse." (Krafft-Ebing, "Psychopathia Sexualis.")

KINDS AND FORMS OF MASTURBATION

In the investigation of the etiology of sexual neuroses we are always compelled to ask the patient whether he has formerly indulged in masturbation, and perhaps in half the cases we obtain a negative answer. A part of these negative answers is made in such a hesitating and non-credible fashion, that the experienced physician can interpret such a "no" unhesitatingly as an affirmative answer. It lies in the very nature of the disease, which injures the character and will; and we must be prepared a priori for the greatest untrustworthiness of the patients' statements in every neurosis, which awakens suspicions of a masturbatory origin. But even when the patient has nerved himself up with the last remnant of energy to make a full confession to his confidential physician, he will still sometimes deny our questions concerning earlier masturbation out of pure IGNORANCE; for according to colloquial usage the layman understands by onanism only *manual* masturbation. So much the more important is it that the physician should be familiar with the various forms of "the vice," since the different kinds of onanism have more or less the same results on the physical and mental condition of the patients.

Following the definition of masturbation given at the beginning of this chapter, we must distinguish the following forms of the habit, which under certain circumstances must be appraised differently in the pathogenesis of the onanistic neurosis.

We shall consider solitary and mutual masturbation, active and passive, manual, instrumental, and psychic, and finally also a variety of sexual abuse, related to onanism—abortive excitements.

The most common kind of masturbation is the solitary, manual self-abuse.

With the aid of erotic conceptions and fancies an erection is voluntarily brought about, and ejaculation is then produced by means of the familiar tactile stimulations (manual friction of the glans and skin of the penis, rubbing of the penis on the abdomen, and pressing between the thighs). Erection can also be produced mechanically from other places, the so-called "erogenic zones."

The urethral mucous membrane, especially the prostatic portion, which is rich in nerves and ganglia, may be the location of the erogenic zone. We know from clinical experience that the introduction of an instrument into the urethra may sometimes be followed by erection and libidinous feelings.

The occurrence of URETHRAL MASTURBATION is explained by the erogenic capacity of this mucous membrane; and we meet this form sometimes in the pathology of the masturbation neurosis.

Objects and instruments of the most various kinds are introduced into the urethra from masturbatory desires. These are mostly advanced neurasthenics, whose tactile sensibility of the penis and glans has suffered severely from years of abuse; but sexual desire and erection may still be excited from the urethra. These cases usually come first to the physician's attention when mechanical injuries of the mucous membrane have been produced by the introduction of instruments, or when with careless handling they slip into the bladder. It is necessary to introduce the instrument deep into the posterior urethra, in order to increase the intensity of the sexual excitation, and then the accident often happens, that the object slips into the bladder and occasions there all the well-known dangerous symptoms of foreign bodies in the bladder. We know cases from our own experience in male masturbators, in which wax-candles, bougies, needles, hairpins, quills, etc., were introduced into the urethra for the purpose of masturbation.

A 45-year-old school porter came to us with a great scrotal and perineal phlegmon. The infiltration was opened by long incisions. After some three weeks a necrotic piece of tissue the size of a goose-egg came off, and investigation of it showed that the whole urethral wall was included in it. A quill ten centimeters [four inches] long and as thick as a pencil stuck in the urethra, which it had pierced and so brought about the infiltration of urine. When the "corpus delicti" was shown the patient, he denied that he had introduced the quill. Healing occurred without stricture.

A painter's model about 60 years old came into the city clinic on account of severe urethral hemorrhage, and confessed that he had himself caused the injury by masturbating with a hairpin, which he had introduced point first.

A gentleman 40 years of age masturbated in an original

way by introducing the Ultzmann endoscope for painting the urethra ("Pinselendoscope"). By means of painting the bulbous urethra he obtained strong erections and ejaculations. In one such attempt, however, the brush broke off. It was extracted with the aid of the endoscope.[1]

The anus and the mucous membrane of the rectum form another erogenous zone.

The erections which we see so often in massage of the prostate, are only partly to be explained in this way. The prostatic tissue, rich in nerves, and the posterior urethra, which are regularly irritated by the massage, are probably to be regarded as a separate erogenic zone. There is no doubt that prostatic massage offers many patients—advanced neurasthenics—a substitute for masturbation; some of our old patients in the city clinic have frankly confessed as much to us.[2]

Krafft-Ebing cites cases of anal "auto-masturbation," and says: "They seem to occur not very rarely and explain passive pederasty." (Garnier, Moll, and Cristiana.)

Masturbation in the society of others occurs both as mutual onanism and as passive onanism.

The former may be homosexual, mutual masturbation between two persons of the same sex, or tribadism, or between persons of opposite sexes.

The last-mentioned, which is a very common resort in fear of genital infection and pregnancy, is frequently met with in "refined" debauchees, to whom coitus in os and inter mammas, etc., forms a much coveted substitute for natural coitus.

This kind of masturbation comes the nearest to normal coitus.

The distinction lies in the fact that not the specific friction

[1] Choppard reports in his "Maladies des vices urinaires" an almost incredible case of masturbation. After a period of ordinary manual masturbation there followed in this patient a period of satisfaction by the introduction of a wooden stick into the urethra. When this means also failed, he resorted to incisions of the glans down to the urethra, and carried these so far, that finally the organ was split down to the pubic bone into two parts (!). This masturbator succeeded still during the next ten years in regularly inducing ejaculations by the introduction of the wooden stick into the remaining portion of the urethra.

[2] An interesting case of rectal masturbation in an old man is reported in *American Journal of Urology*, for January, 1908.

stimuli from the glans penis in the vagina produce the seminal ejaculation, but it requires different and for the particular individual stronger stimuli to awaken the pleasurable feelings that result in erection and finally in ejaculation.

Those cases of "abstract coitus" in which sexually hyperesthetic men obtain their sexual satisfaction by more or less accidental contact with a fully dressed woman, which gives them an erection and orgasm also belong here in part. On the other hand this group may also be classified as psychic onanism (see below).

Such individuals only need to put themselves in an imaginary sexual relation with a female person opposite them in a railway car or a parlor in order to obtain an orgasm and ejaculation. (Krafft-Ebing.)

Another sort of masturbation forms a symptom of the sexual perversion known under the name of *fetichism.*

Separate parts of the woman's body, or sometimes mere objects, such as parts of the woman's clothing, present the adequate stimulus for the origin of libidinous feelings and of orgasm. This morbid fetichism expresses itself in "automasturbation" or manual masturbation on the basis of conceptions which concern the fetich.

HOMOSEXUAL MUTUAL MASTURBATION.

This occurs most often where many young men live together and for external reasons intercourse between the sexes is impossible or very difficult; namely, in schools, barracks, boarding-schools, prisons, in the navy, etc. We have already pointed out the great dangers of this form of masturbation as regards the origin of contrary sexual feeling.

The cases of PASSIVE MASTURBATION have an especial pathologic importance, so far as they do not belong to the just mentioned groups, when the indulgence occurs in early childhood. It is evident from many clinical histories, that some conscienceless governesses and wet-nurses make it a rule to quiet the restless, crying child by stroking its genitals or even by sucking them. There is no doubt that these sexual traumata suffered in earliest childhood have great importance for the child's whole development, and especially for that of its sexual life.

Instrumental masturbation, which is much less important in the male than in the female sex, has been already mentioned under manual solitary onanism. Some observations of anal instrumental masturbation (foreign bodies in the rectum) also belong here, as well as numerous experiences of psychopathia sexualis, in which self-masturbation is performed only by immediate contact and irritation of the organ with the article of female clothing (shawl, stocking, handkerchief, etc.,) which acts as a fetich.

PSYCHIC MASTURBATION.

We have finally to consider a form of masturbation, the importance of which is very much undervalued by our patients and also, unfortunately, by many physicians, although it is not at all inferior in injuriousness to the usual forms of manual masturbation.

Those men commit mental, psychic onanism or ideational masturbation, who can bring themselves to such a state of sensual excitement solely and entirely by force of their imagination, without touching or producing any mechanical stimulation of their genitals, that erection, ejaculation and orgasm all occur.

An objective basis, which aids the lascivious fancy in these cases, is furnished by obscene stories, looking at obscene pictures; but sometimes also the sight of drawings, which excite no erotic ideas whatever in the normal man, can put the sexually hyperesthetic mental masturbator in the highest degree of sensual excitement.

In this form of onanism the imagination alone has to replace all the peripheral stimulations, which in the normal man furnish adequate stimuli for the genital reflex-centers for erection and ejaculation.

The nervous system of the youthful "offender" cannot bear the extreme mental work, used up in this mental masturbation, without serious consequences. Even the immediate effect of the individual act is usually staggering in its results.

Inability to work intellectually or to think, and the greatest weakness and faintness follow each such act. With longer duration of this injurious habit the patients complain sooner than usual of loss of memory, of energy, and of mental elasticity, and come prematurely to the severe forms of sexual neurasthenia. It can indeed not be denied that in men predisposed to neurasthenia the liveliness of their imagination favors the practice of psychic, ideational masturbation. There exists in originally neuropathic men such a marked sexual hyperesthesia that even slight stimuli affecting the sense organs are conveyed by the psycho-sexual cerebral center to the spinal centers, and this causes erection and then ejaculation, or even the latter without the former.

We spoke already on a former occasion of those patients who indulge in the especially dangerous vice of " imaginary coitus."

The meeting with a congenial member of the fair sex enables such mental masturbators, even under the observing glances of the company, by means of imagining the woman disrobed, to bring themselves to the highest degree of sexual excitement, and then by further imagining coitus to obtain a seminal ejaculation and orgasm. The slightest contact with the woman in question, which could hardly be declared unchaste, accelerates the achievement of the final object, ejaculation.

It is usually not far from such practices to the severe forms of spermatorrhea, when diurnal pollutions, seminal emissions with or without erection occur under the same circumstances, although to be sure undersized and unintended.

We should mention here still another form of sexual trauma, which should be regarded in some measure as a masturbatory counterpart of coitus interruptus. We refer to ABORTIVE EXCITEMENTS, conditions of sexual excitement, which do not lead to sexual satisfaction. Daily experience shows us how widespread this vice is among our youth. If we assume, according to recent but perhaps inexact statistics, that of every hundred persons [1] at the age of puberty and older ninety are

[1] In the most recent report Kémény estimates 96% onanists among country pupils.

given to masturbation at least occasionally, we may assume with full justification for nearly all the remaining ten per cent., that they expose themselves, at least now and then, to the above-mentioned injury from abortive excitement. The essential nature of this vice is that its devotees habitually and voluntarily increase their libido to a high degree of sexual excitement, obtaining an erection, but stop the substituted sexual act before the occurrence of ejaculation.

Thus a voluntary interruption in the course of the sexual reflexes takes place, and the interweaving of this voluntary act forms a part of the injury; the other part grows out of the fact that the necessary discharging of the sexual centers in the brain by means of the ejaculation and orgasm is wanting. The libidinous conceptions have led to a certain amount of sexual tension, which should be discharged by the normal course of the genital reflexes.

The cause of these frustrated excitements, which occur as a part-phenomenon of manual and ideational masturbation, and also as a part-phenomenon of normal intercourse, lies in the mistaken conception of the dangers of masturbation; the devotees have the false idea that in this way they do not commit the sin of masturbation; and on the other hand the fear of the consequences of sexual intercourse (pregnancy and infection), and indeed even the fear in irrational people of weakening of the organism by seminal emission in several of our cases, furnish the reason for this abnormality of the sexual life.

EPIDIDYMOTOMY WITH REPORT OF CASES

By Carlisle P. Knight, M.D.

Assistant Surgeon, United States Public Health Service, Stapleton, N. Y.

EXCELLENT success and most gratifying results have been obtained at the United States Marine Hospital, Stapleton, N. Y., with Eckles' operation for epididymitis. The technic described by Eckels,[1] except for slight modifications, has been followed.

In the operation, as I have performed it, an incision is made in the scrotum about 1½ inches below the lower border of the external ring and is prolonged far enough to allow free delivery of the testicle with the tunica vaginalis. The organ is then wrapped in sterile cloths, moistened in warm saline solution, and a small incision is made in the tunica vaginalis which allows any fluid present to escape. The epididymis is next exposed and that portion which appears inflamed is punctured in several places. This relieves the tension by allowing the restricted fluid to escape. Eckels states that for puncturing the epididymis he uses a blunt probe or grooved director. I employ a large bluntpointed needle, making from ten to twelve punctures, and I believe that the needle is better adapted for this procedure, especially when operating under local anesthesia. After the tissues have been thoroughly washed with warm sterile saline solution, the testicle is returned to the scrotum. The tunica vaginalis is then approximated and united with a continuous catgut suture. The scrotum is then united with interrupted silkworm sutures. The skin in proximity to the incision is again painted with iodin solution to insure asepsis, a sterile dressing is applied and the scrotum bridged with adhesive tape to give support for the first few days. Eckels also states that, if pus is present, a longitudinal incision should be made in the epididymis and a few strands of silkworm-gut inserted for drainage. In two cases pus formation was found at operation. I have used the procedure described above, and the results obtained were as satisfactory as in those cases in which only inflammation was present.

Eckels states that the preparation of the patient is the same as that for a general anesthetic, as local anesthesia is not advisable. I have used it, however, for this operation in several of the cases which I report, with absolute success, hearing no complaints of pain, and noting no symptoms of shock. There may

[1] Eckles, Lauren S.: Epididymotomy, *The Journal A. M. A.,* Aug. 16, 1913, p. 470.

be some pain if an orchitis is present, as happened in one of the cases, but with careful handling of the testicle, this symptom can be obviated. For local anesthesia, a 1 per cent. solution of novocain with epinephrin is infiltrated along the line of the intended incision. Twenty minutes later the incision is made and the tunica is exposed, infiltrated and incised, after which the solution is injected into the epididymis, and anesthesia of the part is complete. The procedure of puncturing and, if necessary, incising, is then absolutely painless. Because of the rapidity with which the operation can be performed, from five to ten minutes being the time required, and the absence of pain and shock, the procedure does not seem to warrant the use of the dangerous general anesthetics.

From a study of the cases at this hospital, the points observed almost entirely agree with the conclusions noted in Eckels' article. The only exception is that I am unable to make any deduction as to the probability that there is a smaller percentage of sterility following the disease in those operated on. I agree with him that the operation should be the procedure of choice in the treatment of epididymis and believe that the patients should be operated on as soon as symptoms appear, thereby eliminating the possibility of pus and abscess formation.

REPORT OF CASES.

Case I.—J. M., aged 21, a Swede, seaman, applied at the hospital for admission, Aug. 27, 1913. Patient's previous history was unimportant. A few days before admission he noticed a discharge from the urethra. Gonorrhea was diagnosed. Patient was put on the usual treatment and the case progressed favorably until September 15, when great pain began in the left testicle. Examination revealed an epididymitis. Operation was performed, September 16, under a general anesthetic. Morning temperature on the day of operation was 38.2 C. (100.76 F.), but became normal at the end of forty-eight hours, with patient comfortable and free from pain. Case progressed favorably and recovery was noted Sept. 23, 1913.

Case II.—J. G., aged 40, an American seaman, was admitted to the hospital Oct. 11, 1913. Previous history was unimportant. Gonorrhea was diagnosed. Patient was put under treatment and the disease ran the usual course until October 24, when the discharge stopped abruptly. October 30 the right testicle became swollen and the epididymis became enlarged and very painful. Epididymotomy was performed November 1 under general anesthesia. November 2 pain had ceased. November 6 patient was walking around ward and note of recovery was made.

Case III.—W. H., aged 20, an American seaman, was admitted to the hospital, Sept. 27, 1913. Two weeks previously he noticed a discharge from the urethra and ten days later complained of pain and swelling in the left testicle. Examination revealed gonorrhea complicated by epididymitis. Treatment for the gonorrhea was begun, and palliative measures were employed for the epididymitis. The testicle showed no improvement and on October 8, the patient consented to an operation, which was performed under local anesthesia. Relief from pain was instantaneous, and six days later he was up and about the ward. October 17, patient had fully recovered from the epididymitis. Later, however, an endocarditis developed and he was not discharged until Nov. 22, 1913.

Case IV.—J. H., aged 20, a seaman, was admitted to the hospital, Nov. 14, 1913. Eighteen days previously he had noticed a discharge from the urethra. Two days prior to admission he complained of severe pain and swelling in the left testicle. Examination revealed gonorrhea complicated by epididymo-orchitis. Patient was put to bed and given palliative treatment. Temperature on admission was 39.4 C. (102.92 F.). No improvement was noted in his condition and on Nov. 17 the right epididymis became involved. Temperature at that time was 39 C. (102.2 F.). The next day operation was performed on both testicles under local anesthesia. Twenty-four hours after the operation, patient was resting comfortably except for slight pain which was due to the orchitis on the left side. Pain was gone from the right epididymis. At the end of forty-eight hours temperature was normal and all pain absent. November 21, patient was up and about ward. November 25 wound was healed and recovery was noted.

Case V.—L. A., aged 21, an American seaman, was admitted to the hospital, Nov. 18, 1913. Eight months previously he had first attack of gonorrhea, but had never been cured. The discharge has returned at intervals and lately has been flowing freely. A few days before admission, patient complained of a severe pain in the left testicle. Examination showed a swollen and tender epididymis. He was given palliative treatment until Nov. 23, when he consented to an operation. This was done under local anesthesia. The following day all pain was absent, the swelling reduced and the case made the usual good recovery at the end of six days.

In three other cases operations have been performed under local anesthesia with the same good results, such as absence of pain during operation and the immediate abatement of the symptoms of inflammation.

CONCLUSIONS.

Attention is called to the points which are considered most important in favor of the operative procedure.

1. There is immediate abatement of all symptoms for which the patient seeks relief.
2. The tendency to relapse is nil.
3. The operative procedure is without danger as regards anesthesia, because the general anesthetics can be eliminatd.
4. This operation as compared with the older methods of treatment is one of utmost importance from an economic point of view, not only to the patient, when loss of time from daily labor is considered, but also to the hospital in its economic administration, by greatly diminishing the number of days of treatment.

PROSTATECTOMY UNDER LOCAL ANESTHESIA [1]

By Carroll W. Allen, M.D., New Orleans

IN the operative relief of hypertrophy of the prostate we have in the great majority of cases to consider certain factors which are not, as a rule, involved in other surgical procedures, namely: that of age, as most of the cases requiring surgical relief for this condition have reached or passed middle age, and many of them are infirm or weakened by suffering or infection.

In the old and feeble, prostatectomy is a formidable operation, though not attended by a greater mortality than that following any other major operation in the same class of patients. However, it may even show a more favorable comparison by observing certain methods in the handling of these cases.

Surgical technic has reached such a stage of perfection that in the more commonly performed operations it would seem difficult to suggest improvements in the recognized methods of procedure in typical cases. Improvements will come, but I believe that they will be more in the preparatory treatment, general handling of the case and refinement in details, rather than in the general principles involved in the operation.

One of the notable advances recently introduced as a general

[1] Read at the Thirty-fourth Annual Meeting of the Louisiana State Medical Society, Baton Rouge. *N. O. Med. and Surg. Jour.*, Feb., 1914.

surgical procedure is the anoci-association of Crile. This, I believe to be a factor of great consequence, particularly when applied in old and feeble patients, as it prevents shock-producing impressions from the field of operation from reaching the higher nerve centers.

The two great factors in the production of shock are trauma and hemorrhage. Surgical trauma we cannot prevent, as we intentionally inflict it, but we lessen its shock-producing effect by blocking all nerve endings in the field, by injecting the tissues with weak anesthetic solutions. This is done whether the patient is to have a general anesthetic or not, as Crile has shown that general anesthesia does not prevent shock from trauma.

The method which I wish to present to-day is the result of a gradual evolution in handling cases of prostatectomy. While I had never noticed any marked shock following prostatectomy by former methods, in those cases in which I used the anoci-association of Crile, by resorting to a preliminary injection of the prostate with anesthetic solutions there was an improvement in the results, as these cases showed practically no change in their physical condition after operation.

The control of hemmorhage was accomplished by the logical addition of adrenalin to the injected solution. The absence of all bleeding in cases so treated was most striking, practically no blood being lost at all—just enough to moisten a few sponges; thus there was a decided gain for the patient, the two shock-producing factors being eliminated.

The results of this technic were borne out by a more rapid convalescence of these patients, and this method, combined with a two-stage operation, opening the blader a few days before, under local anesthesia, has enabled me to carry to a successful termination cases of badly infected bladders in feeble patients, which I would have hesitated to operate by any other method.

The continued use of the above method, and its gradual extension, led to the elimination of general anesthesia, until now it is used only from choice and not from necessity, as these cases can be as successfully operated by local anesthesia as can hernia, rectal and many other conditions.

The technic of the procedure is as follows: One hour before operation a suppository containing 10 grains of anesthesin is placed in the rectum to anesthetise this region and prevent any discomfort when the finger is introduced here in elevating the prostate.

At the same time, one hour before operation, a hypodermic of morphine, 1/6 grain, and scopolamine 1/150 grain, is administered to lessen physical disturbances. The operation is begun by opening the bladder under local anesthesia; its walls are then retracted by long, deep, narrow retractors, bringing into view the field of the prostate. Depending upon the size and shape of the prostate, several points are selected for injection on the vesical surface, usually one below the opening of the urethra, near the base of the gland, and one on either side. The needle is passed through the mucosa, with the idea of making the injection between the true and false sheath of the prostate, as it is in this plane that the solution must diffuse around the gland, and it is in this plane that its enucleation is effected. It is here where the large venous plexuses are situated and where the nerve filaments are more easily reached as they pass through to the prostate.

Two or three drams of a 1/2% novocain solution, containing 15 minims of adrenalin to the ounce, are injected at each of the above points. The needle is then passed into the urethral opening and the lateral wall pierced first on one side and then on the other, and similar injections are made at these points.

If the gland is very large, or there is much of a projection above the urethral opening, an additional injection can be made here, otherwise the above will prove sufficient. It is well now to wait two or three minutes for the solution to diffuse and thorough anesthesia to be established before beginning the enucleation. While waiting for the solution to diffuse, the action of the adrenalin is observed in the prostate, which becomes quite pale and bloodless.

In making the injections, should they be made into the substance of the gland itself, no harm will be done, only they are not quite as effective as when injected peripherally between the true and false sheath; any excess of the solution thrown into the gland in this way is removed during its enucleation and not absorbed.

This method may not appeal to all of my audience, as it requires a certain familiarity with local anesthesia before one cares to undertake major operations by its use alone.

I will, nevertheless, urge that even under the general anesthesia you resort to the preliminary injection of the field with a local anesthetic combined with adrenalin as a most potent agent in the elimination of those two most active factors in the production of shock—trauma and hemorrhage.

DEPARTMENT OF SEXOLOGY

SOLON AND GREEK PROSTITUTION

IN every mention of the history of prostitution it is stated that Solon was founder of the system. This is, of course, not entirely correct, though he may be regarded as the sponsor of state regulated prostitution. The authority for the statement is, however, little known. It exists in the work of a Greek-speaking Egyptian of Naucratis, a rhetorician and grammarian, who flourished about the end of the second and the beginning of the third century A. D. His principal work which has come down to us is the *Deipnosophistaa* translated as the *Deipnosophists* and probably meaning "dinner-table philosophers." It consists of a clumsy arrangement of quotations from various authors most of whose works have not been otherwise preserved. It is the chief source of our knowledge regarding the intimate morals and customs of the Greeks. The first edition in book form was issued by the Aldine Press in 1524. An English translation has also been made.

The passage [1] to which reference is made is as follows:

"And Philemon, in his *Brothers*, relates that Solon at first, on account of the unbridled passions of the young, made a law that women might be brought to be prostituted at brothels; as Nicander of Colophon also states, in the third book of his *History of the Affairs of Colophon*,—saying that he first erected a temple to the Public Venus with the money which was earned by the women who were prostituted at these brothels.

"But Philemon speaks on this subject as follows:—

"But you did well for every man, O Solon;
For they do say you were the first to see
The justice of a public-spirited measure,
The saviour of the state—(and it is fit
For me to utter this avowal, Solon);—
You, seeing that the state was full of men,
Young, and possess'd of all the natural appetites,
And wandering in their lusts where they'd no business,
Bought women, and in certain spots did place them,
Common to be, and ready for all comers.
They naked stand; look at them well, my youth,—
Do not deceive yourself; ar'nt you well off?

[1] ATHENÆUS. *The Deipnosophists.* Translated by C. D. Yonge. London. 1854. Vol. 3, pp. 910-911. (Book xiii, par. 25.)

You're ready, so are they: the door is open—
The price an obol: enter straight—there is
No nonsense here, no cheat or trickery;
But do just what you like, and how you like.
You're off: wish her good-bye; she's no more claim on you.

CHINESE PROSTITUTION

A RECENT study [2] presents a digest of most of the available literature on the prostitution system in China. One of the most valuable sources of information was found to be a classic essay [3] by an eminent Dutch scholar who had spent considerable time in China. For the time, 1866, his statements are probably accurate and some of his descriptions are vivid and illuminating.

The training of the prostitutes seems to have been an important affair. "The education of the 'flower maidens' is conducted in a systematic manner. During the first six years of their life they are reared with the greatest care. At the age of seven or eight it is their duty to keep in order the rooms of the older girls. They are richly clothed when they are taken to the flower boats, where they serve tea and smoking materials to the guests. About the age of eleven they learn to sing, and play on the lute and guitar. If any of the girls show a natural aptitude, they teach them writing, arithmetic, painting, and other subjects. This continues until the thirteenth or fifteenth year. The girls must then attempt to win the favor of some rich man by means of coquetry and various artifices. If they have good luck in this their guardian sells their virginity for a large sum of money.

" This happens most frequently at the age of thirteen, when it is called 'trying the flower;' if at fourteen years, 'cultivating the flower;' if at fifteen, 'gathering the flower.' As among the Romans, the day of such an occurrence is a cause for celebration among the Chinese. All the residents in the other prostitution resorts come in the morning to wish good fortune to the young girl. These celebrations continue from fourteen days to two months. After an interval of some days they sell the girl a second time. If she is especially beautiful they allow her a year of rest in order to sell her 'virginity' a second time and sometimes

[2] DOUGLAS C. McMurtrie, Prostitution in China, *Vigilance*, New York, July, 1913.

[3] GUSTAV Schlegel. *Iets over de prostitutie in China*, Batavia, 1866.

even a third. In such instances the girl is called *Ki hang liao ti niu niang*, a 'girl of two times.' After this she takes her place among the inhabitants of the house and is called *tschang ki*."

The article also contains a description of the "flower boats" which are anchored in the Chinese rivers and utilized as houses of prostitution.

STATISTICS OF SODOMY

STATISTICS regarding all crimes in the United States are miserably defective and the results attending an effort to determine the frequency of the offence of sodomy, generally designated as an "offence against nature" is unsatisfactory. We find,[4] however, that on June 30, 1904, there were in American penal institutions 376 prisoners committed for this crime. These prisoners comprised 15.5% of those committed for offences against chastity. Of the total 375 were male and 1 female.

The distribution by states was as follows: New Hampshire, 1; Massachusetts, 20; Connecticut, 7; New York, 62; New Jersey, 12; Pennsylvania, 52; Maryland, 8; Virginia, 3; West Virginia, 1; North Carolina, 4; South Carolina, 1; Georgia, 1; Florida, 3; Ohio, 22; Indiana, 6; Illinois, 20; Michigan, 11; Wisconsin, 6; Minnesota, 8; Iowa, 2; Missouri, 11; North Dakota, 2; Nebraska, 2; Kansas, 4; Kentucky, 6; Tennessee, 5; Alabama, 3; Mississippi, 6; Louisiana, 3; Texas, 29; Montana, 4; Wyoming, 2; Colorado, 5; Arizona, 1; Utah, 2; Idaho, 2; Washington, 8; Oregon, 1; California, 30. It will be seen that the frequency of conviction varies greatly in different localities.

In the figures of crime given for the state of Indiana,[5] which are probably the most complete available, the offence in question is not mentioned. In the Indianapolis police court, however there were[6] two cases of sodomy in 1910 and ten in 1911.

IS THE PROSTITUTE A CRIMINAL?

By Leo N. Gartman, M.D., Philadelphia, Pa.

THE recent reports of different vice commissions and congresses of hygiene are nauseating. Why do not the so-called scientific men profit by their studies and observations?

[4] Prisoners and Juvenile Delinquents in Institutions, 1904, United States Census Bureau, *Special Reports*, Washington, 1907.

[5] State of Indiana, Bureau of Statistics. *Fourteenth Biennial Report for 1911 and 1912.* .Indianapolis, 1913.

[6] *Ibid.*, p. 269.

Why don't they look to the past, and every now and then to other nations, to find by comparison a suitable explanation for the present? I am bewildered by the great amount of stupidity expressed in the reports. The question arises: why is the prostitute a criminal? In what does her crime consist? The answer is very simple. In countries where marriage is a civil contract, the prostitute is not a criminal. It is only in countries where marriage becomes a part of religion that the prostitute becomes a criminal. The outcome of this is: Suppress the prostitute, annihilate this terrible criminal. And to do it successfully, you have to maim, kill, disfigure, divert into other channels, and pervert the normal sex instinct; and then the millennium will come—and no more prostitution. It is this line of thought that nauseates me, and compels me to write the following.

Let us consider this question without religio-moral prejudices, and take up the study of the question, "Is the prostitute a criminal?" from a different point of view.

Let us examine first a few marriage systems. The aborigines of Australia have what may be called a communal marriage system. Each tribe is divided into two, three, or four sections. No man has a right to marry any female of his own section. At the age of puberty, each young man gets a wife from the eligible section to attend to his cooking, tent, etc.; but every woman of the eligible section is legally his wife, and under a number of stipulated conditions, becomes his wife in reality; and he may choose any woman at the time free for a shorter or longer period for his wife. At certain times even this limitation may be over-stepped; and men and women may disregard all restrictions, excepting one: no man may touch a female of his own section. Wives are acquired either by appointment, which comes from the chief, or by exchange of sisters or daughters for wives. The economic conditions are practically nil. Virginity is a bar to marriage, and it is obliterated by a few elderly male relatives before a girl is eligible to marriage. We can easily see that under a free and unbinding marriage system like this, prostitution has no meaning and cannot exist. Even irregularities are rare. Very seldom will a man take a wife from a section he is not entitled to. "If a Panunga man, say, wants a Bulthara woman, he knows perfectly well that it means certain death to both of them; in fact so strictly are the marriage rules adhered to in the normal state of the tribe, that such an idea probably never enters the head of the native." (Across Australia, by Spencer and Gillen, p. 202.)

Next we will take equatorial Africa, where the patriarchal state still exists. Virginity is often obliterated; incontinence is no bar to marriage, because there is no crime in cohabiting with a single woman. If she gives birth to a child or two before marriage, she is a desirable bride, as she has given ample proof that she is not sterile.

Virginity has not yet become a marketable commodity. If a man wants to have the sole use of a female, he pays for her to her parents or relatives, and acquires full right over her. Any relation with her, without his consent, is called adultery, a crime punishable like theft; merely stealing one's private property, and no more.

Prostitution, or organized prostitution in a marriage system like this is impossible. There are no sexually hungry men or women; it is only when a man, in his quest for *variety*, takes a liking to some one's private property—another man's wife—that transgression begins. The punishment in this case entirely depends on the market value of a wife. If the market price is low, a beating of the woman and a small fine for the man will suffice, and the matter is settled. If the market price is higher, the punishment for adultery is severer, but the fine is never forgotten. In some instances the adulterer is compelled to re-purchase the adulterous woman, and she becomes his private property. We may call it divorce and re-marriage. But all I intended to point out is that in this marriage system, with absolute freedom of divorce, prostitution has no place. There is no necessity, no demand, for it, the single woman is free, and even the married woman is not out of reach; pay and you have her; if tired, you can re-sell her. The price seldom falls. The taste for variety thus is easily satisfied.

In this marriage system, bachelors and old maids are absolutely unknown; marriages take place early, as soon as the sex instinct wakens. The primitive man looks at marriage as we look upon feeding. As soon as a child is born, it is fed, and its taste or its likes or dislikes are not consulted. The same view is taken by these people on marriage; as soon as puberty is reached, children are provided with spouses without consulting them. If they are dissatisfied with one another, they have an open door; they separate and re-marry at their own free will. The irregularities that do occur, among this people, mostly take place among married men and women in their quest for variety. The influence of economic conditions is insignificant. In the lowest state, exchange of female for female or abduction takes place. When there is some property, like the implements for the chase, or its products, the products of cattle breeding or agriculture, these are used as means of exchange. So many head of cattle, or so many measures of grain, so many bunches of tobacco for a wife; everybody is suited according to his means.

We will go a step further and consider a more advanced civilization, with an advanced esthetic taste; with more or less accumulation of property in the hands of individuals. The man of means in his quest for *variety* becomes an epicurean in matters of sex. He prefers the young to the old; he prefers the better looking woman to the uglier, and by degrees, the virgin becomes an interesting tit-bit, an especial sweetmeat, something more piquant than it was considered before. There comes a revolution of ideas. Virginity acquires a market price. And instead of destroying virginity before a woman becomes eligible to marriage, parents see that it is preserved intact. The free girl is more or less guarded, and it is again hard and risky to approach her; and it is here that the prostitute makes her first appearance.

A female who has an occupation which consists in gratifying the sexual desires of males for a consideration—how is she treated? In some countries, she constituted the priestess of the temple, and prostitution formed a caste (India). In other countries, she was reasonably respected; even more than a married woman (Greece, Rome). In others, she is tolerated, looked down upon, but still not excluded from society. As a rule, she is not yet a criminal. Prostitution is considered as necessary, and moreover it is considered the best protection of female chastity. As an example of the last, we will take Dahomey.

The king of Dahomey has over seven thousand wives. Every year a new contingent of wives is brought to his harem, and those he does not require any longer are distributed as presents to his favorites. Therefore, there is an artificial scarcity in females. Now let us see what happens there. "In Dahomey adultery is a crime which can only be expiated by life-long slavery or sudden death. Those which we call social evils are here recognized as social necessities. To counteract the only evil of polygamy, namely the inability of the poorer people to purchase wives, the government organizes a body of women who ply their nefarious trade at fixed days at a regulated price, and who add to the royal revenue by paying a tax. This arrangement is certainly indicated; but indecorum is among this people *no vice* at all, since it happens to be conducive to connubial virtue." ("Savage Africa," by Winwood Reade, p. 52.)

More than that. When a rich woman dies, instead of contributing to charity, she contributes to the support of prostitution, and this is considered the most charitable act. When the English government wants to enact a law to which the Dahomeyans object, she closes all the places: then all the men, single as well as married, petition the English government to reopen the houses, and promise that they will submit to the objectionable law, the married men claiming that as soon as these places are closed the safety of their houses is endangered. Greece, and other countries in the Mediterranean, had places specially arranged for strangers and seafaring men, so as to protect their daughters and wives.

Later comes in another factor: rigidity and ceremonies imposed by an established religion, and this makes the marriage tie still more expensive and therefore more solid. When religion comes in a number of more or less expensive ceremonies follow; the high price of the bride and paying the priest are added to expenses for entertaining guests. Marriage thus becomes quite a serious undertaking and is often put off for a few years. The outcome is more prostitution; in fact plenty of it. These conditions are prevalent in China, Japan, some parts of India, Mohammedan countries and among Jews.

In all these marriage systems there are a few redeeming features: First, early marriages between the age of ten and eighteen, or as soon as the sex instinct manifests itself. This reduces prostitution to a considerable extent. Second, the facility with which divorce is obtained. (Divorce is universal.) A married couple who for any possible reason cannot agree, instead of prostituting themselves, divorce and re-marry. One of the very frequent causes of divorce is the love of the human race for variety. The prostitute is not looked down upon, but considered a necessity and reasonably tolerated. She is not made an outcast and the return of the prostitute to her ordinary life is a simple matter. It does not leave a stain on her or on her children. She is not compelled to become an outcast and a prostitute for life.

What do we mean by the term "variety"? It is necessary to understand this. We will have to admit that the normal reproductive instinct has a physiology, though for evident reasons little known to us. There are reasonable indications that the normal reproductive instinct becomes blunted after a shorter or longer time, and requires a new stimulus to bring it again into activity. In the process of survival of the fittest, the individuals who had the faculty of becoming reproductive again and again under the influence of new sexual stimulus, left a larger progeny. On the contrary, those that lacked this faculty became sterile early in life and left a small progeny. Hence, the individuals with the faculty to become rejuvenated under the influence of new sexual stimulus, had the upper hand of the race; and it is this force which the modern anthropologist, who could not help observing it, smilingly dubs "the human taste for variety."

In my opinion, this force is next in importance to the reproductive force itself, judging by the extensive ramifications of its activity. We have seen that when the marriage system is very elastic to accomodate itself to the sexual wants of a nation, prostitution is absent; the stronger the restrictions become the more irregularities take place, and the consequence of restrictions is prostitution. Continuing our line of thought, if we take for example our marriage system, which is absolutely solid, unmovable, unpliable, we should expect the greatest amount of prostitution, and so we have. For the following reasons: First, we do not educate our young men in the spirit of marriage as well as all other countries do; and this ante-marriage education, regardless of economic conditions, produces a great number of bachelors and a corresponding number of bachelor maids, and a state of affairs which stimulates prostitution. Besides, young men often practice masturbation or become addicted to perversions, because they are educated under the ante-marriage régime and absolutely ignorant of sex matters. Divorce, which would in this instance, and in many other instances, act as a preventive, is absent. I may say that the difficulty of separation of the married couple leads, for whatever reason it may be, to their estrangement, and thus becomes one of the greatest factors in the production of prostitution. As to this, the influence of the taste for variety, which is strong in the human race, not being gratified, will produce a tremendous amount of prostitution. Just observe! One-third of the visitors of the prostitutes are *married men;* two-thirds are single. But the married man is much more liberal with his money, and pays so much more for the favors rendered to him by the prostitute, that he becomes the strongest supporter of prostitution; and I have heard time and time again the statement, "that if it were not for the married men, prostitution would be a non-paying occupation." It is not very agreeable to hear these facts, but it cannot be helped. If we want a thoroughly closed marriage system, we must have its inseparable second half, prostitution. We do not like it, but we cannot help it. We would like to have air without the nitrogen, but it does not exist; we would like to insure the existence of the human race without bisexual reproductions, but it is not prepared to suit our religio-moral ideas. We would like to eat meat without slaughtering the cow; but either we will have to give up eating meat, or, if we persist in eating it, the cows will have to be slaughtered. We want a closed, stable, unmovable, inviolable marriage system, then we must have prostitution with it; *one does not exist without the other.* Having a closed holy marriage system, any one that transgresses this law is a criminal against religion and its twin-sister morality. Hence, in Christian countries, the prostitute is an outcast, a criminal; once a prostitute a prostitute for life and for the generation to come; no return, no redemption.

From the foregoing statements it can be seen that the prostitute has more reason to complain than we have to accuse her. And it is this we do not like to admit. But there is another crime imputed to her, that she is the corrupter of our morality and the destroyer of our homes. Let us see how much truth there is in this accusation. We will take a hypothetical case. Imagine that by some miracle, because only a miracle could do it, we get rid of all the prostitutes and free women, and women that have more than one husband, etc., etc. What would happen? A number of sexually hungry males will begin to run about looking for a suitable female. Necessity is the mother of invention. Driven by sexual hunger, this enormous pack of hungry wolves would direct all their ingenuity to overcome the weaker part of the female population. The young, unprepared, unprotected girl in her teens would be the first victim, and chastity would be at a premium. The houses of the married people would be invaded; and wherever a married woman would be found, for any reason dissatisfied with her husband, or on account of her own inconstancy or stupidity, such female would become a prey of the hungry pack and many of them would succumb to this terrific onslaught. Then only we would be able to see that the prostitute is the only protector of the chastity of our young girls, girls that are not prepared by their mothers to be able to protect themselves. Then only would the married man cry out like the people of Dahomey: "Give us back prostitution, the protection of our marriage system and sex morality."

I do not draw on my imagination. I speak from facts. In 1905, Mr. Gibboney succeeded in closing a number of houses of prostitution in Philadelphia. Women were insulted day and night on the streets, on their house steps and even in their houses, many succumbed, and quite a few men were decorated with horns. But th main damage was done to the young girl. I, as well as some other physicians, had never seen so many pregnant young girls as were seen in that short period. According to actual counting, not less than two hundred girls born and bred in Philadelphia were enrolled into the ranks of prostitution. The prostitute is not only an inseparable part of our marriage system, but she is also the wall which protects female chastity, and the sanctity of our homes, as we understand it. She serves like the lightning-rod, who takes up the surplus of unutilized sexual energy and diverts it to harmless channels. She ought to be even excused for her share in spreading venereal disease.

Speaking in an *unbiased* way, the question arises why a strong brainy man can prostitute his noblest part—his brain, and be hardly criticized? Now why can't a female, for whatever reason, sell her body for a consideration without being condemned as a lifelong criminal? Why can one with impunity prostitute his brain, and why cannot another make a living from her body, who while doing so, protects our chastity and homes? Why?

Let us recognize this:—*Until we have founded our marriage system on a purely scientific basis, we cannot get rid of prostitution.*

REVIEW OF CURRENT UROLOGIC LITERATURE

REVUE CLINIQUE D'UROLOGIE

November, 1913

1. **Report of Several Cases of Partial Prostatectomy.**

The authors report seven cases in which a partial prostatectomy was done. The operation performed involved a cystotomy (suprabubic) with removal of the so-called enlarged middle lobe, or the extirpation of adenomatous nodules about the vesical neck. In only one of the patients was there any satisfactory lasting result from the intervention. It therefore appears that in circumscribed lesions of the prostate partial prostatectomy is an operation which can give very satisfactory immediate results, but the final result of which is doubtful.

It makes little difference whether a submucous resection of the fibroma is made or whether the pieces of tumor are removed separately with punch forceps. The question of importance is not the danger of local recurrence from imperfect removal—for any kind of removal can be made sufficiently thorough—but whether new nodules will not develop in the remaining lateral lobes. It is, therefore, clear that the only safe course is to remove the entire gland if the patient is not too old, in good general condition, and with a satisfactory renal elimination. When the subject is not a favorable risk, however, it may be wise, on the contrary to open the bladder and remove the middle lobe alone. Nevertheless, even in the first class of cases it may be necessary to do a partial ectomy especially when the entire prostate is hard and fibrotic and does not present any single enucleable mass. If, nothwithstanding, a total removal is demanded the suprapubic route offers too many dangers and should be supplanted by the perineal method of extirpation.

It is, therefore, wise in any given case to decide in advance whether the prostate has a pericervical fibroma, which can be done by cystoscopy, and whether the gland will be difficult to enucleate, which can be decided, in some measure at least, by rectal examination, for if it is, it will be felt to be small, smooth and of very firm consistency. If the above conditions obtain, the perineal route is the method of choice.

2. **Hypogastric Section in Two Stages.**

In the aged and enfeebled suffering from urinary disturbances requiring hypogastric section Colombino performs the operation in two stages, thus avoiding perivesical and parietal infections.

First stage: Fixation of the bladder (cystopexy). Local anesthesia is produced by injecting the following mixture:

℞ Cocaine hydrochloride	0.05
Adrenalin hydrochloride	0.66
Distilled water	10.00

The bladder is filled with boric acid. The ordinary median incision is made, the peritoneum pushed up, and the bladder fixed to the parietal wall by 8 or 10 sutures arranged in an oval and penetrating only through the muscularis of the bladder. A guide suture is introduced into the center of the exposed organ. The wound is packed wide with gauze.

Second stage: Opening of the bladder.—After 8 days the bladder is firmly united to the parieties and the subcutaneous cellular tissue is protected by a barrier of granulations. The bladder is again distended with boric acid solution, opened with a bistoury by aid of the guide suture, and the desired intravesical manipulations accomplished. A drain is then introduced, fastened to the skin with a stitch, and surrounded with gauze packings. The drainage tube is removed in three or four days and a permanent catheter introduced, if necessary. The second stage can be performed in a short time and may be done under general anesthesia with ethyl chloride.

Indications. The two stage procedure should be done whenever a very infected bladder must be opened in an old or feeble subject. It is indicated, under these circumstances, for removal of the prostate, for the removal of stones, and for severe urinary sepsis with cystitis.

The results, in the ten cases operated on by the author, have been very satisfactory.

3. **Note on a Case of Orthostatic Albuminuria.**

Strominger reports the case of a boy of 15 who complained of lumbar pains and an albuminuria of several months' standing. He also suffered from headaches, had pains in the legs, was anemic and had completely lost his appetite. There was increased sensitiveness to cold.

On examination the patient showed a disproportionate length of the extremities with short trunk and small, thin, chest. The genitals were underdeveloped and the voice thin. He was pale and the extremities cold and blue. There was no bony deformity; the spinal column was perfect. There was no history of infectious disease. A previous examination of a twenty-four hour specimen of urine showed that it contained 0.5 gram of albumen. There were no cellular elements.

The good general condition of the patient, the absence of urinary symptoms or of signs of Bright's disease, and the absence of previous infections led the author to suspect the presence of orthostatic albuminuria. He therefore had the 24-hour output of urine divided into 4 parts, parts 1 and 3 representing the urine obtained while the patient was up, parts 2 and 4 representing that obtained while the patient was lying down. The report came in as follows:

Part 1	contained	0.8%	albumen
Part 2	"	.0	"
Part 3	"	3.0%	"
Part 4	"	.0	"

A complete analysis of the urine showed a normal mineral and nitrogen excretion.

The patient was put on the fresh air cure with general tonic treatment; the milk diet on which he had been kept was discontinued as it only increased the albuminuria. The albumen soon disappeared almost completely and the general condition improved. Strychnine and arsenic were prescribed but the patient dropped from observation.

The author regrets not having been able to determine the coefficient of Ambard in this case as Widal and Javal have reported an orthostatic diminution in the urea excretion.

4. Treatment of Retention in Strictures of the Urethra.

Nin Posadas has used the following procedure with success in cases of retention of urine in strictures allowing of the passage of an armed filiform bougie. After the usual disinfectant procedures he introduces a filiform bougie into the bladder. Then, with a mandrin, he verifies whether the armed bougie is really within the bladder, just as in the Maisonneuve internal urethrotomy. Next he withdraws the mandrin and replaces it by the conductor of the urethrotome which is pushed until it is within the bladder as shown by the escape of urine. The emptying of the bladder proceeds slowly through the lumen of the conductor. When no more urine appears the conductor is withdrawn but the bougie retained for another twenty-four hours. At the end of this period a larger bougie is introduced and the canal thus dilated in the usual manner. Hemorrhage ex vacuo does not occur owing to the slowness with which the urine is withdrawn.

The method may be employed in retentions of prostatic origin. It presents the advantages that:

1. It permits of the introduction on the conductor of an open end catheter which may be left in place in case of necessity.

2. It permits the patient to go about his business instead of confining him to bed.

3. It avoids the danger of false passages, so common in such cases, especially in the hand of the inexperienced.

5. On the Pathology and Therapeutics of Pyelitis.

By pyelitis we understand an inflammation of the kidney pelvis without involvement of the parenchyma. The predisposing causes are mechanical factors and the immediate etiological factor is some bacterium, usually the colon bacillus. The mere presence of microbes in the pelvis, however, is insufficient cause for a pyelitis for bacteriurias are common without signs of inflammation. One of the most important contributing causes is the retention or stagnation of urine.

The frequent occurrence of pyelitis in pregnant women has led to the general impression that the gravid uterus compresses the ureter. Some authors, however, do not believe that compression plays so important a rôle as does the hyperemia of the ureteral mucosa, in its intravesical course, which always accompanies pregnancy and menstruation. It is on this basis that Mirabeau, the upholder of this theory, explains such symptoms as dysmenorrhea, vomiting, cystalgia, which he regards as manifestations of uremia accompanying urinary sepsis.

Of course any kind of intra-abdominal tumor other than a pregnant uterus may press on the ureter causing obstruction to the urinary current with secondary infection. We have also to consider among causes of this condition obstruction arising from within the lumen of the ureter or from disease of its nervous or muscular apparatus. Thus chronic pyelitides have been described as due to ureteral myosites and to ataxia of the ureteral walls.

There are three principal theories as to the manner in which bacteria arrive at the kidney pelvis. 1. Through the blood current. 2. Through the lymphatics. 3. Ascending from the urethra and bladder, either by way of the lumen or through the walls of the ureter. In connection with the last named theory it is important to note that the chief obstacles opposing ascending infection are the force of the urinary current and the tonicity of the ureteral sphincter. It is, therefore, necessary to have increased intravesical pressure due to the presence of some obstruction to the outflow of urine before bacteria can find their way up the ureter.

In this connection one other point is of interest. It has been shown that when the ureter is pressed upon from without its peristaltic movements cease. It is probable, therefore, that this is an additional factor in favoring infection.

Pyelitis is much more frequent in women than in men (about 90% of all cases occur in the former sex). The increased susceptibility of females is due to the incidence of pregnancy and of menstruation, to the shortness of the ureters, to their anatomical relations with the vagina and anus which are rich in bacteria and especially with the neck of the uterus, diseases of which often cause an obstruction to the outflow of urine. Of the two ureters it is the right which is the more frequently diseased, because it lies farther from the spinal column than does the left and is therefore less protected, and because its twists and turns are more marked than are those of the left. Besides, the uterus is more likely to be displaced to the right, and the right kidney is more likely to be ptosed than the left.

Pyelitis may be treated by conservative methods, by surgery, by catheterization of the ureters, or by vaccinotherapy. 1. *Conservative treatment.* This calls for the use of large quantities of fluids: plain or mineralized waters, or milk, to dilute the urine and flush the kidneys. Balsamics are not recommended as they are too irritant, but disinfectants such as salol, urotropin, helmitol, etc., are of real service. The dorsal position with the pelvis elevated has been recommended for pregnant women. 2. *Operative treatment* is not indicated unless the above measures have failed, or unless the patient gets worse or some complication develops such as pyonephrosis, hydronephrosis (infected), stones, renal tuberculosis, etc. In such cases pyelotomy, nephrotomy or nephrectomy may be done. There is much diversity of opinion as to the advisability of interrupting pregnancy for the relief of pyelitis. 3. *In catheterization of the ureters with local treatment* we have a very efficient therapeutic measure. The author has irrigated the kidney pelvis twice a week with a 1:2000 silver nitrate solution. Perhydrol in ¼ to ½ % strength has given very good results. 4. *Vaccintherapy* has so far given uncertain results. The close biological resemblance between the meningococcus and the gonococcus has led to the use of meningococcus vaccine in pyelitides in which the gonococcus was regarded as the etiological factor.

6. Extraction of Foreign Bodies from the Bladder by the Natural Passages.

Lenko summarizes some of the literature of the subject and reports two cases. In the first case a straw was removed from the bladder of a man by introducing a sound to the end of which several pieces of knotted thread were tied. The point of the sound was then revolved within the bladder the thread thus twisting about the straw. When the sound was withdrawn the straw followed after.

In the second case an attempt was made to remove a hairpin from a woman's bladder, with a lithotrite, but as the points were directed forward, the attempt was unsuccessful and a section was necessary.

ANNALES DES MALADIES VÉNÉRIENNES

Vol. VIII, No. 11, Nov. 1913

1. The Value of the Separation of the Upper Median Incisors as a Stigma of Hereditary Syphilis.

In addition to the well-known stigmata of hereditary syphilis and especially the classical dental dystrophies so well described by Hutchinson, Fournier, and Parrot, we have another pointed out by Gaucher. This sign is the separation of the upper median incisors. It may occur in conjunction with other marks of syphilis but most often occurs quite alone. In a patient with a doubtful lesion the finding of this peculiarity should at once raise the suspicion of hereditary syphilis and suggest a careful examination for other signs and a Wassermann test. This is therefore a warning sign of the first importance.

The separation of the incisors may be a dystrophy handed down through several successive generations without reinfection. Gaucher believes therefore that in all cases of separation of the upper median incisors a history of syphilis may be obtained in one of three generations.

2. A Case of Hyperesthesia and of Gustatory Perversion of the Tongue of Specific Origin.

Renault reports the case of a man of rheumatic and nervous disposition who contracted syphilis in 1898. He was very poorly treated, for about 3 months in all. Five years later there appeared some nervous symptoms which promptly disappeared under specific treatment. Seven years after the infection an interstitial keratitis developed which yielded promptly to the same treatment. In the ninth year of his infection the patient complained of small ulcerations of the tip of the tongue and of hypertrophy of the lingual folds on the right side. After administration of 2 centigrams of biniodide of mercury and 2 grams of potassium iodide daily for 10 days the tongue became normal. Two months later, however, the patient again developed a keratitis and the tongue became sensitive without presenting any objective signs other than a slight hypertrophy of the papillae at the point. After 60 daily injections of 1 centigram of mercury cyanide both the eye and the tongue conditions cleared up.

In June, 1910, the patient began to complain of a recurrence of his lingual hyperesthesia which had now begun to involve the entire buccal cavity. This symptom came and went but in the early months of 1912 it became very severe. The patient was now complaining of a burning sensation along the right border and under surface of the tongue. There was much salivation and the subject complained of a bad taste in his mouth as if pepper and mustard was always there.

Physical examination was negative and so the symptoms were ascribed to a neurotic basis and the patient given local mouth washes. As the condition did not improve biniodide of mercury was again given in the dose of 2 cg. daily and in less than 2 weeks the salivation diminished as did the hyperesthesia of the tongue and the perverted taste in the mouth.

The author concludes that it is always wise to think of syphilis in unusual phenomena of any kind which do not yield to the ordinary methods of treatment.

3. A Third Case of Raynaud's Disease of Syphilitic Origin, with Aortitis and Positive Wassermann Reaction.

Gaucher has reported two previous cases of Raynaud's disease cured by specific treatment. In the first case the disease came on during the beginning of the secondary period; in the other, the positive Wassermann reaction was the only indication of a previous unrecognized syphilis.

The present case was a woman of 53 who for the past 30 years was complaining of a painful affection of the hands. For 20 years she had noticed that after a violent emotion, or following exposure to cold she would have a sudden spasm ("stage of syncope") of the fingers of both hands: the digits would assume a dull white or yellowish shade and would become cold and torpid, and at the same time give rise to painful sensations. The patient would obtain relief by plunging her hands into warm water when the spasm would cease but would be followed by a stage of mild cyanosis ("asphyxia") with shooting pains. This would be followed by a complete restoration to normal.

For the last 10 years the patient presented areas of gangrene on various fingers always limited to the terminal phalanges. One of the fingers was amputated. More recently there was marked cyanosis and coldness of the hands. Cicatrices and ulcerations were frequent and the fingers were very tender. The patient complained much of formication, tingling and shooting pains. Sensations of touch and heat were preserved but sensibility to cold had disappeared. There were also trophic changes consisting in striation of the nails, thickening and loss of flexibility of the skin and ankylosis of the terminal joints. At different parts of the body (knees and elbows) were tumefactions or scars of tumefactions which had discharged a thick clayey substance.

Physical examination was negative except for the kidneys (there was a mild albuminuria) and the heart. The left ventricle was hypertrophied and the second aortic sound was ringing. There was abnormal dulness in the aortic region. Functionally there was great dyspnea on exertion culminating in crises of violent substernal pain. The face was pale and the lips cyanosed.

The Wassermann reaction being positive, the patient was put on daily injections of 2 centigrams of benzoate of mercury. Unfortunately the author does not say how much if any improvement followed the administration of the specific medication.

4. **Congenital Syphilis, Probably Atavistic, with Multiple Grave Stigmata and Manifestations.**

The case was one of hereditary syphilis of the second generation ("atavistic" syphilis as-called by the authors). The patient was a girl of 16 who presented a remarkable group of symptoms.

In the first place she presented an ulcerating syphiloma of the pharynx, a very rare and virulent manifestation of late congenital syphilis. In the second place she had interesting eye symptoms, such as a marked grade of congenital myopia (30 diopters or more) with areas of chorioretinitis. This is especially important as Antonelli believes that a congenital myopia or one early acquired, especially if one eye is more affected than the other, represents a rather frequent symptom of hereditary specific disease.

Finally, the patient suffered from a massive deformity of the face due to a hyperostosis or a periostitis with eburneation of the superior maxillae and the malar bones as well as those entering into the floor of the orbit and the nasal cavities. As a result the face assumed a leonine expression. The authors believe that congenital syphilis may give rise to a massive and deforming hyperostosis of the bones of the face representing the beginning of a stage of leontiasis. It may be indeed that certain forms of leontiasis as described by Virchow, may really be syphilitic in origin as has been shown to be the case in that deforming osteopathy called Paget's disease.

MISCELLANEOUS ABSTRACTS

GENITAL TUBERCULOSIS

According to H. CABOT and J. D. BARNEY, Boston (*J. A. M. A.*, December 6), in genital tuberculosis of the male the disease is usually primary in the epididymis, occasionally in the testicles and rarely in the prostate. As the organ primarily involved shows the least resistance. while that of those secondarily affected is far greater and often successful, the operation of choice is epididymotomy. The secondary foci in the testicle can be dealt with locally while that in the prostate should be left to Nature. Operation on the prostate is a radical one and the complete removal of the process is out of the question. One is likely to stir up a hornet's nest and leave things worse than before. The foci in the testicle are generally contiguous to the epididymis and often quite limited; in rare cases they may be more extensive and call for orchidectomy. They advise also the removal of the accessible portion of the vas, up to the brim of the true pelvis, as leaving it may complicate convalescence and give trouble. This done, after the removal of the epididymis through a two-inch incision in the scrotum, by blunt dissection with the fingers up to the external ring where the vas is seized with a clamp pushed up into the sinus, carefully avoiding the canal between the fascia and the fat, and its handle depressed so as to bring its point against the skin where it is pushed out through a half-inch incision. The vas is pulled out, divided, cauterized with phenol, and dropped back. They say: "The operation has seemed to us much superior to that involving a long incision through the scrotum and coverings of the inguinal canal in order to remove an equal amount of the vas. It takes less time in the doing, is equally efficient and shortens the convalescence about two-thirds."

PATHOLOGY OF THE PROSTATE

E. O. SMITH, Cincinnati (*J. A. M. A.*, December 6), notices the imperfect description of the prostate in the text-books, etc., and quotes Lowsley who shows that it develops embryologically from five foci from which the five lobes of the organ start. It reaches its full normal development about the twentieth year and the various lobes normally have no distinct capsulary separation from each other. Its close relation to the posterior urethra renders it subject to infection and the most frequent invader is the gonococcus. This organism may for considerable periods give rise to no serious symptoms but may be lurking and easily called into action. The seminal vesicles are also frequently infected and the prostate is credited with the mischief. It is possible for them to be pathologic with a normal prostate. Tuberculosis of the prostate may be primary but is generally preceded by disease of the kidneys or of the epididymis. Calcareous deposits are not infrequent in late adult life. Many men past 50 years of age have urinary disturbances and the great majority of these are due to pathologic changes in the prostate gland. It must not, however, be taken for granted that this is always the case. The senile changes that occur are given as adenoma fibrosis, and malignant disease. Any one or all three may be present and all the five lobes be affected except that portion below the ejaculatory ducts, the posterior lobe. The middle lobe is the most frequent site of adenomatous growth, the anterior lobe seldom, and the lateral lobes rather frequently. The enlargement of the gland which normally is extravesicular begins to encroach on the bladder and many hypertrophies become so large that they act as a decided rectal obstruction. Sometimes the adenomatous growths form a ring constricting the urethra, troublesome and hard to remove. The so-called prostatic bar is either not prostatic or not a bar. In the first case it is a fibrous bar developed about the internal sphincter from chronic inflammation of the posterior urethra and occurs earlier in life. If of prostatic origin, it is not in the form of a bar but is an enlargement of the middle lobe, changing the shape of the internal meatus from a normal funnel appearance to that of an inverted crescent. There is no true normal prostatic capsule, and the surgical capsule which surrounds the adenomatous growths is the prostate crowded to the side and shows, microscopically, compacted stroma and gland tissue. Not infrequently a patient with marked prostatic symptoms is relieved by a few days rest in bed with free catharsis and continuous bladder drainage. The symptoms were due to venous congestion. Smith does not believe that prostatic hypertrophy undergoes malignant degeneration. Cancer of the prostate begins as such and practically always in the posterior lobe. Tuberculosis of the prostate is usually secondary to that of the seminal vesicles and is seldom found alone.

CHRONIC CYSTITIS IN WOMEN

G. G. Smith, Boston (*J. A. M. A.*, December 6), holds to the view that persistent cystitis in women is not in itself a disease but is the result of pathologic conditions outside of the bladder. This, however, is not the view generally held. He does not contend that simple cystitis never occurs but such cases will generally be cured by a few days in bed, urinary antiseptics and a few irrigations. If it still exists we must look for some other lesion, either in the kidney or ureter, in pelvis or urethra, or in the mechanism by which the bladder is emptied. He has collected the histories of ninety-eight women with cystitis, ward cases or out patients at the Massachusetts General Hospital, and analyzed them according to the pathologic conditions existing. In eight cases a simple cystitis was found. In the others renal infections, non-tuberculous, existed in 61 per cent., renal tuberculosis in 19 per cent., and in the others there was difficulty in emptying bladder, systemic and pelvic infections, or other causes. Every case that was really studied showed a certain or presumptive underlying cause and he maintains that simple cystitis is practically non-existent. Synopses of the cases classified as to the infection from renal sources or from ureteral causes or obstruction are given.

TUMORS OF TESTICLE

Two cases of mixed tumors of the testicle are reported by A. C. Stokes, Omaha (*J. A. M. A.*, December 6). In the first the organ was removed with the iliac lymph-nodes and no recurrence has occurred. In the second patient, operation was performed but the patient died. It was seen late in its history and there were liver metastases. Both cases are considered as of embryologic origin, as shown by the presence of syncytium and the cells of Langhams, the increased amount of muscle and the presence of cartilage, the large embryonal epiblastic cells arranged in alveolar form and the presence of large round cells, degenerating epiblast and chromogenetic cells. From a clinical standpoint the question arises, what is to be done with such growths, and from the evidence gathered it would seem that these tumors, like those of the breast, are at least frequently malignant. Stokes says: "Given a history of trauma some years previously, with a testicle slowly increasing in size, accompanied by rather indefinite pains, continued for several months, one is justified in removing the testicle for malignancy. Some may take issue with this position, but we believe that were this done many lives would be spared, and perhaps a few benign tumors removed. Our two cases illustrate also the two extremes of duration; in one case the tumor was attacked early, and in the other late. Just at what period in the histories of these cases metastasis takes place is not clear. In general it is early, we believe. The simple removal of the testicle is, in our judgment, not indicated, even if a malignant tumor is suspected. Rather the removal of the entire cord and of the retroperitoneal glands along the cord and as far as possible along the iliac veins is indicated, for evidently metastasis takes place frequently along this channel, as shown by the formation of retroperitoneal masses. Clinically it is important to recognize them as early as possible and to do a radical operation on them."

VESICAL TUMORS.

Dr. H. H. Young, Baltimore (*J. A. M. A.*, November 22), from a detailed study of 118 cases of vesical tumor, 93 per cent. of which were malignant, finds that excision as usually carried out is utterly inadequate and recurrence takes place in both malignant and benign cases. The cautery is a very valuable agent, both in suprapubic and intraperitoneal operations, and its thorough use has brought about a cure in some apparently hopeless cases. Cancer of the bladder, except in very extensive cases, is best treated by suprapubic resection of the bladder leaving a wide area around the tumor, the cautery used if possible, ureter transplanted if necessary, and the peritoneum excised when the tumor involves that part of the bladder. Intraperitoneal operations are rarely necessary (except in tumor of the vertex and posterior wall), as an excellent view of the bladder can be had by an extensive median incision, wide separation of the recti, upward displacement of the peritoneum, a long incision into the bladder, and good retraction. Fifty per cent. resorcin or alcohol to kill tumor particles which may have dropped into the bladder also seems desirable but a better plan is to thoroughly cauterize the tumor before beginning the resection. For benign tumors treatment with the high frequency spark seems thoroughly satisfactory but should be vigorously applied. For this purpose in extensive cases the fulgurating sound or a strong spark through an open endoscope or cystoscope, the bladder filled with air, may be very helpful. In apparently hopeless cases destroying the tumors and their bases and adjoining portions of the bladder wall with the Paquelin, hot air, or electric cautery may occasionally give unexpectedly brilliant results. Before treatment it is well to examine an adequate specimen obtained by a cystoscopic rongeur microscopically. A few villi washed from the bladder or obtained by small forceps cannot give a satisfactory diagnosis and he has seen mistakes made this way. Early diagnosis is important as in other situations and he urges strongly the cystoscopic examination in all cases of bladder hemorrhage and sometimes before hemorrhage occurs. It is only within three years that the possibility of often curing benign papilloma of the bladder by fulguration has been learned. It is one of the most brilliant and valuable additions to surgery of recent years. The further proof that cancer of the bladder can sometimes be cured by resection is also another great advance.

SUPRAPUBIC OPERATIONS.

Dr. G. MacGowan (*J. A. M. A.*, November 22) points out certain difficulties in approaching the bladder by the usual longitudinal suprapubic incision from above and advocates a method that he has employed which he has never seen described which largely obviates these troubles. He makes an incision from 3 to 6 cm. long transversely through the skin and superficial and deep fascias to the sheaths of the recti muscles. This is made about 6 cm. above the pubic spine with a slight convexity upwards. When the muscle sheath is divided its edges retract, exposing the body of the muscle. Then the intramuscular septum as it dips down between the recti is slightly nicked below with scissors and rolled back with the sheath on each side, exposing the pyramidal muscles. The space between these is to be sought for and they are to be separated or pressed apart. As soon as this is done the recti muscles can be easily retracted. If the bladder has been previously filled with water or air it then appears in the wound, covered only with a little fatty areolar tissue. Sutures are passed through its muscular coat to hold it in place after the bladder is emptied. The incision into the bladder is then made either transversely or longitudinally. MacGowan prefers the latter. As soon as it is opened from two to four sutures should be inserted through all the coats of the bladder and the rectus muscle or its fascia on each side and the needed operation within the bladder can then be performed. When it is finished and there promises to be some continuous hemorrhage which might interfere with the closing of the wound it is partly closed and a large drainage tube is inserted, large enough not to be clogged with clotted blood. It should be placed so that the eyes will be in the bladder but not permitting its end to touch the bottom of the bladder and thus causing tenesmus or strain. The muscles are then sewed together and the edges of the sheath so that they overlap without tension. The details of this part of the operation are given in full in the paper. For many years MacGowan has used a system of continuous irrigation in suprapubic cystotomies in which the salt solution flowed into the bladder through a catheter in the urethra and passed out through a drainage tube. He later devised a method which seems superior in requiring no expensive apparatus and because it can be managed by ordinary attendants. A catheter a little longer than the drainage tube and about half its diameter but sufficiently large to prevent clogging is introduced through the drainage tube previously mentioned so that the eye of this catheter reaches about 1 cm. beyond the distal end of the drainage tube. The drainage may be continuous or interrupted but he thinks it is best to begin with the latter to prevent lack of attention on the part of the nurses; but after the first 12 hours he uses continuous irrigation. The wound left after this operation does not heal any quicker than that left by the longitudinal incision but it is a funnel-shaped wound from the skin to the bladder and everything is within sight. It leaves a good scar and no weakness in the abdominal wall. MacGowan does not see why the suprapubic operation should be considered so dangerous. He is sure that the wound made by this method would of itself never cause death.

VASOSTOMY.

Dr. W. T. Belfield (*J. A. M. A.*, November 22), says the vas and vesicle will usually hold 4 to 6 c.c. of a non-irritant fluid like 10 per cent. argyrol solution injected through a scrotal vasostomy. When overfilled the sphincter yields and the solution flows usually into the bladder but occasionally forward, escaping at the meatus. Any quantity may then be used for irrigation at the operator's discretion. For days after such filling of the seminal duct, peristalsis occurs as shown by argyrol in the urine. As this is without subjective perception it must be considered a normal function of the vas. In three of Belfield's cases retrograde urination through the vasostomy incision occurred when the impulse to urinate was strongly resisted, and he sees in this a possibly not infrequent cause of recurrent epididymitis and vesiculitis following gonorrhea. The normal peristalsis of the seminal duct also explains, as he shows, the phosphaturia of sexual neurasthenia by the precipitation of the lime salts of the urine by the escaping vesicular excretion. Anastomoses between the dilated extremity of the vas (ampulla) and the associated vesicle are not rare, and as they must afford direct passage of the spermatozoa into the vesicle, this observation seems to prove that the vesicles may not be merely secretory organs, as is supposed, but also reservoirs for spermatozoa. Experience with vasostomy shows that sterility may be due to occlusions of the vas and also to arrest of the functions of the testis through some infectious disease without loss of sexual power. In two of Belfield's patients a chronic colon bacillus of the seminal duct caused a chronic toxemia with continuous high temperature and loss of weight which was relieved by irrigation of the seminal ducts through vasostomy. Infections of the duct from either end may cause a pus tube and toxemia which can usually be successfully treated by vasostomy and irrigation. Some non-irritant solution like 5 per cent. argyrol should be used to test the patency of the entire canal: "Should this reach the urethra in a few minutes (shown by blackening of the urine), collargol solution, 1 to 2 per cent., may be injected. If the argyrol does not appear in the urine, the more irritating collargol should not be used; for it will regurgitate into the scrotal tissues around the cut, and there produce a tender induration which is slow to disappear."

FEVER AS THE ONLY SYMPTOM OF LATENT SYPHILIS.

Within the space of one year Kraus (Wiener Klin. Wochenschrift. No. 49, 1913), had the opportunity of observing at the Wienerwald sanatorium for lung diseases four cases which had been sent in as occult or positive tuberculosis, which ran a more or less continuous fever and which proved to be syphilis. The first case had a history of tuberculous osteomyelitis in youth, the others all had lung signs, fever, emaciation and night sweats. Features which were common to all four cases and finally led to the correct diagnosis were: (1) Continuous fever, lasting for months, irregular in type; (2) Inefficiency of all antipyretic measures;(3) Absence of typical syphilitic lesions (except small gumma of palate, discovered accidently in the first case); (4) History of old luetic infection and positive Wassermann; (5) Exclusion of all other forms of organic trouble; (6) Prompt antipyresis after specific treatment following primary rise in temperature after the first mercurial injection.

In the treatment of these cases the author used enesol by injection, in doses of from 2 to 4 cc. per diem. This drug (hydrargyrum methylarsenicicosalicylicum) comes in phials of a 3% aqueous solution. It is used regularly in the author's sanitarium where tuberculosis is complicated with syphilis.

In conclusion, the author points out that in fevers of unclear origin, in addition to the usual causes, syphilis must also be reckoned with. Great assistance can be had from the Wassermann and probably more from the Noguchi luetin reaction in establishing the diagnosis.

A short bibliography of the recent literature is appended to the paper.

THE AMERICAN JOURNAL OF UROLOGY, VENEREAL AND SEXUAL DISEASES

WILLIAM J. ROBINSON, M.D., EDITOR

VOL. X APRIL, 1914. NO. 4

PROFUSE HEMORRHAGE IN TUBERCULOSIS OF THE KIDNEY: THE USE OF ADRENALIN INJECTIONS AS AN ADJUVANT TO TREATMENT

BY R. P. CAMPBELL, M.D.

Genito-Urinary Surgeon, Montreal General Hospital.

HEMORRHAGE in renal tuberculosis has long been recognized as a prominent and early sign. While not a constant one, it is present in the majority of cases at least during some part of their course, and so much so, that the appearance of blood in the urine should in every instance demand the careful consideration of tuberculosis as an etiological factor. It is occasionally very profuse, and may, as in the following two cases, simulate the hemorrhage of tumor, or of the so-called "essential hematuria" or hemophilic kidney.

1. Miss A. H., (M. G. H.-G. U. 112-13) aet. 35, had always been well until one week prior to her admission to the Montreal General Hospital on July 4th, 1913, when she noticed a sudden appearance of blood in the urine. There were no other symptoms, but the blood was so abundant as to cause clots in the bladder, and a certain discomfort in passing them. The patient lost no weight and felt well. After her admission to the hospital, a slight rise in temperature was discovered, as well as a pulse of 88-92.

Urinalysis showed an acid urine of Sp. G. 1021, dark red with small clots and, microscopically, quantities of red blood cells, with, however, not more than the normally corresponding number of white cells present.

A cystoscopic examination showed the bladder to be distorted and pushed to one side, which was found to be due to a fibroid of the uterus. The bladder wall, beyond a moderate congestion, was normal. The urine from the right ureteral orifice appeared normal, while that from the left spurted as a bloody stream into the bladder.

The left ureter was catheterized and a catheter placed in the right, but owing to the distortion of the bladder, it was impossible to advance the catheter sufficiently to get a satisfactory specimen. Urinalysis of the left urine showed a Sp. G. of 1019, great quantities of blood cells, but no pus cells. Indigocarmin appeared on both sides in three minutes. The patient was observed in bed for one week, and a second cystoscopic examination made, which only confirmed the previous findings.

The slight alteration in functional value of the kidney, as indicated by the specific gravity, was so slight, and the absence of pus cells so remarkable, that due weight was perhaps not given to the slight rise in temperature and pulse, and a diagnosis of Essential Hematuria was made, and an operation undertaken to remedy this by means of decapsulation and fixation. The kidney was found slightly movable, was easily delivered, showed a small supernumerary artery, but was otherwise normal in appearance. The ureter was normal. It was only after stripping the capsule preparatory to fixation, that a small granular patch, the size of one's thumbnail, exactly over the convexity, was found. The kidney was removed and the diagnosis of tuberculosis confirmed by the microscope. (M. G. H. Pathological Laboratory, S 423-'13.)

Recovery was uneventful, except for a slight afternoon rise in temperature for some weeks.

Case 2. W. McM. (M. G. H., G. U. --94. 13) aet 30. Admitted to Montreal General Hospital on July 9th, 1913, had suffered for two weeks with profuse hematuria without any intermission. Previously, there had been no blood or other symptoms beyond a slight frequency of micturition. He had never noticed that the urine was not quite clear. He was confined to bed, and was rapidly losing ground. The previous history of a pleurisy ten years ago, and a chronically inflamed knee five years ago, pointed to a tuberculous condition, and this was confirmed by finding a definite nodule in the right epididymis and nodular infiltration of the prostate and vasa deferentia on both sides, and finally by the discovery of tubercle bacilli in the urine.

A cystoscopic examination showed a fairly normal bladder, blood issuing in spurts from the left ureteral orifice, and no flow from the right. Catheterizatien of the left gave a bloody urine of 1010 Sp. G., acid, with much blood and a few pus cells. Microscopically, this corresponded exactly with the urine taken from the bladder by catheter. The right ureter was catheterized with difficulty, but no flow could be obtained. 4 cc. 4 per cent. indigo-carmin injected intravenously on two occasions did not appear in 30 minutes in either side. A phenolsulphonephthalein test was spoiled through losing some of the urine. There remained no doubt that the left kidney was at fault, but one could not be sure of the condition of the right, and in fact, the right ureter was apparently occluded. Palpation of the abdomen was negative.

In order to determine whether anything could be done with the left kidney, a preliminary exploratory incision was made over the right kidney under gas oxygen anesthesia. It was found large, nodular and tuberculosis with a thick occluded ureter. Nothing further was done, but with the object of controlling the hemorrhage from the left kidney, a catheter was passed up the left ureter, and the pelvis repeatedly washed out with a 1-3000 adrenalin solution. This controlled the hemorrhage at once, nor did it recur. The effect of stopping the drain on the patient was very marked, and he gained strength and colour very rapidly during the next few weeks. For the future, the outlook is, of course, absolutely bad.

These cases would indicate:—

1. That hemorrhage in tuberculosis disease of the kidney may be so profuse as to hide the concomitant pyuria which must be present, and to simulate the hemorrhage of tumor or so-called renal hemophilia.

2. That it may come on as a first symptom of tuberculosis of the kidney or be delayed till the disease has progressed indefinitely.

3. That injections of adrenalin, or of a similar preparation into the pelvis, may be useful as a temporary palliative measure.

SHOULD PATIENTS SUFFERING FROM PULMONARY TUBERCULOSIS BE ALLOWED TO INDULGE IN SEXUAL INTERCOURSE? *

By Dr. Boureille, Paris, France.

SEXUAL intercourse among patients suffering from pulmonary tuberculosis is looked upon with much disfavor, since the excitement is credited with increasing arterial tension and thus favoring hemoptysis. This applies, of course, to both sexes, but is especially true of women, in whom the sexual sphere plays so prominent a part.

All the classic authors protest against sexual relations in the tuberculous, and in every day practice this is the usual advice given by consultants to their patients. When, for non-medical reasons, hospital authorities do not actually house the sexes separately, they invariably recommend absolute abstinence and conjure up before their patients' eyes the specters of impending hemoptysis and of hasty consumption.

This opinion of the medical profession is based on facts of the greatest importance. To be sure, very serious physical damage may result from abuse of the sexual relation. But how about the moral disorders which may be the consequences of abstinence? If there is physical danger in some cases, is there not in others just as much moral danger, with all its physical sequelae?

At my patients' requests I have in several instances had to interfere in this delicate matter. My cases seem all to be built on the same pattern, so great a part do the mental factors and their physical consequences play in tuberculous individuals.

Madame X., residing in the suburbs of Paris, was treated for several years for chronic, caseous, pulmonary tuberculosis. She had been in a sanatorium and had passed the winter in the south. I have been treating her for several months. She is a young, intelligent woman who wishes to be cured, and rigorously follows medical instructions. Her husband, also very intelligent, has been nursing her most affectionately. The union has been a happy one. As is usual in such cases, the husband and wife were taken apart by their physicians and were recommended absolute abstinence from sexual relations.

The patient was treated for two years and had done well.

* Read before the Société de Médicine de Paris, Nov. 22, 1913.

For two years her mode of life had conformed absolutely to directions and sexual abstinence was as complete as had been requested by the doctors. All was well, and the patient, fearing an hemoptysis, was putting up with the above restrictions when she suddenly received the proof of her husband's infidelity. For six months the man had obeyed, and then, not wishing to aggravate his wife's condition, he went to a mistress. Of course, the patient did not see in this infidelity the natural consequence of a medical order against the husband's having sexual relations that he might spare his wife. "Nam sese excruciat," says Petronius, "qui beatis invidet." "Jealous women seal their own unhappiness." And what was the denouément?

In this patient—whose height was 1 m. 60, and whose upper chest measurement was 86-90 cm.—the weight had varied between October, 1912, and the end of July, 1913, from 61 kgs. at the lowest, to 62.2 kgs. at the highest. On July 27, she learned of her husband's faithlessness. On August 8, she weighed 56.66 kgs.; on August 25, she went down to 55.3 kgs. The patient had lost 5.9 kgs. in one month.

The rectal temperature, taken four times daily for a year, never exceeded 37.3° from the 26th of June to the 26th of July, 1913. Throughout the whole of July 26th it remained at 37° the whole day. On the 27th, without there being anything in the pulmonary condition to account for the sudden rise, the temperature jumped to 40° at 2 p. m. and to 40°6 at 5 p. m. The next day the thermometer read 38°2, 38°6, 39°6, 38°4. A few days later, I determined, by auscultation, that there had occurred a recurrence of the lesions which had lain dormant for the preceding two months.

A period of prostration followed, which necessitated vigorous therapeutic measures, and it was only after the twelfth injection of Vallée's antituberculosis serum, and several sittings of free thermocauterization, that the condition seemed to improve. My repeated attempts to calm her also had their effect. On the 24th of September her weight rose to 57.96 kgs., and on the 15th of October to 58.85 kgs., thus showing a gain of 3.55 kgs. since August 25th. The temperature fell little by little and since the first of August it remained between 36°8 and 37°2.

What was my advice on sexual matters when this storm was over? As the patient had taken me into her confidence, I spoke very frankly to her. I prescribed the resumption of coitus with her husband and clearly specified the precautions necessary to avoid the physical disorders which might result. I advised moderation: absolute abstention for some days preceding and following the menses, on the day of and the day following injections of antituberculosis serum, on the days of thermocauterization, and whenever the temperature exceeded 38°.

Undoubtedly this is a delicate matter to handle, but the physician is so often the confessor that he might well seek a remedy for the physical and moral dangers which are unveiled. Do not the secrets of the soul offer the key to the diagnosis and treatment of bodily ills?

In connection with the above case let me present the following which is but one of many similar instances. I saw in consultation, in the country, a young woman of 23 years, married for a year and a half, who was suffering from tuberculosis of the upper third of the left lung. Her general condition was poor, the sputum was loaded with bacilli, and she was running a temperature between 38° and 38°5. My personal knowledge of the couple, their recent marriage, the unavailing efforts of my colleague who had already been talking abstinence for several weeks, all convinced me of the certain failure of repeating the prohibitions against coitus. Neither separate rooms, nor even separate beds were accepted. It was clearly necessary to retire from our extreme position if we were to save the life of this very sick patient.

I represented to the husband the danger of immoderation, even in the slightest degree, for he would thus not only aggravate his wife's condition, but would expose himself to infection. Nevertheless I did permit intercourse, safeguarded by every precaution used in such cases, not only to avoid pregnancy, hemoptysis, and "galloping" consumption, but also to protect the husband against contagion. I saw the husband and wife on several subsequent occasions and reiterated each time my counsels of moderation. I have reason to believe that they were followed. Not only did this patient not become worse, but thanks to thirty injections of Vallée's serum she is now actually on the road to a not far distant recovery.

I am in a position to affirm that in this case, as well as in others just like it which I could report, abstinence from all sexual relations would have resulted in a very serious moral crisis, surely followed by an aggravation of the disease. On the other hand, the very moderate exercise of a normal function was responsible for no disorders whatever.

Physical and moral disturbances arising from sexual relations in tuberculous individuals are not to be scoffed at. The former class of consequences is known to all and the most prominent symptom in the eyes of the patient, viz., hemoptysis, may very well be provoked by irritation of the genitals or by coitus. Plethoric, nervous, excitable, or arthritic patients, big eaters, subjects with high arterial tension, constantly exposed to wind or to weather, hard workers, devotees of hotel life with its social activities, gambling and high living, whether at the sea-shore or at high altitudes, such individuals, when given to sexual excesses, make excellent candidates for hemoptyses. The same causes will produce the same results whether we are dealing with tuberculous subjects who are getting worse or with patients who are improving but insufficiently watched. And it is the woman rather than the man who must fear hemoptysis because of the complicated factors of her sexual life.

The abuse of the sexual function may very well put the patient in danger, but what are the consequences of total abstinence? By no means so simple as may be believed. The man or the woman who has been prohibited sexual intercourse does not *ipso facto* risk any aggravation of his tuberculosis. But let us consider to what dangers the couple become exposed at once. If they live alone, masturbation threatens them; if they live together a prohibition to one party means a prohibition to the other.

If the patient is a man, the wife, by her very nature, will readily restrain herself. On the other hand a healthy man will chafe under an interdiction covering several months or several years. In the case of tuberculous patients who are very ill but who may yet live 2, 3, or 4 years, shall we counsel the absolute suppression of coitus during the entire course of the disease, as I have actually seen done? Or shall we overlook the matter entirely, which is very much worse?

Total abstinence may inflict upon the home the worst possible moral consequences which may in turn be followed by an actual aggravation of the lesions,—and the effect of treatment is but poor indeed in such cases. The physician should foresee this possible outcome.

Can it be a matter of indifference to a sick woman that a medical prescription should be responsible for the entrance of adultery into her home? Or, in general, that a man should in any way injure his wife because of the situation in which her disease puts him?

Such situations open the way to painful discussions and, as far as the woman is concerned, may lead to a severe moral crisis followed by serious physical consequences. In every case of this kind that I was able to follow, the temperature rose from one to two degrees, the auscultatory signs became aggravated, and the general condition became worse. And what prognosis can we give when the aggravation results from a psychic crisis rather than from the virulence of the tuberculous poisons?

Moderate exercise of a normal function, safeguarded by indispensable precautions, will not cause such inconveniences as have been described. Shall we refuse tuberculous patients to have the slightest exercise, as was formerly the custom? We only ask that they be afebrile and we allow them to walk about under supervision. Shall we prohibit our patients from working, as did physicians ten or fifteen years ago? Nowadays work is permitted and even advised in certain well-defined conditions.

Both work and walking are normal manifestations of the exteriorization of the individual, and the reasons must be indeed serious which would call for their suppression. The sexual functions are of the same nature. It is for the physician to decide whether to counsel moderation in tuberculous individuals, or to advise total abstinence, but let us realize that moderation suffices in the overwhelming majority of cases.

The conclusion is obvious, therefore, that the physician must not hesitate to speak of sexual matters to his tuberculous patients. A discussion of arterial tension will pave the way for confidences on this delicate subject. The physician should always lay before his patient the possible consequences of the abuse of sexual relations. But if abstinence should be a source of irritability between two married people he should advise the resumption of coitus and lay down all the necessary precautions for the avoidance or at the least the limitation of possible untoward results.

We may conclude from our study as follows:

1. The abuse of sexual relations in patients suffering from pulmonary tuberculosis is a source of great physical danger.

2. Abstinence from sexual relations may determine a serious psychic upset followed immediately by an aggravation of the disease.

3. Moderation in sexual relations has generally no ill effect whatever.

"Naturae non vincitur nisi parendo," says Bacon in his philosophy,—"not too much, not too little," as I would translate it.

A CASE OF VESICAL PAPILLOMA [1]

By H. Horace Grant, M.D., Louisville, Kentucky.

A FEMALE of thirty had frequently repeated irregularly recurring hemorrhage from the bladder for a year or more. There was little disturbance of the general health except that due to the resulting cystitis. No kidney abnormality could be demonstrated, although the urine contained albumen. However, this was accounted for by the cystitis, there being always a small amount of pus in the urine.

The patient suffered considerably because of frequent micturition and the straining necessary to empty the bladder. Except when quieted by opiates urination was imperative eighteen to twenty times each night. Under the use of sedatives, suppositories and opiates the frequency was reduced to four to five nightly urinations and about the same number during the day.

After the family physician had exhausted customary therapeutic methods without appreciable benefit, he suggested that the patient consult someone else. Cystoscopic examination made two days ago by my son, Doctor Owsley Grant, revealed a papilloma on the posterior wall of the bladder near the left ureteral orifice. It was thought the tumor was larger than a robin's egg, but its exact size could not be definitely determined. However, owing to its approximate size and apparent elevation upon the bladder wall, even allowing for possible error in the cystoscopic examination, it was deemed proper to expose the bladder and ascertain the exact condition.

This morning we exposed the bladder according to a method brought into prominent notice in this country by Dr. Howard A. Kelly. Whether it was an entirely original procedure, or otherwise, there appears some question, but the most important feature, i. e., the method of "stripping up" the fascia and exposing the bladder, is probably original. The modus operandi of Kelly's' method consists in making a large transverse incision through the skin and superficial fascia about an inch above the symphysis pubis, the convexity toward the pubis and the concavity toward the umbilicus, the aponeurosis being divided with scissors to the

[1] Clinical Report before the West End Medical Society of Louisville, Kentucky.

extent of four or five inches. The fatty structures overlying the bladder are thus freely exposed, and the recti muscles being separated, the bladder may be readily brought into view. During the execution of this procedure the bladder was not distended. The viscus was then filled with fluid and a transverse incision about two and a half inches in length made therein.

There was little hemorrhage, the interior of the bladder was clearly seen, the papilloma shaped like a mushroom being plainly visible attached to the posterior bladder wall by a small pedicle. The remainder of the tumor was perfectly free from the bladder surface. The pedicle was clamped with Ochsner forceps and the tumor easily removed. There occurred slight hemorrhage from the pedicle, which was controlled by quilting with catgut after inserting three or four sutures at the base, and there was no bleeding thereafter. However, as there had been previous repeated hemorrhage from the bladder, it was thought wise to practice abdominal as well as urethral drainage. The two drainage-tubes were held together by No. O plain catgut so they could be easily separated. There was no hemorrhage after the operation, and urine was discharged freely, some from the abdominal drain but the greater part through the catheter.

The patient bore the operation exceedingly well except that once or twice the pulse became quite rapid, apparently due to traction upon the base of the bladder while applying the deep sutures in the mucosa between the ureteral orifices. However, after she was returned to bed the pulse improved; it is now not over 80, and she suffers practically no pain. No opiate has been necessary since the operation, the patient partakes freely of water, and is apparently in a perfectly safe condition.

The obscurity concerning the real condition in this case was more apparent than real. Both the family physician and the consultant suspected tumor of the bladder, but were unable to verify the diagnosis, and under all the circumstances the patient quite naturally hesitated about even having a cystoscopic examination made until yesterday. When she consented to the examination and the cystoscope revealed the presence of this tumor, she readily consented to the operation.

Whether this tumor, which is about the size of half a small orange, is malignant or benign has not yet been positively determined, but a section of the pedicle and fragment of the growth have been submitted to the microscopist for examination and report.[2] The fact that the patient suffered little discomfort and that her general health has remained unimpaired induces the belief that the tumor is benign, although papillomata must always be regarded with suspicion and the prognosis is therefore uncertain.

While the patient has at different times had slight elevation of temperature, for the most part it has been normal. For several days prior to the operation the temperature was 99° to 100° F., but her appearance did not indicate any serious condition.

The cystoscopic examination in this case was exceedingly satisfactory. The facility with which the interior of the bladder was exposed by the method of incision outlined, the tumor being plainly seen, and after removal the site of the tumor being clearly observed, render this method of approach exceedingly valuable in operating upon the bladder. However, there is the disadvantage that there results a considerable open space, and if infection occurred it might cause delay in convalescence; but infection should not occur unless urine from an infected bladder be permitted to invade the open area, in which event there might be more difficulty in its control than after employment of the ordinary incision where not so much space remains open.

In facilitating exploration of the bladder the method employed is unquestionably of great value, and the disadvantage mentioned is offset by the many advantages, especially where the bladder is not already infected.

DISCUSSION.

In discussing the foregoing report Dr. J. K. Freeman said that macroscopically the specimen appeared to be a papilloma, but such tumors were suspicious, many of them being malignant. He believed the operation would not have been greatly prolonged, nor any considerable danger added, had the operator excised that portion of the vesical wall to which the tumor was attached. He was especially interested in description of the incision for exploring the bladder, and did not believe it added anything to the danger of the operation. The length of the external incision makes little difference so long as aseptic surgery be practiced. He did not understand the necessity of draining both ways in the case reported, and requested the reporter to explain this in clos-

[2] After careful examination the pathologist reports that the specimens show no evidence of malignancy. The tumor may therefore be classed as a simple papilloma.

ing the discussion. If hemorrhage was controlled the self-retaintaining catheter would have been sufficient, closing the external wound entirely.

Dr. Owsley Grant remarked that on exploring the bladder with the cystoscope it was found the tumor was near the ureteral orifice, and there might have been danger of extirpating this orifice with the tumor had the vesical wall been excised. The method of approaching the bladder described was undoubtedly preferable to any other. The bladder was distended with water, and while air was sometimes utilized instead, he did not believe any better results were obtained.

Dr. H. Horace Grant in closing said that portion of the vesical wall where the tumor arose was not excised, first because the patient's age and duration of the tumor did not indicate malignancy; second, the pedicle was so small that after excision the vesical wall was perfectly smooth. The raw surface was cauterized with themocautery before inserting the sutures to control hemorrhage. Furthermore, he did not wish to add unnecessary risk of future troublesome hemorrhage. Packing of the bladder might have been required had a deep incision been made in the mucosa. Previous hemmorhage from the bladder had been irregular, and while only an ounce or two of blood was lost during the operation, still it seemed wise to drain in both directions to facilitate irrigation of the bladder if hemorrhage recurred. He would have preferred closing the external wound, as suggested by Dr. Freeman, and in the light of the progress the patient has made it would have been safe, but this could not be foretold. The vesical wall was tightly closed around the drainage tube which was afterward employed, in connection with the urethral catheter, to irrigate the bladder.

THE RELAPSES AFTER SALVARSAN *

By Professor Gaucher, St. Louis Hospital, Paris.

IN spite of the frequency of complications arising from the administration of salvarsan and the number of cases where the drug remained without effect, some physicians continue to employ it and some patients accept its use. I think, therefore, it is well to warn both of the dangerous illusions. In what is to follow the treatment by both the old and the new salvarsan is considered. The neo-salvarsan is more dangerous than the old, without being any more efficacious.

And, in the first place, I will retrace the strange history ot this drug born two years ago and whose destiny seemed so glorious. During the first period, that might be termed "the golden age" of salvarsan, the press made an active campaign whose end was simply commercial and the techniques offered were far from scientific. Anyone could contract syphilis and be cured by a single injection!

This first period was of short duration; in the second it was found that one injection did not cure, then that after a number of injections the lesions reappeared and the impotency of the drug was concealed by giving mercury at the same time. By this means the good results could be attributed to salvarsan, which in reality resulted from the mercury and should have furnished to enlightened minds a sufficient proof of the inefficiency of a remedy from which so much was expected.

I will not refer to the grave or even fatal accidents produced by salvarsan; it is sufficient to recall the cases of blindness, deafness, paralysis, arsenical polyneuritis, many instances of which have been put on record. Likewise the many cases of venous thrombosis reported both in France and Germany, and cases of death occuring after the injection of even small doses. In this lecture relapses alone will be considered, coming on nearly always after the use of salvarsan, so that this product must be considered a treacherous one, which, acording to the vulgar expression, "whitewashes the patient without curing him."

The report of a few cases taken haphazard from the records of my service will be the best demonstration of this truth.

* A clinical lecture delivered at the St. Louis Hospital, Paris, and reported by Dr. M. H. Cesbron.

Case I. Female, age 24 years. Syphilitic vulvar chancre in August, 1911. Received three intravenous injections of 30, 40 and 50 centigrams of salvarsan. Chancre rapidly disappeared. Nov. 15, appearance of mucous patches which by December had taken on the cauliflower aspect and resembled syphilides that are met with in women *who have never been treated.*

Case II. Female, age 28 years, mucous patches of the vulva in Oct., 1911. Received three injections of 40, 40 and 60 centigrams of salvarsan. Feb. 2, 1912, very marked roseola. In this respect I would point out that since salvarsan has been employed these returning roseolae are *much more frequent than formerly.*

Case III. Female, age 23 years, chancre and inguinal lymphnodes, Jan. 15, 1912. Received three injections of 15, 30 and 30 centigrams of salvarsan. On Jan. 22, roseola and violent headache.

Case IV. Male, age 35 years, syphilis eleven years ago. In 1900 gummata on the legs, in 1907 ulcerating syphilides. At present has syphilitic keratosis of the right plantar region. Cured by mercury. March 5, 1910, mucous patches of the lips, which were cured. Jan. 23, 1912, the patches have returned. In September three injections of 30 centigrams each were given. Now, two months after treatment, he has ulcerating patches of the commisures and lingual leucoplasia. This proves that *salvarsan does not prevent relapses of stubborn tertiary lesions.*

Case V. Female, had a primary sore on the vulva in Aug., 1911. Was given four injections. In November she presented vulvar ulcerations and edema of the right labium majorum. More injections were administered in Italy, since which the lesions have returned.

Case VI. Female, age 27 years, chancre of the lower lip in Aug., 1910. Three intravenous injections given. One month after, returning roseola and mucous patches.

Case VII. Female, age 19 years, was given three injections of salvarsan for a primary lesion. *One year later* hypertrophic patches on vulva and in labial commisures, alopecia and headache. This case shows *the retarding and aggravating action of salvarsan.*

Case VIII. Male, age 48 years, chancre in Jan., 1911. Feb. 2 the patient was given the first injection of 30 centigrams and then a second one. Since then no treatment. Sept. 6, palmar and plantar papular syphilides appearing *as in an untreated syphilis.*

Case IX. Female, age 20 years, treated irregularly with mercury. In August, 1911, injection of salvarsan. Oct. 30 mucous patches of the vulva and a gumma of the dorsum of the medius. She was given four injections of 20 and 30 centigrams. Two months after the last injection she returned with ulcerating syphilides of the gluteal region.

Case X. Male, age 21 years. In October, 1911, chancre in the upper part of the sulcus of the glans. Three intravenous injections. Two months later the patient returned with an eruption dating back a month. Secondary rose-colored papules, mucous patches, Wassermann reaction positive.

Case XI. Female, age 25 years, mucous patches in mouth in January. In February injection of salvarsan. In March presents a serious iritis of left eye.

Case XII. Female, age 31 years. Syphilis six years ago. *During two months she was given five injections,* the last one a month ago. At present there is an occipital osteoperiostitis, which appeared a week ago. Now, the injections had been given when no accidents were present. Thus *salvarsan does not possess any preventive action.*

Case XIII. Male, 34 years old, chancre in February, 1911. In June, three intravenous injections. No sexual intercourse until Sept. 13. At this time he had mucous patches of the lower lip, ulceration of the glans penis and returning roseola. It is cases such as this one that the partisans of salvarsan speak of as instances of reinfection. Now, this patient had had no sexual intercourse since the injections were given and the case was simply a relapse of the disease after the employment of salvarsan.

Case XIV. Female, age 25 years. In March, 1912, diphtheroid chancre of the tonsil, cutaneous eruption. Three injections of salvarsan. In July, erosive syphilides of the labia minora, left-sided sternomastoid adenopathy, headache.

Case XV. Female, age 33 years. Syphilis two years ago. Three injections given during last year. At present has mucous patches on the tonsils.

Case XVI. Male, 26 years of age, chancre of the nostril in November, 1911. Hypertrophic papula syphilides of the scrotum. Three injections given. Mucous patches three months afterward.

Case XVII. Female, age 23 years. Indurated chancre *on the internal aspect of the left thigh.* Three injections. The lesion retroceded in two weeks. Eight months later mucous patches appeared on the site of the former chancre. Now, this patient had had no sexual intercourse during the interval; and still more it was an extragenital chancre on the thigh. There consequently could not have been syphilitic reinfection, but simply a chancre redux. Now, *the chancre redux, as in the case of returning roseola, was hardly ever encountered before the use of salvarsan.*

Case XVIII. Male, age 32 years. Chancre of the penis and roseola cured for some time past. In August, 1911, four intravenous injections of 30, 60 centigrams. In September mucous patches on the left anterior pillar of the fauces. The patient did not present any lesion at the time of the injections.

Case XIX. Male, age 26 years. Chancre in January, 1912. Was given *twelve injections.* In September he presented, besides the psoriasiform and lichenoid syphilides, which were present at the time the injections were given, some new lesions, namely mucous patches of the lips and tongue and an iritis of the right eye.

Case XX. Female, 28 years old. Indurated chancre of the deltoid region. Injection of 50 centigrams. No accidents for a year, then mucous patches appeared on the tonsils, with acneiform syphilides on the shoulders and alopecia. All these accidents are those observed at the beginning of syphilis and not a year after infection. This is still another proof of the *retarding action* of salvarsan.

Case XXI. Male, age 25 years; indurated chancre in July, 1909. Treated by mercurial injections. In July, 1912, mucous patches. Three injections of salvarsan. In October iritis of left eye.

Case XXII. Male, 38 years of age. Syphilis six years ago. In August, 1911, three injections given for psoriasiform syphilides. A cure resulted. In 1912 cutaneous gummatous syphilides, Salvarsan again employed without results.

Case XXIII. Female, 33 years old. In August, 1911, chancre. At the beginning was given two injections. One year later a generalized returning roseola.

Case XXIV. Female, age 27 years. Syphilis in June, 1911. An injection was given in June, 1912, and soon appeared *a returning roseola one year after the first.*

Case XXV. Male, age 28 years. Chancre in September, 1910. Sept. 12, nine days after, an intravenous injection was given. Nov. 16 the chancre was still present and a second injection was given on Nov. 21; the chancre then disappeared. He returned in January, 1911, and a third injection was given; in June mucous patches still persisted.

Case XXVI. Male, syphilis four years ago. Three injections of 60 centigrams each. Three months later mucous patches.

Case XXVII. Male, syphilis for two years. Two injections of 60 centigrams each. A fortnight later, Wassermann negative. Three months later, mucous patches.

Case XXVIII. Female. On Nov. 4, 1911, mucous patches on vulva. Dec. 12, injection of 30 centigrams. Up to March 29, 1912, was given nine injections. Oct. 31, 1912, erosive mucous patch on the left labium majorum.

The frequency of relapses after the arsenical treatment leads to some most terrible misunderstandings on account of the false security that it gives to patients, and we have unfortunately too frequent examples of *young women contaminated by their husbands who believed themselves thoroughly cured.*

Case XXIX. Male. Indurated chancre of the penis. Three injections of salvarsan. The chancre healed. The patient then married and two months afterwards he developed ulcerating syphilides of the glans penis and buccal mucous patches.

Case XXX. Male, age 28 years. Chancre in April, 1912. Was given six injections of 30, 50 and 60 centigrams in thirty-three days. Total amount of salvarsan administered was 2 grams, 90 centigrams. On June 12, he presented three ulcerating syphilides, the largest one having appeared between the fifth and sixth injection, mucous patches on the tonsils, and a chancriform erosion at the anus. His wife is contaminated.

Case XXXI. Male, chancre of the penis in 1910. For fourteen months he was given injections of gray oil. In March, 1911, circinate syphilides for which he was given three injections of salvarsan. The patient married and infected his young wife. She presents an alopecia and has a positive Wassermann.

I could multiply such cases, and writers of different countries have observed the same relapses. Dind of Lausanne relates a case in which a papular roseola appeared sixty-three days after injections of salvarsan, confirming what I have said about the retarding action of the drug.

Wolf, of Strasbourg, believes that the relapses are constant and that Wassermann's reaction is not influenced by salvarsan.

Dreuw, of Berlin, concludes, as I myself have done, that salvarsan "cannot take the place of mercury, the combined treatment throws a veil over the serious relapses and prevents incriminating the insufficiency of salvarsan. . . . Salvarsan presents no advantage, only danger."

Finger, of Vienna, refers to the frequency of neuro-relapses, which are merely toxic arsenical complications or unrecognized syphilitic accidents.

Trimble, of New York, comes to the same conclusions as myself and even refers to my opinion.

This insufficiency of salvarsan no longer escapes the notice of the patients themselves, for quite recently a syphilitic in Varsovia killed a physician who affirmed that the former was cured, when much to his disgust his symptoms continued. Is not this another unforeseen accident due to salvarsan! Some partisans of the drug point out that often Wassermann's reaction, positive before the injection, becomes negative afterwards and use this as a pretext for lauding the action of the remedy. Without wishing to make a retort to such a fugacious dialectic, I would reply that it is due to the absence of accuracy in the procedures now in vogue. Dr. Desmoulière has, in fact, just communicated to the Institute a new procedure which he devised in my laboratory, and which changes the former statistics. By adding cholesterin to old antigen (extract of heredo-syphilitic liver with the fat removed by ether) in the proportion of one per cent., he obtained an antigen of great sensibility. Then systematically repeating, by means of this antigen, Wassermann's reaction in subjects treated by salvarsan, he obtained positive results in cases which by the older method were proclaimed negative.

It would be quite wrong to believe that this insufficiency of salvarsan has escaped the attention of its most fervent apostles, since they all are preoccupying themselves with the combined treatment with mercury. I would also obtain excellent results by combining mercury with wine of cinchona and phosphate of lime. Would you not find it strange if I should attribute the only merit to cinchona and calcium phosphate? and nevertheless this is what they are trying to do right before us.

It would be superfluous to continue longer the suit of salvarsan, but does this imply that it should never be employed?

Yes, but only in very rare cases, the indications for which I will now give before closing this lecture:

Salvarsan exclusively acts on cutaneous and mucous ulcerations. The cicatrization is perfect, the lesions heal, but they relapse. Salvarsan has no action on visceral syphilis, particularly in tabes; this must be understood once and for all, because there is a tendency to take advantage of these unhappy persons by means of this drug.

Salvarsan may be employed in individuals who do not tolerate mercury or when this drug proves itself insufficient, on the condition that these subjects are not the bearers of any visceral lesion and after the liver, heart, nervous system, eyes and ears have been thoroughly examined. One should always bear in mind that, even in small doses, salvarsan may be dangerous and even fatal in its effects.

A NEW METHOD OF TREATING CHRONIC GONORRHEA AND URETHRITIS SIMPLEX

By Dr. Eduard Bäumer.

THE name "urethritis non gonorrhoica" or "simplex" is misleading in so far as it implies a harmless malady easy to heal. When we leave out of consideration artificial urethritis, such as that caused by injections of irritating antiseptics after coitus, simple urethritis may be divided into two groups. In the first group belong those cases who have never had gonorrhea previously or in whom a previous gonorrhea was completely cured without leaving infiltrations, etc. The course of the disease in these patients is as follows: 2 weeks after coitus a gray, mucous secretion appears at the meatus and the patient complains of a mild itching or burning. The first portion of urine is slightly cloudy; the second, clear. Microscopically, the secretion shows mucus, epithelial and pus cells, and various kinds of bacteria. Even diplococci, superficially resembling the gonococcus, may be present. Even when intracellular. these organisms cannot be regarded as etiological factors, for the normal urethra harbors numerous bacteria, which find favorable developmental conditions during a catarrhal inflammation of the mucosa. Such organisms, which may modify a disease without actually causing it, Casper calls true nosoparasites. On the other hand, the rich flora of the vagina, especially so after menstruation, may actually be the cause of urethritis in susceptible men. This holds especially true for a short, thick bacillus which has given rise to what Finger calls a "bacillus urethritis."

The second class of simple urethritides includes those cases who have had a gonorrhea but in whom the discharge still persists notwithstanding the absence of gonococci. Or else, persons who have had a chronic gonorrhea in the past get up a fresh discharge two or three days after intercourse. In these cases, though gonococci are of course absent, examination with the endoscope or bulb-pointed bougie will reveal the presence of hard and soft infiltrations, even of strictures. Urethritis simplex of the first group may also cause infiltrates, if of long enough standing. Epididymitis and prostatitis may also result.

The usual treatment of this condition with instillations, irrigations, and dilatations of various types gives very unsatisfactory results. Dr. Awerbuch, of St. Petersburg, explains these failures as follows: In chronic inflammations of the urethra, for example, the main change is hyperplasia of the mucosa. This begins in the superficial layers as a mucositis superficialis and then involves the submucosa as well (mucositis profunda). These deep connective tissue hyperplasias cannot be treated mechanically nor by the ordinary bactericidal measures. A drug such as Lytinol, however (about to be described), can revert a mucositis profunda into a mucositis superficialis which can then be readily cured by astringents. Lytinol, which was invented by Dr. Awerbuch, is an iodine compound forming a dark brown solution and miscible in all proportions with distilled water. The original solution (the "Nassovia" Co., Wiesbaden) is 100% strength and can be diluted to any concentration desired.

Bäumer begins with a 5% solution which the patient injects thrice daily, retaining the solution in the urethra 5 minutes each time. At first the secretion increases regularly in amount. The leucocytes increase, whereas the bacteria diminish in number. When the strength is increased to 7.5% and 10% there is slight burning after the injection. In all his cases, after one to three weeks' treatment, the leucocytes disappeared from the discharge and epithelial cells alone were present. To remove this last trace of inflammation a weak astringent solution is all that was required (e. g. 0.75:200 zinc sulfate). Both portions of the urine then became clear and the patients were free of symptoms.

It is not surprising to note this action of Lytinol when we recall the excellent resorptive powers of the ordinary iodine preparations in such cases as lymphadenitis and periostitis. The advantage of the new preparation is that it can be used without danger on so delicate a mucous membrane as that of the urethra. The author admits that his experience with Lytinol has been relatively meagre, that he has observed his cases for too short a period to tell whether the results can be regarded as permanent, and that further tests of the drug should be made to determine its value in urethrocystitis and in cystitis, and that the results should be confirmed by endoscopy and cystoscopy.

CAUSES AND RESULTS OF MASTURBATION

By Victor Blum, M.D.

Assistant in Prof. von Frisch's Urological Department of the Vienna General Polyclinic

AUTHORIZED TRANSLATION. EDITED WITH NOTES AND ADDITIONS BY DR. W. J. ROBINSON

IN devoting here a separate article to the etiology of masturbation we leave out of consideration the fundamental biologic cause of every human sexual act, the SEXUAL IMPULSE per se.

At that time, when the sexual organs show an overpowering tendency to growth and bring about the familiar physical and psychic revolution in the entire organism, the sexual impulse awakes at this period of storm and stress, the youth is impelled to sexual acts with more or less violence according to his age, race, climate and character. This impulse represents the fundamental cause of every sexual activity in general, and it leads to masturbation, when the cardinal factors unite to bring about that vice; namely, hereditary predisposition, education, and eventual accessory causes.

We will consider the etiology of masturbation from this point of view, since onanism and the severe traumata to the nervous system growing out of it arises only through the co-operation of all these factors.

The nervous and neuropathic tendency, which is so often made responsible for the origin of all sorts of neuroses and psychoses, is really an *undefinable disposition to nervous affections*, and consists of a lessened resistance to all sorts of injuries attacking the nervous system. It is an ancient and daily re-proved experience, that the children of neuropathic and psychopathic parents may inherit a nervous constitution, so that nervous affections develop under the influence of certain agents upon the nervous system.

The laws of heredity are not yet sufficiently established for us to be able to give the reason why both normal and neuropathic children can come from the same parents.

From the hereditary constitution there results a series of characteristic traits which play a most important rôle in the neuropathy which we are just about to consider—masturbation.

The temperament of the individual, which already in early childhood in many cases must be regarded as a markedly sensual disposition, is a resultant of the inherited constitution and various external influences, to which the person was subject in early youth. Schwartz says on this point: "It is proved that the children of lascivious parents fall victims more easily to the temptations of sensuality than do others. Our intellectual capacities can be transmitted to posterity; in this way we bring with us at our birth the germs of our good as well as our bad qualities." (Dissertation sur les dangers de l'onanisme. Thèse de Strasbourg, 1815.)

Temperament is further affected by climate and race. The greater sensuality of the Southerners, of the Jews, etc., is well known.

It is clear that masturbation is made much easier in a precociously developed, sensual temperament. Thus we see that some children, as a result of a morbidly increased and precocious sexual impulse, already show a disposition to masturbation in the fact that in them many perceptions and ideas, which remain for other persons sexually indifferent, acquire a connection with the sexual sphere.

The other influences, which assail the youthful spirit and lead to the development of a particular temperament,—in this case a sensual one—are the effect of its environment, of social conditions, of the power of example, the first education by the nurse, who is sometimes chosen too thoughtlessly.

To these are added the results of a wrong education during the years of boyhood. The favorite aim of precocity in modern education of children seems to be the most injurious. The imagination is provoked to unbridled excitement through the precocious development of an active mental life, and the child's attention is directed to a group of ideas which should be kept away from the youthful mind for a long time to come. The neglect of physical culture, of exercise in the open air, of bodily exercises and active games, all contribute to the injurious results of our mistaken system of education.

But when the boy approaches the age of puberty then all these injurious features of modern education assert themselves to an increased degree. The development of the generative organs goes on unconsciously but unceasingly, and through the revolution in the entire organism new ideas and sensations press upon the mind of the adolescent, and his attention is now directed continually to his sexual organs, and his imagination revels unfettered among conceptions of a sexual nature.

The path hence to masturbation is a short one. Especially at night the temptation to masturbate comes overpoweringly, when no supervision can divert or control the flight of the imagination.

The best remedy against these excesses of the imagination; namely, bodily exercises and physical movements carried to the point of severe fatigue, is almost always neglected in the education of our modern youth. As Trousseau says: "In the present state of society we occupy ourselves only with the understanding, the intelligence, because it rules the world; it is cultivated in hot-house fashion, to obtain precocious but weak and juiceless fruits, without taking any thought as to what the forced, maimed plant, exhausting itself in its fruit, will become." [1]

The mistaken education at home and at school is also to blame for the spoiled and pampered nature of many youths. Their will-power is so small that they can make no serious resistance to the storm of their sexual impulses. They fall victims to the first temptation to onanism, which overtakes them in the long hours of idleness.

Dietary errors are also often to blame for masturbatory practices among our growing youth. The injurious effects of alcohol, above all, and also of coffee, tea, and tobacco, of an abundant meat diet, and of stimulating spices are still not

[1] The great value of physical exercise admits of no discussion. But its effectiveness as a panacea against masturbation and the manifestations of the sexual impulse I question very much. Only too often, it seemed to me, did physical exercise have the contrary effect.—W. J. R.

sufficiently appreciated. The congestive effect of these substances upon the abdominal organs is well known, and yet these foods, condiments, and stimulants still appear without discrimination in the dietary of the adolescent!

We have until now attempted to bring the "vice" of self-pollution into etiologic relation with hereditary defects and mistakes in education. Much more might well be said concerning these points, but we will confine ourselves to these suggestions.

But the actual or exciting causes of masturbation have a great, perhaps the greatest importance.

These often stand in close relation to errors in education and in manner of life, but can also develop their injurious action at any period of life, if an exciting cause for masturbation is furnished by some local affection of the genitals or other external reasons.

Thus we often find in the social relations the condition which favors the origin of masturbation. In a part of the cases it is the wealth of the family with its accompanying wasteful luxury, which may lead to masturbation. And here the above-mentioned errors in the diet of the children and adolescents is a contributory factor.

The entire freedom from care, in which such children grow up, the frequent opportunities for unbridled flights of the imagination make the boys weak-willed and devoid of energy; they develop an inclination to falsehood and secretiveness, which, as is well known, greatly favors onanism.

The luxurious manner of living of our modern metropolitan families is the reason why masturbation occurs so much more frequently in the large city than in the country. Not nearly so many sexual allurements offer themselves to the imagination of the growing youth in the country, and thus his sexual impulses may be much longer restrained. The rural life with its physically exhausting labor and exercise in the open gives enough diversion to the imagination, and in this way protects the country people at least in part from masturbation. But of course there, too, the greatest excesses in vice may occur through seduction and mental infection. [The greater purity of the "country" is now being questioned by those competent to judge.]

But great poverty also furnishes equally great dangers to the sexual development. The promiscuity of the sexes and the undisguised intimacy of the family life turns the child's attention early to the sexual realm. The bad example of older, corrupted children, which younger ones are liable to meet at any time unhindered by the lack of supervision, does the rest in weakening their resistance to the incitement to masturbation.

Thousands of observations have shown how great the danger is of seducement to masturbation; for example, there are many recorded cases of the infection of a whole school class and a whole division of soldiers with the vice of onanism.

Merely to avoid ridicule, the charge of "cowardice," many boys succumb to the seduction of their corrupted comrades.

Among the social causes of masturbation we must also include those cases, which occur everywhere, where normal sexual intercourse is made impossible to adolescents and men. The vice thus breaks out in epidemics in cloisters, prisons, on board ships, and in boarding-schools.

Certain kinds of occupation may also be the exciting cause of masturbation. So horseback and bicycle riding were given as the direct cause by many. We must of course suppose a certain degree of increased nervous excitability, if we are to believe that these occupations, which belong to the better class of sports, are the primary cause of masturbation. We have already expressed our opinion on this point on another occasion (morbid seminal losses).

The cause of masturbation may lie in some cases in a morbid imagination. AN EXAGGERATED FEAR OF VENEREAL INFECTION FROM ILLICIT INTERCOURSE HAS MADE MANY A MAN A MASTURBATOR. It is, as the proverb says, especially "burnt children, who dread the fire." And we have repeatedly noticed that men, who had been finally cured of an obstinate gonorrhea, preferred "safe" masturbation to the dangers of illicit coitus. I have especially observed this among medical students and physicians.

(To be continued)

DEPARTMENT OF SEXUAL PSYCHOLOGY

BY DOUGLASS C. MCMURTRIE

NOTES ON SEXUAL PSYCHOLOGY

EXCEPTIONAL CASE OF PSEUDOHERMAPHRODITISM

BENDA describes [1] a case of pseudohermaphroditism occurring in a two-months-old child who was christened with a male first name. No doubt regarding the sex of the child was occasioned because the external genitalia showed no abnormality other than that no testicles could be felt in the scrotum. For the age of the child the penis was approximately normal, being about 4 cm. in length. The prepuce was ample, completely enveloping the head of the penis. The urethral orifice was small. The scrotum was normal; the raphé scroti fully closed.

The child was, however, of female sex. When the region of the pelvis was explored in post-mortem examination a complete set of female sexual organs was disclosed. These were fully formed in practically every respect. Tubes, ovaries, and uterus were all present.

The condition is termed pseudoarrhenism, which might be defined as "apparent approach to the male." Benda considers the case under consideration as the classic example of this anomaly, which belongs to a class previously recognized by Fibiger.[2] The present case, however, represents the most extreme degree of paradoxical sexual development, in that there are coexistent external male and internal female organs of normal morphology. The present case represents a standard example of pseudoarrhenism, while the earlier case of Fibiger manifested a slight degree of hypospadia, *i.e.*, congenital opening of the urethra on the under side of the penis.

To just the degree to which the penis through hypospadia departs from the male type, it takes on the appearance of female genitalia. To just the degree in which the vulva, through defective growth of the nymphae and excessive development of the clitoris, approaches the male type it departs from the appearance of the female genitals. The conclusion of all other investigators is verified that never can double sex exist in a human organism.

The appearance of incipient male external genitalia on a fe-

[1] C. Benda. Fall von Pseudohermaphroditismus femininus externus (Pseudarrhenie). *Berliner klinische Wochenschrift*, Berlin, 1914, li, 66-69.

[2] Johannes Fibiger. Beitrage zur Kenntniss des weiblichen Scheinzwittertums. *Virchows Archiv*, Berlin, 1905, clxxxi, 1-51.

male has been denoted as pseudoarrhenism. The accentuation of the clitoris to such a degree as to approach the appearance of male genitalia—the opposite condition—is denoted as pseudothelism (*Pseudothelie*). Both these conditions may, of course, exist in varying degrees.

Benda's case is clearly one of the most remarkable instances of pseudohermaphroditism yet recorded.

FERTILIZATION TIME AND INCEPTION OF GESTATION

It is universal practice to reckon the period of gestation in the female from the date of the cessation of the last menstrual discharge. In all cases it is impossible to diagnose the existence of uterine pregnancy until the fourteenth day after the date on which the first menstrual discharge held in abeyance by the occurrence of pregnancy should have made its appearance. Furthermore, in cases of diagnosis at such an early stage, the size and consistence of the pregnant uterus is always, to all intents and purposes, the same.

Adducing these facts, Oliver finds,[3] however, that the time of impregnation shows no corresponding regularity. He points out that we are forced to conclude either that fertilization time bears a definite and fixed relation to menstruation, or that gestation begins at a definite and fixed time in the human female. By one or other interpretation alone is it possible to account for the unvarying size of the uterus at the time already referred to.

Oliver continues as follows: "The belief prevails that the ovum which is fertilized in the human female is more commonly that belonging to a past than that belonging to an on-coming menstruation, and yet in support of this tenet no substantial evidence can be adduced. If indeed this hypothesis were tenable we should be obliged to admit—and this is impossible—that the gestation period for an ovum fertilized a few days before an expected menstruation is shorter than for an ovum fertilized immediately after a menstrual period; for in both cases we reckon the duration of gestation from the date of the cessation of the last menstrual period, and most authorities consider that fertilization and vitalization—otherwise the inception of gestation—are in a measure synonymous terms. Now in my opinion there is good reason to believe that the ovum which is fertilized is never that of

[3] James Oliver. Fertilization time and the inception of gestation in women. *Edinburgh Medical Journal,* 1914, n.s., xii, 49-52.

a past but always that of an approaching menstruation, and that fertilization takes place at any time during the intermenstrual period, except, perhaps, during the thirty-six or forty-eight hours preceding menstruation, because then, menstruation having begun to assert itself, this function cannot be inhibited by another physiological influence." Another consideration is that many women conceive while menstruation is held in abeyance by lactation. In such instances, of course, the ovum fertilized can only be that of an on-coming menstruation.

Several analogies in the animal and vegetable worlds are cited to show the independence between fertilization and the inception of gestation. Grains of wheat which have lain in the tombs of the Pharaohs for more than two thousand years have germinated when placed advantageously in the soil. The fertile egg of the hen may be kept under very ordinary conditions for ten or more days and be then incubated and "it is noteworthy that the incubation period for the egg begun to be hatched twelve days after it is laid is the same as for the egg begun to be hatched on the day it is laid. In the case of the human egg there is good reason to believe that a similar condition obtains, and that gestation does not necessarily follow directly on fertilization, but depends on some extrinsic or maternal influence." Oliver ventures to "hazard the opinion that this influence is probably a vascular one, and that it comes into play at or about the time when in the ordinary course of events the preparation for the first inhibited menstruation would have asserted itself." In brief, therefore, the conclusion is that gestation must begin at a definite and fixed time in the human female, this time being independent of the exact date of impregnation.

CONCEPTION AND MENSTRUATION

Miller has also concluded [4] that the ovulum of the first suppressed menses is the one embedded holding that no post-menstrual embedding occurs. Menstruation is merely the relief of the hyperemic uterus and has nothing to do with conception. He considers the most favorable time for conception to be the tenth day before the onset of the approaching menses. On this basis the standard duration of pregnancy should be reduced nineteen days. An excellent bibliography on the corpus luteum is appended to the article.

[4] John Willoughby Miller. Corpus luteum, Menstruation und Gravidität. *Archiv für Gynäkologie,* Berlin, 1914, ci, 568-619.

COMPARATIVE BIOLOGY OF MOTHER AND CHILD

Mother and child have been found [5] by Fellenberg and Doll to be independent biological entities. As a result of extensive research they concluded that antibodies and other biological characters did not pass to the fetus or the nursing infant. The fetus is regarded as an individual entity with its cell-chemistry complete.

PROGRESS IN ATTITUDE REGARDING SEX

In an exhaustive history of medicine,[6] Garrison, discussing the attitude toward the sexual instinct during the modern period, makes the following observations: "Another characteristic development is the exhaustive or intensive study of sexual psychology, with which modern writers, from scientific students like Krafft-Ebing and Havelock Ellis, down to insane men of letters like Nietzsche and Weininger, have been vastly preoccupied. The atmosphere of the present time, its art, poetry, fiction, and drama, is saturated with sexualism. Poets like Goethe, Swinburne, and Walt Whitman did much to dispel the ancient theological nightmare of the sinfulness of normal sexuality in men and women, and were forerunners of the scientific view that the instinct, guided by proper ethical restrictions, is an all-important part in normal human development which has to be either recognized or reckoned with. Schopenhauer wrote on the subject with bitter and unsparing realism, and latterly women of such high repute as Rahel Varnhagen, Ellen Key, and Helen Putnam have considered the matter from a higher viewpoint, on account of its importance in connection with such problems as the proper hygiene and well-being of growing children, the growth of prostitution and commercialized vice, the social enslavement of women in crowded communities, and other degradations of a purely industrial age. In Germany, several periodicals are devoted to the sexual instinct alone, and the problems of biological teaching of school-children in these matters is under consideration. On the pathological side, there is the question of sexual perversion and the crimes resulting from it, for which, in young, healthy frontier communities like the United States, no special provisions had been necessary in criminal procedure until the crowded conditions of modern cities brought the unsavory subject to the surface."

[5] R. v. Pellenberg. and A. Doll. Ueber die biologischen Beziehungen zwischen Mutter und Kind. *Zeitschrift für Geburtshülfe und Gynäkologie*, Stuttgart, 1913, lxxv, 285-319.

[6] Fielding H. Garrison. *An Introduction to the History of Medicine.* Philadelphia and London, 1913, p. 609-610.

THE PHENOMENON OF EXHIBITIONISM

The sexually pathological addiction of exhibitionism must be a phenomenon of frequent incidence to judge by reports from various sources. Only recently there came to my attention an incident which took place in a moving-picture show. A man of about fifty years of age, evidently a person of position and education, was located three seats away from an attractive girl of about twenty-one. From the first he seemed very nervous and would move first one seat nearer the girl and then back again. Finally he summoned the necessary "nerve" and moving over near her, he unfastened his clothing and took out his genitals in such a way as to exhibit it to her. He made no other move and said nothing, being content, as is usual in such cases, with the abnormal gratification he derived from the observation of his act.

The young woman who witnessed the performance immediately got up and left the theater. Complaints are hardly ever made in such instances for obvious reasons, the principal ones being the modesty and fear of publicity by the witness.

Another case which came recently to my attention concerned a laboring man employed in a village community by the owner of property adjoining a convalescent home for children. This man on several occasions when opportunity offered would expose his genitals to the view of the little girls at the home. The matron of the home reported the matter several times to the man's employer, but the latter did not regard the affair as serious and took no steps to prevent the occurrences. It was only by drastic threats to secure the arrest and conviction of the offender that any improvement was effected. The attitude of the employer in this case is interesting as being fairly typical of the ideas of a large class of people. Such occurrences are regarded as "dirty tricks" but they can hardly be convinced that their commission constitutes a criminal act.

In this connection I may relate a personal experience at the time I was nine or ten years old. I was on an elevated railroad train, sitting in one of the cross seats. An Italian laborer came and sat down opposite me and I soon observed that he had his clothes unfastened and a large erect penis protruded in full view. Naturally I did not know what it all meant but intuition classified it as abnormal and, frightened, I hurried from the train at the next station.

The subjects of this anomaly usually choose as its objects

or witnesses young or ignorant persons who are liable to be exceptionally impressed by its manifestations. It is highly probable that the degree of gratification gained by the exhibitor may bear a direct ratio to the degree of impression of the witness or witnesses. The social harm wrought by such performances lies largely in the indelible memory of the occurrence left in the mind of the innocent observers, and it is principally on this account, as well as for general considerations of public decency, that all possible measures be taken to suppress this nuisance.

REVIEW OF CURRENT UROLOGIC LITERATURE

JOURNAL D'UROLOGIE

Vol. IV, No. 5, November 15, 1913

1. Non-toxic Antigonococcic Vaccine Applied to the Treatment of Gonorrhea and its Complications.

The authors have succeeded, after a year and a half of experimentation, in eliminating the toxicity of antigonococcic vaccines by growing the organisms on special media, and in conserving their beneficial properties by the employment of a special solution. They have thus produced a stable, non-toxic vaccine with which they have treated about 200 cases, comprising 24 cases of ophthalmia, 25 of orchitis, 3 of rheumatism, and 127 of acute or chronic urethritis. All the complications of gonorrhea and the pain of the urethritis are relieved after almost the first injection. The discharge persists for some time but is completely arrested by seven or eight injections combined with local lavages of weak permanganate solution.

One-half cubic centimeter of the vaccine is diluted with one and a half c.c. of physiologic saline and injected intramuscularly or intravenously. Subcutaneous injection is painful and should be avoided. Each dose of the vaccine corresponds to about 3 billion bacteria. In the acute stages inoculations are made every day or every second day. In chronic cases every two to four days are the intervals recommended.

The preparation may be procured on application to the authors.

3. Wounds of the Bladder by Impalement (Concluded).

Complications: Certain symptoms may become so severe as to merit the term complications. Thus hemorrhage may require tamponade. Moreover, when the wound is small the urine may be obstructed in its escape and, dissecting up the perineal planes, cause infections of more or less severity. Finally, ascending infections may arise directly from introduction of septic matter or indirectly from rupture of the intestines.

Sequelae: (a) Foreign bodies in the bladder may be either pieces of clothing, debris from the pale or material from the rectum. When not too large these foreign bodies may be passed per urethram. Otherwise they form the nuclei for secondary calculi; these begin to give symptoms generally as late as ten to fifteen months after the impalement. (b) Vesical fistulae may be either vesico-rectal (most common), vesico-perineal, or vesico-vaginal. Spontaneous closure may occur in from eight to fourteen months. Intervention may help but is especially indicated where foreign bodies prevent closure.

Prognosis: This varies according as the peritoneum is involved or not. When the peritoneum is penetrated the non-operative mortality is 80%, whereas the operative mortality is only 30%. When the peritoneum is not involved the mortality is only 4%.

Diagnosis: It is of the first importance to decide whether the pale has penetrated the peritoneum or not. In addition to a very careful investigation of the conditions of injury, of the wound, and of the pale, the patient himself must be most carefully watched for the development of the characteristic signs of peritonitis. If it can be positively established that urine has not been recently voided or expelled through the wound, a "dry" catheterization is strong presumptive evidence of intraperitoneal rupture. The injection of carefully sterilized air may aid in the diagnosis.

After deciding whether the peritoneum is injured or not, the surgeon may next proceed to establish the exact nature of the injury sustained by the bladder. Here it is important to know whether the bladder itself has actually been damaged as hematuria or urinary leakage may result from rupture of the urethra. Catheterization will establish the differential diagnosis.

Treatment: When the peritoneum is perforated immediate laparotomy is indicated; the vesical and rectal wounds should be sutured, foreign bodies removed, the peritoneum cleansed, drained, and the patient put up in Fowler's position and given routine peritonitis treatment. If the wound is extraperitoneal it should be carefully cleansed and disinfected, under anesthesia, if necessary. Fortunately, infection rarely occurs in these cases. If urine escapes through the wound, the introduction of a permanent catheter is indicated. This procedure gives the added advantage of allowing of frequent lavages of the bladder which are of especial service in cases where there is a communication between the rectum and the bladder.

In this group of cases, as a rule, it is only the complications which demand intervention. Thus purulent collections may require evacuation by hypogastric section but in most instances surgical operation is indicated for the common sequelae of impalement: viz., fistulae, and secondary calculi.

It should be a rule never to dismiss a case of vesical injury as cured until a thorough cystoscopic examination has been made. In this way the presence of foreign bodies can be recognized and their early removal accomplished.

The author summarizes 85 cases of injuries to the bladder by impalement thus far reported in the literature, including one personal case.

4. A Case of Double Hypospadic Urethra.

The patient was a young soldier who came to consult Worms because of a purulent discharge from his penis coming on after a suspicious intercourse. There was no burning on micturition nor nocturnal erections. At first blush the glans appeared normal, but on separating the lips of the meatus no urethral opening was present. Two centimeters below, however, at the base of the glans and in the median line was found the true meatus in hypospadic position. It was through this aperture that urine was voided and that spermatic fluid was ejaculated. A number 16 sound passed readily into the bladder.

Between the two meati and equidistant from each was a small pinpoint aperture through which a droplet of pus exuded on pressure. The pus contained gonococci. This small opening was proved to be the orifice of a blind accessory canal, 5 cm. in length, which extended first in front of, then above the spongy urethra. The prepuce was rudimentary below; on the dorsal surface it formed a hood of large proportions. There were no other abnormalities.

Despite irrigations with permanganate, followed by instillations of silver nitrate, the discharge persisted for three weeks and was even complicated by a mild attack of arthritis. The true urethra was never infected.

A review of the literature showed that in almost all cases the supernumerary or "false" urethra was situated above the true urethra. Pathogenetically this condition arises from the fact that the urethra does not close uniformly from behind forward but the balanic portion situated in front of the base of the glans closes last. As a result, during a certain period of development, the urethra possesses two openings, one at the apex of the glans (normal meatus), the other at the base. When this primitive condition persists hypospadias results, and if, in addition, the normal meatus ends in a cul de sac and the balanic part of the urethra develops independently of the spongy portion we have an accessory urethra as in the case reported.

Clinically, the hypersusceptibility of the accessory canals to infection and their resistance to treatment are noteworthy. As regards treatment of chronic infection, extirpation may be tried but is not to be recommended. Sectioning the tissue between the two canals and thus forming a common urethra is a preferable procedure.

5. Diagnosis of Ureteral Calculi.

The case reported by Weisz is of interest because of the faulty information given by the X-ray. This examination seemed to show a calculus in the right ureter. On cystoscopy the right ureteral meatus was edematous and pouted to such a degree as to suggest a ureterocele. At first the ureter could not be catheterized but finally a No. 6 instrument was introduced and a very purulent urine obtained. It was then thought that the catheter had slipped by the stone which was located in a pouch and had caused a ureteritis.

At operation no calculus was found. Post mortem examination showed that the right kidney was in a state of calcareous tuberculosis. Apparently a small piece of this diseased tissue had passed down the ureter near its termination in the bladder and had given rise to the deceptive X-ray shadow. The true condition of the kidney was not shown in the plates because of the thick panniculus adiposis surrounding the organ. At no time did the urine contain tubercle bacilli. The guinea pig inoculation was negative.

6. Resection of Diverticula of the Bladder.

Marion recommends the following procedure:

1. *Preliminary catheterization of the ureter on the side of the diverticulum.* This can be done either before the operation, through the cystoscope, or during the operation when the bladder is laid open. If necessary, indigocarmin may be injected subcutaneously to aid in locating the ureter orifice.

2. *Incision of the bladder.* The patient is in the reclining posture. Median abdominal incision, 8 to 10 cm. in length. Peritoneum is pushed up. Two guide sutures introduced into the bladder. Incision into the bladder. Introduction of new guide sutures higher up. Stripping the penitoneum from the bladder. Enlargement of bladder wound, introduction of Legueu's self-retaining retractor, digital exploration of the diverticulum and catheterization of the ureter if not previously effected.

3. *Stripping the bladder from the prevesical tissues on the side of the diverticulum.* The bladder wall is held by the guide sutures and the stripping is done with the fingers protected by a piece of gauze. This procedure is carried out until the base of the pedicle is exposed.

4. *Incision of the stripped (freed) bladder wall.* The cut is made at right angles to the original bladder incision down to the orifice of the diverticulum.

5. *Stripping (freeing) the diverticulum.* With one finger inside the sac the surgeon keeps constantly working it out into the wound (as in a hernia sac) while with the other hand he dissects off the surrounding tissues on the lateral and posterior aspects. During this procedure great care must be exercised to spare the ureter.

6. *Resection of the diverticulum.*

7. *Reconstruction of the bladder wall by suture in two planes.* A layer of fine catgut sutures involving the whole thickness of the bladder wall except the mucosa, covered by a layer of heavier catgut taking in only the muscularis.

8. *Partial closure of bladder; drainage of urine and of the prevesical space.* The median bladder wound is closed in two planes about a large elbow drain. The prevesical space is drained with another tube and gauze strips if necessary.

9. *Partial closure of the abdominal wound. Post operative treatment.* The prevesical drainage is kept up until the discharge ceases. The vesical drain is removed a few days later and replaced by a permanent catheter which is retained until the bladder closes. Lavages of the bladder or of the prevesical space may be required to promote healing.

7. Combined Treatment of Certain Bladder Tumors.

In large tumors (size of a nut or peach) of the bladder Heitz-Boyer proposes a combined two-stage operation as the procedure of choice.

1st stage. A hypogastric section is made and the bladder opened as for a prostatectomy. The pedicle of the tumor is seized with a curved clamp, ligated, and removed. The entire procedure can be carried out in from five to ten minutes under local anesthesia if necessary. The incision is then partially closed and a large hypogastric drain inserted. After forty-eight hours the large tube is replaced by the series of progressively smaller tubes as used by Marion (described in the preceeding number of the *Journal d'Urologie* and previously abstracted in this journal). At the end of eight or ten days a permanent catheter is introduced into the urethra and at the end of two or three weeks the bladder is closed and the patient cured of this intervention. The patient may leave his bed after the third or fourth day.

2nd stage. Two weeks after the bladder wound is closed the endoscopic destruction of the tumor stump may be undertaken. This is done by a special "sparking" modification of Beer's high frequency method as described by Heitz-Boyer and Cottenot in previous papers.

(Cf. "Nouvelle méthode de traitement endoscopic des tumeurs de vessie." *Congrès français d'Urologie,* Paris, 1911). One or two sittings suffice for the complete destruction of the stump. Two or three weeks should then be allowed for the sloughing of the necrotic, cauterized, base and then a confirmatory cystoscopy may be undertaken.

By adopting the above two-stage procedure surgeons will not have to face the danger of severe hemorrhage resulting from excision of the base of the tumor after the one-stage radical operation.

8. Antiseptic Treatment of Gonorrhea: Choice of Drug, Dosage, and Intervals of Lavages.

Janet relies mainly upon potassium permanganate, less on protargol, for the cure of his gonorrhea cases. Permanganate furnishes the basis for his treatment. He lavages with strengths of 0.1 to 0.2 gram per 1,000 in the acute stages, 0.25 per 1,000 in the subacute stage, and 0.3 to 0.35 per 1,000 in the stage of apparent cure. Strengths of 0.1 to 0.15 per. 1,000 should not be exceeded in the beginning because it is essential to produce as little reaction as possible, and they should be returned to whenever the posterior urethra is penetrated for the first time as it is important to spare the patient pain in order that the bladder may be penetrated. When acute signs diminish and the bladder may be entered with care the strength is gradually increased to 0.20 gram per 1,000 and two and three days later to 0.25 per 1,000 which is the routine strength and with which cure can generally be effected. If gonococci and shreds still persist in the discharge after the third week the strength may be increased to 0.3 or 0.4 g. per 1,000 or even higher but the stronger solutions should be followed by boric acid irrigations.

In some cases permanganate seems to lose its effect. Here it may prove necessary to substitute protargol in strengths of 1 to 5 grams per 1,000. Rapid cure may follow this change, or else permanganate may again be resorted to with good results.

It is very important to lavage at regular and definite intervals. Janet irrigates twice a day during the acute stage. After from 3 to 6 days he irrigates once daily. These daily irrigations (and Sunday should not be omitted) are to be kept up until the discharge has ceased entirely, until the first glass is no longer cloudy, and until gonococci and filaments have both disappeared. When this point is reached it is wise to give two more daily injections, then two at thirty-six hour intervals and still another forty-eight hours later. If the above symptoms return, another course of daily lavages should be instituted.

9. Use of the Twisted Bougie in Catheterization of the Ureter.

The catheterization of the ureter obeys the same laws as the catheterization of the urethra and if the ureteral sound is arrested by a kink, a stone, a diverticulum or a stricture it means that the lumen is eccentric and will be catheterized more readily by an elbow instrument than by a straight one. Nogués has therefore devised a supple catheter, size 14 or 15, with an open end through which a whalebone bougie can be introduced. This bougie is 6 to 8 centimeters longer than the sound, and is provided at one end with a hard rubber rod, 2 centimeters long, which can be moulded into any desirable shape such as a bayonet or cork-screw.

The technique is as follows: The bougie is greased and is run into the catheter until both ends coincide. The instruments are then introduced into the cystoscope and up the ureter until the obstruction is met with. The catheter is then withdrawn 10 to 15 millimeters and the assistant is asked to push the bougie. As soon as the rubber rod escapes from the catheter it assumes the shape previously given it. The bougie is then manipulated with a back and forth as well as with a rotatory motion and the chances of finding the eccentric lumen are thus very much increased.

In case these efforts fail, a new bougie with a still differently shaped rubber tip may be introduced through the catheter.

The Use of Urotropin in Dermatology.

Otto Sachs (Wiener Klinische Wochenschrift, No. 49, 1913) reports beneficial results from the internal administration of urotropin in doses of from 4 to 6 grams a day. Of 82 cases of herpes zoster treated in this manner 78 were cured and 4 improved. Formaldehyde is spit off and has been recovered from the skin lesions. The action of urotropin may be regarded as specific in this condition since the affected lymph nodes decrease in size, the burning pains in the herpes region disappear, and the accompanying severe neuralgia is relieved. Local treatment is entirely unnecessary. The results of urotropin therapy in 29 cases of erythema exudativum multiforme et bullosum were not quite so brilliant since recurrences were not prevented. In impetigo contagiosa and eczema impetiginosum the urotropin treatment constitutes a great step in advance since all local treatment—especially awkward bandaging—is unnecessary, the hair of the scalp and beard does not have to be sacrificed and even very extensive lesions can be healed up in ten to fourteen days.

BOOK NOTICES

GENITO-URINARY DISEASES AND SYPHILIS. By Edgar G. Ballenger, M.D., Adjunct Clinical Professor of Genito-Urinary Diseases, Atlanta Medical College; Urologist to Westley Memorial Hospital; Genito-Urinary Surgeon to Davis-Fisher Sanatorium, Atlanta, Ga., assisted by Omar F. Elder, M.D. The Wassermann Reaction by Edgar Paullin, M.D. Second Edition Revised. 527 pages with 109 illustrations and 5 colored plates. Price $5.00 net. E. W. Allen & Co., Atlanta, Ga.

The book before us is a satisfactory conventional text-book on venereal diseases. It presents nothing new or original, but the teachings are conservative and dependable. We regret to say that we cannot share the authors' enthusiasm about the rapid cure of gonorrhea by the sealing in of arygrol in the urethra for several hours. And we also regret to say that the proofreading has been rather carelessly done. But nevertheless the volume makes a satisfactory text-book on genito-urinary diseases and syphilis.

A MANUAL OF CLINICAL DIAGNOSIS BY MEANS OF LABORATORY METHODS for Students, Hospital Physicians and Practitioners. By Charles E. Simon, B.A., M.D., Professor of Clinical Pathology and Experimental Medicine at the College of Physicians and Surgeons, Baltimore, Md. Eighth edition, enlarged and thoroughly revised. Pp. 809, illustrated with 185 engravings and 25 colored plates, $5.00. Lea and Febiger, Philadelphia.

A thorough revision of a useful and comprehensive work. The book is divided into two parts, the first part being devoted to technical questions and the second to the application of laboratory findings to diagnosis. This revision incorporates the more modern methods of investigating the existence and extent of renal disease, the newer technique of the Wassermann reaction, the complement fixation test for gonnorrhea, the protective ferments of Abderhalden and other recent additions to the field of laboratory diagnosis.

THE AMERICAN JOURNAL OF UROLOGY, VENEREAL AND SEXUAL DISEASES

WILLIAM J. ROBINSON, M.D., EDITOR

VOL. X | MAY, 1914. | No. 5

EXTRAGENITAL CHANCRES IN WOMEN.

By DR. JEAN BOBRIE, Paris.

IN his work "Les Chancres Extragénitaux," Professor A. Fournier, from a study of the statistics, divides primary lesions into the following cases as regards their site and frequency:

Genital chancres, 93 per cent. of cases.
Perigenital chancres, 0.67 per cent. of cases.
Extragenital chancres, 6.33 per cent. of cases.

In publishing these figures—representing as they do men, women, and children, seen by him in his private as well as his hospital practice—Professor Fournier insists on the fact that the figure 6 to 7 per cent. for the frequence of extragenital chancres represents a minimum which is far below the truth, for the following reasons:

1. Because of their unusual location many of these chancres escape attention and remain unrecognized.

2. A certain number of these chancres (such as those of the tonsil, for instance) are not diagnosed as such even when submitted to a medical examination.

3. There are certain chancres, such as those of the eye, for which patients will not consult a syphilologist, but an oculist.

Now that the microscope often establishes the specific nature of primary lesions of atypical appearance, and when the course of events also proves them to have been the portals of entry, it seems of great interest to determine the incidence of extragenital primary lesions in women occurring during the past ten years.

Our statistics are restricted purposely to the female sex, for woman, who has often done nothing to fear infection, is held by her husband and by society at large in a state of ignorance, which her previous education, her more or less proper notions of modesty, and the popular prejudice against sexual hygiene, will by no means tend to enlighten. Moreover, the primary lesion is so often overlooked in women that Desprès, writing in *Arch. Gén. de Méd.*, Jan., 1869, went so far as to deny that in the female sex the hard chancre is the primary lesion of syphilis. In the presence of doubtful symptoms one must therefore explore every inch of the patient's body most minutely, and it is to prove this necessity that we now publish statistics covering all diseases of women observed in the service of Professor Gaucher from October 1, 1902, to March 1, 1912, both in the "Salle Henri IV" and in the "Policlinique de l'hôpital Saint-Louis."

We have classified primary lesions as perigenital and extra-genital, and we have also included for comparison, statistics published by Professor Fournier in 1897, based on 10,000 cases, and some of those published by Rudolf Krefting in 1891, based on 2,196 cases.

Up to March 1, 1912, Professor Gaucher saw 24,097 patients afflicted with various diseases, of whom 2,912 were syphilitic women. Of these 2,912 patients 762 came for the treatment of specific lesions which were too old for investigation or direct examination to reveal any trace of a primary lesion. Of the remaining 2,158 patients there were 801 who came for the treatment of recent syphilitic symptoms, but in whom even the most careful objective examination failed to reveal any trace of a primary lesion, nor did they themselves have any knowledge of one. It was only in 1,357 patients, therefore, that there was any evidence whatever of the existence of a primary lesion and in 175 of these we had only the patients' word for it and this was so indefinite that we could place no reliance whatever on such data.

Thus there remained but 1,182 patients in whom the situation of the chancre could be definitely established and it is from this group that we have prepared our figures. That is to say, in women, where specificity is so often overlooked, more than half the cases do not appear in any statistics whatever.

1. *Genital Lesions.* Of the 1,182 patients, 834 presented primary lesions of the vulva. In this group are included 13 chancres of the clitoris. This gives us, for genital chancres, properly so-called, a percentage of 70.55. The corresponding figures in R. Krefting's statistics are 81.50 per cent.; in Professor Fournier's, 93 per cent.

2. *Perigenital Lesions.* These occurred in 35 cases. Only 10 of these were chancres of the cervix uteri; 5 patients had

chancres of the meatus; in 4 cases the chancre was on the vaginal wall. The inguinal region and the skin of the inner aspect of the thighs were the seats of chancres in 11 instances. Five chancres occurred in the perineal (ano-vulvar and perianal) region. This gives a total percentage of 2.96 for perigenital chancres. Fournier's figures are 0.67 per cent.

3. *Extragenital Lesions.* These occurred in 326 patients. Chancre of the anus—which Fournier saw 77 times—was found in 55 cases of this series. Chancres of the buccal region were much more numerous. There were four chancres of the mouth. The upper lip was the seat of 57 initial lesions, the lower lip of 45. There was thus a total of 102 labial chancres in this series, whereas R. Krefting reports 142, and Fournier 567. We saw ten chancres of the tongue, Krefting 11, and Fournier 75. Chancres of the tonsil occurred in 97 of our women. Krefting saw 58, and Fournier 69 such cases. As regards primary lesions of the gums, there were 5 cases in our series, one in Krefting's, 11 in Fournier's. In both Fournier's and our statistics there was but one chancre of the buccal mucous membrane.

There were 16 initial lesions of the face. Six women had chancres of the chin. Krefting saw a similar case and Fournier 54 such. Fournier reports 18 chancres of the nose; we have only seen seven. Two of these were on the cutaneous surface of the nose; one was on the nostril; one on the Schneiderian membrane; three on the the nasal septum. There were 3 chancres of other parts of the face: once on the cheek, once at the left preauricular region, once on the chin. One patient was seen with a chancre of the hairy scalp. Krefting mentions two cases of this kind, and Fournier has seen three.

Fournier has seen three chancres of the neck. We have seen two, one of the nape, and one of the right carotid region.

Nineteen of our patients had primary lesions of the breast; another had a chancre of the sub-mammary fold, and still another had one of the chest wall a little below the breast. In his series, Krefting had 58 cases, while Fournier had nineteen. We have also seen a primary lesion of the back and two chancres of the axilla.

Among lesions of the upper extremity we saw a chancre of the wrist and four chancres of the fingers, all in midwives. There was one chancre of the thumb, one of the index finger, one of the left middle finger and one of the right ring finger. R. Krefting reports 4 chancres of the fingers, and Fournier has seen 49, of which 30 were contracted in the line of professional duty.

In the abdominal region we saw a primary lesion of the umbilicus.

In the lower extremity we met with a chancre of the knee, one of the left calf, one of the heel, and one of the interdigital space.

The relative frequence of the various groups of primary lesions met with in women in Professor Gaucher's service from October, 1902, to March I, 1912, may be summarized in the following table:

Of 1,182 primary lesions:

Genital chancres formed..........	70.55%
Perigenital chancres formed.......	2.95%
Extragenital chancres formed......	26.50%

Professor Fournier found that of 10,000 primary lesions:

Genital chancres formed..........	93.00%
Perigenital chancres formed........	0.67%
Extragenital chancres formed......	6.33%

Finally Rudolf Krefting found that of 2,916 primary lesions:

Genital chancres formed...........	81.5%
Extragenital chancres formed.......	18.5%

The discrepancies between our statistics and those of the other authors seem to us deserving of explanation.

In the first place we must keep in mind that their researches were carried on with syphilitics of both sexes and that in men the existence of an unsuspected primary lesion is a great rarity.

If our percentage of extragenital chancres was based on the entire number of women with recent syphilis examined in Prof. Gaucher's service during the period indicated, we would find that of the 2,158 patients 15.105 per cent. had extragenital chancres, that is to say a proportion intermediate between that of Krefting and that of Fournier. But in women, to deceive whom all lengths are taken, the chancre is often overlooked, not only by the subject but by the physician as well, who may be consulted too late to find even the slightest trace of the lesion. For this reason we have been obliged to eliminate 801 cases, or 37 per cent. of our material, because even the most careful examination made in the secondary stage failed to reveal the localization of the initial lesion, originally overlooked. Nevertheless, as a matter of fact, these very chancres must have in all probability been situated in the genital zone, for anywhere else they would have attracted the attention of the majority of these 801 patients.

In the second place we must consider that recent bacteriological discoveries have enabled us to classify as chancres innocent-looking ulcerations which contained treponemes and which were followed in 3 to 5 weeks by a roseola and by other typical secondary manifestations without our being able to find any other possible portal of entry. Whence, for example, the relatively great frequency of tonsillar chancres in our statistics, where we report 97 cases whereas Krefting mentions 58 and Fournier 69. Similarly, we have been able to find only 26 cases in the first 12,000 patients registered in the "polyclinique" records, whereas in the remaining 12,000 cases there were 71 chancres,—an increase corresponding to the increased knowledge of the treponeme and its more ready recognition bacteriologically.

We may note in passing that there are extragenital localizations of the initial lesion which have disappeared. Thus we have not seen a single instance of a chancre of the arm, formerly so common at the time of arm to arm vaccination and of vaccinal syphilis.

From our researches on the localization of the primary lesion in the female sex it seems to follow that in women, where the primary lesion so often passes unperceived (37 per cent. of cases), the chancre, when it is discovered, is extragenital once in every four cases (26.5 per cent.).

The multiplicity of localizations for these extragenital lesions should incite the physician to look for them everywhere. He should make a very guarded and discreet, and at the same time most minute investigation without allowing a square inch of accessible skin or mucous membrane to escape his eye. Naturally his first attentions will be directed to the genital region and it is unquestionably there that the primary lesion will most often be found.

The physician's task is here especially difficult, for with women, most frequently married, the question arises more often than with their consorts, as to the etiology of the syphilis (husband or lover?) and an imprudent word may have the most serious consequences. The doctor's embarrassment will be less in the case of an extragenital chancre. It being possible, in this event, to explain the contamination innocently, there is nothing to prevent him from disclosing to those interested the true nature of the disease and from taking from the very outset any prophylactic and therapeutic measures which may be necessary.

THE PRACTICAL VALUE OF POSTERIOR URETHROSCOPY.

By Dr. Max Roth and Dr. Theodore Mayer.

CONSIDERABLE experience is necessary for the correct interpretation of the pictures obtained by posterior urethroscopy. Thus we must learn to attach much more significance to plastic appearances than to color changes in the urethral mucosa since the latter depend on local hyperemias and anemias resulting merely from the presence of the instrument. Moreover, accidental trauma may give rise to an appearance resembling an ulcer, and small hemorrhages may simulate granulations or polypi. It is therefore essential to repeat the examination on different occasions so as to avoid possible doubt as to what has been actually observed.

The first and perhaps most important cause of pathological findings in the posterior urethra is gonorrhea. Here we may have either a "soft" infiltration (comparable to that found in the anterior urethra) in which the internal sphincter is swollen and the colliculus inflamed and presenting one or more projections, or a "hard" infiltration resulting in stricture formation, which is much less common. Proliferative changes represented by the formation of raspberry-like polypi are frequent occurrences at the verumontanum. In chronic posterior gonorrhea such changes were present in two-thirds the cases examined and, what is more, they were present in almost the same proportion in those clinically cured of the condition.

Objective symptoms such as persistent discharge, terminal hematuria and hematospermatorrhea *may* or *may not* be associated with the above pathological conditions. Conversely these conditions may exist without any symptoms whatever, and in 46 per cent. of the cases without the existence even of any antecedent gonorrhea.

The authors also found numerous abnormalities in the urethras of patients suffering from symptoms of sexual neurasthenia such as erections and pollutions. Thus in many cases they observed a gaping of the utriculus and ducts. This was probably due to a lowered muscular tone of these passages. They also found various types of prolapses of the mucosa and of granulomas in the membranous urethra. However, they do not regard these changes as the cause of the symptoms (pollutions, etc.) but rather as the result or the accompaniment thereof. In support of this view they point to the favorable results obtained by therapy—such as internal medication—which is not directed toward the relief of the local conditions, as well as to the failure of local treatment in some cases. In all such cases the authors feel that there is an unsatisfied libido which causes an increased sexual irritability resulting in masturbation, this in turn producing congestion of the parts and the pathological pictures above described. Erections and pollutions may result from a general psychopathic constitution without any local changes whatever.

Similar findings in the posterior urethra have been described as the cause of sexual impotence. That this condition results from the exhaustion of a previously overexcited erection center, as suggested by Finger, is not accepted by the authors. The "somatic" (i. e. local lesion) basis for impotence has been much overdone and they feel that the cure of a case by local treatment proves nothing more than that the *psyche* is influenced by local therapy suggestion. If the above theory is correct, impotence should follow an enormous number of cases of gonorrhea, for the sequence of enlarged colliculus is very common indeed. The real basis for this condition is not an enlarged colliculus but a functional weakness of the central and peripheral nervous systems—a neurasthenia. Suggestion will often effect a cure where local cauterization fails, and the reason the latter is sometimes effectual is that it opens up the way for, and multiplies the number of centripetal nervous stimuli to the sexual centers, the colliculus being the most favorable point for the stimulation of the sexual nerve organs. Just as was the case in regard to objective symptoms, polypi and other lesions may exist at the colliculus without causing any subjective impotence whatever.

By first subjecting all patients to general measures, and not proceeding at once to the local treatment, the authors were enabled to divide their cases into two classes. The first consisted of real sexual neurasthenics who complained of indefinite symptoms: burning in the testicles, feeling of heat and pressure in the urethra, tearing in the inguinal canal, etc. In 80% of these subjects the posterior urethra was pathologically altered as in gonorrhea. In these men the sexual symptoms were merely a part of an outspoken general neurasthenia. General measures, or local applications which did not in any way affect the pathological picture often caused a cure. The benefits of cauterization, etc., were but temporary. The second class comprised those who com-complained definitely of frequency, urgency and pain during urination. In 60% of these cases there were pathological changes in the posterior urethra and here they were actually the cause of the symptoms, for their removal was in the great majority of instances followed by a permanent cure.

The authors conclude that though modern endoscopy has thrown much light on many difficult problems it has led us to overestimate the importance of the local lesion, especially in cases of sexual neurasthenia.

SYPHILITIC REINFECTION

By Dr. A. Dupuylatat.

CONTRARY to the current opinion, syphilitic reinfection does occur. It is important however to distinguish this condition from secondary or tertiary chancriform lesions. In order for there really to be reinfection Fournier has laid down the following conditions:

1. A hard chancre with indolent adenopathy followed by a roseola or some other secondary manifestation, such as headache, transient alopecia, mucous patches. Nowadays when the treatment of syphilis is so intensive from the first, it is not absolutely necessary to demand a history of secondaries especially if the presence of spirochetae was established in the original lesion.

2. A complete silence (i.e., absence of symptoms) for several years. At the present time it is not necessary to wait as long as this, for the patient's system, being more energetically treated after the first infection, is more rapidly sterilized and is therefore so much the sooner able to present the symptoms of a new infection.

3. A new hard chancre following a suspicious intercourse and accompanied by a characteristic adenopathy, followed in its turn, after a few weeks by a roseola or other secondary manifestation. Here also it is not essential to await the appearance of secondary signs for these may be diminished or completely abolished by the early institution of treatment. Besides the postponement of medication may seriously jeopardize the patient's chances of recovery.

4. A "confrontation." This is valuable when it can be obtained. An example will explain the meaning of this term. Thus a case has been reported of a man with a primary lesion on the

right side of the penis, "the woman in the case" having mucous patches on the left labium majus.

While of course accepting Fournier's four rules as fundamental, the author believes that we have to-day still other aids to diagnosis. In the first place, there can be no question of reinfection unless the second lesion is located at a different point from the original chancre; otherwise there might always be raised the objection of chancre redux. In the second place, a sufficient time must elapse between the two infections for the evolution and healing of the secondary as well as of the primary lesions,—and this space must elapse whether the secondary manifestations actually appear or not. These points being granted, the author insists on the following conditions, which in connection with those laid down by Fournier, ought to suffice for a positive diagnosis of syphilitic reinfection:

1. *Clinical study of the chancre.*—After an incubation period of from fifteen to thirty days the chancre appears in two different aspects according as it is located on the skin or on the mucous membranes. On the skin the chancre spreads out, becomes projecting and crusted over, often resembling an ecthyma. There are no sharp borders and the edge is indurated. On the mucosa the ulceration is more apparent than real, the borders are thick, regular, without the polycyclic outline of a herpes. The base of the chancre is red and shining and is covered by a diphtheroïd membrane.

2. *Microscopic study.*—The demonstration of the treponema eliminates soft chancre and chancriform tertiary ulcerations where the organism is but rarely found. In secondary chancriform lesions, on the other hand, spirochetes are present in much greater numbers than they are in chancres.

3. *Primary adenopathy.*—This always accompanies the chancre. It is absent in chancriform syphilides where there is usually a general adenopathy. Herpetic lesions have no adenopathy, whereas soft chancres have bubos.

4. *A study of the Wassermann reaction.*—In general the Wassermann reaction is always positive in syphilis. Should it become negative after treatment it can often be restored by an intravenous injection of 606. This is known as the biologic reactivation of the Wassermann reaction or the reaction of Milian-Gennerich. It should be borne in mind that the Wassermann reaction is negative at the time of the appearance of the chancre

and only becomes positive a few days thereafter. On the other hand, it is always positive in secondary manifestations. These facts will therefore enable us to differentiate between a primary lesion and a chancriform secondary one, if we investigate the Wassermann reaction at the beginning of the lesion in question. It should be noted, however, that a positive Wassermann may be found in hereditary syphilis.

5. *The history of infection.*—Of course the history of previous infection and of recent suspicious intercourse is important. Auto-inoculation should be carefully distinguished from reinfection. The former may be direct or indirect. Direct auto-inoculation is illustrated by a case in which a chancre of the lip follows a chancre of the tongue after a three weeks' interval. Indirect auto-inoculation would be where the patient would carry the virus from his penis to his lips by means of his fingers. In all cases of auto-inoculation the second chancre appears from two to three weeks after the first. There should therefore be no confusion with reinfection since in this case a space of time must elapse between the two chancres sufficient for the normal evolution of secondary symptoms,—at least two months.

CAUSES AND RESULTS OF MASTURBATION

By Victor Blum, M.D.
Assistant in Prof. von Frisch's Urological Department of the Vienna General Polyclinic

AUTHORIZED TRANSLATION. EDITED WITH NOTES AND ADDITIONS BY DR. W. J. ROBINSON

(Concluded from April)

The desire to prevent conception also leads not rarely to masturbation, when for various reasons the more popular method of interrupted coitus is not desired. Mutual onanism plays a very large rôle in the illicit intercourse of young people. The enlightenment given by teachers to young people at puberty, which warns them in a perhaps exaggerated way of the dangers of venereal infection and of conception, often lead them direct to masturbation, either self-masturbation or the mutual variety.

A further cause of masturbation, or rather a cause for continuing masturbation, is "imagined" and psychic impotence. Neuropathic individuals, who have convinced themselves by reading the popular-scientific literature, although without foundation, that they are and must always be impotent, become so hypochondriac and lose their self-confidence to such a degree that they do not dare to attempt natural intercourse with a woman, since no art of persuasion can convince them that they will be able to carry out coitus normally.

And if the sexual power has actually suffered severely from masturbation or other sexual abuses, and the patient has always experienced the same wretched fiasco at each attempt at coitus, then he usually prefers masturbation to another disgrace.

And actual experience teaches that habitual masturbators may be impotent with the most seductive woman, while the pleasure of their lonely hours still brings them full satisfaction of their sexual need. The ability to masturbate often outlasts the ability for coitus in such neuropaths for many years.

It is a disputed question whether sexual continence may become an exciting cause of masturbation or not. [It is no disputed point with us: we answer it unhesitatingly in the affirmative.—W. J. R.]

It need not necessarily become so; that is proved by the countless observations of perfectly chaste men, in whose mental life the sexual sphere, as a result of a rational physical hygiene, takes a subordinate place.

It is certain, however, that chastity requires great energy, a complete control of the will-power and the temperament. Especially sensual natures will hardly ever possess this power, and will sooner or later succumb to the temptation of the vice. But it should be the task of a rational method of education so to steel the youth's will-power by means of physical hygiene, sports, and exercise in the open, and to divert the imagination so far from the natural impulses, that the youth could never fall a victim to masturbation, this vice which mocks at ethics and esthetics.

Plenty of opportunities will be given in metropolitan life to weak-willed and unresisting persons to let the imagination revel in forbidden ways. Lascivious, graphic exhibitions, "shameless" and sensually exciting statues, obscene literature, which generally does not fail in its well-calculated attraction, can at any time furnish the exciting cause to masturbation, and has thus made many a youth, until then innocent, the hopeless slave of habitual onanism.

These obscene exhibitions will always excite anew the imagination of the weak youth, and by representing in imagination these once perceived situations the habit of masturbation develops to a vice.

According to the statements of some authors certain drugs and foods, which cause a congestion of the sexual organs, also sometimes become a direct cause of masturbation. These are pepper, nutmeg, vanilla, truffles, caviar, strong alcoholic drinks, absinthe, and saffron.

Such an effect is also ascribed to certain perfumes. (Pouillet mentions as such "benzoin, patchouli.") The action of these odors is probably only through associations, by means of which the perception of the perfume leads to the excitement of the cerebral sexual centers.

Here belong further all the drugs designated as aphrodisiacs; namely, cantharides, strychnine, cocaine, phosphorus, cannabis indica, opium, nux vomica, aloes, ergotin, atropine, blatta orientalis (Rohleder). [With the exception, perhaps, of cantharides and strychnine, the other drugs are in no sense aphrodisiacs. Too many drugs have been considered aphrodisiacs, which are quite worthless in this respect.—W. J. R.]

Some authors also report that an especial sexually exciting influence is to be ascribed to various internal diseases.

It is always asserted that pulmonary tuberculosis is often the cause of conditions of sexual excitement, which under circumstances can lead to immoderate masturbation. We still lack a satisfactory explanation, why in spite of the steady decline, the sexual power and libido can be not only unweakened but often considerably increased. Fürbringer says that there are here probably peculiar stimulating factors, which under circumstances overcompensate the dominating force of the cachexia.

In the excellent work of Rohleder concerning masturbation we also find diabetes mentioned as an occasional cause of masturbation. He is of the opinion that the well-known tendency of the skin of diabetics to eczema—especially on the genitals—and the characteristic pruritus pudendorum leads to manipulations of the genitals and so to masturbation.

This is not correct in our opinion. As we have already explained in the chapter on impotence, certain forms of diabetes are just the cause of sexual impotence as a result of the loss of the libido. I remember especially two cases with marked genital pruritus (one had an extensive, chronic eczema of the penis and scrotum), who suffer from complete extinction of the sexual desire. Onanism may then result only exceptionally from diabetes; Rohleder gives no figures for his observations in this matter.

But the assertion of this author that leukemia, in which disease priapism from thrombosis of the corpora cavernosa was repeatedly observed, leads to masturbation, is entirely wrong. Rohleder writes: "It is certain that masturbation is caused by this [leukemic] priapism." So far as we can discover from the literature on this subject, however, and from our own observations, in not a single known case of leukemic thrombosis of the corpora cavernosa is anything reported concerning masturbation resulting.

In addition to the internal diseases, we have still to report on masturbation resulting from mental diseases and organic cerebral and spinal diseases.

Very often the first signs of a mental disease show themselves in a greatly increased propensity to seek sexual satisfaction, especially to masturbation. It is, to be sure, often very difficult here to distinguish cause from effect; is the masturbation merely a symptom, an effect of the psychosis, or does it appear as a provoking cause of the psychosis? Masturbation plays an especially important part in the psychoses of youth, hebephrenia and dementia præcox. Here as well as in the "periodical psychoses" there occurs, usually episodically, a period of increased libido with obscene fancies, deliria and masturbation. There likewise occur frequently in dementia paralytica periods of overpowering, impulsive sexual desire, which for external reasons do not result in normal sexual congress but in masturbation.

The elsewhere referred to attacks of erethism in the early stages of tabes dorsalis become occasionally a direct cause of masturbation, especially when the patient cannot save himself in any other way from the tormenting attacks of priapism.

Myelitis can also occasionally excite an inclination to onanism.

Then further the functional neuroses, hysteria, neurasthenia, hypochondria, and epilepsy may be regarded as exciting causes of masturbation. We have already explained in the general considerations preceding this chapter our views regarding the pathogenic significance of the "nervous constitution" and hysteria and neurasthenia for the origin of onanism.

To avoid repetitions I will merely refer to those conditions, and only remark here that the weak will, common to and characteristic of all these neuroses, greatly favors the origin of masturbation.

Certain morbid conditions of or about the genital organs may be an occasional cause of masturbation.

Irritations of the skin from eczema, cutaneous pruritus, urticaria, scabies, prurigo, etc., can sometimes by the immoderate itching, and the resulting scratching and pulling, especially in children, both boys and girls, be the exciting cause for manipulations of the genitals and so of masturbation. The unfamiliar pleasurable sensation on the one hand and the temporary removal of the annoying itching and formication on the other, impresses itself so deeply on the child's consciousness, that later with different intention new manipulations are repeated again and again, and the habit of masturbation is acquired.

Too long a prepuce and congenital narrowness, which lead to accumulation of smegma, to balanitis and tormenting itching, are met in many of these youthful "sinners." It sounds rather forced, when it is claimed that this lengthening of the prepuce in these little masturbators is the effect of masturbation!

In nervous children the first occasion for masturbation may be given by irritations of the rectum and anus. Parasites, oxyuris, chronic rectal catarrh, anal eczema and hemorrhoids may all be such occasional causes of masturbation.

The state of sexual excitement in the adult, which causes masturbation, may be produced by inflammation of the urethra, especially in its posterior part and in catarrh of the prostate.

We know that the time during and after a gonorrheal infection of the urethra and prostate is a critical one as regards the origin of masturbation.

The physician's order of long continued sexual abstinence produces a genital erethism; the irritation of the sexual centers by the chronic inflammation of the posterior urethra and its treatment with caustic agents, massage and passage of sounds, and finally postgonorrheal neurasthenia, are all contributory factors, which working together sufficiently explain the origin of masturbation after gonorrheal urethritis.

We have already mentioned the fact, that the fear of renewed infection may be a further psychic reason, which causes the patient to decide in favor of masturbation as against natural coitus.

PESTERING THE PROSTITUTE

By Henry Bronson Hollen, M. D., Chicago, Ill.

SOME time ago the Chicago Tribune came out with an editorial on the passing of our late lamented state's attorney; it wound up as follows:

"It is gratifying to recall that his last public act in this community was the wiping out of the segregated district."

Now, this is a pretty bit of speech but one that is perfectly empty and unwarrantable. Congratulations are not in order yet. We have yet to see that the wiping out of the segregated district has bettered the city any. It is only an experiment, as the mayor frankly admits—an experiment which the thorough student of vice conditions knows full well cannot possibly succeed. Nothing in the past, or in the present, is there to encourage in us the hope of success.

When the people of Chicago finally awaken to this fact they will have no right to hold Carter Harrison accountable. He was opposed to it from the very beginning, and only yielded to the insistency of several factions, bent on reform, when it got to be positively burdensome. When he finally gave in he said softly to himself:

"Well—if they want it so let them have it so, and we'll see what we'll see. Anything to stop this awful clamor—it is getting on my nerves."

So at last an order issued from his office sanctioning the proposed invasion of the district; and the police rushed in and emptied the brothels in no time.

"Where shall we go?" queried the affrighted population in unison.

"Go to hell—go anywhere—we don't care where you go—only get out of here," was the reply of the officers.

And they went; some weeping, some protesting, some scoffing. But not a few of these prostitutes laughed, laughed heartily, as if they considered the intrusion as a huge joke—they whose philosophy directs them to give no heed to the things of tomorrow and to drown incipient sorrow with a drink or two or three. They went in every direction, the hundreds of them and thousands in fact, just as thistles are cast about when the wind blows hard, and as hornets scatter when some small boy pokes a stick through their nest.

This happened less than a year ago. At this time the segregated district was quite well defined and orderly, although not regulated with any great seriousness. Several desirable rules were being enforced: the girls were not allowed to solicit by word of mouth or by gesture; they were not permitted even to show themselves at their windows; they were obliged to wear skirts reaching well below the knees; and the connections between resort and bar were closed. There was comparatively little disturbance. The resort-keepers were generally in for doing a "nice, quiet business." In many places there was no venereal disease; the majority of girls were compelled to undergo a weekly medical examination and enjoined to keep themselves clean, in order to retain an established patronage. The most disreputable places had been weeded out. On the whole, conditions were not half bad.

But the reform factions were not content either to let well enough alone or to attempt to perfect the system of regulation in vogue. No—they clamored loudly for an absolute wiping out of the entire district.

"We are on a new tack," they cried. "No compromising with vice for us. We are going to clean it out entirely."

The most of them were actually so simple-minded that they believed it possible to legislate the prostitute out of existence.

"Just enforce the laws and we will have no prostitutes," was their assertion, made in the self-satisfied, cocksure manner of reformers.

Really, such simple-mindedness is mirth-provoking; and then, again, in our more sober moments, it is pathetic.

The lesser fools, who are in the minority, will concede that "prostitution and kindred evils cannot be absolutely eradicated" but they strenuously object to "vice which flaunts itself in the very face of the community." The principle upon which they act is that it is better to spread vice evenly and thinly over a large area; then it will be less noticeable than if bunched in one locality.

As for this onslaught on the prostitute being "a new tack," that is preposterous. It is nothing of the sort. The tack is an old one—so old that it is quite rusty. Repeatedly, in every period, they have tried to exterminate the prostitute. The cruelest weapons that devils personified could devise have been used to this end.

But the end was never accomplished; nor will it be till the very pattern of our social fabric is changed.

The sudden and violent suppression of "the social evil" results always in still greater evils. Harass the prostitute, and she will turn from plying her trade openly to plying it secretly, with all the cunning and persistency of the driven female. And we know that vice-diseases must and do multiply under cover.

To think that the wiping out of a segregated district will benefit a community is ridiculous. It only disperses the corrupting forces. The girls have to live somewhere; they are not effaced by this measure. The few who leave for more tolerant fields are very soon replaced by others.

"Birds of a feather flock together," is the old saying. It's true. Let alone and unmolested, the vicious will naturally collect; and so collected, in little worlds of their own, will demoralize good people less than if they were scattered. In the first instance, only those who seek will find them—only the one who so chooses need meet them.

What are the conditions in Chicago at present? They are exactly as might have been expected—worse than before. We find that the prostitute has invaded respectable neighborhoods, where, up to now, she was never seen. Our virtuous wives and children are now obliged to come in close contact, in the streets and public places, with this new demoralizing element. In the very midst of respectability she plies her trade—very cautiously to avoid being caught—and who will question that she is doing more genuine harm, clandestinely, than when she operated in the open, under the eyes of the police and the medical inspector?

And is the segregated district (that was) really clean? No—it is not. The dozens of orderly resorts are deserted and dark but the re-opened "saloon resort" is seen on nearly all the corners, catering ostensibly to thirst-requirements but harboring, in the rear or above, a force of low-brow girls. Also we see several restaurants and tea-rooms and tobacco-shops (new features here) which, to the sophisticated, are secret resorts. A pedestrian, in this locality, is now solicited every few paces; one man reported that eight different girls stopped him in one evening, and that he saw a group of four prostitutes at a certain transfer corner, soliciting males who got off the car! Before the "wiping out," soliciting was a thing unheard of and unseen in the district. A notorious dance hall (really a club of prostitutes of the worst order) is still open.

We may now expect gonorrhea and syphilis—"the pestilence that stalketh in the darkness"—to be more prevalent than ever; and our virtuous women to fall victims to the depredations of unmarried males, who do not care to take the trouble of locating the secret resorts nor the risk of being arrested during raids upon such resorts. Only last week one place was raided by the police and eleven of both sexes arrested; and this place was located in a first-class residential neighborhood!

It is a fact that the proportion of virgins in any community diminishes rapidly following the outlawing of the prostitute. Again and again this has been observed. In old Paris, for example, the open brothels were suddenly abolished. What happened? "Two years later the tradesmen complained that they were having the greatest difficulty in guarding the chastity of their wives and daughters against the enterprises of the military and the students; and they begged the authorities on this account to re-open the brothels, which was done."

Not yet can the factions of reform see the folly of their ways. The experiment, according to the mayor's last message, is to be continued.

"It is certainly worthy of a thorough test," he says, "and will be given it. If it works out satisfactorily a notable advance will have been made, while the benefits to the cause of morality will be incalculable."

But it is clear that Carter Harrison is not a bit sanguine as to the result. He feels in his heart what the posted investigator knows absolutely, viz., such an experiment has never succeeded and never can succeed!

REVIEW OF CURRENT UROLOGIC LITERATURE

ZEITSCHRIFT FÜR UROLOGIE

Vol. VIII, No. 1, 1914

1. The Practical Value of Anterior Urethroscopy. By Franz Blumenthal.
2. The Practical Value of Posterior Urethroscopy. By Max Roth and Theodor Mayer. Appears as special abstract.
3. A New Method of Treating Chronic Gonorrhea and Urethritis Simplex with Lytinol after Dr. Awerbach of St. Petersburg. By Edward Bäumer. Appears as special abstract.
4. A Further Contribution to the Sealing-up Abortive Treatment of Beginning Gonorrhea. By Edgar G. Ballenger and Omar F. Elder.

1. Practical Value of Anterior Urethroscopy.

Blumenthal describes the various instruments; the indication for the use of each; the reliability of the results obtained; the applications of the procedure in acute and chronic gonorrheas, respectively. He then compares endoscopy with other methods of diagnosis such as the use of sounds and bougies, and finally takes up the therapeutic results obtained by the means under discussion. In his opinion the chief advantage of endoscopy is that it enables us to definitely prove the presence of gonococci where all clinical symptoms of gonorrhea are lacking. His conclusions are as follows:

1. Irrigation-urethroscopy (with the Goldschmidt instrument) and dry-urethroscopy (with the Valentine-Luys apparatus) have each their own field of usefulness. The former is adapted especially for the diagnosis of tumors, papillomata, diverticula, and tuberculous and syphilitic processes; the latter, for the recognition of superficial changes in the mucous membrane, glands, and crypts.

2. There are two possible sources of error which must be considered in the diagnosis of superficial changes in the urethral mucosa. In the first place, we must bear in mind the fact that in different individuals there is a wide normal variation in the color, luster, and size of the urethra; in the second place, the introduction of the instrument itself is responsible for many changes.

3. In acute gonorrhea, endoscopy in general is not to be recommended. Occasionally, however, it can be employed for the differentiation between chancre, herpes, and gonorrhea, and for the diagnosis and treatment of localized foci of infection.

4. In the subacute stage it is not wise to postpone endoscopy too long, in order that the early diagnosis of local foci and their special treatment may be commenced forthwith.

5. In chronic urethritis this procedure is always indicated, but we

must beware of too much prejudice in its favor. It is a most useful method when employed in conjunction with the others that are at our service, but it can play us false and mislead us grossly when we rely too much upon it alone to the neglect of other reliable procedures.

4. **A Further Contribution to the Sealing-up Abortive Treatment of Gonorrhea.**

After four years' experience with their method, the authors are very enthusiastic over the results obtained. If the patient begins treatment within 24 or 48 hours after the onset of the discharge, the gonorrhea can often be rapidly cured by the sealing up within the urethra of a 5% solution of argyrol once a day for about 5 days. The best sealing material is non-contractile collodion, U. S. P. In order to effect a cure: (1) the argyrol must come in contact with the entire portion of the urethra which has become infected and in order to accomplish this, treatment must be begun early; (2) the medicament must be retained within the canal at least 6 hours a day.

Factors interfering with or preventing cure by this method are: (1) The spread of the infection to parts inaccessible to the injected argyrol; (2) sexual intercourse during the incubation period, especially shortly before the appearance of the discharge; (3) an extended incubation period; (4) any treatment such as irrigation or instrumentation before the institution of the sealing-up treatment. The authors have used this method in about 650 cases, the length of treatment varying from 3 to 6 days. It makes no difference whether the urethritis is caused by the gonococcus or by some other organism. Under favorable conditions they have cured 90% of their cases in 5 days. They always order provocative measures on the 6th day, such as the drinking of beer, to bring on a return of the discharge in case the patient is not cured. If the latter is the case the flow reappears in from two to four days and runs the typical course of a gonorrhea. Even should the abortive treatment fail there is no danger to be feared from its employment. When the method works, both the gonococci and the discharge disappear after one or two treatments. The authors advise the learner of this method to try it first in cases of chronic gonorrhea as there, also, no harm can arise from its employment.

Technique.—The patient empties his bladder and lies on the operating table. The penis is scrubbed up and wrapped in a sterile towel. A small graduated urethral syringe is then employed to inject 25 minims of a 5% argyrol solution into the urethra and the meatus is pinched together when the syringe is withdrawn. The meatus is now sealed with one or two strokes of a camel's hair brush dipped in collodion, the argyrol being pinched back in the urethra until the collodion is completely hardened. It is not wise to inject more than 25 minims as the danger of escape is thereby increased. The patient may then go about his business, provided his work is not heavy, and is cautioned not to drink anything whatever until the collodion is removed. This may be accomplished after 6 or more hours by moistening the collodion with cotton dipped in acetone, or better still, by originally sealing a strip of cotton (in part only) under one end of the collodion dressing, thus furnishing a convenient handle for the removal of the seal. This strip of cotton should not project over the meatus as otherwise the argyrol may escape. After the dressing is removed the patient should be ordered to drink at least a litre of Lithia water in order to flush out the canal thoroughly before bed-time. The next morning, however, fluids should again be restricted to a minimum.

Five per cent. solutions are quite strong enough to produce the results desired. Toward the end of the treatment, 2 and 3 per cent. strengths may be employed. In any case the argyrol must be made up fresh daily, as a stock solution is less effective and may cause irritation.

When gonococci are still demonstrable after the third or fourth treatment and the first portion of urine is still cloudy, there is little hope for a cure by the abortive treatment.

Patients should be told to come for treatment early in the morning so that in case the seal is unsatisfactory it can be repeated the same day. Moreover they should be cautioned to return immediately the argyrol escapes, so that valuable time is not lost in the treatment.

ZEITSCHRIFT FÜR UROLOGIE

Vol. VIII, No. 2, 1914.

1. Congenital Cysts of the Penile Raphe. By Gustav Fantl.
2. A Metal Spiral for the Pezzer Catheter. By Jonathan Paul Haberern.
3. Nephrectomy in Bilateral Tuberculosis. By Robert Bachrach.
4. The Prognosis in Nephritis. By H. Holweg.
5. Reply to the Above Paper of Dr. Holweg's. By H. Strauss.

1. Congenital Cysts of the Penile Raphe.

Fantl had the opportunity of observing, in the course of a few weeks, four cases of this rare condition. He describes his findings in detail and gives the result of histological studies in two of the cases. One of the latter was a mucous cyst, the other an epidermoid cyst.

The author then takes up at length the embryology and pathogenesis of this condition and concludes as follows:

1. Abnormalities of the raphe cannot be explained by the current theories of its origin.

2. The raphe develops independently of the closure of the urethral canal.

2. A Metal Spiral for the Pezzer Catheter.

Haberern finds that the part of the catheter outside the body often becomes kinked by the dressings or movements of the patient, thus interfering with proper drainage. He therefore employs flexible metal spirals made of new silver wire, which he slips over the catheters thus rendering the latter firm and always patent. He lays down the following requisites for such spirals:

1. They must be of light build so that their weight does not inconvenience the patient.

2. They must be made of a material which does not react with the rubber of the catheter.

3. They must present an absolutely smooth surface and must adapt themselves to every change in the shape of the catheter.

4. They must be readily sterilizable, both alone, and when fitted onto the catheter.

5. They must be of moderate cost.

The author's heaviest spiral, which is adapted for a 30 Charrière catheter, weighs only 1.85 grams. These spirals have given very satisfactory service and may be used to reinforce rubber drainage tubes introduced into any cavities or wounds anywhere in the body.

3. **Nephrectomy in Bilateral Tuberculosis.**

Bilateral renal tuberculosis is now not to be regarded as an invariable contraindication to nephrectomy. More and more frequently one kidney is removed when the remaining organ is deemed capable of carrying on the excretory functions. No radical cure is expected of such a procedure but actual palliative results have been obtained. Bachrach reports five cases of neprectomy in bilaterally diseased kidneys. The first case died soon after the operation, but this occurred at a date when our functional and clinical tests were not so well developed as they are at present. The other four patients are still living and all showed an immediate improvement after the operation: the temperature dropped, the general condition improved, and the patients gained in weight. The second case is now two and a half years postoperative, has gained 17 kg. and feels subjectively well, but his bladder is diseased and he excretes cloudy urine of low concentration from the remaining kidney. The third case was operated on a year ago, has slight bladder complaints, but is able to work. The fourth and fifth cases, who were operated on a few months ago, have both become fever free and have improved unmistakably as far as the bladder symptoms are concerned. Whether the lives of these patients have been lengthened remains to be seen, but it is at least certain that they have been relieved of their distressing symptoms.

The author concludes that a palliative nephrectomy is indicated in bilateral renal tuberculosis:

1. When fever is present, caused by a mixed infection in the more diseased kidney.

2. When the bladder is severely inflamed by the elimination of large amounts of pus.

3. When the primarily diseased organ is so far gone that its functionating no longer figures in the excretory economy.

When ureteral catheterization is impossible, cryoscopic examination of the blood, followed by an exploratory examination of both kidneys, with or without ureteral catheterization through the open bladder, can give very valuable information.

4. The Prognosis in Nephritis.

In 1911 Hohlweg pointed out that an increase of the rest nitrogen in the blood offers a very bad prognosis in uremia cases. In 1912 Strauss wrote a paper saying that work that he had published 10 years before showed exactly the same thing. He looked over his original tables and in 1913 wrote a second paper in which he claimed, according to Hohlweg, that he had for more than ten years regarded a high rest-N figure as of unfavorable prognostic import.

Hohlweg's point is that Strauss could not have formed the same conclusions from his material available in 1902. Moreover if he had formed them why did he wait from 1902 to 1911 to publish them?

5. Reply to the Above Paper of Dr. Holweg's.

Strauss quotes from his original paper of 1902 to the effect that "in uremia there is generally a very big increase in the rest nitrogen." Although he did not at that time publish the fact, he has already long since had the impression that a high rest-N figure is of severe prognostic value. He never however *recommended* its determination for prognostic purposes, until later, when he gave Hohlweg and others full credit for having suggested the idea. Strauss says that he looked over his old tables again not to see whether he could prove an unfair priority on such a basis, but in order merely to confirm by cold figures a general impression that he had long carried. He has no desire "to adorn himself with others' feathers" and feels that his position is secure anyway as it is admittedly owing to his original work that the present world-wide interest in the determination of the rest-N was aroused ten years ago.

ANNALES DES MALADIES VÉNÉRIENNES

Vol. IX, No. 1, January, 1914

1. The Skin Reaction in Syphilis. By R. Burnier.
2. Papular Syphilides Unmodified by Treatment with "606." By L. Giroux and Mlle. Patte.

The Skin Reaction in Syphilis.

1. Burnier first takes up the cutaneous reactions performed with the aid of materials obtained from various syphilitic organs such as the liver and lungs. He then takes up at considerable length Noguchi's

luetin, describing its preparation, the normal reaction obtained therewith, and the three types of positive reaction: the papular, the pustular, and the torpid. He next presents an excellent series of 24 tables summarizing the results obtained with this method by different authors in various types of syphilitic and non-syphilitic disease and adds a table of his own. He then gives a comparative table based on about 1500 cases contrasting the results obtained by the luetin test with those given by the Wassermann reaction.

The table is as follows:

	Luetin positive in	Wassermann positive in
Primary syphilis	33% of cases	72% of cases
Secondary syphilis	47% of cases	80% of cases
Tertiary syphilis	79% of cases	80% of cases
Latent syphilis	65% of cases	59% of cases
Heredo-syphilis	70% of cases	69% of cases
Tabes	49% of cases	64% of cases
General paresis	59% of cases	60% of cases

It appears from the above evidence that the Wassermann test is more constant than the luetin reaction in primary and secondary syphilis, especially when there has been no treatment. The skin reaction is practically as valuable as the Wassermann in tertiary syphilis and in heredo-syphilis, whereas it is more constant in latent syphilis and in syphilis under treatment. In fact Noguchi believes that the luetin test is far less affected by treatment than the Wassermann reaction. It is not unusual to observe that after active treatment both the clinical signs and the Wassermann reaction (blood as well as cerebrospinal fluid) become negative, whereas the cutaneous reaction persists. Conversely, there are cases in which the Wassermann is positive and the clinical symptoms straightforward, in which the luetin test is negative. In such instances it suffices merely to give energetic treatment, such as an injection of salvarsan, and the situation becomes completely reversed.

The author then goes into the theories concerned with the nature of the luetin reaction. He summarizes his paper as follows:

1. Luetin often gives a negative reaction in primary and secondary syphilis.

2. The reaction is generally positive in active tertiary lues. Next in order are heredo-syphilis, latent syphilis, treated syphilis, and parasyphilis.

3. On the other hand, there may be a positive reaction in non-syphilitic diseases, as gonorrhea, soft chancre, lupus erythematosus, lupus vulgaris, pityriasis rosea, and eczema.

4. The skin of certain syphilitics, most often in the tertiary stage, reacts positively with emulsions of other microbes (gonococci, colon bacilli, staphylococci) or with tuberculin.

It therefore seems difficult to admit the absolute specificity of luetin in the diagnosis of syphilis.

2. Papular Syphilides Unmodified by Treatment with "606."

The case we report to-day is but another confirmation of what our master, Professor Gaucher, has long been teaching in his service, namely, that although 606 may in certain cases favorably and rapidly influence the ulcerative lesions of syphilis its action may be insufficient or negligible against some of the other manifestations of the disease.

Case (No. 30502 in the "clinique" records)—Miss X, cook, 27 years old, admitted to the "policlinique des maladies cutanées et syphilitiques," Aug. 12, 1913, complaining of violent headaches lasting since May. The pains were most marked in the occipital region and lasted the whole day with a severe paroxysm at night which prevented all sleep. About two weeks after the outset of this condition the patient had a sore throat for a few days but she could not recall ever having had any vulvar lesions.

On the tenth of June she discovered three lesions on her face. They were red and itched, and were located, respectively, on the right upper eyelid, on the forehead near the root of the nose, and on the ala of the left nostril. A few days later similar sores appeared on the hairy scalp and on the lower part of the face near the naso-labial folds. Then toward the end of the month there rapidly developed an eruption involving the trunk and thighs and extending as far as the knees but avoiding the legs and upper extremities, and consisting of small itching red spots, pin-head in size. An extensive lesion occupied the side of the left chest. Ultimately the lesions became more numerous and more extensive and stopped itching. The persistence of this eruption and of the headache caused the patient to seek relief at the Saint-Louis hospital where she informed us that her friend had had an ulceration of the penis for several months.

Examination of the patient disclosed a generalized papular cruption of the face and body. The lesions were round, infiltrated, and copper-colored. There were no sores on the vulva or in the throat. The patient was put on daily injections of 10% mercury benzoate, 2 cc. being given at a dose. She kept up treatment faithfully until the 26th of August, on which date examination showed that the lesions were much improved, having become paler and less infiltrated. On the 9th of September the patient had an intestinal reaction with bloody stools. Treatment was suspended for several days. By this time she had received 29 injections, the lesions were considerably modified, the infiltration was scarcely perceptible, and the headaches had ceased definitely for some time past.

On September 10, tormented by her enteritis, she asked to be admitted to the hospital. Our service being closed, she entered the

"Salle Gibert," under the direction of Dr. Tibierge. This time she received five intravenous injections of 606. They were given at weekly intervals, the first two doses being 0.45 gram, the last three 0.6 gram. After each injection she had intense headaches which came on in a few minutes, persisted for 48 hours, and were accompanied by severe depression. The lesions were not modified by the new treatment. The patient confirmed this failure herself and returned to see us on October 19, three days after the last salvarsan injection. At this time her face showed faint red spots, the remains of the original eruption. On the rest of her body were slightly infiltrated scattered papules. These lesions had retained the same aspect that they presented after the original treatment given on our service. There were no other sores, either of the vulva or of the mouth. The patient was at once put back on the daily injections of mercury benzoate. By November 4, after a series of 17 injections, the lesions were much improved. The trunk showed only non-infiltrated macules. The face lesions had paled considerably and were hardly visible.

In short, here was a case of a patient afflicted with a generalized papular syphilide, in whom treatment with 606 had no other effect than to cause severe headaches after each injection. The lesions, which had been much improved by the benzoate, were quite unaffected by this new treatment, and it was only the resumption of the daily benzoate injections which rapidly and profoundly influenced the disease.

ANNALES DES MALADIES VENERIENNES

Vol. IX, No. 2, February, 1914.

1. Hereditary Syphilis and Infantile Encephalopathies. By L. Babonneix.
2. Chronic Aortitis of Acquired Syphilis. By Drs. Gaucher and Brin.
3. Chancre of the Upper Eye-lid. By Jean Bobrie.
4. Chancriform Gumma of the Corpus Cavernosum. By Georges Lemos.

1. Hereditary Syphilis and Infantile Encephalopathies.

Babonneix reviews the entire subject of infantile encephalopathies in the light of our newer methods of diagnosing syphilitic infection. He divides his study into three chapters: I) Clinical; II) Anatomical; III) Therapeutic results.

Chapter I. The Clinical Types of Infantile Encephalopathies.— There are two forms, viz.: motor syndromes and intellectual syndromes. The motor syndromes may be either occasional (episodic), such as convulsions or epilepsy (whether symptomatic or essential), or else permanent. Under the permanent syndromes we have the spasmo-paralytic group, including infantil spasmodic hemiplegia, and the cerebral diplegias and Little's disease. In support of the specific nature of this condition we have to consider the *etiologic* evidence, for these cases have occurred in hereditary syphilis of the first and second generation, the *clinical* evidence, for Little's disease occurs in the premature, in families where there are many miscarriages, and is often associated with presumptive and often with positive signs of syphilis. Furthermore, at autopsy specific lesions of unquestioned authenticity have been discovered, the Wassermann reaction is often positive, and, finally, specific treatment often gives splendid results. Lastly, we must include among the motor syndrome group certain cases which show athetosochoreiform movements.

Under intellectual syndromes the author includes cases of arrested mentality, imbecility and idiocy. Meningitic idiocy is almost always of specific origin, whereas mongolian idiocy is less often so and amaurotic family idiocy is never specific. On the other hand syphilis plays a capital rôle in the production of hydrocephalic idiocy.

Chapter II. The Anatomic forms of Infantile Encephalopathies.—There are six principal varieties, namely: 1) Chronic meningoencephalitis; 2) Cerebral sclerosis with possible subsequent atrophy; 3) Tuberous sclerosis; 4) Porencephaly; 5) Various cerebral malformations besides porencephaly, such as hemicephaly, microcephaly, cerebral hernias, multiple anomalies, etc.; 6) Hydrocephaly. The clinical evidence for the specificity of these conditions is similar to that previously stated for Little's disease; the laboratory evidence is as follows: 1) Spirochetes have been found in the cerebrospinal fluid and pia mater of cases of hereditary syphilis; 2) The Wassermann reaction in 330 young idiots examined was positive in 51 cases, that is in 15.4%; 3) The brain of a child who suffered from epileptic crises and who had a positive Wassermann reaction showed a large cyst which was probably the result of an old syphilitic lesion; 4) Many authors have obtained positive Wassermanns in cases of hydrocephaly.

Chapter III. Therapeutic Considerations.—Many cases have have been cured or improved by specific treatment. Among these have been instances of convulsions, of aphasia, of infantile cerebral hemiplegia and of Little's disease. However, it is in cases of inflammatory tertiary hydrocephalus that the best results have been obtained. It is therefore wise in all infantile encephalopathies to think of hereditary syphilis as the etiological factor even though there may be another apparent cause such as trauma from obstetric forceps, for even here the tissues may be already "prepared" by an underlying syphilis.

2. Chronic Aortitis of Acquired Syphilis.

Clinically, from 55 to 60 per cent. of cases of chronic aortitis are due to syphilis. On the other hand from 70 to 85 per cent. of the cases show a positive Wassermann reaction. In other words, considering that a negative reaction does not always rule out syphilis, chronic aortitis should be considered a parasyphilitic disease just as much as tabes and general paresis. The male sex is more frequently affected than the female: nine cases out of ten in the authors' series. This is explained by the greater frequency in men of the exogenous intoxications (tobacco, alcohol).

Pathologically, the lesions may be spread throughout the entire length of the aorta (diffuse aortitis), or they may be localized in certain places, which is more common. The chief localizations, in the order of their frequency, are: the arch of the aorta, the abdominal aorta just above its bifurcation, lastly, the thoracic aorta at its origin. Macroscopically, syphilitic aortitis may assume the diffuse subacute form when the lesion is in the process of evolution, or the fibrous form when it is complete. In the subacute diffuse form of aortitis the vessel is not externally changed nor is its calibre sensibly augmented. On opening the lumen there are seen numerous plaques from 2 to 5 cm. in diameter varying in consistency from the "soft" to the "hard" variety. In the fibrous form of aortitis, on the other hand, the aorta appears, externally, to be uniformly much dilated. In this variety moreover the plaques are more irregular in shape and are all of the "hard" variety. Microscopically the subacute form is distinguished by a massive cellular infiltration of all the layers of the aorta, with active proliferation of the normal elements, whereas the fibrous form is characterized by the excessive development of connective tissue which comes gradually to replace the normal structure. Pathologically, it is of importance to distinguish the above lesions from those of simple atheroma, and this is sometimes difficult, but the discovery of the spirochetes in the wall of the vessel will always clear up the diagnosis.

Symptoms.—Pain may be strictly localized to the aortic region and consist rather of a sense of constriction and oppression. At other times it may be very severe and accompanied by marked anxiety, and may radiate especially along the left upper extremity. Here we are in reality dealing with attacks of angina pectoris and these may be due to an associated syphilitic sclerosis of the coronaries. Dyspnea is also a prominent symptom. This may come on only after exertion, or in paroxysms at night (so-called aortic pseudo-asthma), or more rarely it may be constant. Longcope believes the dyspnea of chronic syphilitic aortitis to be moderate but that it is characterized by coming on after only the very slightest exertion. As a matter of fact, much of the dyspnea may be due to the associated pulmonary, myocarditic and especially renal lesions. Other symptoms of this disease are cough, palpitation, vertigo. The facies are not characteristic.

Physical Signs.—In one-half the author's cases inspection and palpation revealed dilatation and pulsation of the aorta above the suprasternal notch and of the subclavian arteries above the clavicles. Percussion reveals an increase in the transverse aortic dulness. Auscultation may reveal nothing if the lesion is diffuse or above the semilunar valves, but the signs are marked if the aortic valves are affected. Thus the first sound may be exaggerated or prolonged owing to the impact of the blood against the rigid aorta. Modifications in the second aortic sound are much more common. There may be simple accentuation or a distinct metallic quality. This clanging second aortic may be regarded as almost pathognomonic of chronic aortitis. A systolic murmur is due to an actual or, more rarely, to a relative stenosis of the aortic valve; a diastolic murmur is practically always indicative of insufficiency. Radioscopic examination serves to establish a uniform dilatation of the aorta and to rule out aneurysm. The pulse is usually firm and sustained but where insufficiency exists it is of the Corrigan variety. The tension is almost always raised to 180 or 200 at the least.

The course of the disease is slow and insidious. Recovery is very rare. Numerous complications, such as sclerosis of the coronaries, aneurysm, obliteration of the large vessels, may supervene. There are four chief clinical forms of the disease: 1) Diffuse aortitis. This may give no symptoms or else cause a variable degree of dyspnea, accentuation of the second aortic and marked hypertension. This form often yields to treatment. 2) Aortitis of the semilunar valves. This condition is characterized by the association of valvular signs with those of the aorta proper, and evolves more like a cardiac than like an arterial lesion. It is not modified by specific treatment. 3) Supra-semilunar aortitis. This is associated with coronary sclerosis and gives rise to anginal attacks. It is fortunately favorably influenced by specific treatment. 4) Abdominal aortitis is characterized by spontaneous or pressure pains along the course of the aorta, most marked above the umbilicus and radiating in every direction; by gastro-intestinal crises with repeated vomiting, hyperacidity, and diarrhea; by painful epigastric pulsation. There is objectively marked dilatation of the aorta and increased mobility, and there is increased tension in the dorsalis pedis which may exceed the pressure in the radial by 20 to 30 mm. The prognosis in this type is always grave as there are generally associated supradiaphragmatic aortic lesions.

The diagnosis is made from the clinical signs above mentioned, by the X-ray, and by the Wassermann reaction. Treatment of the condition is both symptomatic and etiologic. Symptomatic treatment calls for the use of counterirritants, of amyl nitrite, of morphine. Etiologic treatment is directed, of course, against the underlying syphilis. Mixed treatment is best and must be persevered in, even if there are no immediate results. The authors have adopted the following procedure: On each of ten successive days they inject 2 centigrams of the benzoate of mercury. During the next ten days the patient receives potassium iodide at the rate of 2 grams a day. During the remaining ten days of the month the patient rests. This course is repeated every month. In each of the ten cases observed there was a marked improvement in the symptoms and in some cases in the general condition as well. There was practically no change in the physical signs.

3. **Chancre of the Upper Eyelid.**

Bobrie reports the case of a man who had a chronic inflammatory lesion of the right upper eyelid. While the wound was still open he had extra-conjugal intercourse and contracted a chancre of the penis. At the same time he developed at the site of his eye lesion, an indolent, painless erosion, 2 by 3 cm. in size, which presented an indurated base, and was associated with a painless enlargement of the right preauricular gland. Spirochetes were demonstrated in the palpebral lesion. A secondary roseola developed.

4. **Chancriform Gumma of the Corpus Cavernosum.**

Lemos reports the case of a man who had had for six weeks a slowly growing deep ulceration of the penis. The lesion was 4-5 cm. deep, its orifice was located at the bottom of the glans, to the left of the frenum. The lesion was bounded externally by the overlying skin, internally by the corpus spongiosum, and above by the left corpus cavernosum. The walls of the ulcer were red and the base was formed by an adherent false membrane; there was a moderate non-fetid discharge.

The diagnosis lay between a gumma and a phagedenic chancre. The author decided in favor of the former for the following reasons: (1) There was no inguinal adenopathy. (2) The patient presented no other evidences of tertiary syphilis but gave a history of chancre ten years previously. (3) The ulceration commenced as a slight erosion and developed slowly without local reaction and without subjacent induration. (4) A chancre would have been followed by secondary lesions, which was not the case. The lesion healed slowly under mixed treatment.

JOURNAL D'UROLOGIE

Vol. IV, No. 6, Dec. 16, 1913

1. Staphylococcemias of Urinary Origin. By F. Legueu. P. 893.
2. Intravesical Technique in the High-Frequency Treatment of Tumors of the Bladder. By Maurice Heitz-Boyer. P. 907.
3. Treatment of Soft Chancres with Solutions of Argyrol. By M. Ravary. P. 915.
4. Functional Examination of the Two Kidneys when Ureteral Catheterization is Impossible. By Eugène Pirondini. P. 919.
5. Where Shall We Stop in the Treatment of Gonorrhea? By Jules Janet. P. 971.
6. A New Graduated Ureteral Sound for Radiography. By O. Pasteau. P. 975.

1. **Staphylococcemias of Urinary Origin.**

The urinary tract may present two different manifestations of staphylococcemia. (1) It may be the localization of a general staphylococcus infection. Thus a furuncle, an anthrax or grippal infection or an angina may cause a perinephric phlegmon or a descending pyelonephritis. A vesiculitis or prostatitis may even result. (2) On the other hand the primary focus may be in the urinary tract and thence spread throughout the entire system. Thus the urethra, bladder, or kidney, may be the starting points for such infections.

The author reports two new experiences. The first was that of a man of 48, who suffered from severe attacks of pain in the right kidney region. The diagnosis was made of a low-grade pyelonephritis, possibly caused by a calculus. Cystoscopy was attempted and after this, signs of severe sepsis supervened. The right kidney region was explored, a perinephritic phlegmon opened up and the kidney found to be studded with miliary abscesses. The organ was split open and drained. Staphylococci were recovered from the pus. For a time the condition improved but soon the patient got up bilateral parotid abscesses which had to be opened and numerous subcutaneous infections on various parts of his body. From all these, as well as from the blood, staphylococci were isolated. Following this the patient recovered, gained weight, and remained well until the following year when he developed an osteomyelitis of the tibia. After this, more abscesses developed bringing the total number up to fifty-four. Finally the patient developed a pyarthrosis of the left knee to which he succumbed. Staphylococci were recovered every time that cultures were taken.

The second patient also complained of pains in the right side. The attacks were accompanied by anuria and followed by the passage of large quantities of urine. The condition was at first attributed to a right inguinal hernia which was operated on and was followed by relief for four years. The pains returned suddenly, however, and a cystoscopy was done which revealed the presence of calculi in the bladder. Catheterization of the ureters showed a depressed function on the right side. The corresponding kidney was explored and stones removed from the calices. After the operation the patient did poorly, became septic, ran a constant temperature, and had frequent chills. A blood culture was taken and showed staphylococci. Abscesses formed under the right scapula and in the presacral region, both containing staphylococci. Despite the use of electrargol, cacodylate of soda and two preparations of auto-vaccines, the patient died about 3 months after the operation. Autopsy revealed the presence of a parietal thrombus in the inferior vena cava. This was probably the immediate point of departure for the systemic infection. Smears from the thrombus also revealed the presence of staphylococcus.

3. Treatment of Soft Chancres with Solutions of Argyrol.

Ravary had occasion to treat a large chancre of the soft variety, the size of a 50 centime piece. The lesion had been subjected to all the ordinary therapeutic measures applied in such cases but without avail. Microscopic examination of the sero-purulent discharge revealed the presence of the Ducrey bacillus in great numbers. The Wassermann reaction was negative. It occurred to the author to use dressings of 20% argyrol. He prepared circles of sterile gauze which he saturated with this solution, placed them over the exposed glans, and retained them in position by drawing the prepuce back over them. The end of the penis was wrapped in dry cotton to prevent soiling. The patient was directed to change the dressing after each urination.

On the following day, the ulcer had lost its sanious aspect and had dried up to such an extent that it was impossible to obtain enough discharge for microscopic examination. Investigation of scrapings established the complete absence of Ducrey bacilli. On the fifth day the wound was entirely healed.

A large bubo which complicated the condition was treated with dry cups applied three times in succession at intervals of five minutes. By the fourth day of this treatment the bubo was sensibly diminished in size and showed no tendency to suppuration. By the end of the second week it had shrunk to the size of a pea.

The author reports two other cases, one of which was complicated by the appearance of a hard chancre after the soft chancres had been cured. The author has had no opportunity to try the argyrol treatment in the large phagedenic ulcerations of the penis but is convinced that they could be cured much more rapidly by argyrol than by any other method of treatment such as aero-thermo-cauterization.

5. Where Shall We Stop in the Treatment of Gonorrhea?

If we stop treatment too soon the gonococci will attack new foci and a cure will be all the more difficult; if, on the other hand, we prolong treatment unnecessarily we may produce a discharge due to irritation which will persist just as long as we treat it. It is obvious that repeated microscopic examinations of the discharge and of the shreds for gonococci will give us the best answer to the question. If no gonococci are discoverable, if the patient feels subjectively well, if the discharge ceases, and the urine is practically clear we may safely stop treatment. A very favorable sign, according to Janet, is when, on separating the lips of the meatus, they open progressively from before backward like two leaves of moist paper.

The aspect of absolute cure varies with the methods of treatment employed. If we employ the antiseptic method we can rest assured that in case a cure is not effected the discharge will reappear generally in 48 hours—surely by the end of seven days. Janet therefore waits 8 days before giving the beer provocative test—which is generally negative—and 3 days after that allows intercourse with a condom, the latter being for the protection of the female partner.

Balsamic treatment is very deceptive as to whether a cure has really taken place or not. This method merely dries up the discharge which reappears just as soon as the dose of the balsamic is diminished.

The "laisser couler" treatment is similarly unreliable, for the patient, tired of the long wait, often allows the discharge to dry up spontaneously. In such instances, there is only too often an incomplete auto-immunization and a chronic discharge is the unfortunate result. Unlike the Germans, Janet does not treat the chronic discharge which persists after the disappearance of the gonococci. In the overwhelming majority of cases this catarrhal flow ceases just as soon as treatment is stopped, so that the author absolutely disregards it for one month at least.

JOURNAL D'UROLOGIE

Vol. V, No. 1, Jan., 1914.

1. The (Ureo-secretory) Constant as Applied to Nephrectomy for Tuberculosis. By F. Legueu.
2. The Movable Kidney Syndrome: a Clinical Contribution. By Giusseppe Bolognèsi.
3. Incrustating Cystitis. By J. François.
4. A Case of Impaling Wound of the Bladder and Rectum, Operation, Death from Pelvic Cellulitis. By Ch. Lenormant.
5. Lesions of the Vesical Mucosa in Purpura Hemorrhagica as Seen by the Cystoscope. By C. Bruni.
6. Aspiration in the Treatment of Chronic Urethritis. By A. Cariani.
7. A Technical Point in Catheterizing the Ureters. By Augusto Brandao Filho.

2. **The Movable Kidney Syndrome: a** Clinical Contribution.

Bolognèsi reports twenty-eight operative cases. Of these only eleven had pain, with or without crises; two showed nervous phenomena; two presented symptoms of atony of the gastro-intestinal tract; one had both nervous and gastroenteric complaints; three cases showed atony of the digestive tract with appendicalgia; two had compression of the ductus choledochus with biliary retention and probable biliary lithiasis; and finally one case presented peculiar digestive disturbances, represented especially by a complete and persistent anachlorhydria. As regards the anatomical condition of the abnormally movable kidney there were three cases in which there was obstruction to the outflow of urine (intermittent hydronephrosis) and three others in which there were inflammatory lesions of the urinary passages (catarrhal pyelonephritis, catarrhal pyelocystitis).

The author concludes from his clinical observations that the symptoms of movable kidney are too varied for classification in the three classic groups, viz.: the painful group, the nervous group, and the gastro-intestinal group. In fact the manifestations of this condition may be so diverse that—more often than is generally believed—one may be led into an erroneous clinical diagnosis, especially if he makes but a superficial physical examination.

Especially noteworthy are the two rare cases of compression of the bile ducts and the case of anacidity, all three of which were relieved after operation. In every one of the twenty-eight cases the technical result was perfect, the author employing the technic of Remedi in performing the nephropexy. Moreover the clinical diagnosis was confirmed in every one of the reported cases since there was not only an immediate, but also a permanent, amelioration or absolute disappearance of the morbid symptoms.

3. Incrustating Cystitis.

Incrustating cystitis is an ulcerating inflammation, more or less localized, of the bladder wall with deposits of phosphate of lime on and below the surface. As regards etiology, the author has found from a study of sixteen cases that the condition occurs in middle life and with equal frequency in men and women. The disease is, in the great majority of cases, preceded by a chronic cystitis of several years' standing, occasionally by an acute cystitis, sometimes of puerperal origin. The chief symptoms are the following:

1. Pain toward the end of urination. There may be tenesmus.

2. Great urgency and frequency of urination.

3. Terminal hematuria. This, like the two preceding symptoms, is not influenced by rest or movement.

4. Urinary changes. The urine is cloudy, alkaline in reaction, with an ammoniacal odor. There is a gelatinous deposit, and the microscope shows pus and blood cells as well as calcium phosphate crystals.

5. The bladder capacity is reduced to from 30 to 100 cubic centimeters.

6. A pathognomonic symptom, when it is carefully observed, is the excretion of calcareous concretions during a vesical crisis. These masses are yellowish-white, flattened, with irregular borders. Their attached surface is irregular and downy, whereas the side facing the bladder cavity is smooth and polished. Such plaques were passed in only four of the sixteen cases reviewed.

There are two complications which may supervene in this condition that are worthy of note: retention of urine (where there is no enlarged prostate) and pyelonephritis.

Cystoscopy reveals at least two characteristic types of incrustation. The first is the *flat* or *sheet* incrustation which throws no shadow. There are usually several plaques, silvery white in color, of an irregular and downy aspect, with lacerated margins and resembling for all the world thin layers of cotton pasted on the vesical mucosa. The second type is the projecting incrustation which may be compared to a white sponge dropped into the bladder. This form, of course, throws a shadow and may be mistaken for a stone or tumor. Further cystoscopic characteristics of this condition are the multiplicity of the lesions (4 to 10 in number) and the intense inflammation of the vesical mucosa about the incrustations. Their favorite location is the trigone, the ureteral regions, the vesical neck, the prostate, or on the bar bordering the prostatic pouch after a prostatectomy.

Microscopically, three distinct zones can be established. 1. A superficial zone of necrosis with accumulations of phosphatic deposit. 2. A middle zone of infiltration. 3. A deep zone of submucosa or muscularis which becomes more and more normal as we recede from the surface. The pathogenesis is simple. There is an acute exacerbation of a chronic cystitis with ulcer formation. The necrotic membrane remains attached to the deeper parts and collects upon itself the phosphate deposit resulting from the bacterial decomposition of the alkaline urine.

The prognosis is grave. The condition never clears up spontaneously and does not yield to medical treatment. As regards diagnosis, it is well to bear in mind that flat incrustations may be confused with fibrinous deposits and leucoplasias. The deposits can generally be ruled out by examination after a lavage, whereas the leucoplasias can be recognized by the microscopic discovery in the urine of the characteristic epithelial cells which compose them. Moreover incrustating cystitis is seven times more frequent than leucoplasia. Projecting incrustations may be confused with calculi or with tumors. Calculi are more regular and are mobile. Tumors should afford no difficulty unless covered with fibrin, in which case a biopsy will relieve all doubt.

Treatment should be directed against ulceration and alkaline decomposition of the urine. Medical treatment consists in internal antiseptics, vesical lavages and instillations, and fumigation with iodine. Surgical treatment consists in curettage either through the natural passages (in women) or after a cystostomy, and in excision with suture of the wound thus produced. The last procedure, when supplemented with deep curettage of the small incrusted ulcerations and cauterization of the wound with tincture of iodine, is the method of choice. After the operation it is essential to keep the bladder clean by irrigations in order to prevent recurrence.

4. A Case of Impaling Wound of the Bladder and Rectum.

In view of Gerard's recent comprehensive article on wounds of the bladder by impalement (Journ. d'Urol. IV, 4, 5, 1913, abstracted in two numbers of this Journal), the following single case reported by Lenormant is of interest. A farmer of 26 was driving a power-rake when he fell off the seat, one of the steel teeth penetrating his perineal region. He immediately began to bleed from the anus and urine flowed from his wound. The point of perforation was to the left of the anus, no urine was obtained from the bladder on catheterization. At operation, which was done on the following day, it was found that the pale had torn the subperitoneal part of the rectum on the left side, had lacerated the pelvic cellular tissue and had perforated the bladder at the bas-fond, below the reflection of the vesico-rectal peritoneum.

There was a great extravasation of urine into the prevesical and left latero-pelvic cellular spaces but the peritoneal cavity was not entered. Despite the triple drainage—of the bladder, the rectum, and the perineal wound—a pelvic cellulitis set in, the patient gradually became more and more septic and succumbed to a generalized bronchopneumonia one month after the accident.

From a study of this case Lenormant feels that Gerard has greatly underestimated the seriousness of extraperitoneal wounds of this nature, and that instead of advocating abstention from all intervention in such cases the author would insist on operation with almost the same urgency as in peritoneal affections. The author asks whether, in such wounds as this, where the rectum has been torn, it would not be wise to perform a colostomy, thus diverting the feces from the wound, in the same manner as the urine had been diverted by cystostomy. He cites a case of gunshot wound of the rectum in which this procedure was carried out with success.

5. **Lesions of the Vesical Mucosa in Purpura Hemorrhagica as Seen by the Cystoscope.**

Bruni's patient, a man of 31, noticed that after a period of high fever, lasting a few days, he began to pass bloody urine. The hematuria was of the total type but there were no other local or general symptoms or signs whatever. Cystoscopy, however, revealed a striking picture. All over the vesical mucosa, scattered at irregular intervals, there were numerous spots, some round, others irregular in shape. Their color varied from red, through reddish brown, to violet, bluish, and dark blue. There was no local zone of reaction. Their size varied from that of a flea-bite to that of a fifty-centime piece. These spots were clearly due to an extravasation of blood but there was no local cause visible and there had been no previous instrumentation.

A careful examination of the patient then revealed a purpuric eruption on the arms and legs; there was also slight bleeding of the gums. The diagnosis of purpura hemorrhagica was then made and the vesical condition was explained on this basis.

[*Editor's Note:* It is much to be regretted, in view of the excellent description of the local lesions and the beautiful plate accompanying the text, that the author has not presented a more complete clinical picture of the condition. Presumably the glands and spleen were not enlarged, else they would have been noted in the physical examination, but there is no statement that the blood was ever investigated. A full blood count with determination of the coagulation time and estimation of the blood platelets was certainly indicated. We have thus no definite proof that the condition was not one of sepsis with bleeding tendency (cf. onset with fever) or one of the classical forms of "blood disease."]

6. **Aspiration in the Treatment of Chronic Urethritis.**

Cariani describes his urethral aspirator which he presented before the Congress of Urology held in Rome in 1908. He therefore claims priority over Bronner who described his instrument in 1911 and whose last paper appeared in the Revue Clinique d' Urologic, 1913, and was abstracted in this Journal. Cariani feels that both aspiration and lavage in a vacuum can be much more successfully carried out by his instrument than by Bronner's. He believes moreover that the results obtained with aspiration in chronic urethritis are in direct relation with the perfection of the instrument, the precision of the technique, and the type of inflammation.

In chronic blennorrhagic urethritis with persistent discharge aspiration gives brilliant results, but when used alone in the other forms of urethritis it only moderately affects the secretion and the pyuria. Even here, however, it exerts a favorable influence on the urethral infiltrations, rendering them softer, and assists dilatation of the canal. On the other hand, when associated with dilatation, with instillations, and with lavage, the aspiration method may give excellent results.

7. A Technical Point in Catheterizing the Ureters.

Filho advocates the following technic in employing the Albarran cystoscope:

After introducing the instrument and locating one of the ureter mouths, the left for example, catheterize not with the corresponding catheter, but with the opposite one, that is, with the right catheter if the beak of the instrument is pointed upward.

When the catheter is introduced sufficiently up the left ureter the "deflector" is lowered and the cystoscope is turned with the beak directed upward so that the latter swings in the superior semicircle of the bladder. After finding the right ureter opening and catheterizing with the remaining sound, the beak of the instrument is again directed upward, the catheters not being crossed, and the instrument withdrawn.

In this manner we may remove the cystoscope without traumatizing the inferior wall of the posterior urethra, thus safeguarding the important organs that lie in this region.

REVUE CLINIQUE D'UROLOGIE

January, 1914.

1. Periurethral Adenoma (Hypertrophy of the Prostate). By B. Motz.
2. Recurrent Calculi of the Bladder. By Michel Pavone.
3. Penoplasty in Destruction of the Greater Part of the Penis as a Result of Phagedenic Ulcerations. By J. Brault.
4. Treatment of Tumors of the Bladder, Especially Papillomas, by Electrocoagulation. By Drs. Lepoutre and d'Halluin.
5. Contribution to the Study of the Limits of Operability (by Nephrectomy) in Renal Tuberculosis. By J. Abadie.
6. Pathology of the Seminal Vesicles. By M. Palazzoli.

7. Sexual Disturbances of Psychic Origin. A Clinical and Psychological Study. By A. Wizel.
8. Note on the Use of Iodin in the Treatment of Rebellious Urethritides. By B. Motz.

1. Periurethral Adenoma.

Most present-day authors agree with Motz in his conclusions concerning the origin of prostatic hypertrophy. The author has done considerable histological and pathological work on the subject and finds as follows:

1. Contrary to the opinion of Thompson and Launois, according to whom sclerosis is responsible for prostatic hypertrophy, it has been shown by the author that it is really a new formation of glandular tissue which characterizes hypertrophied prostates, and that the development of this tissue really bears a certain relation to the conservation of the vessels.

2. Moreover, in a paper published in collaboration with Perearnau the author has established:

a) That the newly developed masses have their origin in the peri-urethral glands, that the true prostate plays no role whatever in the formation of prostatic hypertrophy but that on the contrary it is more or less atrophied, pushed to the periphery, and constitutes the surgical pseudo-capsule.

b) That prostatectomy by the hypogastric route is merely an enucleation of the benign tumor, of the peri-urethral adenoma which is possible owing to the plane of cleavage which is formed between the tumor and the true prostate.

c) That it is the conservation of the ejaculatory ducts which are crowded to the periphery together with the prostate, which explains the retention of sexual power in certain prostatectomized individuals.

2. Recurrent Calculi of the Bladder.

Pavone finds that neither the operation of hypogastric section nor that of lithotrity can prevent the recurrence of vesical calculi, for this depends entirely on the persistence of the general and local causes of lithiasis. Thus of 52 cases operated on by the author by section there have been 5 recurrences, whereas in 1839 lithotrities there were 92 recidives,—that is to say 10% after section, and almost 5% after lithotrity.

We may hope to prevent the recurrence of vesical calculi by carefully observing all the rules of diet, hygiene, and medication applying in each special case. As regards treatment by operation, lithotrity, owing to the improvements lately introduced into the technic, is the procedure of choice in the great majority of cases, whereas section is the operation of necessity. Moreover, the indications for lithotrity correspond to the contraindications for section. The surgeon should be prepared to practice the one method or the other, according to special indications.

3. **Penoplasty in Destruction of the Greater Part of the Penis as a Result of Phagedenic Ulcerations.**

Brault describes a satisfactory result from performing an autoplasty with two V-flaps thus freeing—or "exhuming," as he calls it—the portion of the penis which remained. He first makes sure in such cases that the phagedenic process is thoroughly under control whether by thermocautery or other local measures, or by the use of 606, etc., if the process is on a syphilitic basis. He then anesthetizes the patient, and prepares two V-flaps, one on the abdomen, above the pubic arch, with the apex pointing upward, and the other involving the scrotum and adjacent parts of the thighs, with the apex of the V pointing downward. In this way the stump of the penis is freed, by cutting the suspensory ligament if necessary, and a sheath is formed for the organ. The raw surfaces are sutured together. At subsequent sittings an existing hypospadias may be corrected and the penis shaped more accurately if desired.

In the case reported, that of an Algerian cavalryman, the anatomical result, at least, was good. Erections, also were satisfactory and painless. The author does not state whether complete sexual power was restored.

4. **Treatment of Tumors of the Bladder, Especially Papillomas, by Electrocoagulation.**

The authors report five cases of papillomata treated by electrocoagulation. In three of the cases the intervention was actually curative to the same extent that an extirpation would have been after hypogastric section. In the fourth case reported recurrences were destroyed little by little. A surgical intervention in this case was out of the question. The patient will have to be followed in order to see whether anything short of a total cystectomy can save him. In the fifth case the authors were able to observe the cessation of hematuria and progressive diminution in the size of the tumors. In this case however a section would have been preferable (large papillomata limited to one portion of the bladder complicated by a diverticulum rendering endovesical manipulations difficult), but the writers hesitated to perform this operation without the active coöperation of the patient.

Electrocoagulation offers the advantages common to all endovesical operations, the chief of which being the avoidance of successive sections as far as the patients are concerned. Moreover the subjects do not have to give up their occupation during the course of treatment.

Of all endovesical methods electrocoagulation seems so far to be the method of choice because it is the simplest, the easiest to execute, and the least harmful in its immediate consequences. The only disadvantage of the method is the necessity of a large number of sittings. Moreover the method should not be used in very big papillomata. Nevertheless this rule may be set aside in special circumstances, such as in the authors' second case, which shows that very good results can be obtained even in a rather large tumor.

5. Contribution to the Study of the Limits of Operability (by Nephrectomy) in Renal Tuberculosis.

Abadie hopes that her contribution will help solve the problem: "Up to what point are we justified in removing a kidney known to be tuberculous with a hope of cure?" The case she reports is that of a woman who for 3 years had suffered from hematuria and from lumbar pains worse on the left side. The corresponding kidney was increased in size and tender on palpation. Endovesical separation of the urines showed the left kidney to be functionating poorly and disclosed the presence of tubercle bacilli in the urine from that side. A nephrectomy was proposed and declined.

When seen again the patient had fever, the local condition was the same but the woman had become pregnant, had enlarged cervical glands, and had signs of congestion at the right apex. The pregnancy resulted in a still-birth. The diagnosis of tuberculous pyonephrosis of the left kidney was now made, nephrostomy performed, much pus evacuated, and drainage instituted. A second separation of the urines was now done and showed that the right kidney was still functionating normally. An extracapsular nephrectomy of the left kidney was then attempted but found impossible so that the organ had to be removed intracapsularly piecemeal. The wound healed kindly, however, no fistula resulting. Four years later the patient was in good health, had returned to her work, her other tuberculous lesions had healed, and her urine, injected into a guinea pig, caused no tuberculosis.

The author concludes from this case that even in the presence of a generalized tuberculosis (unless the pulmonary condition is far advanced) we may hope for a radical cure by nephrectomy, provided always that the other kidney is capable of carrying on the functions of excretion.

6. Pathology of the Seminal Vesicles.

It is impossible to do justice to Palazzoli's article in an abstract of ordinary length. The author feels that the seminal vesicles have been neglected by anatomists, physiologists, and pathologists alike. In this installment he begins with a comprehensive historical section and then proceeds to take up the macroscopic anatomy of the subject. He accepts Picker's classification (XIVth session of the XVIIIth International Congress of Medicine, London, 1913) of the various types of seminal tubules and agrees that the different forms of disease follow the changes in shape of these organs. The article is freely illustrated, the figures borrowed from Picker being especially interesting.

8. Note on the Use of Iodin in the Treatment of Rebellious Urethritides.

Motz describes the advantages of the iodin treatment of rebellious urethral lesions of non-gonoccocal nature. Up to the present, the drug has been used exclusively by direct application through the urethroscope. The author hopes to do away with the necessity for the constant introduction of this instrument by using the iodin in the form of instillation or injection. It is the soft superficial infiltrations of the anterior or posterior urethra which finally yield to the iodin—but not to any other—treatment.

Motz employs three formulae for the tincture of iodin, made up as follows:

A. Strong solution:—

Iodin	1.00
Potassium iodid	0.50
Alcohol (60%)	40.00

B. Medium solution:—

Iodin	0.75
Potassium iodid	0.50
Alcohol (60%)	40.00

C. Weak solution:—

Iodin	0.50
Potassium iodid	0.50
Alcohol (60%)	40.00

The strong solution is only to be used in instillations into the anterior urethra of subjects whose mucosa has become keratinized. The medium solution is to be used for instillations into the anterior and posterior urethra. The weak solution is to be used for instillations or even for injections into the anterior urethra. Instillations should be made with a half c.c. of the solution; injections with 3 c.c. The strong and weak solutions cause only temporary discomfort. The inflammatory reaction is minimal. In order to determine the sensitiveness of the urethra it is wise always to commence with the weak solution, applied every three or four days.

The author has also employed Lytinol, a complex compound of iodin, benzol, and aluminium, introduced by Dr. Awerbuch of St. Petersburg (See Zeitsch. für Urologie, VIII, 1, 1911, article by Bäumer, abstracted in this Journal). This substance is very useful in superficial, non-gonococcal infections. Its use is to be preceded by a copious antiseptic lavage. Motz always insists upon this before commencing any form of iodin treatment. He prefers 1:2000 potassium permanganate as a disinfectant for this purpose. Lytinol may be used either in the form of an injection or as a permanent dressing. In the former case 4 c.c. of a 30% solution may be retained in the canal for 2 or 3 minutes. As a permanent dressing, on the other hand, a 5 to 10% solution of Lytinol may be employed for a period of two to three hours. Lytinol mixes readily with water and it is the aqueous solution which is made use of.

THE AMERICAN JOURNAL OF UROLOGY, VENEREAL AND SEXUAL DISEASES

WILLIAM J. ROBINSON, M.D., EDITOR

VOL. X JUNE, 1914. No. 6

THE DIAGNOSIS AND TREATMENT OF EARLY MALIGNANT DISEASE OF THE PROSTATE

By HUGH H. YOUNG, M.A., M.D.[1]

Associate Professor of Urological Surgery, Johns Hopkins University, Baltimore, Md., U.S.A.

THE subject which has been allotted to us would seem to be intended to include both carcinoma and sarcoma of the prostate, but as no case of early sarcoma has ever been reported (to my knowledge), and as I have personally only seen a few cases—and all late—I have decided to confine this paper—which must of necessity be abbreviated—to the subject of early diagnosis and radical cure of cancer of the prostate.

In order to arrive at an idea of the symptoms and findings on which an early diagnosis of cancer of the prostate can be based, I have carefully collected all of the cases of cancer of the prostate which might be considered as being early cases when admitted. I find among my records twelve such cases, which may be divided in three classes, viz.:

I. Those in which the only pathological process present is cancer; six cases.

II. Those in which cancer is associated with hypertrophy or benign adenoma; five cases.

III. A case of chronic prostatitis with small area of cancer in it.

Class I furnishes the most satisfactory group for study, and we find the following:

Age, between 60 and 64 years	1 case
Age, between 65 and 69 years	2 cases
Age, between 70 and 74 years	1 case
Age, between 75 and 79 years	1 case

Duration of symptoms before admission:

6 months . . .	1 case
1 year . . .	3 cases
2 years . . .	1 case
3 years . . .	2 cases

The initial symptoms were as follows:

Frequency of urination	1 case, duration	2 years
Difficulty of urination	1 case, duration	1 year
Urgency of urination	1 case, duration	1 year
Pain in penis during urination . . .	1 case, duration	1 year
Frequency and difficulty of urination . .	2 cases, duration each	3 years

Subsequent symptoms were present as follows: pain in the penis and perineum came on two years later in one case. None of the other five patients suffered at all from pain. Hematuria was never present in any of the six cases.

In one case the catheter life was begun eighteen months after the initial difficulty of urination, and was followed for eighteen months before admission. The other five patients had never used the catheter.

There were apparently no other symptoms present in these six cases, and a consideration of those presented shows that there was nothing diagnostic or even suggestive presented. The surprising thing is that in four of the six cases symptoms had been present for periods of two years or more. The fact that careful pathological examinations of the lateral and median portions of these prostates failed to reveal any benign adenomatous hypertrophy seems to point to carcinoma as being the sole cause of the obstructive symptoms in these cases.

The complete absence of hematuria at any time shows, as I have pointed out before, the error of expecting this as an early symptom. It is distinctly more common in benign hypertrophies (except possibly late in the disease).

Class II. The five cases in which cancer and benign hypertrophy existed together in the same prostate were as follows:

Case I, age 60 years, beginning with frequency 3 years before.

Case II, age 69 years, beginning with frequency 6 months before.

Case III age 75 years, beginning with sudden complete retention 10 months before.

Case IV, age 78 years, beginning with frequency 4 years before.

Case V, age 67 years, beginning with frequency and difficulty 2½ years before.

In Case I there was pain in the end of the penis before and during urination, and in Case V a sciatica. In none of the others was there ever any pain present. Hematuria did not appear in any case.

Regular catheterization was necessary in Case V for one year; in Case II for ten months, and in Case IV for four months. In Case I supra-pubic drainage became necessary three years after onset.

Class III. The case in which chronic prostatitis was present along with a nodule of cancer, was a man, 61 years of age, who had for fifteen years had symptoms of irritation in the deep urethra and attacks of frequency of urination. Catheterization was never necessary, and hematuria and pain were never present.

In conclusion, it seems from a study of the above early cases (and other later cases) that the symptomatology of cancer of the prostate in the early stages is almost identical with that of benign hypertrophy, so that we must look entirely to a careful physical examination to furnish suspicion of cancer.

The examination. There was nothing in the appearance of any of these twelve patients to suggest malignant disease; they were not emaciated, nor were they suffering pain, with the exception of four cases, and in these it was not severe. The urine was free from blood in all cases.

In the six cases not associated with hypertrophy the size of the prostate was described as considerably enlarged in three cases, moderately enlarged in two cases, and slightly enlarged in one case. The surface was smooth in two cases, rough in three cases, nodular in three cases. Here we have in six cases conditions which should always make one suspicious of cancer; for the benign adenomatous prostates, unless associated with considerable inflammation or with calculi of the prostate, are nearly always smooth, though they may be lobulated. The consistence was described as very hard in all of the six cases not associated with hypertrophy, and in some was said to be "stony hard." In five cases both lobes were involved, but in one case the left half of the prostate was normal. In this interesting case (in which an urgency of urination had been present one year) the right lobe was enlarged, very hard and rough, the induration extending to the median line, where it ended abruptly, forming a straight edge well elevated above the normal left half of the prostate. The lower portion of the right seminal vesicle was involved as was the posterior part of the membranous urethra. The contrast between the two halves of the prostate here was most sharply defined. In one case there was a hard nodule in each lobe, which was otherwise soft on each side. Two years later the whole prostate was rough, irregular, very hard, and greatly enlarged. In the other four cases, although in two symptoms had been present only one year, the prostate was completely invaded by cancer on both sides, although the vesicles were mostly free.

The five cases associated with hypertrophy are interesting:

In Case I (J. T. Y., No. 463) the prostate was considerably enlarged, smooth, rather hard in consistence. Microscopic study showed benign hypertrophy associated with prostatitis on both sides with only one small area of cancer in prostatic tissue which was the seat of prostatitis.

In Case II (T. C. S., No. 2750), in which symptoms had been present only six months, the left lobe was only slightly enlarged, smooth, and elastic. On the surface of the right lobe there was a prominent lobe 1 cm. in size, which was quite hard, but seemed elastic on pressure. (This proved, however, to be entirely cancerous.) The right lobe was otherwise very little enlarged, and the seminal vesicles were not indurated, but nevertheless cancer was present in the lower portion of the left seminal vesicle. The left lobe when removed was found to be a benign hypertrophy, the right being cancerous.

In Case III (W. J. R., No. 1779), the prostate was moderately enlarged and generally indurated (but not stony), with three very hard nodules present, one in the median line near the apex, one at the upper end of the left lateral lobe, and one near the apex of the right lateral lobe. Seminal vesicles negative. At operation a layer of cancer beneath the posterior capsule was found on the left side, beneath which was a benign hypertrophied lobe, on the right side and also in the median portion benign hypertrophied lobes were removed.

In Case IV (J. R., admitted June 26, 1905) the prostate was moderately enlarged, smooth, the right lobe was elastic and only slightly indurated. Operation showed a posterior layer of cancer, with a hypertrophied lobe beneath. The left lobe was smaller and softer, and proved to be benign hypertrophy.

In Case V (E. G. W., No. 206) the prostate was considerably enlarged, smooth, but very hard. Examination showed a posterior subcapsular layer of cancer, with benign hypertrophy in front of it on both sides.

A review of these five cases shows that the presence of hypertrophy of the lateral lobes generally gives an elasticity to the prostate on deep pressure which is very deceptive. In these cases a small layer or nodule of cancer lying between the capsule and an hypertrophied lobe may be compressible on deep pressure. More delicate palpation, and particularly palpation upon a cystoscope in the urethra, will often show the real induration of the local carcinomatous area.

These localized areas of induration or nodulation should always be suspected, and subjected to early perineal operation.

The case characterized by a small nodule of cancer in a prostate which was the seat of a chronic prostatitis of fifteen years' standing, showed, on rectal examination, a prostate smooth, slightly indurated, and not tender. The small nodule was not detected, and was only found accidentally when the stained sections of the tissue removed were examined.

The clinical examination of the seminal vesicles in these twelve early cases shows no definite invasion of these structures. In one case only was there an induration for a short distance in the region of one vesicle, but subsequent pathological examination (after radical operation) showed that the carcinoma had not penetrated the seminal vesicle as supposed but lay between it and the excised trigone, an area of cancer 1 cm. long being present. In the two other cases in which the radical operation was carried out, only the juxta-prostatic ends of the seminal vesicles and vasa deferentia were invaded.

The vesical mucosa was normal in all of these cases, and no invasion of the trigone was present as shown by the cystoscope and at operation.

The seven cases in which no coexistent hypertrophy of the prostate was present showed, on cystoscopic examination, only a small median bar, with no intravesical enlargement of the lateral lobes. In one case the median portion formed a small sessile lobe, and one case showed both a median bar and a slight right lateral enlargement.

The characteristic picture, then, in early cancer of the prostate is a small bar, unaccompanied by marked lateral intravesical enlargement.

In one case a carcinomatous constriction of the prostatic urethra was present, requiring dilatation before cystoscopy was possible, but there was no evidence of ulceration of the urethra in any case.

In later cases stricture of the prostatic urethra is not an

uncommon finding, and is to be considered very suggestive of cancer.

The *diagnosis* of early carcinoma of the prostate is principally based on the finding of great induration in a portion of the prostate, as shown by our cases. It may occur as one or more small nodules, or lobules which may be prominent or imbedded in the prostatic tissue, but apparently always palpable per rectum. In later cases one whole lobe, or both lobes, may be involved, but the disease apparently remains well encapsulated for a fairly long period, and the line of progress is upward, beneath the fascia of

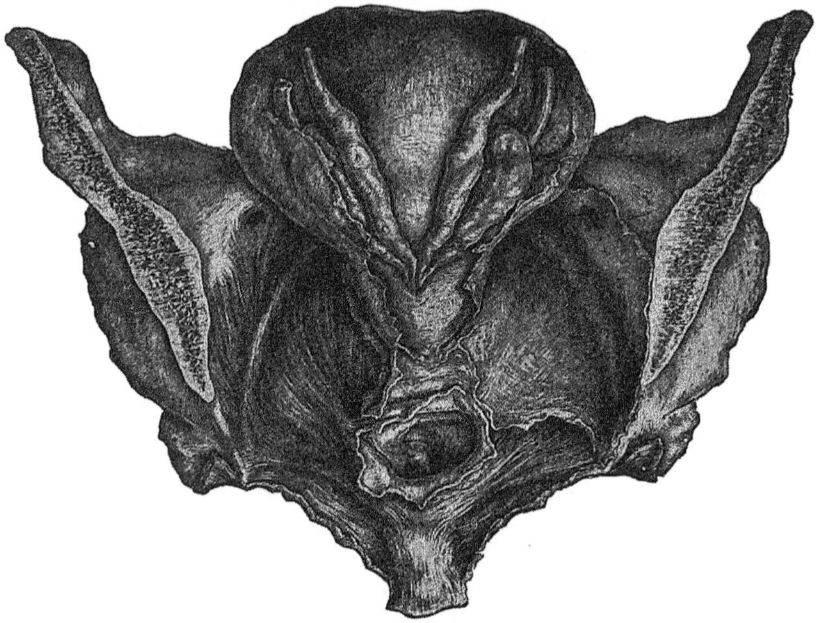

FIG. I. The aponeurosis of Dénonvilliers, which covers the posterior surface of prostate, seminal vesicles, and vasa deferentia: here partly removed to show these structures. (After Deaver.)

Dénonvilliers (which forms the posterior capsule of the prostate and seminal vesicles, Fig. 1), the ejaculatory ducts and the structures between the lower ends of the vasa deferentia and the bladder being invaded after the cancer-cells pass beyond the limits of the prostate. Induration immediately above the prostate and easily palpable, with a finger in the rectum and a cystoscope in the urethra, as a hard subtrigonal thickening is of great diagnostic value. In later cases this "intervesicular plateau" of induration becomes more and more pronounced, but it is remarkable how long the upper portions of the seminal vesicles and vesical mucosa are free from invasion.

A careful study of about 200 cases of carcinoma of the prostate—most of them in advanced stages—shows that ulceration of the vesical mucosa and intravesical tumour outgrowth are both quite rare except, possibly, extremely late in the disease. The same thing is true of the rectum, which I have found ulcerated and invaded in very few cases. The two layers of Dénonvillier's fascia (the remains of a peritoneal process which extends to the perineum in fetal life, and which probably have separate systems

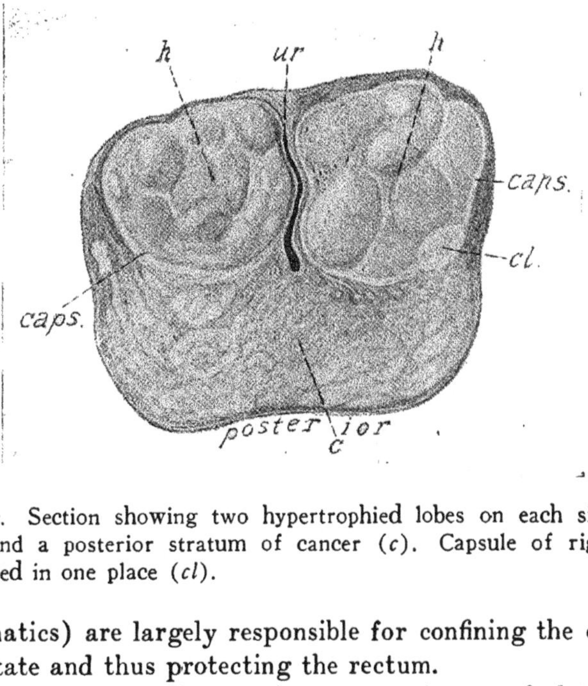

FIG. 2. Section showing two hypertrophied lobes on each side of the urethra, and a posterior stratum of cancer (*c*). Capsule of right lateral lobe invaded in one place (*cl*).

of lymphatics) are largely responsible for confining the cancer to the prostate and thus protecting the rectum.

Another remarkable fact is that carcinoma of the prostate is characteristically not a very ulcerating form of the disease, as evinced by the rarity of the ulcer of the urethra, bladder, and confinement of the progress of the disease in most cases for a long time to the tissues between the rectum and the bladder—although the involvement there may be great.

To recapitulate, marked induration ("stony hardness") either localized or diffuse in the prostate is to be suspected in men past 50 years of age, particularly when there is no history of a long-standing chronic prostatitis (and even sometimes then, as shown by one of my cases, in which a small nodule of cancer was found in a lateral lobe, the seat of chronic prostatitis).

The absence of hematuria is not specially a symptom of cancer of the prostate. Pain, while suggestive, is also often absent in early cases, though generally present and almost pathognomonic later on.

The presence of benign hypertrophy of the lateral and median portions of the prostate, which occurs in half of the cases, should not lead to error, but one must remember that the elasticity of the soft adenomatous masses may often rob the posterior nodule or layer of carcinoma of its sensation of induration to the finger in the rectum particularly on deep pressure. The cancer generally lies in a subcapsular stratum back of the hypertrophied lateral lobes as shown in Fig. 2.

I have several times been deceived in cases where the cystoscope showed large intravesical lobes, and although the rectal finger detected marked induration immediately beneath the capsule in some portion of the prostate, yet the prostate as a whole was so elastic as to persuade one that the whole process was benign. It is only by being continually suspicious of marked induration, even if confined to a small nodule, that early diagnosis can be expected and radical cures obtained.

The Radical Cure. In October, 1905, the writer published in the *Johns Hopkins Hospital Bulletin* an operation for the radical cure of cancer of the prostate. Since then further details and cases have been furnished in other articles.[1]

In the first communication on the subject a thorough study of the literature was presented which showed that whereas various operations had been employed in cancer of the prostate, no systematic radical procedure, coupled with plastic repair of the defect produced, had ever been recommended.

The plan and scope of the operation was based on pathological studies which showed that if a radical cure was to be expected the seminal vesicles and most of the trigone, with the intervening tissues, would have to be excised in one piece with the whole prostate (capsule, urethra, internal sphincter, cuff of bladder, and part of membranous urethra).

The eight years which have elapsed since our first publica-

[1] *The Johns Hopkins Hospital Reports*, vol. xiv, 1906; *Annals of Surgery*, December 1909; *Annales des maladies des organes génito-urinaires*, 1910; *Transactions of the International Association of Urology*, London, 1911.

tion have only added further proof of the correctness of the assertions then made, viz., that the carcinoma of the prostate was prevented, for a more or less considerable period, from spreading downward or posteriorly by the firm capsule and the pelvic fascias of Dénonvilliers, and that the first line of invasion beyond the prostate was into the space immediately above the prostate be-

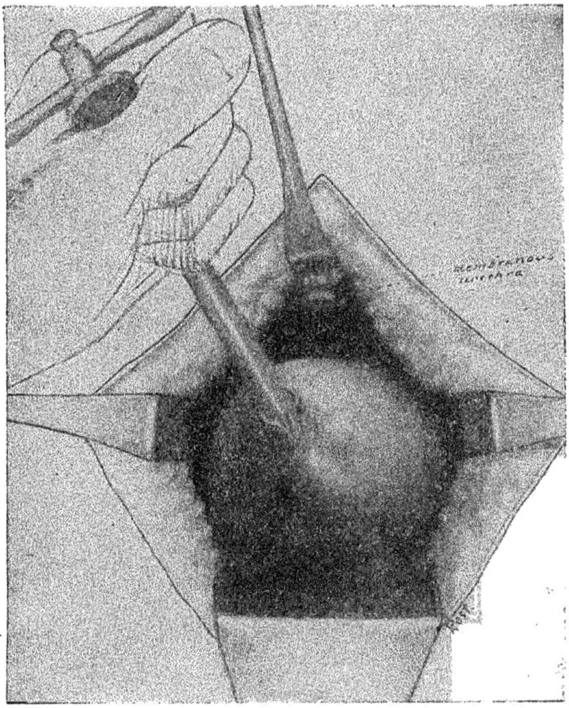

FIG. 3. Transverse section of membranous urethra—anterior and posterior surfaces of prostate freed.

tween the trigone and the seminal vesicles, and the fascia of Dénonvilliers, which covers them.

Technic of the Radical Operation. The patient is placed in the exaggerated lithotomy position, and an inverted V perineal incision made, as in the operation for simple hypertrophy of the prostate, the successive steps of which are followed until the tractor has been inserted through a urethrotomy wound of the membranous urethra and the posterior surface of the prostate has been exposed, largely by blunt dissection. If there is then any doubt in the mind of the operator as to the malignant nature of the disease, an incision is made through the capsule and a section of the prostatic lobe removed for examination, frozen sections being made if necessary to establish the diagnosis, when either the simple prostatectomy for hypertrophy or the radical operation for cancer can be performed as the case requires. In the case of cancer the next step after exposing the posterior surface of the prostate is to free

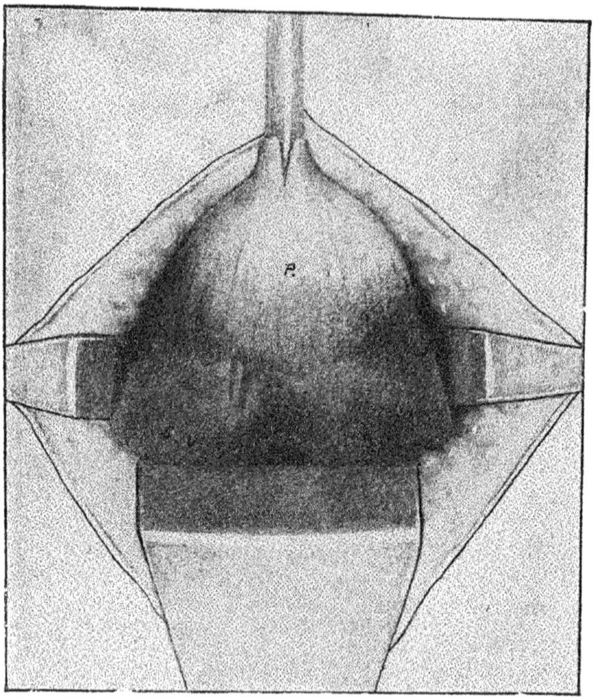

FIG. 4. Exposure of seminal vesicles from behind.

the lateral adhesions of the prostate and also the seminal vesicles as much as possible by blunt dissection; then the membranous urethra is divided in front of the tractor, as shown in Fig. 3. The handle of the tractor is then depressed markedly and the pubo-prostatic ligaments are divided with scissors close up to the anterior surface of the prostate, efforts being previously made to push away the anterior plexus of veins by blunt dissection. Fairly abundant hemorrhage usually follows, and should be controlled as much as possible by clamps and then a gauze pack, which should be held tightly against the posterior surface of the pubes and the triangular ligament by means of a retractor. The seminal vesicles should be freed further (Fig. 4).

The prostate is drawn outward as far as possible, thus exposing the anterior surface of the bladder, which should be punctured, as shown in Fig. 5, just above the prostato-vesical juncture. This wound is now enlarged on each side by scissors, the line of division being close to the prostato-vesical juncture, until the trigone is exposed, as shown in Fig. 6. With a scalpel a

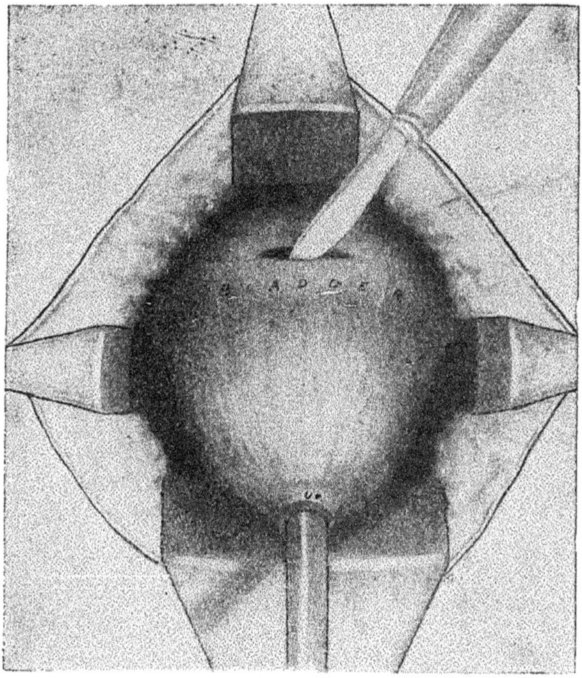

FIG. 5. Incision into anterior wall of bladder just above prostate.

curved incision is made across the trigone, thus leaving the upper angles of the trigone intact, and being careful to do no injury to the ureters. By blunt dissection the seminal vesicles are then exposed, as shown in Fig. 7, and the vasa deferentia picked up with a blunt hook and divided with scissors as high up as possible. (In doing this it should be remembered that the vasa deferentia pass around the lower end of the ureters.) The deeper attachments of the seminal vesicles are then freed, and the mass, consisting of the prostate, urethra, cuff of the bladder, seminal vesicles, and about 5 cm. of the vasa deferentia, removed in one piece. Hemorrhage is again encountered in the last step above described, owing to the fact that the prostatic plexus of veins, which passes up along each side of the prostate, is closely attached to the lateral border of the seminal vesicle; but this can easily be controlled by ligatures or long clamps. The bleeding which comes from the vesical wound is controlled by the subsequent sutures, which are placed so as to anastomose the bladder with the membranous urethra, and completely close the vesical wound. This is

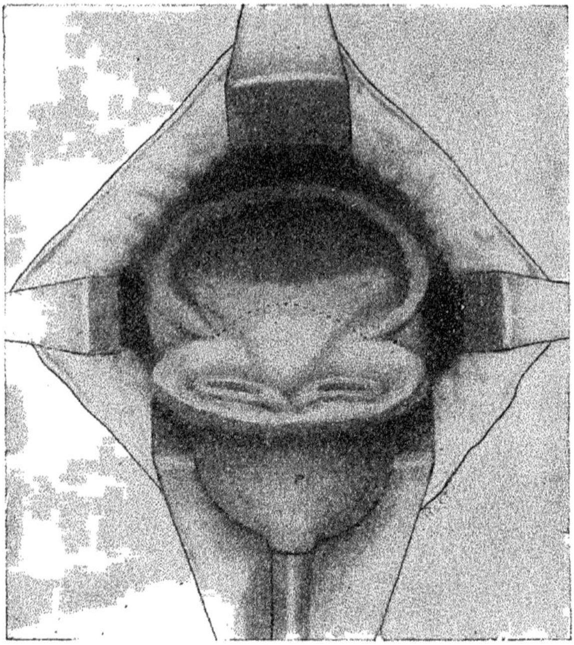

FIG. 6. Exposure and division of trigone.

readily accomplished, as shown in Figs. 8 and 9. As seen here, the anterior wall of the bladder is drawn down and fastened to the stump of the membranous urethra by means of interrupted catgut sutures. After forming the anastomosis with the urethra a considerable vesical wound is left posteriorly, but it is easily closed by transverse sutures. I have found it best to use an occasional suture of silkworm gut in order to take care of the tension which is present. The ends of these are left long enough to emerge from the wound, so that they can be removed two or three weeks later. A retained rubber catheter, which should be inserted before the vesico-urethral anastomosis is made, is fastened to the glans penis with adhesive plaster. After placing light gauze packing in the depths of the wound the levator ani muscles are approximated with two or three interrupted sutures of catgut, so as to protect the rectum again post-operative necrosis, and the external wound is almost completely closed with interrupted sutures of catgut. In some instances I found it difficult to place ligatures around hemostatic clamps which were deeply placed, and have therefore not removed the clamps, but allowed them to emerge

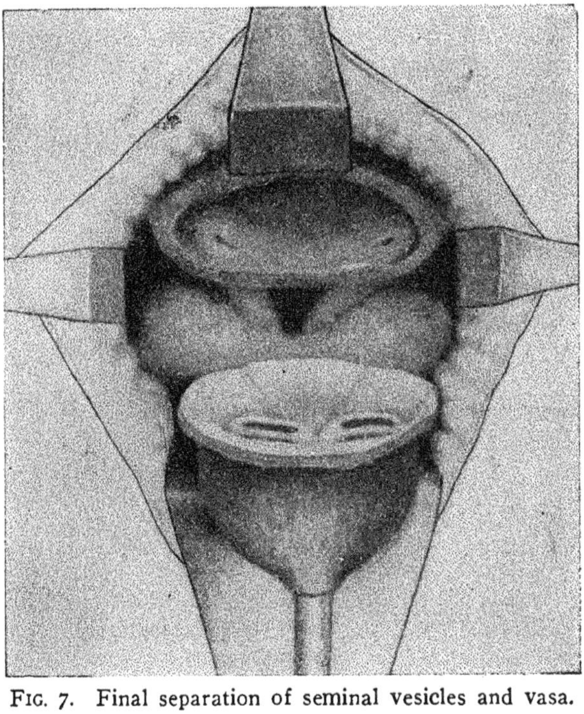

FIG. 7. Final separation of seminal vesicles and vasa.

with the gauze packing from the anterior angle of the wound (they were removed twenty-four hours later). If careful attention has been given to the prevention of hemorrhage and an infusion has been begun early in the operation, there should be little or no shock.

The treatment during convalescence is very similar to that employed after perineal prostatectomy, viz., water in abundance, urotropin, the patient allowed to sit up as soon as possible, daily irrigations of the bladder with small amounts of boracic acid solution. The gauze packs are removed in two or three days, and the urethral catheter in a week, but the silkworm-gut sutures are allowed to loosen and no attempt is made to extract them forcibly for about three weeks. No difficulty is experienced in getting a good approximation and wound healing, and little or no stricture formation has been encountered at the point of vesico-urethral anastomosis. Sounding is not necessary. My patients have all had incontinence, but none have had persistent fistulæ.

The cases on which I have carried out this procedure are as follows:

Case I. *Carcinoma of prostate. Radical operation. Excision of entire prostate, seminal vesicles, ampullæ of vasa deferentia and cuff of bladder. Recovery. Lived nine months. Died of perivesicular infection following litholapaxy.*

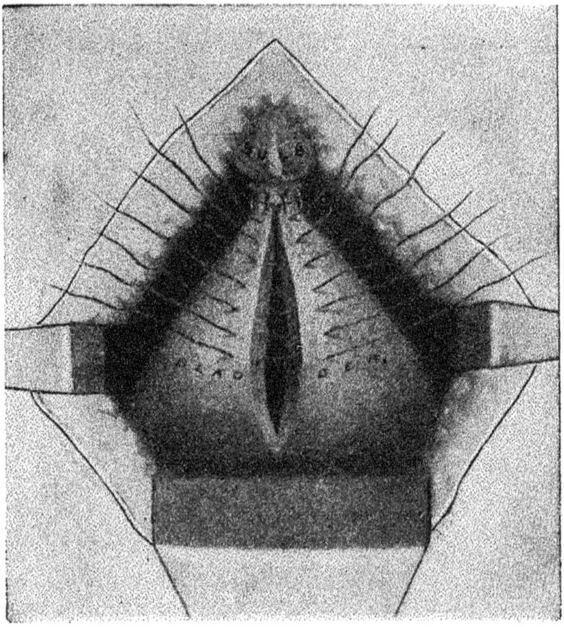

FIG. 8. The anastomosis of anterior wall of bladder to urethra has been made. The rest of vesical opening is being closed.

E. J. G., S. No. 15929. Aged 70; married. Admitted April 1, 1904. Eleven months ago patient began to have pain in the urethra at the end of urination. During the next three months the pains increased and he began treatment with an osteopath, receiving prostatic massage. He grew steadily worse and soon began to have pain in the perineum and thighs. Four months ago consulted a surgeon who performed a Bottini operation with partial benefit. He now has to void every fifteen minutes and severe pain is constantly present. On rectal examination the prostate is considerably enlarged, irregular, nodular, hard, and the capsule is apparently adherent to the rectum. The right seminal vesicle is palpable, apparently distended but not indurated. In the region of the left seminal vesicle there is an oblong mass of induration continuous with the prostate, but the upper end of the seminal vesicle seems free. Catheterization is very difficult, filiforms being required. Residual urine 400 c.c. The cystoscope shows no intravesical enlargement of the lateral lobes and only slight elevation of the median portion of the pros-

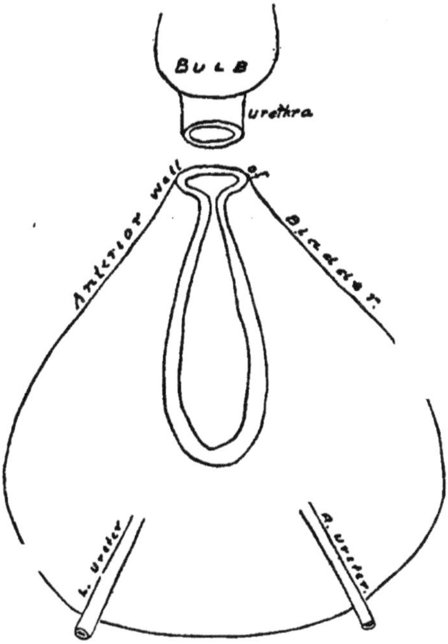

FIG. 9. Diagram showing plan of vesico-urethral anastomosis.

tate. Diagnosis of carcinoma was made on marked induration of the prostate extending into the region of the left seminal vesicle and the absence of intravesical enlargement. After preliminary treatment (catheter, hydrotherapy, etc.), the radical operation was performed. Specimen removed is shown in Figs. 10 and 11.

As shown here, the seminal vesicles, intravesical and subtrigonal tissues were removed in one piece with the prostate and membranous urethra. No difficulty was experienced. There was

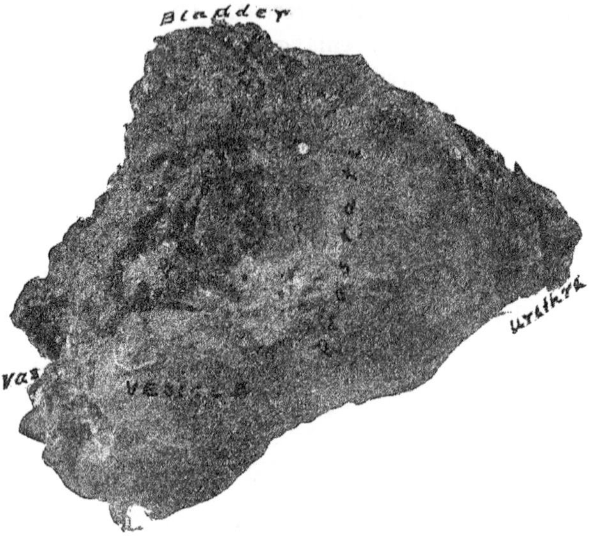

FIG. 10. Photograph of specimen, Case I. Side view.

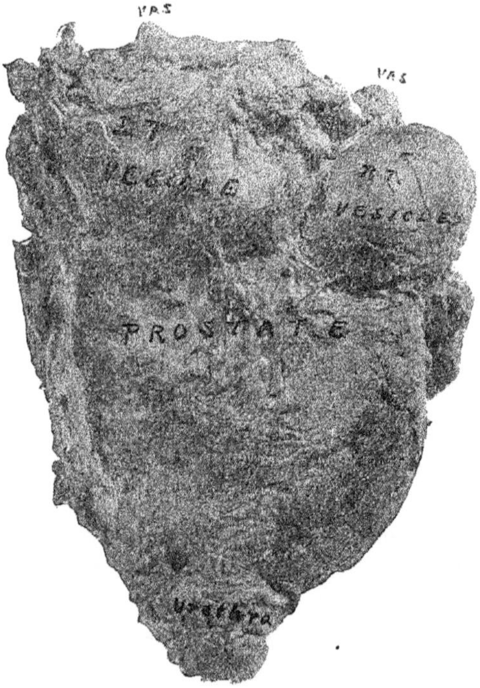

FIG. 11. Photograph of specimen, Case I. Posterior view.

only a moderate amount of hemorrhage and the anastomosis between bladder and membranous urethra was easily performed, silk sutures being used (a mistake to do so). A large rubber catheter was fastened in the urethra and the patient was returned to ward in good condition. The specimen (which, along with the operation and microscopic examination, is described in full in the *Johns Hopkins Hospital Reports*, vol. xiv, p. 506) showed adenocarcinoma of the entire prostate, which had extended into the tissues beneath the anterior portion of the trigone adjacent to the ejaculatory ducts and seminal vesicles, but had not penetrated into their cavities. In the muscle of the anterior part of the trigone several lymphatics containing cancer cells were seen, but at the upper limit the tissues seemed healthy everywhere.

The convalescence was satisfactory but slow. In two weeks the patient was walking about and all the stitches had been removed (apparently). Only a little urine came through the perineum. On the sixteenth day the perineal fistula was healed completely and urine came freely through the penis. On the twenty-third day the patient was discharged from the hospital in good condition. At night he could hold his urine for several hours until the desire to urinate came on, when he arose and voided. Did not wet the bed at night. During the day urine dribbled away.

December 22. Patient improved steadily for five months, the intervals between urinations becoming long and incontinence gradually diminishing. In October he began to suffer pain at the end of the penis during urination. He has now incontinence during the day, but none at night. A silver catheter meets an obstruction about the triangular ligament, but filiforms pass with ease and dilating followers are easily introduced. A stone is felt in the bladder and the cystoscope shows two small calculi in a shallow pouch on the right side of the bladder and, just behind the triangular ligament, a small stone attached to a silk suture which was easily seen.

December 23. Operation. Litholapaxy. Two stones in the bladder were easily crushed and evacuated, but to engage the calculus which was attached to the ligature it was found necessary to pass through the urethra a long curved clamp with which the ligature was withdrawn; but in doing so a tear was made in the mucous membrane. Following the operation there was tenderness in the suprapubic region and an extensive perivesical infection developed from which the patient died one month after the operation.

Autopsy showed the bladder contracted, but excellent union between it and the urethra. There was no evidence of recurrence in the bladder or region of the prostate, and no glandular metastases were to be made out; but just back of the bladder a small indurated area, about 1 cm. in size, was present, and a section of this showed carcinoma. There was present a large perivesicular abscess cavity.

Note.—This case showed the necessity of using some other form of suture material than silk, and for the next case catgut alone was employed (also to my regret). It was interesting to note that although the specimen showed after the operation that the prognosis was not good because the lymphatics above the prostate were involved, at autopsy, almost ten months after the radical operation, only a very small area of carcinoma was present (about 1 cm. in diameter and in the tissues back of the bladder, which was healthy), and the patient had been entirely relieved of the severe pain and the obstruction to urination.

Case II. *Carcinoma of the prostate involving the lower portion of the seminal vesicles. Radical operation. Death six weeks later—nephritis. Autopsy showed no remaining carcinoma.*

W. R., S. No. 16675. Aged 64; married. Admitted September 14, 1904. Onset with increased frequency of urination three years ago. Complete retention of urine for the first time three weeks ago. On admission patient voided ten to twelve times during the day; no pain present. No history of hematuria. Has lost very little weight. For the past week catheterization has been necessary.

Rectal. The prostate is moderately enlarged, smooth, hard, but not nodular. There is no enlargement or induration in the region of either seminal vesicle, but in the space between the two there is a distinct plateau of induration extending between 1 and 2 cm. above the limits of the prostate. Above this the tissues feel soft. No glands. Rectum negative.

Cystoscopic. A catheter passes easily. Bladder capacity 300 c.c. The cystoscope shows a slight intravesical enlargement of the median portion which is continuous with an elevation of the anterior part of the trigone. Lateral lobes very slightly enlarged. Mucosa normal. With finger in rectum and cystoscope in urethra there is induration beneath the trigone and considerable thickening of the sub-urethral portion of the prostate. The diagnosis of carcinoma was made upon induration, sub-urethral thickening, and the absence of intravesical hypertrophy.

September 23. Total excision of prostate, seminal vesicles, 5 cm. of the vasa deferentia, most of the trigone. When the trigone was exposed palpation showed an indurated condition of the trigone which seemed to extend up to the two ureteral orifices. It was thought advisable to excise both ureteral papillæ and a portion of the posterior wall of the bladder immediately above the trigone. The upper part of the intramural portion of the ureter on both sides was left undisturbed. The anastomosis between the bladder and membranous urethra was easily performed, care being taken not to include the partially excised ureters in the suture.

Examination of the specimen showed that the seminal vesicles and upper portions of the vasa deferentia were normal, and that the trigone, which seemed indurated, contained no carcinoma (*Johns Hopkins Hospital Reports*, vol. xiv, p. 511), and that it was unnecessary to excise the ureteral papillae. Catgut was alone used as a suture material.

Convalescence. Patient convalesced poorly; nausea considerable. The wound broke down completely, leaving a large unhealthy cavity. At the end of three weeks he began to fail gradually, and died on November 8, forty-six days after the operation.

Autopsy. Anatomical diagnosis—perineal wound diphtheritic, cystitis, ureteritis, and pyelitis. Chronic diffuse nephritis, cardiac hypertrophy, and dilatation. Chronic myocarditis, endocarditis, and emphysema of the lungs. Chronic perihepatitis, splenitis, and pancreatitis. The anterior wall of the bladder was found to be continuous with the urethra, sutured portion in this region having united. The posterior sutures had broken down. The right ureteral orifice was covered by a small calcareous mass. The left ureteral orifice could not be found. Acute ureteritis was present on both sides, evidently an ascending infection. Careful examination failed to reveal carcinoma anywhere in the pelvic tissues or in other portions of the bladder. Numerous microscopic sections were made and showed no evidence of carcinoma.

Note.—From the careful study of the specimen removed at operation and the autopsy it is evident that the malignant disease had been completely removed. The excision of the upper portion of the trigone and lower ends of the ureters was not necessary and probably led to the ascending renal infection which caused the death of the patient. The use of catgut proved a mistake, as it led to a rapid breaking down of the wound. The prognosis for a radical cure in this case should have been excellent.

Case III. *Cancer of the prostate involving the seminal vesicles and anterior part of the trigone. Radical operation. Recovery. Restoration of urination through urethra. Patient apparently well for nearly three years. Died over three years after the operation. Autopsy showed recurrence.*

S. R. B., Of. No. 829. Aged 65; widowed. Admitted February 4, 1905. Onset four years ago with increased frequency of urination, which has gradually increased until he now voids every few minutes. Never hematuria nor complete retention of urine. For two years pain in the left hip and knee. Constant pain in the back, perineum, and rectum. No loss of weight.

Rectal. The prostate is considerably enlarged, smooth, very hard. In the upper end on each side is an indurated mass occupying the area of the seminal vesicle and between the two is a small indurated plateau. It is apparently easy to reach above the area of induration everywhere. The rectum is negative. No enlarged glands.

Cystoscopic. Residual urine 500 c.c. Moderate median bar, slight lateral enlargement. No clefts. No evidence of involvement of the trigone. Vesical mucosa normal. With finger in rectum and cystoscope in urethra considerable sub-trigonal and sub-urethral thickening felt.

The diagnosis of carcinoma was made on the great hardness, involvement of the seminal vesicles, absence of intravesical prostatic outgrowths and pain.

February 16. Radical operation. The lower end of the left ureter was unintentionally removed with the specimen and it was found loose in the space behind the bladder. This accident was due to the use of straight scissors instead of curved ones while dividing the wall of the bladder, the incision going up much too high on the left side. The incision across the trigone was made with a knife and the lower end of the right ureter was spared. The divided left ureter was transplanted into a higher portion of the bladder by simply pushing a sharp clamp through from the inside and drawing the ureter into the bladder, where it was held by two intravesical catgut and one extravesical silk sutures. The bladder was easily drawn down and anastomosed with the stump of the urethra and the rest of the wound closed with alternate catgut and silkworm-gut sutures, one end of each of the latter sutures being left long so as to project from the wound to facilitate subsequent removal.

Examination of the specimen showed that the left ureteral ridge and 1.5cm. of the lower end of the left ureter had been removed with the trigone, prostate, prostatic urethra, seminal vesicles, and 4 cm. of the vasa deferentia in one piece. Sections of the upper portion of both seminal vesicles were negative for carcinoma, but the vasa deferentia were filled with cancer-cells near the upper limit, and although the bladder muscle was negative the fat immediately beneath it showed small cancer-cells. Microscopically the specimen is adeno-carcinoma, in places carcinoma solidum.

The convalescence was satisfactory with the exception of a severe pressure slough on the back, due to a hard sand-bag at operation. The perineal wound healed in about two months. During the day there was incontinence, but at night he was able to retain 450 c.c. of urine and to arise and void without wetting the bed. No stricture present.

March 12, 1906—Letter: 'It is now thirteen months since operation. I now weigh 167 pounds, appetite and digestion good. Fistula is healed. Urine passes through penis, but I have no control during the day.'

April 15, 1908—Letter from son: "Father died March 29. For some time he has had symptoms of interstitial nephritis. He never did have any positive symptoms of recurrence. His bladder never troubled him at all other than from a little catarrhal condition. He complained greatly of pain in the sacral region, chest, shoulders and legs.

"Autopsy showed the bladder studded with many hard nodules and much thickened. Both kidneys were filled with pus. The retroperitoneal and bronchial glands, both kidneys and ureters showed metastases. Liver, spleen, stomach, and intestines were normal."

Remark. This case would now be classed as one very unfavorable for radical cure on account of the extensive involvement of the seminal vesicles and intervesicular space. The examination of the tissues removed showed that an early recurrence was to be expected. The fact that the patient lived nearly two years in comparative comfort was surprising.

Case IV. *Carcinoma of the prostate and lower part of the intervesicular region. Radical operation. Apparent cure. Lived 6½ years after operation. Autopsy. No recurrence or metastases.*

J. E. D., Of. No. 930. Aged 64; married. Admitted May 12, 1905. (See p. 517, *Johns Hopkins Hospital Reports*, vol. xiv.) Onset one year ago with straining at urination. After one week the symptoms disappeared and he remained comfortable until seven months ago. The catheter then withdrew 16 ounces of residual urine, and after that he was catheterized once a day and treated by prostatic massage by an osteopath. For two months he had used a catheter twice daily. Suffers no pain. Sexual powers normal. No hematuria.

Rectal. The prostate is considerably enlarged, more in the left lobe, which is hard but not stony, smooth, very tender. The right lateral lobe is moderately enlarged, oval, smooth, elastic, not tender, indurated, but not so hard as the left. Neither seminal vesicle is apparently indurated, but on the left side several indurated cords are felt above the prostate. No glands; rectum negative.

Cystoscopic. Residual urine varies between 100 and 400 c.c. No stricture. The lateral lobes are very little intravesically enlarged and the cleft between them is shallow. In the median portion there is a small sessile rounded lobe with a shallow cleft on each side. Trigone and vesical mucosa negative. With finger in rectum and cystoscope in urethra the beak is easily felt; no subtrigonal thickening, but by turning the beak to the left a distinct increase in the thickness of the left seminal vesicle is felt. Diagnosis, carcinoma.

May 16. Radical operation. Palpation of the prostate when exposed showed that it was very much harder than seen in hypertrophy. Radical operation was carried out without difficulty; the ureters were not injured. The trigone was excised to within 1.5 cm. of the ureteral orifices. One large gland adjacent to the left seminal vesicle was removed. Wound closed with catgut and silkworm-gut sutures. No shock.

Examination of specimen. The prostate with its capsule and urethra, both seminal vesicles, vasa deferentia for a distance of 3.5 cm., cuff of the bladder 2 cm. wide in the region of the trigone, have been removed in one piece. Microscopic examination shows adeno-carcinoma. The seminal vesicles and vasa deferentia are invaded near the prostate, but are free higher up. The trigone has not been invaded. The prostatic urethra is healthy.

Convalescence. The patient reacted well. The urethral catheter was removed on the seventh day. The silkworm-gut sutures were not pulled out until the twenty-fourth day, and on the thirty-ninth day the perineal fistula was completely closed and urine passed through the penis, but without control.

August, 1907. Patient reports for examination. Feels well. Weight 196 pounds. Has incontinence night and day. No pain or other discomfort. The urine is clear, no infection present. Careful examination of the rectum shows no recurrence.

September 15, 1909—Letter: "I am free from pain, weigh 195 pounds, and am in excellent health. I am partially able to retain urine at night, and get up once to void. During the day I have complete incontinence and wear a urinal. Urine flows out freely without pain. No hematuria, no rectal disturbance or constipation. Sexual desire is present as much as ever, but I have no erection and am consequently unable to have intercourse."

On March 18, 1911, I received a letter from his physician, Dr. W. R. Tyndale, saying that for six months the patient had suffered with pain in the chest, and examination showed evidence of myocarditis.

A letter from Dr. H. C. Moffit of San Francisco, dated August 29, 1911, stated that the patient had "an extensive osteoarthritis of the spine," that " it was first thought possible that the malignant prostate might have led to spinal metastasis, but that this could be very definitely ruled out by the course and character of the changes." "X-ray plates fully confirmed this."

The patient died of cardiac dilatation on October 25, 1911, at the age of 71 years. A careful autopsy, including the spine, was made, the diagnosis of osteo-arthritis confirmed, and malignancy excluded.

O this question Dr. T. B. Beatty of Salt Lake City writes me on January 30, 1913: "There was no evidence of malignant involvement of the rectum or prostatic region, nor had there been any pain, tumor, or other symptoms of the same previous to death. The autopsy showed osteo-arthritis of the dorsal vertebræ with complete ankylosis. The condition was not malignant, and there were no metastases or local recurrence."

Remark. The physicians quoted are men of high standing

in American medicine, the case was very thoroughly studied, and I have every confidence in their report. It would therefore seem justifiable to claim that this patient had remained completely cured after the operation for radical cure of cancer of the prostate six years and five months before.

Case V. *Carcinoma of the prostate and seminal vesicles. Radical operation. Death from shock. Autopsy showed extensive unrecognized peritoneal and deep glandular metastases.*

M. G., Of. No. 1052. Aged 75; widower. Admitted September 25, 1905. Onset eight months ago, with increased frequency and difficulty of urination which have rapidly increased. Now has severe pain in the bladder, rectum, membranous region, left thigh and knee. He has lost 16 lb. in weight and is very weak. Has not had complete retention of urine, but voids every twenty minutes.

Rectal. The prostate is moderately enlarged, is hard, but not stony, and slightly elastic. The right seminal vesicle is not enlarged nor indurated. The left vesicle is negative, but the left lobe of the prostate extends farther up than the right, and the induration may involve the lower portion of the seminal vesicle. Above the prostate, between the seminal vesicles, the tissues are firm, and on the right side several hard cords can be felt along the pelvic wall. No enlarged glands are made out and the rectal mucosa is soft and not adherent.

Cystoscopic. A Coudé catheter cannot be introduced owing to obstruction at the apex of the prostate. A small silver catheter passes with ease and withdraws 80 c.c. residual urine. Bladder capacity 360 c.c. The cystoscope shows the median portion of the prostate moderately enlarged in the shape of a bar, and extending upward and to the left is an elevation of the trigone which is somewhat irregular; but the mucosa is intact. There is no ulceration or tumor to be seen in the bladder. The lateral margins of the prostate are a little irregular, but not intravesically hypertrophied. With finger in rectum and cystoscope in urethra there is considerable induration beneath the trigone and the sub-urethral portion of the prostate is considerably thickened.

Remark. It is evident that the trigone is invaded, but owing to the absence of induration in the region of the seminal vesicles the radical operation is thought to be advisable.

October 13. Radical operation. Excision of the prostate with its capsule and urethra intact, a portion of the membranous urethra, cuff of the bladder, nearly all of the trigone, including

5 mm. of the left ureter, both seminal vesicles and about 5 cm. of the vasa deferentia, all in one piece. When the prostate was freed examination showed no extension of the disease above the upper portions of the prostate, and the seminal vesicles seemed to be healthy. On exposing the trigone it was found elevated and reduplicated in a mass continuous with the median portion of the prostate and extending up to the region of the left ureter, which could not be seen. The line of incision was carried across the trigone just below the right ureteral orifice, above the ligamentum interuretericum, and just above the rounded elevation of mucous membrane seen at the upper left-hand corner of the trigone. The left ureter could not be seen, but later examination showed about 5 mm. of the left ureter had been excised, the orifice being situated in the prominent mass above described. The upper end of the left seminal vesicle was very adherent to the peritoneum, and in freeing it a portion of the peritoneum was removed. It was found thickened and evidently involved. The patient lost more blood than usual, and at the end of the operation, which was more prolonged than usual, the etherizer reported his pulse as weak, but not very fast. Very soon, however, the respirations became alarming. He had been given 500 c.c. saline infusion during the operation and at the end was transfused with 700 c.c. Under this treatment his pulse became fairly good, but his respirations grew worse and he died about two hours after the operation.

Autopsy showed an extensive involvement of the peritoneum and numerous metastatic lymph-glands in the pelvis and along the great blood-vessels.

The operative and autopsy findings in this case were very unexpected. Rectal examination seemed to indicate that the disease had not spread far beyond the prostate, the seminal vesicles apparently being healthy. The appearance of the trigone, however, should have warned us against attempting a radical excision, because, although not ulcerated, the irregular elevation evidently meant infiltration. There was, however, nothing to indicate that the disease had spread into the peritoneal cavity, and, in fact, this case is unique in this respect as we have found no similar case.

Case VI. *Carcinoma of the prostate. Seminal vesicles not invaded. Radical operation. Recovery. Well six months later.*

L. A., No. 2166. Aged 68; widower. Admitted April 8, 1909. For one year the patient had frequently suffered with imperative urination, during which the desire would come on suddenly, and urination was very frequent. For several days after an attack he would be normal for three or four days. During the past month urination has been extremely frequent, so that he has begun to wear a urinal. Now voids very frequently night and day.

Examination. Patient is well preserved; no general glandular enlargement.

Rectal. The prostate is enlarged on the right side. The left lateral lobe is normal in size, smooth, very slightly indurated. The right half of the prostate is rough, irregular, markedly indurated, the induration extending to the median line and there ending abruptly, forming an almost straight declivitous edge. The induration on this side extends forward for about 3 mm. along the membranous urethra and backward to the junction of the seminal vesicles and vasa deferentia. The seminal vesicles and vasa deferentia can both be easily felt, but are apparently not more than slightly indurated and not enlarged. No enlarged glands. No intravesicular mass. Rectum negative.

Cystoscopic. Retention of urine complete. Bladder capacity 650 c.c. The cystoscope shows a small rounded median bar with no sulcus on either side. The lateral lobes are slightly thickened and the whole prostatic margin a little irregular, with some swelling of the mucous membrane produced by the retention catheter. The trigone is not elevated nor enlarged. With finger in rectum and cystoscope in urethra there is no sub-trigonal thickening, but there is a definite increase in the sub-urethral portion of the prostate, and the left lobe is considerably indurated.

April 21, 1909. Radical excision of prostate, seminal vesicles, and cuff of bladder. The tractor was inserted without difficulty and the prostate exposed easily. It was very hard, particularly the right lobe, which was stony. An incision was made and the capsule gaped widely and did not bulge nor show spheroids as in benign hypertrophy. A section was taken for microscopic study (stained frozen sections) and report was received that it was very dense fibroid tissue. The usual conservative perineal prostatectomy was then carried out, two small lateral lobes and a small median bar being enucleated. The tissue removed showed no spheroids, was very firm, fibrous, with small yellowish areas scattered throughout, and so thoroughly suggested carcinoma that a second section was obtained and showed definite carcinoma. Radical operation was then begun and carried out without much difficulty. The upper portion of the trigone was left intact, both ureters having been left intact. Anastomosis was easily completed with alternate catgut and silkworm-gut sutures. Condition of patient excellent. Infusion on return to ward.

Convalescence. The patient convalesced slowly and the fistula was very slow in completely healing. He was discharged on the seventy-second day in good general health, with complete incontinence.

October 26—Letter: "I have gained much in weight; have no pain. Incontinence is still present."

January 27, 1913—Letter: "My health is very good. I have no pain, but a burning in my bladder, and incontinence of urine night and day. Have never used a catheter." Now four years since operation.

ANALYSIS OF THE SIX CASES ON WHICH THE RADICAL OPERATION WAS PERFORMED

The ages of the patients were 70, 64, 65, 64, 75, and 68 years respectively, and symptoms had been present 11 months, 3 years, 4 years, 1 year, 8 months, and 1 year respectively. Physicians had been consulted and treatment given 8 months before in one case, and 7 months before in another. In both of these cases an osteopath was employed who gave prostatic massage, thus losing valuable time. One case was subjected to a Bottini operation 6 months before admission. In all cases sufficient symptoms were present to warrant rectal examination by which a diagnosis could have been made long before the patient applied for treatment with us.

The onset symptoms were difficulty and frequency of urination in all cases except Case I, in which the first symptom was pain in the urethra. Three patients, II, IV, and VI, had never suffered any pain. In the other three cases pain either local or referred was a prominent symptom. On admission, urination was extremely frequent and difficult in all cases except Case IV, in which a catheter was used twice daily.

The prostate was described as considerably enlarged in 3 cases, moderately in 2 cases, and slightly enlarged in 1 case. Marked induration was present in all cases, involving the whole prostate in 4 cases. In Case IV one lobe was indurated, but less so than the other and distinctly elastic. In Case VI the marked induration was confined to half of the prostate, the other half being very slightly indurated.

The seminal vesicles were found on rectal examination to be free from infiltration or induration in 4 cases (II, IV, V, and VI). An area of induration between the seminal vesicles was present in Cases I, II, III, and V. The catheter showed 400, 300, 500, 400, 80, and 600 c.c. residual urine respectively.

The cystoscope showed a slight elevation of the median portion in 5 cases (I, II, III, V, and VI). In Case IV there was a small, definitely rounded median lobe with a shallow cleft on each side.

The lateral lobes were scarcely at all enlarged intravesically in every case. There was generally not even a sulcus between them in front, but in 2 cases it was shallow. The vesical mucosa was everywhere intact, but the cystoscope showed, in 2 cases, an elevation of the trigone, which involved only the anterior portion in Case II. In Case III the trigone was considerably elevated and irregular, extending out on the left side as far as the ureter. In 4 cases the trigone was negative.

At operation, the lower ends of both ureters were intentionally excised for a short distance in Case II, the operator thinking that the disease had reached this point. This was a mistake, as it was afterwards found that the induration was inflammatory in character. In Case V the lower end of the left ureter was involved and had to be excised. This patient died of shock, and autopsy showed that while the seminal vesicles were free, the disease had traveled into the peritoneal cavity. The cystoscopic evidence of elevation of the whole trigone should evidently militate against the radical operation, as shown by this case. In Case III the lower end of the left ureter was unintentionally divided by scissors in making the division along the left lateral wall of the bladder. Anastomosis was made high up and no inconvenience resulted (the patient living three years). In 5 cases the operation was carried out with apparent success and without shock, but a study of the specimen removed showed carcinoma near the upper limit in 2 cases (I and III). In Case V (patient dying of shock) autopsy showed extensive carcinoma of the peritoneum and retroperitoneal glands, although the bladder and seminal vesicles were free from invasion. In Case I the patient died nine months after the operation as a result of traumatism and infection, in attempting to remove a stone adherent to a silk suture. Autopsy showed a very small area of recurrence back of the bladder. In Case III the patient lived over three years in comfort, but autopsy showed metastases in various parts of the body, the bladder and urethra, however, being free from ulceration. In Case II in which the patient died six weeks after the operation from ascending renal infection, as a result of the intentional but injudicious division of the two ureters, extremely careful examination of all the pelvic tissues at autopsy with numerous sections taken for microscopic study failed to reveal any evidence of carcinoma, and it seems probable that the disease had been completely eradicated. Two patients have apparently been cured. One died six and a half years after the operation, and the other is well four years after the operation. In both of these cases the specimens showed that the disease had not reached the upper line of excision.

As a result of the experience gained in these six cases it may be said that the operation should not be attempted where the infiltration extends more than a short distance beneath the trigone as determined by the cystoscopic examination with the finger in the rectum and the cystoscope in the urethra; nor where the upper portions of both seminal vesicles are involved; nor where an extensive intervesicular mass or indurated lymphatics or glands or involvement of the membranous urethra or muscle of the rectum shows that the disease is manifestly too far progressed; that the ureteral papillae should be left intact with sufficient tissue below them to ensure proper suture and to leave their openings free from constriction, 1 or 2 cm. above the wound; that hemorrhage should be carefully checked (by hugging the capsule, injury of the periprostatic plexus may be largely avoided); that silk should never be used and catgut only when occasional stitches of silkworm gut are employed to hold the tissue together in making the urethro-vesical anastomosis; that when the operation is attempted early it can be performed without much danger or great difficulty, and with excellent chance of cure; that only three of the six cases above recorded were suitable for the radical operation and that in all of these the disease was apparently completely removed.

RADICAL CURES BY PARTIAL PROSTATECTOMIES

Two cases, in which small nodules of cancer were completely removed in the course of perineal prostatectomy for supposed benign hypertrophy have been radically cured, and therefore deserve reporting here.

Case VII. J. T. Y., No. 463. Aged 60; married. Admitted September 24, 1903. Onset two years ago with frequency of urination. Suprapubic drainage six months. Prostate considerably enlarged, smooth, rather hard in consistency. The seminal vesicles not palpable, but both lateral lobes extend upward and are quite closely adherent. The cystoscope shows two lateral lobes. With finger in rectum and cystoscope in urethra there is very little median enlargement.

October 4, 1903. Operation. Perineal prostatectomy. Lateral lobes were surprisingly small and adherent, but were apparently completely removed. No median lobe present. The wound healed well but urination was never free.

December 6, 1907. General health excellent. Urination difficult. Residual urine 760 c.c. The cystoscope shows large intravesical lateral lobes (same as before operation—evidently not removed).

Rectal examination showed cicatricial induration, but no carcinoma of prostate or seminal vesicles.

Operation. Perineal prostatectomy. The rectum was very adherent and a small tear was made into it. Two considerably enlarged adenomatous hypertrophied lateral lobes easily enucleated. No evidence of carcinoma. Rectum sutured. (Good result.)

Remark. Study of the tissue removed at first operation showed everywhere benign hypertrophy except in one small area which was definitely carcinomatous, but apparently completely excised (Fig. 12). (See *Johns Hopkins Hospital Reports*, Case IX, p. 556.)

October, 1909—Letter: "I enjoy good health—urination fairly free. No pain." Now six years since the lobe containing cancer was removed.

February 1, 1913. "My health is still good. Urination free."

Pathological Note.—The lateral lobes show typical benign adenomatous hypertrophy, with the exception of one portion, probably the posterior aspect, which shows prostatic gland tissue with periacinous inflammatory infiltration. In a portion of this area of prostatitis is a small nodule of carcinoma about 2 mm. in diameter, a section of which is shown in Fig. 12.

The second case is as follows:

Case VIII. J. H. McI., No. 1898. Aged 61; married. Admitted May 19, 1908. Has suffered with prostatic trouble, irritation, and frequency of urination for over fifteen years. Three years ago began to have difficulty and pronounced frequency of urination, which has gradually increased and he now voids every two hours and six times at night. Never passed a catheter. No hematuria. Pain in neck of bladder. The prostate is a little broader than normal, slightly indurated, smooth. Seminal vesicles negative. Prostatic secretion contains pus cells. Urine clear.

Cystoscopic. Residual urine 60 c.c. Bladder capacity 300 c.c. The cystoscope shows a small rounded median bar. Bladder negative. Diagnosis chronic obstructive prostatitis.

May 21, 1908. Perineal prostatectomy. When the capsular incisions were made the wounds gaped widely, as if on tension. The lateral lobes were small and removed each in one piece. The median portion was larger than normal and excised through the left lateral cavity. Urethra and ejaculatory ducts preserved. Internal sphincter tight, but easily dilated. Examination of bladder negative.

Convalescence. On removal of tubes on day after operation the patient was able to retain his urine for a short length of time, but urine did not come through penis until the fourth day. Perineal fistula closed on the twelfth day. Patient discharged on the fifteenth day, able to retain urine for three hours.

September 15, 1909—Letter: "I void naturally about every four hours and twice at night. No pain. General health good. I regard the operation as most successful."

October 1, 1909—Letter from physician: "Rectal examination shows no evidence of carcinoma. Patient is well."

February 1, 1913—Letter: "I regard the operation as entirely successful. I void urine naturally about every four hours, have no pain, and consider myself cured."

Pathological Note.—Microscopic examination shows that the tissue removed at operation is chronic prostatitis. No adenomatous spheroids seen. A small area (3 × 4 mm. in size) is seen in one section which is definitely carcinoma. The outline of the malignant area is irregular, and consists of densely packed epithelial cells, which grow wildly and spread in lines of infiltration into the surrounding prostatic tissue. The tissue surrounding the cancerous area shows a chronic prostatitis, and the cancer seems to have been completely excised with it. The picture presented is much the same as shown in Fig. 12 from Case VII.

REMARKS ON THE TWO FOREGOING CASES.

It is interesting to note that in both of these cases the carcinoma was found in areas which were of a chronic prostatitis, and not adenomatous hypertrophy. They presented none of the characteristics of Albarran's "epithelioma adenoide." In both cases the area was completely excised with the chronically inflamed lateral portions of the prostate, and, by good luck, completely,

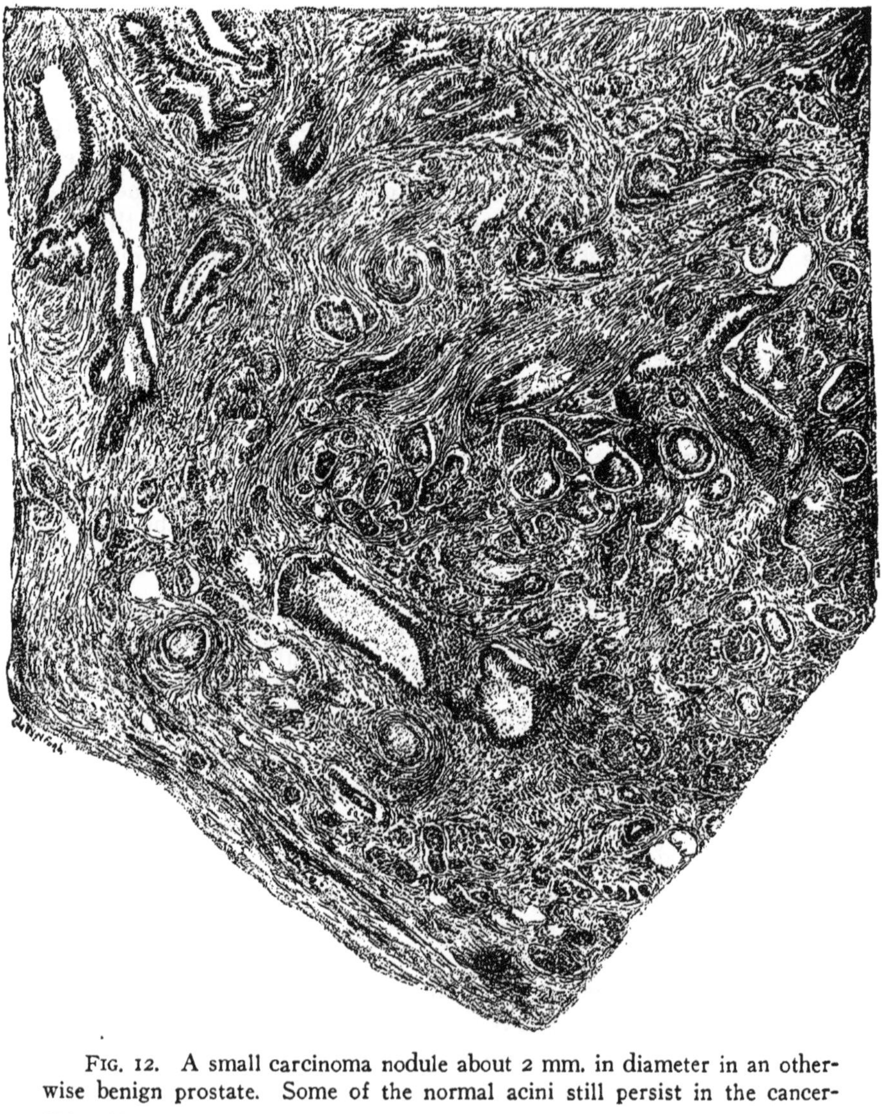

FIG. 12. A small carcinoma nodule about 2 mm. in diameter in an otherwise benign prostate. Some of the normal acini still persist in the cancerous area.

as shown by the cures which have now stood for ten years and five years respectively in the two cases.

The operation of conservative (partial) perineal prostatectomy has been shown to produce, in advanced cases of cancer of the prostate, wonderfully fine functional results—maintained as long as the patients have lived in most cases. The discovery of this fact came accidentally as a result of operations performed on supposedly benign prostates, which proved to be malignant.

At a meeting of the International Association of Urology in London, 1911, I presented the results obtained in 34 cases, which were as follows:

Class A. Perfect functional result as long as the patient has lived, 10 cases (three patients having lived 3½, 2½, and 2 years respectively).

Class B. Patients still alive and completely relieved, 12 cases (the time elapsed being over a year in 8 cases).

Class C. Patients completely relieved for a time, with partial recurrence of obstruction later, 3 cases.

Class D. Good immediate result; recurrence of obstruction requiring catheterization (4) or suprapubic drainage (3) in 7 cases.

There were only two deaths (6 per cent.). I have now (April, 1913) had 52 cases with two deaths (the same as before). Recent reports show that the good results shown above have been generally maintained. Of the 12 patients who were included in Class B two have since died, but remained relieved of the obstruction. Three are still alive and well (10, 5, and 3 years respectively). One is still alive after 4½ years, but had to return to a catheter life eight months ago. No report was received from eight cases.

During the last two years 16 cases have been operated upon (with no deaths), and I have just heard from 10 of them. Of these, all have been relieved of the obstruction except one, who has had to return to a catheter life. Two died within six months of cachexia.

The results in recent years have been even more satisfactory than before, and I now feel justified in carrying out the procedure of conservative perineal prostatectomy on almost all cases of cancer of the prostate which are too advanced for a radical operation, and in whom the frequency and difficulty of urination are considerable and a catheter life difficult or painful.

APPENDIX

A description of the principal steps in the operation of conservative perineal prostatectomy seems desirable here, as many of the steps are the same as for the radical operation for cancer of the prostate.

POSITION OF THE PATIENT.

The exaggerated dorsal position of the patient is the most satisfactory, and the perineal board devised by Halstead is admirably suited for this purpose. The perineum should be so

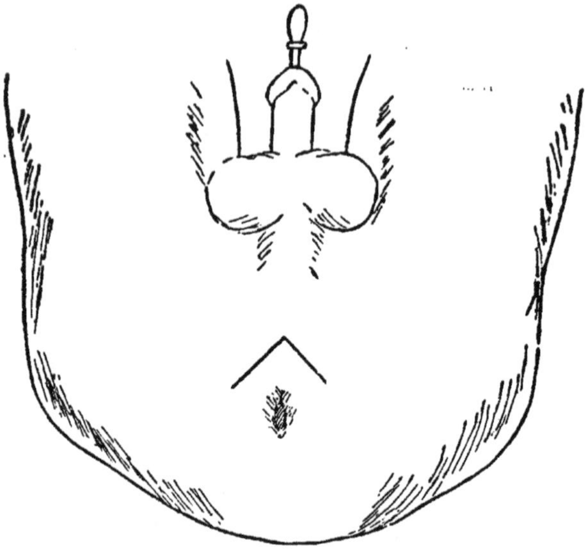

FIG. 13. The inverted V cutaneous incision.

elevated that it is almost parallel with the floor, thus allowing excellent retraction of the rectum and splendid exposure of the posterior surface of the prostate. After placing the patient upon the table, before elevating the thighs, a No. 24 F sound should be inserted into the posterior urethra, to be used subsequently as a guide for urethrotomy. If the operator waits until the patient is placed in the urethrotomy position, he will frequently find it difficult to introduce the sound through the triangular ligament.

CUTANEOUS INCISION.

The inverted V cutaneous incision unquestionably gives a much better exposure than a median incision. The apex should be just over the posterior part of the bulb, about 2 inches in front of the anus, and the lateral branches directed outward and backward parallel to the ischiopubic ramus, each about 2 in. in length, as shown in Fig. 13. The incisions are carried through the skin, fat, and superficial fascia, and then by blunt dissection with the handle of the scalpel and the index finger of the left hand the space to each side of the central tendon is opened up. In this way it is very simple to open up by blunt dissection very quickly a space on each side reaching as far as the triangular ligament. In so doing the levator ani is pushed backward and outward on each side and the transverse perineal muscles are pushed forward.

EXPOSURE OF THE MEMBRANOUS URETHRA.

The bifid retractor is inserted as shown in Figs. 14 and 15. Traction upon this instrument gives an excellent exposure of the

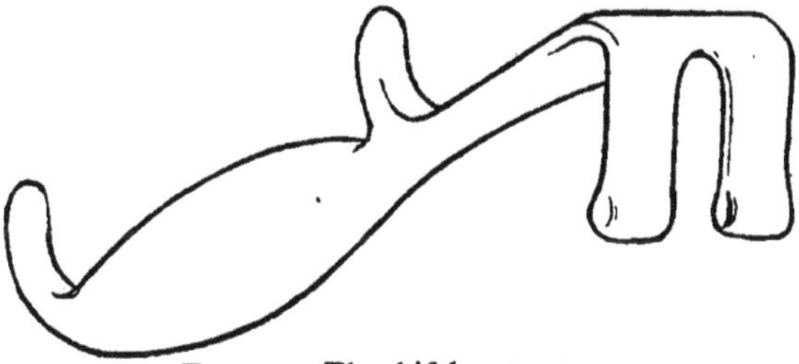

FIG. 14. The bifid retractor.

narrow band of central muscle and tendon and greatly facilitates the division close to the bulb without injuring this hemorrhagic structure. After the central tendon has been completely divided and the posterior surface of the bulb freed, it is well to insert a grooved retractor (Fig. 16), by which the bulb and triangular ligament and external sphincter are drawn upward and a better view obtained of the recto-urethralis muscle, which lies between the two branches of the levator ani and covers the membranous urethra, toward which it draws the anterior wall of the rectum. In dividing the recto-urethralis muscle care should be taken not to injure the rectum, which is often drawn forward so that it lies almost in front of the membranous urethra. It nearly always covers the apex of the prostate. As soon as the recto-urethralis has been thoroughly divided it is easy by blunt dissection to push the rectum backward and thus obtain a good view of the membranous urethra, the bulb being drawn forward along with the muscular structures of the triangular ligament. The membranous urethra is then opened upon the sound (Fig. 17) and the edges picked up with artery clamps, being sure to secure the mucous membrane. A straight sound is then inserted into the bladder through the urethral wound (an assistant having withdrawn the sound from the anterior urethra), to open up the way

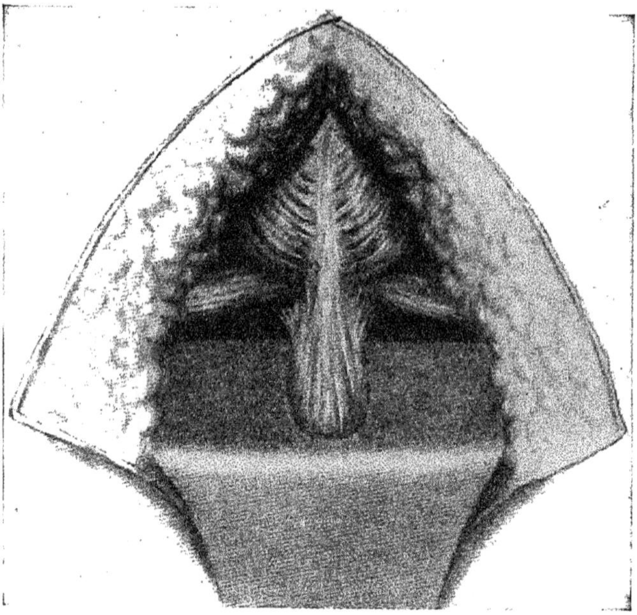

FIG. 15. Showing the bifid retractor in use. The bulb, transversus perinei, and central tendon exposed.

for the prostatic tractor,—and in these cancerous cases it may be necessary to stretch the contracted posterior urethra considerably with a glove-stretcher before it is possible to insert the tractor into the bladder through the perineal urethrotomy wound.

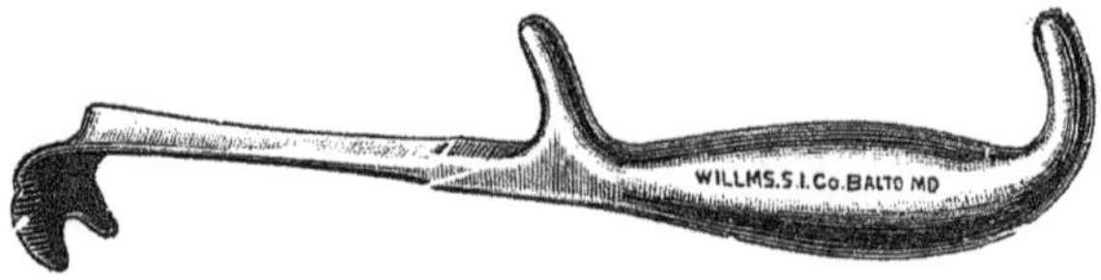

FIG. 16. Retractor grooved so as to surround the membranous urethra and retract the triangular ligament and bulb.

Owing to the rectangular shape of this instrument (Fig. 18) it is sometimes difficult to insert. Sometimes it is well to begin its introduction with the beak turned backward, and then to rotate the instrument 180 degrees before carrying it into the bladder. After the instrument has penetrated into the prostatic urethra it is generally advisable to remove the anterior bulb retractor, and thus allow the shaft of the tractor to be carried farther forward. As a rule, little difficulty is experienced in

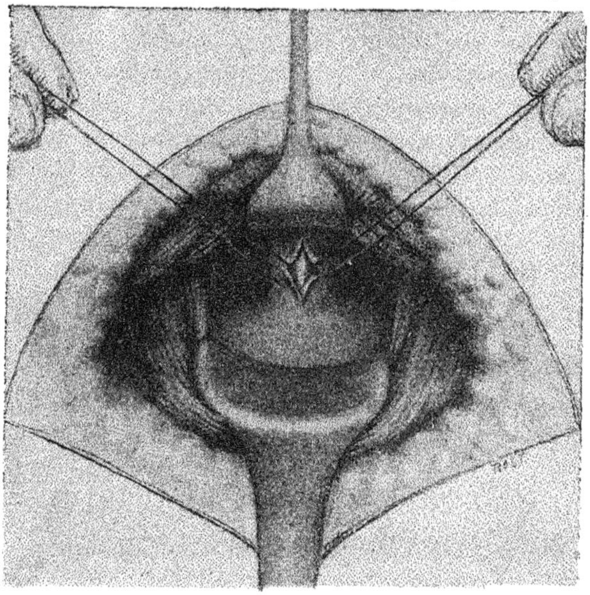

FIG. 17. Opening of urethra on sound preparatory to introduction of tractor.

inserting the tractor if one has been careful to secure the edges of the mucosa of the membranous urethra. After reaching the bladder the blades of the tractor are opened out by means of the external handles (Fig. 19), and after being fixed in this position by means of a set screw, traction is made upon the prostate, and the further separation of the rectum from the posterior surface of the prostate made. After dividing the recto-urethralis muscle and exposing the apex of the prostate, one generally finds it necessary to use the knife to divide a layer of fibrous tissue which lies behind the posterior surface of the prostate. After this (the posterior layer of Dénonvilliers's fascia) has been divided the rectum can be more easily pushed backward, and one enters, generally with ease, into the space between the two layers of Dénonvilliers's fascia, and the smooth glistening surface of the prostate is exposed. When this layer is properly exposed, no difficulty is generally experienced in rapidly freeing the entire posterior surface of of the prostate and seminal vesicles, a good view of which is obtained at once by the insertion of a broad angular retractor posteriorly.

INCISION OF CAPSULE.

Lateral retractors are so placed that with posterior retractor drawing the rectum backward and the prostatic tractor drawing the gland outward a splendid exposure of the posterior surface of the prostate is obtained. An incision is then made through the capsule on each side of the median line for almost the entire length of the posterior surface and about 1.5 cm. deep. These incisions are about 1.8 cm. apart behind and 1.5 cm. apart

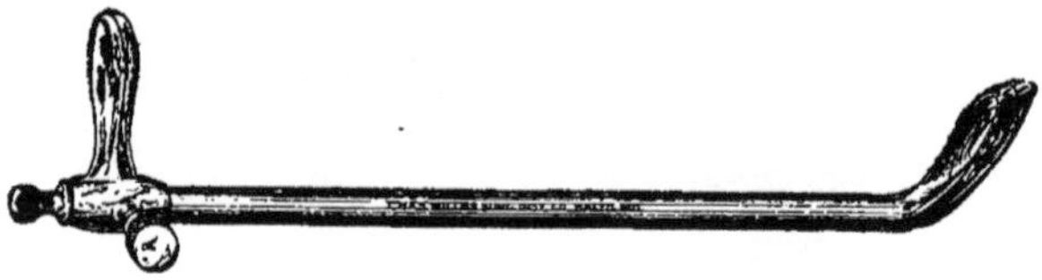

FIG. 18. Prostatic tractor closed.

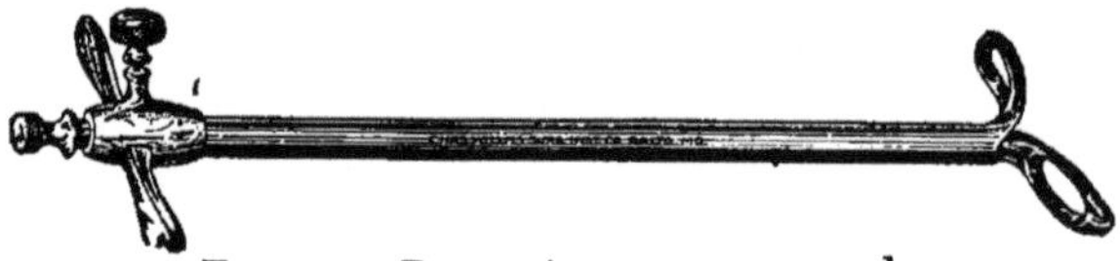

FIG. 19. Prostatic tractor opened.

in front, as shown in Fig. 20. The bridge of tissue which lies between them contains the ejaculatory ducts and the floor of the urethra.

The lateral lobes are then each completely removed, much of this being done by the blunt dissector. When the deep portion is reached—that is, at the base of the seminal vesicle and the bladder—it is often necessary to use a sharp periosteal elevator or a curette in order completely to remove all of the carcinomatous prostatic tissue in that region. The entire lateral mass of prostatic tissue usually comes away in one piece, but in those cases in which the cancer is confined to the posterior subcapsular layer in front of which is a hypertrophied adenomatous lobe, the latter is usually separately enucleated. After the two lateral cavities are emptied the median portion of the prostate is next attacked. This is indicated in Fig. 21, in which the median portion is shown diagrammatically, caught with a sharp hook. It should be our object here to excise this median sub-urethral portion without injury of the ejaculatory ducts which lie behind it (in order thus to avoid epididymitis), and with as little injury to the urethra in front of it as possible. For this purpose an instrument which we call a "punch" has been very satisfactory in that it forces out into one of the lateral cavities

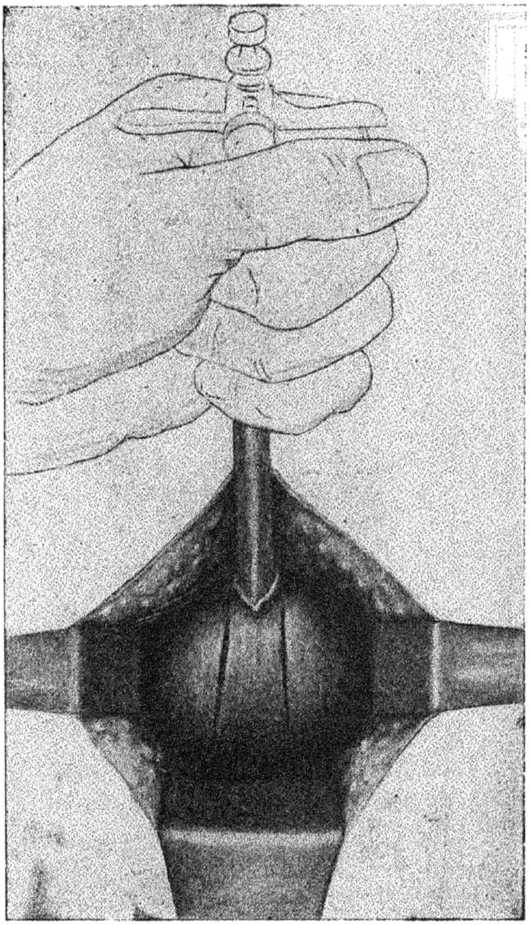

FIG. 20. Tractor introduced, blades separated, traction made exposing posterior surface of prostate. Incisions in capsule on each side of ejaculatory ducts and urethra 1.5 cm. deep.

a large mass of median portion. Remaining tissue can be removed with scissors, curette, or rongeur. If a rounded middle lobe is present it may be drawn down and removed through a lateral cavity (Fig. 22). It is then advisable to remove the tractor and dilate thoroughly the external prostatic orifice with a large forceps after removal of the tractor. The finger is then inserted through the urethra and an examination of the vesical neck made. As a rule the sphincter will be found tight, or often sclerotic, and thorough dilatation should be made. If there remains any prostatic tissue in the median portion or elsewhere around the orifice this can easily be enucleated or excised, using the finger as a tractor. In some cases carcinomatous infiltration continuous with the median bar and extending beyond the trigone is felt and it may be advisable to remove this more or less completely (which can usually be done with ease with a curette working upon the finger in the bladder against the trigone as a guide).

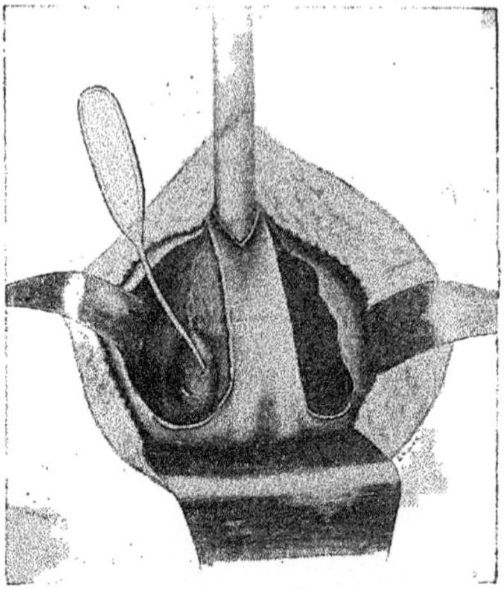

FIG. 21. Showing removal of a fibrous median bar.

Care should be taken not to tear a hole in the urethra or bladder; but it is a remarkable fact that although not infrequently the urethra has been torn into laterally or posteriorly during some of my operations, and in a few cases a small portion excised, the healing in all these cases has been entirely satisfactory, and there has been no evidence of intraurethral or intravesical ulceration or tumor outgrowth through the rent. If a globular median lobe is present this is usually easily enucleable as in cases of benign hypertrophy. The rest of the operation is similar to that for benign cases: a large two-way drainage tube through the urethra into the bladder, continuous irrigation begun at once, the lateral cavities packed each with strips of iodoform gauze, the levator ani muscles drawn together in front of the rectum with a single suture of

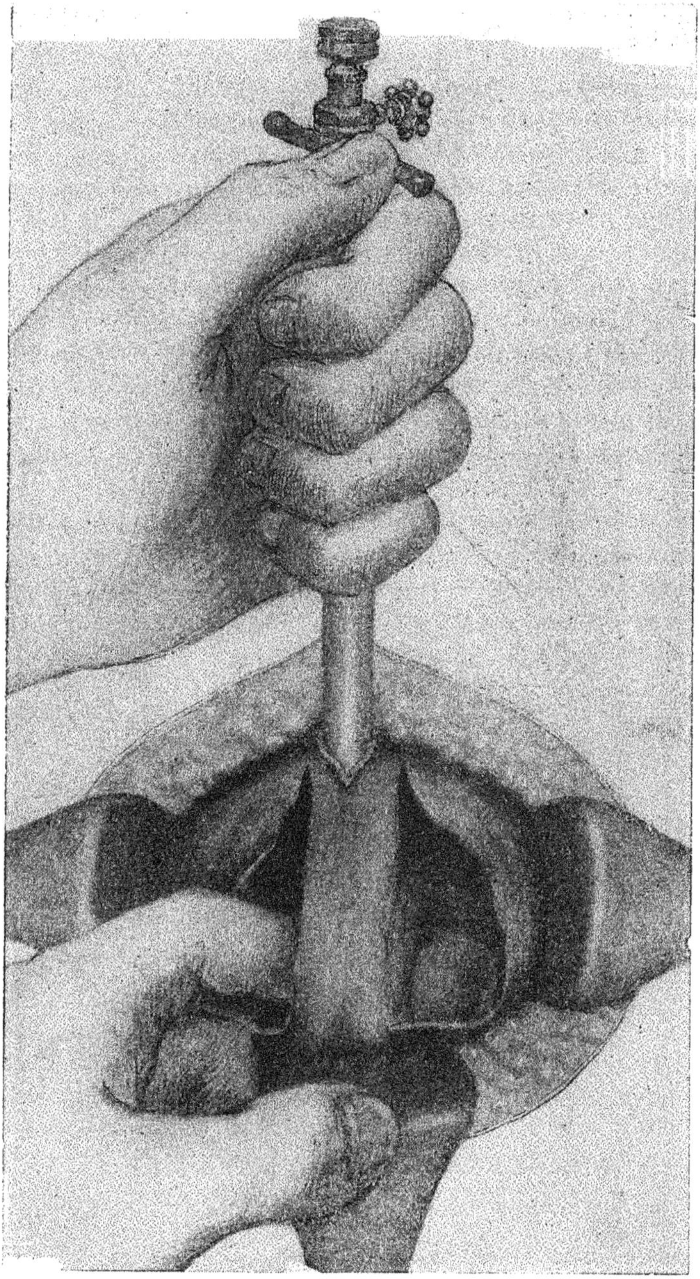

FIG. 22. Showing technic of delivery of a rounded middle lobe into the left lateral cavity.

catgut, and the skin approximated on one side by interrupted sutures of catgut. If the patient is very weak an infusion is often begun at the beginning of the operation, but usually we wait until the return to the ward. From 500 to 800 c.c. are generally given beneath the breasts. Continuous irrigation, begun on the operation table, is continued in the ward and, as the hemorrhage becomes less, the rapidity of the flow is cut down. In this way very little trouble is experienced in keeping up the irrigation for twenty-four hours. The patient is given water to drink as soon as possible and an effort is made to make him take as much as he can. The gauze is generally removed on the morning after the operation, and the tubes during the afternoon when all bleeding following the removal of the gauze has ceased. On the following day the patient is usually put in a wheel-chair and taken out-of-doors and as a rule the convalescence is as rapid as we see after perineal prostatectomy for benign hypertrophy. In fact, owing to the small size of the cavity the closure of the fistula and restoration of normal urination are usually somewhat quicker, as shown by reference to the detailed report elsewhere of cases treated by perineal prostatectomy.

DEPARTMENT OF SEXUAL PSYCHOLOGY.

NOTES ON THE PSYCHOLOGY OF SEX.

By Douglas C. McMurtrie, New York.

VI.

AN INDIGENOUS AMERICAN SEXUAL PHENOMENON.

Many of the studies which we may make in the field of sexual science must be, to a certain degree at least, eclectic or synthetic. There are, however, certain sources of information which are distinctly American, for the study and record of which the foreign scientists might properly look to us.

One of the most interesting phenomena in all sexual science has been widely manifested among the Indians, the indigenous inhabitants of the United States. Yet this native phenomenon has never been studied nor comprehensively described in the English language. The only extensive mention of it has been in German. I refer to the berdache.

THE BERDACHE.

In many of the tribes of North American Indians there existed a person known as the *berdache*. This individual from youth or early manhood dressed as a woman and assumed the duties and customs of the squaws. The Indians as a general thing believed that he assumed his manner of life as the result of a revelation to him in a dream, but there was, of course, some deeper reason. With the idea, however, that his practices were due to "divine dispensation" he was not usually regarded with contempt but, on the contrary, often occupied a position of some distinction in the tribe. He was frequently regarded as "medicine," that is, possessed of especial powers. Some tribes held an annual ceremony which centered around him.

The early ethnological observers designated these individuals as "hermaphrodites" but this was due, of course, to their own misconception. Where detailed examinations have been made the berdache has been found to be of normal anatomical configuration.

In reports where the sexual nature and practices of the berdache are described it is evident that he is a pederast. He lives the domestic life of a squaw but his social relations are with men, and many have been known to marry men.

The material bearing on this interesting phenomenon is extremely widely scattered and is difficult of location. I have, however, been undertaking a compilation of it, and several references are presented herewith, while others will appear in this series from time to time.

It will be safer not to draw any final conclusion regarding the exact nature of the berdache's sexual characteristics until all the available data have been consulted. The items are, however, of much interest, and indicate clearly a species of sexual inversion.

COURTSHIP BY A BERDACHE.

One of the fairly early reports [1] concerning a berdache runs as follows:

" Some time in the course of the winter, there came to our lodge one of the sons of the celebrated Ojibbeway chief, called Wesh-Ko-bug (the sweet), who lived at Leech Lake. This man was one of those who make themselves women, and are called women by the Indians. There are several of this sort among most, if not all of the Indian tribes; they are commonly called A-go-kwa, a word which is expressive of their condition. This creature, called Ozaw-wen-dib (the yellow head), was now near fifty years old, and had lived with many husbands. I do not know whether she (*sic*) had seen me, or only heard of me, but she soon let me know that she had come a long distance to see me, and with the hope of living with me. She often offered herself to me, but not being discouraged with one refusal, she repeated her disgusting advances until I was almost driven from the lodge. Old Net-no-kwa was perfectly well acquainted with her character, and only laughed at the embarrassment and shame which I evinced whenever she addressed me. She seemed rather to countenance and encourage the Yellow Head in remaining at our lodge. The latter was very expert in the various employments of the women, to which all her time was given. At length, despairing of success in her addresses to me, or being too much pinched by hunger,

[1] JOHN TANNER. *A narrative of the captivity and adventures of John Tanner (U. S. Interpreter at the Saut de Ste. Marie) during thirty years' residence among the Indians in the interior of North America.* Prepared for the press by Edwin James, M.D. New York, G. & C. & H. Carvill, 1830.

which was commonly felt in our lodge, she disappeared, and was absent three or four days. I began to hope I should be no more troubled with her, when she came back loaded with dry meat. She stated that she had found the band of Wa-ge-to-tah-gun, and that the chief had sent by her an invitation for us to join him. He had heard of the niggardly conduct of Waw-zhe-kwaw-maish-koon towards us, and had sent the A-go-kwa to say to me, 'My nephew, I do not wish you to stay there to look at the meat another kills but is too mean to give you. Come to me, and neither you nor my sister shall want anything it is in my power to give you.' I was glad enough of this invitation and started immediately. At the first encampment, as I was doing something by the fire, I heard the A-go-kwa at no great distance in the woods, whistling to call me. Approaching the place, I found she had her eyes on game of some kind, and presently I discovered a moose. I shot him twice in succession, and twice he fell at the report of the gun; but it is probable that I shot too high, for at last he escaped. The old woman reproved me severely for this, telling me she feared I should never be a good hunter. But before night the next day we arrived at Wa-ge-tote's lodge, where we ate as much as we wished. Here, also, I found myself relieved from the persecutions of the A-go-kwa, which had become intolerable. Wa-ge-tote, who had two wives, married her. This introduction of a new inmate into the family of Wa-ge-tote, occasioned some laughter, and produced some ludicrous incidents, but was attended with less uneasiness and quarreling than would have been the bringing in of a new wife of the female sex."

THE WOMAN DANCE AMONG THE MUSQUAKIE.

In a study of the folk-lore and customs of the Musquakie Indians, Miss Mary A. Owen records [2] a ceremony in which the berdache was concerned.

"The Woman Dance (*I-coo-coo-ah*). This is a most extraordinary and disagreeable ceremonial or function, or whatever you choose to call it. Perhaps I would better say was than is, for at present there is no one to start the I-coo-coo-ah. Until a year or two ago, there were a few men in the tribe who dressed in women's clothes and lived in wigwams apart from the others. They were said to be the unfortunates who had failed to strike the war-post the first time they attempted it, or had in some other

[2] MARY A. OWEN. *Folk-lore of the Musquakie Indians of North America.* London, 1904.

way failed to come up to the standard of manliness. They were worthless creatures, nearly always drunkards, and always uncombed, unwashed, and arrayed in rags. They did no work, made no visits, never spoke to a woman. They passed their time in gambling with one another, singing indecent songs, and dozing and dreaming from the effects of swallowing tobacco-smoke or, when they could get it, whiskey. They were considered 'good medicine' for the tribe; and the women insured a share of it by leaving cooked food and bundles of wood at their doors when no one was observing. Once a year, a feast and dance was given them, at which some of the young men of the common people took them by the hands, danced with them, insulted them by pretended love-making, and finally gave them presents of old clothes begged or bought from the squaws. While the dance was in progress, the on-lookers of both sexes kept up a continual clapping, and shouted '*I-coo-coo-ah*' and '*Hoo-hoo, henow-chee-chee.*' The reason the dance is not given at the present time is that these make-believe *henow-och* (women) are no more to be found in camp. The last appointees refused to accept the place, and an unwilling incumbent would be 'bad medicine.' "

LESBIAN LOVE AND THE LEXICOGRAPHERS.

Lesbian love as the designation of love relationships between women is widely used and its meaning is universally understood, at least by all persons at all versed in sexual science. Yet the standard dictionaries which list medical terms and certainly those of a medico-psychological character take no notice of the terms relating to sexual inversion in women.

The exact sexual characteristics of Sappho—from whom and from whose home city, Lesbos, the sexually inverted phenomenon in the female has derived two of its terms—are in some dispute among historical authorities, but the literary and scientific acceptation of the terms is in no dispute whatever. There seems therefore to be little excuse for their omission by the lexicographers.

Being interested in the definitions which might be given I recently looked up the terms referred to in several large lexicographical works. The results were of some interest.

Under the adjective *lesbian*, Murray, in the Oxford Dictionary,[3] fails to note its association with the homosexual love of

[3] JAMES A. H. MURRAY. *A new English dictionary on historical principles.* Oxford, 1908, vol. 6, p. 207.

women. The main definition is "of and pertaining to the island of Lesbos." There is mentioned the *lesbian rule*, a mason's curve of lead which could be bent to fit the curves of a molding, but there is no reference to *lesbian love*.

The Century Dictionary, the most extensive American lexicographical work, omits any definition of *tribade* or *tribadism*. It also fails to especially identify [4] the adjective *lesbian* with love relations between women. In the course of the definition of the word "*Lesbian*, adjective and noun," it is remarked: "From the reputed character of the inhabitants and the tone of their poetry, *Lesbian* is often used with the implied sense of 'amatory' or 'erotic.' ".

TRIBADISM IN A FRENCH DICTIONARY.

The subject has received more attention in the French works. Larousse defines both *tribade* and *tribadism*. In translation his entries run as follows. " *Tribade*, (Greek, *tribas*, from *tribo*, I rub), woman whose clitoris is developed to an exaggerated degree and who misuses those of her own sex." [5] And of tribadism: "*Tribadisme*, vicious practices of tribades." [6] Augé, in an edition [7] of one of the Larousse works, notes among other meanings, the use of the adjective *lesbienne* substantively as a synonym for tribade.

EVIDENCE ON A QUANTITATIVE BASIS OF SEX.

All zoological evidence points to a quantitative rather than a qualitative basis of sex. An additional datum on this point was recently presented [8] before the meeting of the American Society of Zoologists. The study concerned the doves of a sex controlled series, reciprocal cross of *T. orientalis* x *S. Alba*. The young hatched early in the summer were nearly all males and young hatched from eggs later in the season were nearly all females. Females hatched early in the season, that is nearest to male-producing conditions, were found to be more masculine in their sex behavior than their own sisters hatched late in the season from

[4] *Century Dictionary*, New York, [1911], Vol. 5, p. 3417.

[5] PIERRE LAROUSSE. *Grand dictionnaire universel*. Paris, n. d., Vol. 15, p. 482.

[6] *Ibid.*, Vol. 15, p. 483.

[7] CLAUDE AUGÉ. *Nouveau Larousse illustré*. Paris, n. d., Vol. 5, p. 652.

[8] OSCAR RIDDLE. A quantitative basis of sex as indicated by the sex behavior of doves from a sex controlled series. (Abstract). *Science*, Lancaster, Pa., 1914, n. s., xxxix, 440.

eggs produced under the strongest female producing condition. Two full sisters hatched from the two eggs of a single clutch most strongly contrasted with one another, the bird from the first or male-producing egg of the clutch usually taking the part of the male to a full 100 per cent. Masculinity was determined by the number of times in which they functioned as males in copulation.

The injection over a period of one month of extracts and suspensions of ovarian tissue into the more masculine of the females last referred to, with simultaneous injections of testicular extract and suspension into the more feminine of the pair, succeeded in some cases in very strongly reversing the sex behavior of the pair. The effect persisted more than twenty-five days after the last injection. The behavior itself, and the effects of the extracts were recorded on moving picture films.

The following conclusion was drawn: "These two results together with our very abundant data on the storage metabolism of the ova of these forms, and the initial fact of sex control itself, strongly indicate that the basis of sex is a fluid reversible process; that the basis of adult sexual difference is a *quantitative* rather than a *qualitative* thing."

PROSTITUTION IN PALESTINE.

Palestine holds a peculiar interest to the student of prostitution by reason of the fact that the universal prototype of the prostitute, Mary Magdalene, was a native of the country. The academic accuracy of this characterization is seriously questioned but the popular conception is firmly established.

A study [9] of the prostitution system in Palestine has recently appeared. Many of the brothels are located in grottos or caves on the outskirts of the cities, and the conditions in them are extremely insanitary. There is the merest pretense of medical inspection which is actually a farce. The prostitutes are either Moslems or Jewesses, but the latter are usually domiciled within the city limits.

[9] DOUGLAS C. MCMURTRIE. The prostitution system in Palestine. *Lancet-Clinic,* Cincinnati, 1914, cxi, 475-476.

REVIEW OF CURRENT UROLOGIC LITERATURE

ZEITSCHRIFT FUR UROLOGIE

First Supplementary Number, 1914.

Proceedings of the Deutsche Gesellschaft für Urologie. Fourth Congress.

1. Urology as a Science and Branch of Instruction. By L. Casper.
2. Biology of Infections of the Uropoetic System. By A. Von Wassermann.
3. The Scientific Basis of Vaccinetherapy in Urology. By G. Michaëlis.
4. Vaccinetherapy in Urology. By Richard Volk.
5. Vaccinetherapy in Urology with Special Reference to Coli-Infections. By C. Schneider.
6. The Diagnostic and Therapeutic Value of Sera and Vaccines for the Treatment of Gonorrheal Diseases. By Paul Asch.
7. Note on the Treatment of Local and General Complications of Gonorrhea with Antimeningococcus Serum Injections. By P. Herescu and L. Strominger.
8. Vaccinetherapy in Cases of Chronic Non-gonorrheal Disease of the Urinary Tract. By Alfred Zinner.
9. The Indications for Suprapubic Prostatectomy. By Dr. Thelen.
10. Prostatectomy in Insufficient Kidney Function. By Max Waldschmidt.
11. Prostatectomy for Prostatic Hypertrophy. By Paul Steiner.
12. The Surgical Treatment of Prostatic Atrophy. By Paul Steiner.

2. Biology of Infections of the Uropoetic System.

The uropoetic system is in close relationship with the gastro-intestinal tract. It is therefore not very surprising that the colon bacillus, which makes its home in the gut, should invade the urinary tract. It is a wonderful thing, however, biologically, that this organism, which is a harmless parasite in the former location, should act as the cause of serious disturbance in its new home. This is due to the fact that the gastro-intestinal tract, in adults, if not so much in children, has gotten up a local immunity to the colon bacillus, whereas the urinary tract is normally sterile and has no such resistance. Should the latter system get up an immunity to the organism, the bacillus may be excreted as a harmless parasite and cause what we call a bacteriuria. This superficial infection is of little significance but a deep infection may at any time arise from an ascent of the same organism from the bladder to the kidney pelvis, or from a variation in the strain of the colon bacillus and a substitution of a variety to which the urinary tract has not been gradually accustomed.

It is important to distinguish the deep from the superficial forms of infection because in the latter vaccinetherapy is of no avail, whereas in the former, where the blood elements have already been called into play, vaccintherapy may be of the greatest service. The same is true in gonorrheal infections. In this example, a urethritis can be in no wise modified by vaccines, whereas gonorrheal epididymitis or arthritis may be cured by such treatment.

3. **The Scientific Basis of Vaccinetherapy in Urology.**

Michaëlis presents clearly and fully the underlying principles of immunology and vaccinetherapy. It is impossible in a special abstract to take upthe general topics that he discusses. Suffice it to say that he explains the meaning of immunity, its active and passive forms, the classic theories of Metchnikoff, Pfeiffer, and Wright, the difference between opsonins and tropines. He then points out how Wright has used killed vaccines instead of the attenuated vaccines of Pasteur and Jenner, explains the "Opsonic Index" with its negative and positive phases, in which connection he enters into Ehrlich's side chain theory, and then lays down the rule that in a severe general infection small doses are indicated, whereas in a mild localized infection, large doses of the vaccine should be injected.

As regards the bacteriology of urinary infections, Michaëlis points out that in many bacteriemias the organisms may cause an infection of the urinary passages. Thus from one-quarter to one-half the typhoid cases excrete bacteria in the urine. The author has examined 160 cases bacteriologically and has found the colon bacillus, alone, or in combination with another organism in 80% of the urines. Tubercle bacilli were found in 5 cases, twice in combination with staphylococci. Owing to the numerous forms of coli which exist it is absolutely necessary to use autogenous vaccines of this organism. In other types of infection, of course, autogenous vaccines are always preferable.

4. **Vaccinetherapy in Urology.**

Volk concludes his paper as follows:

1. The American reports of favorable results from passive immunization with gonococcus serum demand further confirmation.

2. Not only gonorrheal complications but various other infectious diseases are fit conditions for vaccinetherapy especially when the latter is combined with the older methods of treatment.

3. Determination of the opsonic index is in general unnecessary. Careful clinical observation is sufficient.

4. The modus operandi of vaccinetherapy is not yet cleared up. Increase of the bacteriotropic power of the serum is probably not the chief factor.

5. Acute urethritis is not fit for vaccine treatment, prostatitis and folliculitis are more amenable, whereas epididymitis, funiculitis,

and arthritis are most likely to be cured. A good polyvalent vaccine is the best preparation for gonococcus cases, but an autogenous vaccine may be used when the former is lacking.

6. The other urinary infections are more amenable to vaccine treatment the sooner they are attacked. Especially favorable results are obtained in coli and staphylococcus infections. At least the subjective disturbances are improved or entirely relieved. In these cases the preparation of an autogenous vaccine is indicated.

7. Untoward effects are not to be feared from vaccinetherapy. Therefore this method of treatment may almost always be undertaken.

8. Diagnostic inoculation is apparently of value in gonorrheal diseases and should be tried out in infections of other nature.

9. The combination of vaccinetherapy with other methods was in general of value. It is still doubtful whether local treatment similar to that with the Histopin of Wassermann can give useful results. We look to chemotherapy for a cure for certain conditions such as the pyelogenous bacteriurias and the bacteriurias of typhoid and cholera.

5. Vaccinetherapy in Urology with Special Reference to Coli-Infections.

Schneider concludes that vaccinetherapy marks a distinct advance in our methods of treating infectious processes of the urinary tract and that its harmlessness recommends its adoption in all acute and chronic cases. Whenever possible, vaccine treatment should be combined with local measures as the pathological changes caused by the disease demand the use of both methods.

6. The Diagnostic and Therapeutic Value of Sera and Vaccines for the Treatment of Gonorrheal Diseases.

Although American authors have reported good results with antigonococcus serum in gonorrheal epididymitis and arthritis and in gonorrheal affections of the female genitalia, this method has not met with much success in Europe. On the other hand, owing to the morphological and biological similarity between the gonococcus and meningococcus, French and Roumanian writers have suggested the use of antimeningococcus serum in such cases. The serum is injected at intervals of from 6 to 10 days, in doses of 20 and more c.c., intragluteally. Asch's results with this treatment, in gonorrheal arthritis and epididymitis have been only fair.

Asch is particularly interested in vaccinetherapy. He has tried out a half dozen stock preparations of polyvalent (heterogeneous) gonococcus vaccines. He uses both small (5 million) and larger (25 million) beginning doses according to the type of case but does not believe that there is any advantage in the intravenous administration of the vaccine as recommended by Bruck and Sommer. He prefers intramuscular injections and has observed no ill results from their employment. He has treated 22 cases of gonorrheal arthritis in this manner, and believes that gonococcus vaccines are the best means of treating this condition. In 36 cases of gonorrheal epididymitis the results were also good but did not, in his opinion, begin to approach those obtained by electrargol injections given in the manner he has advocated.

In acute prostatitis Asch is able to record some favorable results but in acute gonorrhea, of course, there was no effect whatever from vaccines. In peri- and para-urethral abscesses and infiltrations there have been some cures, but in 3 cases of rectal gonorrhea no effect was observed.

As regards the diagnostic value of gonococcus vaccine injections, Asch is by no means convinced that a rise in temperature always means gonorrhea. Moreover an examination of the urethral discharge after such an injection cannot be relied upon to give definite information as to the absence or presence of gonococci in the urethra. The author has, however, devised a method which he regards as a great aid in the diagnosis of latent specific urethritis. He makes an intramuscular injection of 50 million killed gonococci (75 to 100 million in very old cases) after having made a careful clinical and *endoscopic* examination of the patient. From one to three days later he endoscopes again and if gonorrhea is present is often able to discover the typical pathological changes in the urethra. This method is of great value in deciding whether the patient is in a contagious state and should always be carried out before allowing a suspect to marry.

The combination of vaccine injection and endoscopy is also of value in recognizing "gonorrhea carriers." Such persons show no manifest clinical or endoscopic symptom of their condition. Yet their urethral mucosa harbors gonococci. After a single injection, however, the endoscopic picture becomes characteristic and in some instances even a latent gonorrhea may be converted into a manifest one.

7. Treatment of Local and General Complications of Gonorrhea with Antimeningococcus Serum Injections.

The authors have treated 21 cases by this method. There were 14 cases of blennorrhagic arthritis, one of arthritis and ophthalmia, one of sciatica, one of gonococcal septicemia, one of gonococcal uretero-pyelitis, one of gonococcal meningitis two of gonococcal epididymitis.

The arthritis cases were all improved. Indications for the use of the serum are the acute condition, severe pain, much swelling, and fever. Ten or twelve days after the first injection the pains had disappeared, the swelling had diminished, and there was restoration of joint mobility. The ophthalmia, the sciatica, the uretero-pyelitis, and the meningitis cases were all improved. On the other hand similar results were not obtained in the cases of epididymitis, for the pains did not disappear so soon or so completely.

The injections were given either subcutaneously at the outer aspect of the thigh or intra- or periarticularly. There was generally very little pain or inflammatory reaction at the point of injection. Forty to sixty cubic centimeters of the serum were injected in all, the entire amount being subdivided into doses of 10 c.c. at each sitting. The intervals between injections were 2, never more than 3, days. The fever resulting from each introduction of serum was regarded as a direct indication for the repetition of the dose, for the authors feel that had they waited for a normal temperature they would have invited the occurrence of anaphylactic symptoms.

8. Vaccinetherapy in Cases of Chronic Non-Gonorrheal Disease of the Urinary Tract.

In order to establish definitely whether vaccinetherapy has any effect on urinary infections Zinner has made a careful study of 15 cases in which non-vaccine treatment had proved absolutely without result. When vaccinetherapy was begun no other local or general treatment was used with it. From this study, Zinner concludes as follows:

1. Healing, in a bacteriological or clinical sense, was not achieved.

2. In chronic cases of non-gonorrheal infections of the urinary tract which have proved refractory to all local and general therapy, vaccines alone can effect considerable improvement, but vaccinetherapy should be supplemented by the older methods of treatment.

3. Temperature reactions after the injections are not necessary for a cure. In fact very high temperatures should be attributed to an overdosage and are generally followed by a longer or shorter period of aggravation of symptoms.

4. In general, larger doses of staphylococci can be used than of colon bacilli.

5. It is of the first importance that in all cases of bacterial infection of the urinary tract, ureteral catheterization be done in order to establish whether a renal focus is present. If this should be the case, only the bacteria recovered from the ureter urine should be used for the preparation of the vaccine, since otherwise we cannot exclude the entrance of bacteria into the bladder from the urethra, and since we do not know just what changes in virulence colon bacilli may undergo in the bladder.

6. Careful intravenous injections are harmless. In severe cases they may be able to effect more rapid changes in the clinical picture.

7. Finally, vaccinetherapy, when carefully carried out, is harmless and should be employed in subacute as well as in chronic infections of the urinary tract after a careful localization of the process has been made. This treatment may work where the other clinical methods have failed but should always be supplemented by these where necessary.

9. The Indications for Suprapubic Prostatectomy.

In the first stage of prostatic hypertrophy, characterized by congestion and inflammation of the gland, hygienic and dietetic measures are as a rule sufficient for relief, and the attacks of acute retention can be overcome by occasional catheterization or in the worst cases by puncture of the bladder. Only when carcinoma is suspected or when the night's rest is too much disturbed, should prostatectomy be carried out so early in the disease.

It is only in the second stage of chronic bladder insufficiency, and in the third stage of chronic retention with catheter life, that the operation is to be seriously considered. Even in such cases the author first begins with a conservative method of treatment and attempts to improve the bladder tone with the use of the permanent catheter. Only when such measures fail, does he advocate operation. Cases of chronic retention with distention of the bladder offer the greatest difficulties in deciding as to their operability. In such instances it is the author's custom to carefully empty the bladder by systematic catheterization and to overcome by every possible means the threatening danger of urinary infection. When this is done he determines the contractility of the bladder musculature and the renal sufficiency, and when these are unsatisfactory he warns against operation. Other contraindications are arteriosclerosis and severe constitutional diseases.

The author then goes on to discuss at length the explanation of the clinical picture of obstruction associated with prostatic atrophy. In these cases also, cure can be accomplished by prostatectomy or in some instances the same result may be achieved by the removal of a small projecting portion or by the division of a muscular band or by the excision of scar tissue.

10. Prostatectomy in Insufficient Kidney Function.

Waldschmidt prefers as a rule to do the one stage operation, but in cases of renal insufficiency the two stage procedure opens a means of relief to a much greater number of sufferers. As tests of kidney function the author mentions phloridzin and indigocarmine injections with determination of the time of excretion, and the estimation of the freezing point of the blood. The last-named he considers the most reliable method as it gives definite and accepted limits of operability. Sometimes the freezing point level can be raised above the danger line by systematic catheterization (permanent catheter where necessary) and in a still greater number of cases by a preliminary sectio alta under local anesthesia. In this way an appreciable restoration of the kidney function takes place and the secondary operation can be undertaken at a later date with increased chances of ultimate success.

12. The Surgical Treatment of Prostatic Atrophy.

There are now 22 reported cases of prostatic atrophy, including five of the author's. As regards the etiology Steiner believes that gonorrhea is at the bottom of all cases. Not only does operation reveal an indurating periprostatitis but histological examination reveals the inflammatory origin of the condition. There is a hypertrophy of the connective tissue and muscle elements and a destruction of the glandular constituents of the prostate, associated with the presence of a large number of corpora amylacea in the acini. In the diagnosis of prostatic atrophy we must be very careful to rule out disease of the central nervous system, especially tabes. Rectal palpation reveals the presence of a sinking in of the prostatic bed, and if at the same time a sound is introduced into the urethra, one receives the impression of the sound being immediately beneath the examining finger. Cystoscopy shows the bladder outlet to be flat or concave instead of convex. Trabeculae are rare, but dilated veins are present. The author's five cases were all prostatectomized with splendid results. He therefore recommends ectomy for the relief of this condition.

MISCELLANEOUS ABSTRACT

Dangers of Injections Into the Kidneys.

Pyelography by use of collargol injections and the roentgenogram has come into favor to a considerable extent in this country chiefly through the writings of Braasch and the reports of the Mayo clinic in none of which, says J. M. Mason, Birmingham, Ala. (*Journal A. M. A.*, March 14), has he found reference to any injurious effects with the use of the method. He reports two cases of his own observation in one of which the patient suffered intensely from pain, nausea and vomiting and had a slight rise of temperature for four days. When the kidney was removed five days later its surface showed numerous nodules with black discoloration beneath the capsule. On section each nodule proved to be the outer surface of an infarcted area, deeply stained with collargol and the different infarcted areas showed different degrees of inflammation. No collargol remained in the kidney pelvis. A few days later a patient with renal tumor—a hypernephroma—was injected with collargol, care being taken to use a smaller quantity and to stop at the first appearance of pain and leave the catheter in the ureter until it was thought the collargol had all drained away. No special constitutional effects were noted but on removing the tumor ten days later, there were found a few of the discolored nodules on its surface and the same black infarcts on section. The kidney contained a quantity of precipitated collargol. The microscopic examination by Dr. E. M. Mason showed wide-spread collargol deposit in the kidney substance, collargol stained deposits and granular casts throughout the tubules and many of the malpighian corpuscles showed collargol masses within the capsule of Bowman. No definite evidence of inflammatory reaction was seen in the collargol-containing tubules outside the necrotic areas but in some areas tube-casts both stained and unstained are more numerous than one would expect as a result of the primary condition.

Mason also gives a description of the microscopic appearance of a kidney showing similar conditions from the laboratory of Dr. Mallory of Boston, who attributed them to pushing the catheter too far and entering a calix into which the fluid was injected under pressure. Mallory mentions having seen one other case of damage to the kidney from collargol injection. Mason reviews the literature and comparing the findings says that we are able to show by the pathologic conditions that a definite sequence of events follows injection of the renal pelvis, if the intrapelvic pressure is raised beyond a certain unknown point. The pelvis is overfilled and the injected material, together with any infectious matter in the pelvis passes up into the convoluted tubules and glomerated capsules, and may be followed by rupture of the tubules and production of infarcts or abscesses. Whether or not the collargol has any irritating or cauterizing action in the process is in dispute. Mason gives a summary of the experimental work of Voelcker, Oehlecker, and of Strassmann and in endeavoring to account for the difference between the pathologic observations of the latter and those of others, he thinks it may be due to the lesser pressure employed. The cases he presents, he says, show that damage may result from conditions not entirely under our control in the injection of the kidney and that such are contra-indicated in the presence of infection and where the integrity of the kidney has been impaired by injury or disease. The article is illustrated.

BOOK NOTICE

NIERENPHYSIOLOGIE UND FUNKTIONELLE NIERENDIAGNOSTIK IM DIENSTE DER NIERENCHIRURGIE UND DER INTERNEN KLINIK. By Dr. Victor Blum, Privatdocent in Urology in the University of Vienna. Pp. 121. Franz Deuticke's Verlag, Leipzig.

Dr. Victor Blum is doing good and careful work in genito-urinary pathology, and in this monograph of 120 pages the author gives us an excellent resume of the relationships of renal physiology and functional renal diagnosis to the surgical and medical diseases of the kidneys. The volume is illustrated and a good bibliography adds to its value.

ZUR ANATOMIE DER PROSTATAHYPERTROPHIE. By Prof. Josef Englisch, Vienna. Verlag Dr. Werner Klinkhardt, Leipzig.

This is a reprint from the Folia Urologica of 120 pages and presents in a concise way our latest knowledge of the anatomy of this still little known and somewhat mysterious gland, the prostate.

THE AMERICAN JOURNAL OF UROLOGY, VENEREAL AND SEXUAL DISEASES

WILLIAM J. ROBINSON, M.D., EDITOR

VOL. X JULY, 1914. No. 7

LOCAL ANESTHESIA IN ROUTINE UROLOGICAL PRACTICE.

By MAXIMILIAN STERN, M.D., New York.

IN this paper it will be my aim to set forth briefly the advantages of local anesthesia as an aid in routine urologic practice. While it is true that many urologists employ solutions of anesthetic drugs to some extent to facilitate their work, it is equally true that but a comparatively small number do so habitually, reserving them for those hypersensitive cases in which it is actually imperative.

The use of local anesthetics in urology, and for that matter for nearly all other surgical purposes, has not made more rapid progress because of the many grave sequelæ and minor disagreeable manifestations of cocaine absorption, this being the drug generally employed.

Owing to the delicate structure of the tissues of the genito-urinary tract manipulation here should be performed only after anesthetization, and in view of the rich vascular supply of these tissues and their high absorbing power it is important that the drug selected be as little toxic as possible.

Although cocaine acts as an efficient anesthetic in the urethra in those able to tolerate it, there are many valid objections to its use, other than its toxicity, which make it unsuitable for application in this field. Its constricting effect on the capillaries and the resulting blanching of the mucous membrane make any examination of the parts impractical, as the picture would be misleading in the extreme. This effect upon the mucosa also militates against its use prior to medication of the urethra because of the diminished action of any drug applied to a membrane already shrunken by cocaine.

The minimum strength of a solution of cocaine necessary to produce sufficient anesthesia would be one per cent. At least two drams of this would ordinarily be employed, this representing the capacity of a rather small urethra. The amount of cocaine contained in two drams of a one per cent. solution is 1.2 grains. This is much in excess of the safe dose, which has been placed at about one-third grain. In a urethra of larger caliber more would be necessary to introduce the solution into the posterior urethra by means of anterior injection, which has proved to be the easiest and best method of application. Two grains is often required, and on account of the free absorption taking place from the urethral mucosa it is evident that where such amounts are necessary this is not the drug of choice.

Urologists who use cocaine in their routine work, therefore, see many instances of cocaine poisoning and the author can testify that this is a common and disagreeable occurrence. Besides those patients who have a real idiosyncrasy toward the drug there are others who because of increased vascularity of the membrane, greatly enhancing its absorptive capacity, become giddy, weak and cyanotic. The occurrence of these symptoms during a treatment requires its immediate termination. Stimulation and rest must be resorted to and the patient allowed to leave with the treatment either uncompleted or not even begun. Hertzler cites a case in which death followed the urethral injection of two drams of a two per cent. solution of cocaine. Of course, the length of time such a solution is allowed to remain in the urethra is an important consideration. Cocaine, however, is a drug unsuitable for general urethral work, and as we are in possession of many substitutes which are more or less efficient, it behooves us to employ the one best adapted for our routine work.

Among the drugs used in place of cocaine is quinine and urea hydrochloride. This, in a stronger solution than two per cent., is an efficient anesthetic, but has the disadvantage of causing severe burning immediately after its injection, which lasts quite a few minutes. It also seems to be less effective than other drugs for topical application or contact anesthesia than for the infiltration method.

A local, anesthetic drug, to be adapted for genito-urinary work, should possess certain properties which are so essential as to render the absence of any one of them a real contraindication to its use. It must not produce ischemia, for the color and vascular state of the urethra and bladder mucosa are of prime importance in determining any departures from normal. It must be sufficiently active to produce a satisfactory degree of anesthesia in about five minutes and permit of being used in adequate amounts without causing toxic symptoms. It must not be irritating to any degree on immediate contact with the mucosa. These requirements have best been met by alypin, which I have selected in my work for the past three years to the exclusion of other local anesthetics, all of which have been more or less disappointing.

Symptoms of shock are seen so frequently in very trivial urological proceedings, even those requiring no anesthetic, that operators in this field look upon such manifestations as natural to the work because of the close association of the genito-urinary tract with the vital centers. Now, in view of the fact that cocaine adds to the already existing predisposition to shock, it would seem to be directly contraindicated in this field. Prior to the time that I began to employ alypin in my daily work it was common for me to have to relieve symptoms due to the use of cocaine. This has been entirely eliminated by the newer drug, and up to the present time, after thousands of injections, no disagreeable symptoms have been seen.

While indicated in every field of urethral work where a local anesthetic is required, I have thought it of interest to discuss in some detail the application of alypin in two of its most frequent indications:

IRRIGATIONS.

In the use of both the Janet and Valentine methods it is recommended that the irrigating fluid be allowed to exert gentle pressure against the contracted compressor urethræ muscle, so as to cause it to tire and relax, thus allowing the fluid to penetrate into the posterior urethra and bladder. While this gentle and continued pressure many times facilitates posterior irrigation, it always does so at the expense of more or less pain and trauma. A burning sensation and frequency of micturition nearly always follow, even when non-irritating solutions are employed. These symptoms are more often due to the force exerted against the cut-off muscle than to the character of the solution used, though much more severe when an irritating fluid must be employed. In either case it is not justifiable to undertake this procedure without first overcoming the spasm of the compressor muscle except where perfect relaxation is possible, and even then it would be much better to anesthetize when an irritating fluid is to be employed in order to allay the consequent strangury, which in itself injures the delicate mucosa at the vesical neck and is often the sole cause of terminal hematuria.

In gonorrheal involvement of the posterior urethra, with severe symptoms, we are often at a loss to know just how to attack the inflamed area owing to the presence of strangury, tenesmus and bleeding, either terminal or with each effort at micturition. The gentlest measures must be employed as well as the most unirritating gonocides. Hot or warm water in a continuous flow is found efficient and agreeable, as are also mild organic silver salts, such as sophol. But we are confronted here with the difficulty of getting the solution into the posterior urethra through a sensitive and spasmodic constrictor muscle. The Janet method is out of the question, as any degree of force in the stream of fluid against the resisting muscle would be extremely painful and might directly cause more or less profuse hemorrhage. What then will be the best method of treatment? The use of antiblennorrhagics, together with rest, diet, and hot sitz-baths are of real value and quite often constitute the sole treatment during the acute stage. This is probably because of the difficulty of employing local treatment. Were the advantages of local anesthesia in the urethra more commonly appreciated this condition would be found to yield to mild treatment and the patients would be made quite comfortable from the start. With a good non-toxic anesthetic drug we are able to overcome the tonic spasm of the compressor urethræ, reduce the constant desire to micturate, and can instill a gonocidal solution, such as one of sophol, without causing the patient the slightest discomfort. It must be borne in mind, however, that though we have caused the constrictor to yield, we must not take advantage of the temporary abatement of the symptoms to resort to harsh methods. The vascular engorgement still exists and any additional injury to the mucosa, however slight, will cause bleeding which, though rarely dangerous, is always disagreeable to the patient, while much more soreness will be felt when the effects of the anesthetic have passed. The same reasoning must guide us in the selection of the solution for instillation or irrigation. Should we employ an irritating salt of silver, which is the most common mistake, we would only aggravate the existing inflammation and possibly occasion sufficient edema and swelling to interfere with the passage of the urinary stream. Should this occur the catheter would have to be resorted to, which, though used with extreme care, would constitute a real hardship for the patient, besides exposing him to the danger of prostatic or seminal vesicular infection.

TO FACILITATE THE PASSAGE OF INSTRUMENTS THROUGH THE COMPRESSOR URETHRÆ.

The normal urethra, and especially its posterior portion, is extremely sensitive to contact with solid objects. The compressor muscle is excited to immediate and spasmodic contraction, and only patients accustomed to such treatment, and many "neurasthenics" in whom the membranes are more or less anesthetic, can tolerate manipulation of these parts without the use of local anesthetics.

It is this spasmodic contraction of the compressor which is so frequently mistaken for stricture and which yields so readily to the instrument after an anesthetic solution has been allowed to bathe the parts for a few minutes. Those patients who by long experience have learned to control this muscle so as to relax it sufficiently to permit of instrumentation are often subject to painful erections occurring while the instrument is *in situ*, requiring its hasty withdrawal. This is probably the direct result of irritation of the spinal centers due to stimuli emanating from the floor of the prostatic urethra in consequence of the pressure of the instrument. In a case previously reported, the author, while looking through the cysto-urethroscope into an unanesthetized posterior urethra, saw two distinct jets issue from the ejaculatory ducts. In this case perfect control of the cut-off muscle permitted easy passage of the instrument and rendered the examination a painless one except that erection and orgasm occurred, which would have been avoided had an anesthetic been employed.

In the average patient this region is extremely sensitive to the sensations of heat, cold, pressure and pain, and without precautions being taken to guard against it they will writhe and groan so as to make examinations in the posterior urethra or bladder well-nigh impossible. Cystoscopic examinations and treatments through the cysto-urethroscope, such as fulguration, puncture, aspiration and injection, are all more or less possible without local anesthesia, but can never be done with the completeness and ease permitted by its use.

INSTILLATIONS INTO THE POSTERIOR URETHRA.

Instillations into the posterior urethra, a common form of medication and one designed to reduce inflammatory conditions in that region, is nearly always followed by frequency of urination and strangury, which tend to counteract the beneficial effect of the treatment. Were the tissues rendered insensible sufficiently long to permit of the wearing away of all sensations incidental to this procedure, all untoward symptoms would be eliminated and the benefits of the treatment completely secured. This applies as well to dilatation of the urethra either anteriorly or posteriorly, and while making it incumbent upon the operator to exercise his tactile sense more intelligently, the patient being unable to inform him of the degree of distention, it will insure a treatment free from all sequelæ due to irritation.

It will, therefore, be seen that in this branch of surgery, where so much local instrumentation is required, the use of local anesthesia becomes a most valuable adjunct in routine work, and, if the comfort of the patient is considered, an absolute necessity.

In office operations, such as circumcision, meatotomy, and the incision of abscesses, an anesthetic drug capable of being sterilized by boiling and of being employed liberally in effective solutions without fear of toxic effects, is a necessity which, if met, renders this work easy of accomplishment and gratifying to the patient.

In conclusion I would state that the qualities most looked for in a local anesthetic are found in alypin, and though at present it is being employed more by urologists than other practitioners, I see no reason why it should not meet the requirements of local anesthesia in other fields.

RATIONAL TREATMENT OF ACUTE GONOCOCCAL EPIDIDYMITIS

By I. Gonzalez Martinez, M.D.

Director of the Insular Laboratory of Biology, San Juan, Porto Rico.

THIS question which I propose to treat is not one that has ever caused serious discussion. On the contrary, for a great many years, acute gonococcal orchi-epididymitis has had a classic treatment which no one, general practitioner nor specialist, has dared to change to this date. Rest in bed, suspension of the local treatment for urethritis and revulsive and antiphlogistic medication are the three basic indications of the present therapy for this troublesome complication of gonorrhea. Against this routine practice, full of dangers for the diseased testicle and other organs synchronously involved in the inflammatory process, I desire to voice an opinion and to propose a more rational method of treatment, more in harmony with the latest acquisitions of science. Inasmuch as it is not my purpose to discuss *in extenso* or to consider under all its phases gonococcal orchi-epididymitis, but shall occupy myself with only that most practical question—its local treatment, I shall naturally omit a great deal with reference to the clinical description of the malady so that I may lay special stress on those things which serve as a basis for my argument. Before going fully into the question itself and in order that the foundation of my ideas may be better understood I believe it necessary first to consider, if only in a superficial manner, some details of descriptive anatomy and pathologic histology which are important to recall so that I may clearly explain with them, as with a diagram, the much discussed pathology of acute gonococcal orchi-epididymitis.

We all know that the male urethra is a closed canal measuring 18 to 20 centimeters long from the neck of the bladder to the anterior extremity of the glans. Modern surgeons divide the urethra in two sections, the anterior or extrapelvic and the posterior or intrapelvic urethra; the triangular ligament, urogenital diaphragm or median aponeurosis of the perineum being the resistant lamina which serves as a boundary for this division. The posterior urethra, which includes the membranous and prostatic urethrae, lies then immediately behind the triangular ligament, between that aponeurotic membrane and the neck of the bladder; it is about 5 cm. long and is that portion of the urethra which plays the most important rôle in the pathology of the urethral orchi-epididymitis. In fact, between the membranous portion of the posterior urethra and the neck of the bladder lies the prostatic urethra, measuring two and a half to three centimeters in length in a normal individual and more in those with a hypertrophied prostate; and in this zone, as can be seen in Figure 1, taken from Testut, we find the *genito-urinary crossroad* of

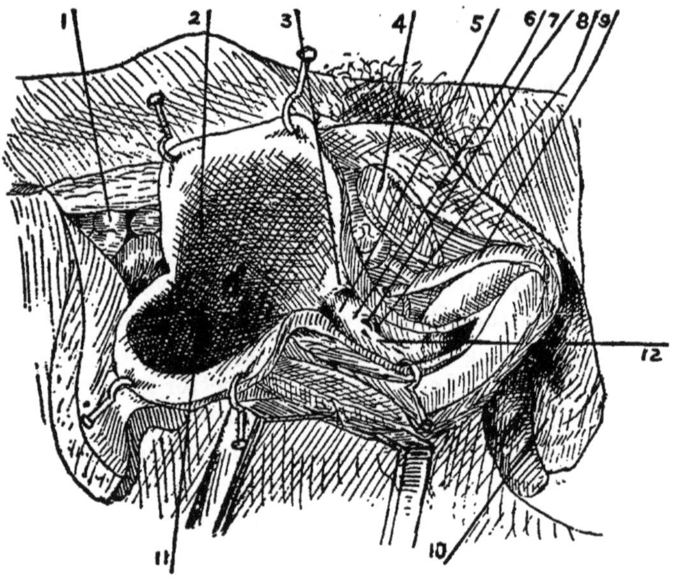

FIG·I

1—Intestines. 2—Bladder (cut open). 3—Neck of the bladder. 4—Pubis. 5—Prostatic urethra. 6—*Veru montanum* and the *genito-urinary crossroad* where the sinus pocularis (7), the ejaculatory ducts (8), and the prostatic ducts (12) come together. 9—Deep dorsal vein of the penis. 10—Penis. 11—Orifice of the ureter.

Guepin, formed by the orifices of the ejaculatory ducts, on both sides of the verumontanum, the prostatic utricle or *sinus pocularis* in the middle and the excretory ducts of the prostatic acini all around. In this *prostato-genital crossroad*, and at a common orifice, that of the ejaculatory ducts, begin the common excretory canals of the seminal vesicles and the terminal *ampullae* of the vas deferens, this last extending to the epididymis of the same side. (See Fig. II.) The urethra is lined throughout its whole length by columnar epithelium, excepting the fossa navicularis and the meatus which are covered by squamous epithelium. The mucous membrane of the anterior portion has a great many follicles and triangular depressions, known as the glands of Littre and the lacunae of Morgagni, respectively, and in these crypts the gonococcus lodges itself in chronic anterior urethritis. Around the verumontanum, as we have seen, a great number of prostatic ducts empty, and, due to the great vascularity and irregularity of structure of this part, it is a fertile ground for the development of chronic inflammations, especially those of gonorrheal origin.

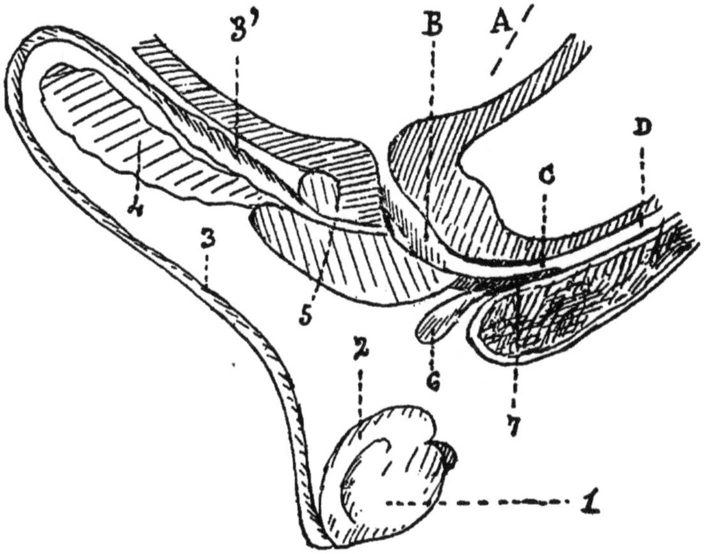

FIG II

1—Testicle. 2—Epididymis. 3—Vas deferens. 3—Terminal ampulla of the vas deferens. 4—Seminal vesicle. 5—Ejaculatory duct. 6—Cowper's gland. 7—Excretory duct of Cowper's gland. A—Bladder. B—Prostatic urethra. C—Membranous urethra. D—Spongy urethra.

Besides this, a great number of anatomo-pathological observations carried on by skillful investigators have conclusively proved that, even though it is not always possible to demonstrate macroscopically the presence of inflammatory processes in the vas deferens, seminal vesicles, prostatic gland and ejaculatory ducts, microscopic lesions of this nature are constant during a gonorrheal orchi-epididymitis; and whether it be a simple irritative desquamation or a profuse desquamation with or without a leucocytic infiltration and fatty degeneration of the epithelial cells, the fact remains that these findings are conclusive proof of how the inflammation and microbic migration progress and invade those regions. In the epididymis the inflammation and irritation begin at the tail and then extend to the body and head. Sometimes, however, they remain stationary at the tail. The periepididymal cellular tissue also becomes involved in the inflammatory process; it becomes infiltrated, increases in volume and almost entirely covers the testicle, like a cap. The inflammation rarely ends by suppuration and more rarely still does it extend to the testicle itself.

Now that I have gone over the most interesting of the anatomic and pathologic points, let us see what is the mechanism by which the orchi-epididymal complication arises in the course of a gonorrheal urethritis. It does not seem pertinent to discuss theories that have not been generally accepted, or the experimental and anatomo-pathologic facts that have been raised to prove them. I refer to the theory of extension by the lymphatic channels presented by Sappey in 1876 and defended by Pilven and Rollet, and to the theory of funicular phlebitis of Desprez, Guepin and Lozé.

On the other hand, I shall consider the theory of extension through the arterial tree, especially since recent investigations by Rey,[1] (along which line Dr. Biamon and I have started a series of experiments) tend to show that the presence of the gonococcus in the blood stream is more common than is generally supposed. According to this theory gonococcal epididymitis is a local manifestation of a gonorrheal septicemia, the gonococcus, carried by the blood stream, becoming lodged in the epididymis in the same way that it becomes lodged in the synovial membrane of an articulation, in the endocardium or in the meninges.

I am very far from accepting this conclusion, and I would not accept it even after finding the gonococcus in the blood of patients suffering from epididymitis, because I believe that, in view of anatomic facts, the arterial tree would carry the gonococci with greater ease to the testicle itself than to the epididymis, and that, although it may clearly explain the pathology of orchitis following parotitis, typhoid or varioloid, it does not explain gonorrheal epididymitis. On the other hand, the presence of the gonococcus in the blood stream during a gonorrheal epididymitis is not an argument in favor of extension by the circulatory tract, inasmuch as a gonorrheal septicemia can coexist with an epididymal in-

[1] Ch. Rey.—"La culture du gonocoque dans le sang circulant."—*Annales de Dermatologie et Syphiligraphie,* 1912. Paris.

flammation of purely local origin. To accept such criterion it would be necessary to demonstrate the presence of the diplococcus of Neisser in all cases of gonorrheal orchi-epididymitis. This is a process that I consider as a local complication of another local process, posterior urethritis; and therefore the urethral theory is the only one that clearly explains the mechanism of its production. Everything is in favor of my way of thinking. The anatomy of the organs involved, clinical observation, manual exploration and the laboratory all coincide in proving the simultaneous occurrence of prostatitis, vesiculitis, deferentitis and epididymitis.

In 1894, Humber and Lucas [2] had already shown the co-existence of vesiculitis and epididymitis in 47% of their cases. And if we take into account that the diagnosis at that time was established by clinical means only, which are not sufficient to demonstrate latent and aborted prostatitis and vesiculitis, it can be understood how far below the real are these figures, so far below that I can say that they only represent 47% of the actual number. In fact, I have sufficient reasons to maintain that in all cases of epididymitis there is also acute, subacute or chronic prostatitis more or less clearly evident; since there can not be an epididymitis without a prostatitis, because in order that the gonococcus may reach the epididymis it must necessarily pass by the vas deferens and it can not enter this duct without previously passing through the prostate and ejaculatory ducts. In the same way that an acute gonorrheal prostatitis can not be conceived without a previous posterior urethritis, just so is an inflammation of the epididymis impossible without inflammation of the organs that precede it in anatomical order, especially if it is a process that extends by continuity of tissue rather than by the circulatory vessels.

The fact that gonorrheal epididymitis rarely appears during the first days of a urethritis but that as a rule it shows itself after the second week, between the third and fifth, when the acute symptoms have subsided and the process seems to be coming to an end, but when the infection has really run the whole length of the anterior urethra and passing the barrier afforded by the triangular ligament invades the pelvic portion of the urethra and the *prostato-genital crossroad*, presents an argument in favor of my opinion; as it can be easily understood how from this *prostato-*

[2] G. Lucas.—"Resultats du toucher rectal daus 285 cas d'epididymite blennorrhagique."—Paris, 1894.

genital crossroad through the ejaculatory ducts and vas deferens, the gonococcus will have easy access to the epididymis.

Again, the microscopical analysis of the urinary sediment has shown me that in all cases of gonorrheal epididymitis there are constantly present desquamated epithelical elements from the prostate, ejaculatory ducts, prostatic ducts and seminal vesicles; in other words the sediment presents all the evidence of the presence of inflammation in those organs.

Rectal touch, systematically practiced, will also show in a great number of cases an increase in volume of the terminal ampulla of the vas deferens as well as an abnormal sensibility of this part; it will also discover a prostate which is more or less tender, often swollen and presenting all the evidences of inflammation.

Lastly, a microscopical examination of the products obtained by pressure through the rectum upon the prostate gland and seminal vesicles will show, almost invariably, the presence of polynuclear leukocytes and gonococci, together with desquamated epithelium corresponding to the mucōsa. And, in cases in which this direct and extemporaneous microscopical examination fails, a bacteriological analysis of cultures of those secretions in special culture media will demonstrate the diplococcus of Neisser.

Hence, there is no doubt that gonorrheal orchi-epididymitis is always preceded by an inflammation, acute or chronic, more or less latent or manifest, of the prostate, seminal vesicles and vas deferens; and it is, therefore, a local complication of a posterior urethritis, caused by the direct extension of the virus through the above named organs to the tail of the epididymis; being also indisputable that it is from the posterior urethra, prostate and vesicles that the bacteria and toxins which start the inflammation come.

There are several predisposing causes that contribute to the development of this inflammatory process, namely: traumatisms, endourethral maneuvers, athletic exercise, forced marches, violent shakings and efforts, coitus, masturbation, sexual excitement, high pressure irrigations, caustic injections, badly handled catheterization, preëxistent inguinal hernias and varicoceles, testicular anomalies and alcoholic excesses.

These facts stated, upon which I shall base the reasons for the treatment I recommend, let me now briefly review the clinical aspects of the condition. Acute gonorrheal orchi-epididymitis does not always present the same symptoms nor does it always have the same beginning. Although true that its clinical aspect is not usually serious, there are times, as I have seen in some cases, in which the general reaction is so violent and the local symptoms are so intense that they may produce well founded alarm. At other times, the disease develops and progresses without causing any trouble to the patient and may be so benign as to make him think that he can dispense with any treatment.

As changes in the clinical picture will necessarily involve changes in the technique of my treatment, though this be fundamentally the same, it is well to have present in our minds these changes in making this brief symptomatic description.

Acute gonorrheal epididymitis does not usually become apparent before the third or after the fifth week of the acute urethral process. But please bear in mind that I do not refer to the epididymitis which occurs in the course of a chonic urethritis, as these, brought about, as a rule, by sexual abuse or intra-urethral maneuvers for therapeutic or diagnostic purposes, come on shortly after the exciting cause has been brought into play and manifest themselves months or even years after the beginning of the gonorrhea. Although this complication usually comes on suddenly and is not often preceded by prodromes, there are some cases in which there may be some malaise, slight fever, anorexia, and slight pain in the inguinal region; these signs giving warning of the extension of the inflammation to the epididymis. In fact, acute pain and swelling of the epididymis, localized in the corresponding scrotal zone, soon make their appearance; the urethral discharge, if present, ceases; micturition becomes frequent, the urine becomes turbid, and fever rises to 38°C. and 39°C. followed by cephalalgia, gastric disorders, constipation and at times vomiting. The swelling and the pain go hand in hand, while the one increases the other becomes intensely acute, radiating to the lumbar region, abdomen, inguinal region and thighs; it becomes exacerbated by pressure, even by the least contact. The epididymis enormously enlarges, covering the testicle like a cap, and the scrotum becomes reddened and edematous. The tunica vaginalis of the testicle reacts to the neighboring irritation with a slight exudation, the vas deferens is sensitive and enlarged and at times there develops in the cord a violent funiculitis. Rectal touch is usually able to confirm the concomitant inflammation of the prostate and the seminal vesicles; this is also evidenced by the frequency of nocturnal seminal emissions of a puriform and sanguinolent spermatic fluid.

From the second day the subjective acute pain begins to remit, but the fever and the pain on pressure continue as long as the increasing intensity of the inflammatory process lasts. This condition of affairs usually lasts from five to seven days, but as a rule it begins to decrease from the fifth day on. The temperature falls, the inflammation decreases, the appetite is better, there is a rapid return of strength and general good feeling and the patient can usually be considered cured at the end of three weeks, although there will remain as a relic an induration of the tail of the epididymis.

Acute gonorrheal epididymitis ends in this way, going to a rapid resolution. It is but rarely that it goes on to suppuration and more rarely to gangrene. Sometimes, however, after the patient is well, when he has already gone back to his work, the epididymis becomes inflamed again, or there is an inflammation of the epididymis of the opposite side, or of both epididymes at the same time; these varieties being known as *repeating, balancing* and *double* epididymitis.

I have already mentioned the fact that this disease does not always present the same clinical picture, but that it shows various clinical types. I have just described the acute type, which is the most common. There is also an *abortive* type without any general symptoms and characterized by a simple induration of the globus minor of the epididymis. This type which, as a rule, does not inconvenience the patient in any way, may at times be accompanied by a serious funiculitis, as occurred in one of my cases. In the *sub-acute* type, of relative frequency, the symptoms are very slight and the patient can usually attend to his business from the first day. The *painful* type of Gosselin and the *grave* form with hyperpyrexia or a peritoneal reaction are very exceptional.

Acute orchi-epididymitis is second in frequency among the complications of gonorrheal urethritis. According to the highest authorities it complicates 15 to 20% of all gonorrheas, and although true that, due to the advances made in antigonococcic therapeutics, the percentage of this complication has been lessened, it is just as true that in some cases it is impossible to avoid it no matter how careful the treatment. Such cases, however, are not an argument against the well demonstrated fact that very often the occurrence of epididymitis is due to errors or carelessness in the local treatment.

The fact that on various occasions, both in the hands of general practitioners and experienced specialists, acute epididymitis has occurred following the instrumental explorations of the posterior urethra, irrigations with silver salts, urethro-vesical washings, or catheterization in subjects having recent or old strictures, posterior urethritis or chronic prostatitis, was no doubt one of the chief reasons for considering as contraindicated the continuation of local treatment of urethritis during acute gonorrheal epididymitis, and why the legendary treatment by rest in bed together with poultices, ointments and ice bags should have acquired such vogue, both in Europe and America. Having had the opportunity of using this filthy and uncomfortable method (Case II and III) and of comparing it with a total abstinence of all treatment (Case II, second attack, and Case XII), limiting my measures to rest in bed together with complete suspension of the testicle by means of a bridge of adhesive plaster, or by means of the suspensories of Horand-Langlebert and the athletic supports of Johnson & Johnson or of Bauer & Black, I have found that the first mentioned has no advantage over the last method; as I noticed that it did not shorten the course of the disease nor did it avoid suppuration, when this had to occur (Case III) nor, what is most important, did it lessen the pain any more than did a good suspension of the testicle.

When I compare these methods with those of Delbet and Perrin, which I have often used, their inferiority is made manifest. With the latter I can lessen the duration of the process to about ten days and can allow my patients to walk about at an early date even in the most severe cases. I can also often abort a case when I have the opportunity to interfere early. With the more ancient methods, the disease lasts about three weeks and the patient will be troubled by a persistent induration and sensitiveness of the epididymis long after he is cured. And so, leaving aside all those treatments which have as a basis immobility associated with the local use of drugs over the diseased part, such as the use of revulsives like a 10% solution of silver nitrate, poultices of linseed flour and tobacco (3:1) as recommended by Guiteras, ointments of ichthyol (20 to 50%) and guaiacol (5 to 15%), fomentations of lead water and laudanum, or the famous ice bag, I shall limit myself to describe the method I use, which imitates in part the methods of Delbet, Du Castel and Perrin. Although I keep the basic principles of each one of these surgeons in my method, I have, notwithstanding, introduced such marked modifications in the technique of their application, and have associated with them other therapeutics measures of such importance, that I can well consider my method to be a very much improved modification of theirs.

In 1896 Paul Delbet showed in a very interesting article[3] that, contrary to the general opinion, the local treatment of urethritis with irrigations of potassium permanganate during the course of an acute gonococcal epididymitis, instead of being harmful, was highly beneficial as it shortened the duration of the disease and at the same time helped to suppress the primary cause. A year later (1897) I began to experiment with Delbet's method and obtained such good results that for a long time after, and whenever the circumstances allowed it, I used it in preference to any other.

In some cases when I was unable to attend the patients personally because of reasons of economy or of professional secrecy, or of their living too far from my office, so that it was impossible to subject them to a daily treatment, I was compelled to resort to the classical method of antiphlogistics, rest in bed and cessation of the direct treatment of the urethritis. I have believed it convenient to mention some of these, in the relation of cases given below, to compare them with those treated by the methods of Delbet and Perrin and with that which I now advocate, so that my readers may be better able to judge the therapeutic value of each. Of the twelve case whose clinical history I give below, two (Cases III and VIII) were treated by the classical method exclusively; one (Case II) was treated during the first two attacks in the same way but during the third attack by Delbet's method; three (Cases X, XI and XII) were subjected during the first few days to the classical treatment and later to the method I recommend. In cases I and IV Delbet's method was used exclusively while cases V, VI, VII and IX were treated by mine alone.

Since 1897 I have treated 118 cases of gonococcal epididymitis and in the majority of these cases I did not suspend the treatment of the causal urethritis, but in 37 cases this treatment was not used, having been substituted *a fortiori* by one or other of the several modifications of the classical treatment. It is in-

[3] Paul Delbet.—"Cinq cas d'orchites blennorrhagiques traitees par les lavages au permanganate de potasse."—*Annales des Maladies des organnes genito-urinaires,* 1896. Paris.

teresting to note that three of those 37 cases ended in suppuration, and that in one of these three cases there was a vaginal empyema with a real suppurative orchitis (Case III), while in the remaining 81, in which the treatment of the urethritis was not suspended, none showed such complication.

Keeping in mind the fact that gonococcal orchi-epididymitis is only a complication of the acute urethro-prostato-vesiculitis, which extends by way of the vas deferens, I usually proceed as follows:

(a) I begin a systematic treatment of the posterior urethritis by means of copious urethro-vesical irrigations with a weak solution of potassium permanganate.

(b) Every day at the time of the urethral irrigation, I massage the prostate and seminal vesicles.

(c) I order the patient to wear a suspensory bandage of the Horand-Langlebert type or, if this is not at hand, the triangular bandage for athletes of Johnson & Johnson or that of Bauer & Black.

(d) I do not require rest in bed, on the contrary my patients can attend to their usual business after the second day.

(e) I give a saline purgative on the first day and then try to keep the bowels free by means of mild laxatives or hot enemas.

(f) I give two grams of sodium salicylate daily, as an antiseptic and sedative.

(g) If the pain is too intense I recommend the use of one centigram of morphine by hypodermic injection or the use of suppositories of morphine and antipyrine.

(h) If it does not improve by these means but becomes intolerable, then I resort to the heroic measures recommended by Guiteras in his excellent treatise on "Urology"[4]: light touches with the Paquelin thermo-cautery over that portion of the scrotum that covers the inflamed epididymis.

(i) I order the patient to take a sitz-bath at a temperature of 40° to 59°C. at least once in twenty-four hours.

If the patient was under my care prior to the onset of the epididymitis, one of two things was being done: either I was treating him for acute gonorrheal urethritis or I was treating him for a chronic urethral process, posterior urethritis, prostatitis, stricture, etc. In the first instance I would simply continue to use the irrigations of potassium permanganate that I

[4] Ramóu Guiteras.—"Urology," 1912.—New York.

had been using for the urethritis, and in addition give a daily prostatic massage. In the second instance we would change the bi- or tri-weekly séance for daily treatments and would substitute the other special measures for urethro-vesical irrigations with potassium permanganate and also a daily prostatic massage. When the subject has not been under my care prior to the onset of the attack of the epididymitis, I throw aside any therapeutic plan that he may have been following, if there was any, and immediately begin with the irrigations and prostatic massages.

For these urethro-vesical irrigations in the course of an epididymitis I prefer the "Record" bladder syringe to the fountain syringe, because in the first it is the intelligent hand of the surgeon capable of appreciating the least resistance that pushes and guides the piston in its descent, while in the irrigators by hydrostatic pressure it is the unconscious force of gravity that gives impulse to the liquid column which must force the muscle of Wilson and enter the bladder passing through the posterior urethra. With the "Record" syringe the surgeon knows all the time the degree of contraction or relaxation of the membranous sphincter and is in a position whereby he can avoid overdistention of the urethra and the traumatisms which follow excessive pressure, as he can stop as soon as he notices the least resistance. The irrigation apparatus shows the contraction too late, frequently provokes spasms, and in this way is liable to cause tears of the mucosa and thus aggravate the inflammatory process. The syringe I use has a capacity of 100 c.c. and has a metallic plunger and a canula which ends in a pyriform dilatation. It is thus capable of being adjusted to obstruct the entrance of the urinary meatus. When this canula is not at hand it can be replaced by inserting an olive of rubber, Einhard model, into the anterior extremity of the ordinary conical canula.

At the beginning of the treatment with the urethro-vesical washes, if I have to deal with nervous subjects or with persons suffering from an acute epididymitis, it is my custom to first anesthetize the anterior urethra and bulbar region with a 2% solution of alypin, or with cocaine hydrochlorate, novocain or stovain of the same strength. I let this solution act on the mucosa for five minutes, compressing the distal extremity of the glans with the thumb and index fingers of the left hand, while with the right hand I lightly massage the urethra until I can get a few drops of the liquid into the membranous region of the canal. This done it becomes very easy to wash the posterior urethra, the sphincter will not resist and I can pass 200 c.c. of the permanganate solution into the bladder without any trouble. As a rule I employ a solution weaker than 1 to 4000. I empty the first 200 c.c. injected by asking the patient to urinate. Then I inject 100 c.c. more. Then I massage the prostate, asking him to urinate again and finally inject another 200 c.c. that will be emptied as before.

When I massage the prostate I do not ask the patient to bend forward but instead, following Legueu[5] I prefer the lithotomy position as it is my belief that this is more decorous, less troublesome for the patient and allows me to make a better and more complete exploration as well as a better massage. It will not be amiss to say here that with the exception of cases of prostatic abscess, which rarely complicates epididymitis, the massage of this gland must be practiced with energy and patience, as this is the only way, avoiding poor attempts, that one will be able, as Perrin says,[6] to express into the urethra the purulent contents and microbic colonies hidden in the glandular acini and canaliculi. It is important to keep the testicles immobile and suspended against the pubes during the course of the affection as it is the best way I know to avoid and to relieve pain. As we are seldom able to obtain in this country suspensories of the Horand-Langlebert pattern and as it is somewhat difficult for the patient to put on these suspensories by himself, I use in their stead, imitating Guiteras, athletic support bandages or if these can not be obtained than I use a simple T bandage. Following our distinguished professor of the New York Post Graduate School, I place a thick covering of absorbent cotton over each testicle and on top of this oiled silk (B & B) and then cover the whole with the bandage. Proceeding in this manner I obtain at the same time an excellent suspension of the testicle, the antiphlogistic and sedative action of the moist heat developed and conserved by the layers of cotton and oiled silk and also protect the testicle against any traumatism. Thus, as I am able to keep the organ immobile in this artificial bed, which is also warm and soft, the patient need not be subjected to an uncomfortable stay in bed and it also allows him to attend to his urgent business after the first day. Of course there are cases in which this is not possible because of the epididymitis being accompanied at the

[5] Legueu.—"Traité d'Urologie."—Paris, 1910.

[6] Th. Perrin.—"Diagnostic et traitement des affections chroniques les plus fréquents du canal uretral et de la vessie."—Paris, 1907.

start by hyperpyrexia, excessive pain, intense cephalalgia, nausea and vomiting, all of which require the bed *a fortiori;* but these are exceptional cases, and even after the second day when with appropriate treatment the general symptoms have subsided, the patient may leave bed whenever he is protected as already mentioned.

I have said that in all cases I try to keep the bowels free by means of enemas and laxatives, and only have to add that this measure not only combats the gastro-intestinal disturbance which accompanies or precedes the epididymal inflammation, but it also exerts a highly beneficial action in carrying the inflammatory process of the prostatic gland towards resolution.

Among the drugs to be given internally I prefer sodium salicylate, not only because it quiets the pain and lowers the temperature present during the first days, but also because in combination with urotropin it is the best medication for the accompanying prostatitis and urethro-cystitis. I give 2 grams daily, divided into four 50 centigram doses, one every four hours, and prefer the stable solutions prepared by various reputable manufacturers, as they are not only of guaranteed purity but are easy to take.

In most of the cases, these measures are sufficient to rapidly modify the course of the epididymitis and bring it to a complete resolution in a few days, the average duration being about twelve days. But in other instances the intensity of the process is such that I have to adopt more heroic measures. The patient is compelled to remain in bed. Local pain is agonizing. Fever rises to 40°C. And to be able to control the situation I give aspirin instead of sodium salicylate, inject one centigram of any morphine salt and then employ *effleurage* on the scrotum covering the diseased epididymi, just grazing the skin with a Paquelin thermo-cautery with the lamina at white heat, or by means of a large galvano-cautery. Forty-eight hours afterward the patient is usually able to get up and the epididymitis then follows the course of an ordinary case.

When the symptoms on the part of the prostate are very evident I recommend the daily use of sitz-baths at a temperature as high as the patient can bear it, and if possible I would also use rectal douches at 45°C. with canula having a double stream; Guiteras type or any other similar one.

In some acute cases which develop in the course of gonococcal urethritis, and in all cases of repeated epididymitis or whenever it complicates chronic gonorrheal affections, I recommend the use of antigonococcic vaccines, autogenous or polyvalent, pure or mixed with staphlococcus, streptococcus or colon bacilli, depending on the result of the bacteriological analysis of the urethral secretions or of the products of the prostato-vesical massages.

With this method of treatment, I can obtain in less days than by P. Delbet's or by Perrin de Laussane's method, of which it is an advantageous modification as it takes care of both the local and general condition of the patient, rapid and sure cures with very little suffering, a thing that could not be accomplished by the classical method, and I may at times abort a beginning epididymitis.

We must not forget that although, as a rule, the treatment of gonococcal orchi-epididymitis has always been highly satisfactory from the standpoint of relief of symptoms, it is necessary that we should exert ourselves in trying to obtain complete cures, to avoid further recurrences and with them the possibility of secondary tubercular implantations, to which matter Casper[7] says, the urologists have not been paying the proper attention. That is why I am opposed to the famous ice bag, and in general to all measures which endanger the vitality of the testicle.

Summary of Cases.

CASE I. (1897.)

Acute gonorrhea—Acute epididymitis.

C. F., 26 years old, married, clerk. Came to my office three days after a suspicious coitus, with all the symptoms of a beginning acute gonococcal urethritis. I immediately began to treat him with urethro-vesical irrigations with potassium permanganate, following Janet's method then in vogue. Twelve days after all the discharge had ceased and the urine in both the first and second glasses was clear, but the urine of the first glass still contained thick, heavy filaments. The patient then took a chance on another love affair and had such bad luck that his anterior urethra ruptured in a bad motion made during the coitus. Profuse hemorrhage resulted. Permanent sound was used for 48 hours. When I took out the sound the discharge began again; this I did not treat locally for fear of distending the broken mucosa. Three days later, preceded by prodromes consisting of

[7] Leopold Casper.—"A Text-book of Genito-urinary Diseases."—Philadelphia, 1906.

general malaise, pain in the inguino-abdominal region and fever, an epididymitis appeared accompanied with funiculitis, hyperpyrexia, cephalalgia, vomiting and intense pain in the left cord and epididymis. I immediately instituted again the urethro-vesical washes with permanganate solutions varying in strength from 1 to 10,000 to 1 to 5,000. I prescribed a purgative of magnesium citrate, two grams daily of sodium salicylate, and applied a thick covering of absorbent cotton under a T bandage to suspend the testicles and keep them immobile. After 48 hours the patient got up and was able to attend to his duties.

Results:—Four weeks later he was cured of the epididymitis and the posterior urethritis by irrigations, dilatation with Beniquet sounds and silver nitrate instillations. As a reminder, he kept for a long time a persistent induration of the tail of the epididymis.

CASE II. (1898–1901.)

Chronic Gonococcal Urethritis—Repeating Epididymitis.

L. M., 23 years old, single, clerk. He first came to me about the middle of the year 1898. He then had an acute gonorrhea in full blast. He was unable to come to my office daily to be treated by copious irrigations, so I subjected him to the classical treatment, prescribing for the first few days salicylate and sodium bicarbonate and later frequent injections of the anterior urethra with a solution of potassium permanganate, 1 to 2500. One week later I was summoned to bis home and found him in bed with severe pain and great swelling of the left testicle, moderate fever and complete cessation of the urethral discharge. As it was impossible, in this case, for private reasons, to use Delbet's method, I followed the old therapeutics of rest and ointments. I prescribed a 10% ointment of vaseline and guaiacol, rest in bed, a saline purgative, and two grams of sodium salicylate daily. On the second day the pain began to lessen but the inflammation progressed up to the sixth day and my patient was unable to leave the bed for the first week nor could he return to his business before twenty days had elapsed. When I discharged him the indurated zone of the epididymis was as large as a chestnut, and to hasten resolution I advised him to envelop the testicle with iodized cotton, every twelve hours.

I did not see this patient again for a year, when he came back because of a second epididymitis. Internally I used the same treatment as before but did not use any drugs locally, limiting myself to advise rest and the use of a Horand-Langlebert suspensory. After 36 hours the pain began to abate and six days later the patient was able to get up, returning to his business on the eighth day. Three weeks later I advised the need of curing the urethritis so as to avoid future recurrences, and taught the patient the technique of the urethro-vesical irrigations that he might practice them daily. A month later he thought he was cured and became careless with his urethral treatment. He continued to deceive himself in this way for a year and a half when one day the urethritis reappeared, due to sexual excesses. This time he attempted to cure it with patent medicines but when three days later the epididymitis reappeared on the same side as in previous years, the patient came to see me. He was willing to submit to my treatment in full and therefore came to my office every day for treatment. Rectal touch revealed a chronic prostatitis. I immediately began with the urethro-vesical irrigations with potassium permanganate, and as in the previous attack I suspended his testicles in a suspensory similar to Langlebert's. This time my patient did not have to remain in bed or to keep away from his business. He was rapidly cured of the epididymitis and the posterior urethritis. The irrigations were continued for a month and were then substituted by instillations with silver nitrate and modified catheterizations with Beniquet sounds every three days. Ten weeks later he was perfectly well and reacted negatively to Neisser's test.

CASE III. (1903.)

Sub-acute gonorrhea. Suppurative epididymo-orchitis. Empyema of the tunica vaginalis.

Young man, 24 years old, single, merchant, came to me with a sub-acute urethritis. Microscopical examination showed the presence of the gonococcus in the purulent secretion from the urethra. The urine was turbid in both glasses, although more marked in the first. He complained of a sensation of weight in the perineum, frequent urination and a certain amount of tenesmus after urination. I made a diagnosis of sub-acute posterior urethritis, and instituted Janet's method of copious washes with potassium permanganate but used solutions weaker than 1 to 4000. The patient improved rapidly, the urine of both glasses becoming clear although it still contained heavy filaments, the heavy sensation in the perineum disappearing and urination becoming more regular. But the patient was somewhat careless and he did not follow the treatment to the letter. About the fourth week of treatment the urine became turbid again, and a few days later an epididymitis appeared with all its classical symptoms. My patient went to bed and was unwilling to continue the treatment of the urethritis. I prescribed suspension of the testicles, 33% ichthyol ointment, sodium salicylate internally, laxatives and rest in bed. The pain disappeared quickly, but the inflammation continued even after the fever had gone. Twelve days later the pain returned but this time more pronounced over the gland than over the epididymis. Fever reappeared, being preceded by chilliness, and was of the intermittent type accompanied by sweating. It was the beginning of abscess. The patient was unwilling to have it incised just yet and I was compelled to wait until fluctuation became manifest. I then made an incision, deeper than usual, evacuated the pus and put in gauze drainage. Immediately the fever disappeared, his appetite became keen and his good humor returned. Everything seemed to be returning to the normal, but as the wound in the scrotum tended to form a fistula and fever, sweatings and pain, although of moderate intensity, reappeared at certain hours from the third day, there was no doubt that there was retention of pus. I injected a 1 to 4000 solution of bichloride of mercury into the fistulous tract of the drain, and while I massaged and carefully expressed the diseased organ to favor the expulsion of the retained products, I noticed the presence of seminiferous tubules in the pus. I had, therefore, a real suppurative orchitis before me, that had opened into the vaginal sac producing an empyema, and which I had mistaken at first for a deep abscess of the scrotum. I decided to intervene on the following day, and using local cocaine anesthesia, I operated together with two colleagues. I made a large incision, divided the tunica albuginea, carefully curetted and then placed a gauze drain. The results of the operation were very satisfactory. Shortly afterwards the patient was allowed to go.

CASE IV. (1903.)

Sub-acute gonorrhea. Epididymitis.

J. M., 30 years old, clerk, called me on account of a painful inflammation of the right testicle that had kept him in bed since the previous day. He had an acute epididymitis in the course of a gonorrhea, also acute, which began 4 weeks before. I immediately began the urethro-vesical irrigations, prescribed a purgative of sodium sulphate and two grams of salicylate internally, and placed a T bandage over both testicles. I practiced the first irrigations in the patient's home. Three days later he returned to his business and a month later he was pronounced cured of both the epididymitis and the urethritis.

CASE V. (1910.)

Sub-acute gonorrhea. Acute epididymitis.

A. A., 18 years old, student, came to me the sixth day after the beginning of an acute urethritis; microscopical examination showed it to be due to the gonococcus of Neisser. Urethro-vesical irrigations were used. During the first days of the third week, the urine of the second glass became turbid and, at the beginning of the fourth day, an epididymitis of the left side appeared with high fever, intense pain, constipation and cephalalgia. He was not able to come to my office. I then continued the permanganate irrigations in his home and at the same time began the systematic and daily massage of the prostate gland. I prescribed Seidlitz Chanteaud, one dose to be taken every morning, two grams daily of sodium salicylate and an athletic support bandage. Two days later the patient was able to continue the treatment in my office. Two months later he was pronounced cured of his urethritis, having reacted negatively to Neisser's test several times.

CASE VI. (1910.)

Sub-acute urethritis. Epididymitis.

M. R., 24 years old, single, clerk, had a gonorrheal urethritis for four months which he had been treating himself by means of balsams and astringent injections. He came to see me because of an exacerbation of the process. Microscopical examination confirmed the clinical diagnosis. Physical exploration also revealed the presence of a chronic prostatitis and of an epididymitis that had begun two days before. I advised urethro-vesical irrigations, prostatic massage, suspension of the testicles and sodium salicylate. The patient did not go to bed, attended to his business and was rapidly cured of his epididymitis without any induration remaining. Four months later he was completely cured of his gonorrheal process. Neisser reaction negative.

CASE VII. (1910.)

Acute gonorrhea. Acute epididymitis.

S. P., 19 years old, clerk, came to me the twelfth day after having felt the first symptoms of a urethritis. Discharge was abundant, examination for gonococci positive and the urine of the second glass slightly turbid. I began urethro-vesical irrigations, followed by marked decrease in the suppuration. On the eighth day the urine of the second glass became more turbid and the patient complained of pain in the right inguino-abdominal region radiating toward the testicle. I explored the prostate and found it very sensitive as were the terminal ampulla of the vas deferens and the right epididymis. On that same day I practiced prostato-vesicular massage which I continued daily for two weeks and I also recommended wearing an athletic support bandage. The epididymitis was aborted. The patient did not have to stay in bed, and six weeks later I considered him cured after having reacted negatively to Neisser's test.

CASE VIII. (1910.)

Acute gonorrhea. Balancing epididymitis.

S. C., 22 years old, chauffeur, came to see me on account of epididymitis on the left side. For five weeks he had been suffering from acute gonorrhea, for which he had been treating with a quack, who advised and sold him some secret injections and some beverages also of secret formula. The pain and the inflammation had begun three days before coming to my office, and were now causing him intolerable suffering. This patient was unable to come to my office and it was impossible for me to go to his house. On this account I was forced to employ the classical treatment and so prescribed him a 33% ichthyol ointment, an athletic support bandage and sodium salicylate. A month later he came back with epididymitis on the right side. A month later the inflammation returned to the left side. I have lost sight of him since then.

CASE IX. (1910.)

Chronic urethritis. Stricture. Chronic prostatitis. Urethral process becoming acute. Acute epididymitis.

A man 59 years old. Since 1909 I had been treating him for a chronic urethritis complicated by stricture and chronic prostatitis. He came to the office with much irregularity and too little constancy and progressed very slowly toward cure. During that time he had two recrudescences of the urethritis, due to transgressions in the diet prescribed and to imprudent erotic ventures. During the last acute process, the prostate played a very important rôle and our patient complained of tenesmus, frequent, painful and difficult micturition, and a sensation of heaviness and of the presence of a foreign body in the rectum. I treated the prostatitis with urethro-vesical irrigations of protargol, hot sitz-baths and sodium salicylate internally. The patient did not improve. On the sixth day an epididymitis developed on the left side. I immediately abandoned the protargol and began 1 to 10,000 permanganate irrigations preceded by prostatic massage, and ordered the patient to wear a suspensory. He immediately began to get better. The patient did not have to remain in bed and could attend to his many and troublesome occupations. Twelve days later the epididymitis was completely cured.

CASE X. (1910.)

Acute gonorrhea. Acute prostatitis. Epididymitis.

E. B., 32 years old, married. A month ago he contracted acute gonorrheal urethritis which by the blunderings of a *practicant*, in whose hands he had placed himself, was carried by the point of a catheter to the posterior urethra. The prostate became violently inflamed, compelling him to go to bed and to send for his physician. The prostatitis was treated as usual by rest in bed, hot enemas, hot sitz-baths, antiseptics internally and suspension of all local treatment while the fever and the acute symptoms persisted. In the course of the prostatitis there developed an epididymitis that was also treated by the classical method. The patient improved of both processes slowly.

In the last days of June, 1911, I returned from the United States and the physician of E. B. sent him to me for treatment.

Microscopical examination of the pus revealed the presence of the gonococcus. Study of the urinary sediment showed that there was an intense desquamation of the cells of the prostate, prostatic ducts, ejaculatory ducts, seminal vesicles, urethra and neck of the bladder; together with an abundance of pus globules, some red corpuscles and spermatozoa. Clinical examination showed a turbid urine in both the first and second glasses, and also a very sensitive and voluminous prostate. The epididymis as large as a dove's egg, was very sensitive to the least touch.

Very little purulent discharge passed through the urethra. On the same day I began copious urethro-vesical irrigations with a permanganate solution and daily massage of the prostate and seminal vesicles. The patient became better rapidly. The prostate and the epididymis decreased considerably in size. The subjective symptoms disappeared. A month later the induration in the epididymis was gone and the prostate returned to its normal size; but there were still many filaments in the first glass of urine. The patient practically discontinued treatment, only following it for periods of a week every 3 or 4 months, and for this reason the chronic Neisserian process in the urethra and prostate persists.

CASE XI. (1911.)

Acute gonorrhea. Epididymitis.

H. C., 28 years old, single, clerk, came to see me at the beginning of an acute gonococcal urethritis. Copious urethro-vesical irrigations were instituted. At the end of the third week there began an inflammation of the left epididymis. I immediately practiced the first prostatic massage after injecting the first 100 c.c. of the permanganate solution. I made the patient urinate and continued the irrigations. I recommended him to wear an athletic support bandage. During the four days that followed he did not come to the office, as he was being treated by the family physician, who was opposed to continuing the local treatment and prescribed rest in bed and ichthyol ointment. On the same day that the patient returned to me I again instituted the massages and urethro-vesical irrigations. The results were very good; three weeks later I considered him cured, after having reacted negatively to Neisser's test.

CASE XII. (1912.)

Hypertrophied prostate. Acute prostatitis. Epididymitis.

S. F. L., 48 years old, merchant, had been suffering from an acute prostatitis for a month, being treated by the family physician following the usual routine. I saw him in consultation. He complained of frequent and difficult urination and of vesical tenesmus. I recommended the use of a 20% solution of "gomenol" in oil besides continuing with the treatment his physician had established. Fifteen days later the patient felt well enough to come to my office, where his physician kindly sent him. I took charge of his treatment and began to practice massage of the prostate and irrigation of the posterior urethra with silver nitrate, twice weekly. After the sixth séance, he complained of pain and swelling of the right epididymis. Being unable to come to my office on account of distance I treated him by rest in bed, 30% ichthyol ointment, suspension of the testicle with an athletic support bandage and sodium salicylate internally. Twelve days later the epididymis was still as large as a dove's egg, very sensitive to pressure and bothered the patient a great deal. Arrangements were made to do the urethro-vesical irrigations and prostatic massages at the house. The following day I began with a very weak solution (1 to 1000) of argyrol, which he did not stand very well, but it immediately began to improve. The size of the epididymis diminished rapidly, the symptoms of prostatitis and posterior urethritis disappearing almost altogether and the patient is at present progressing to rapid recovery.

REVIEW OF CURRENT UROLOGIC LITERATURE

ZEITSCHRIFT FUR UROLOGIE.

Second Supplementary Number, 1914.

Proceedings of the Deutsche Gesellsschaft für Urologie, Fourth Congress, Berlin.

1. Bladder Stones, their Origin, Prevention, and Treatment. By S. P. von Fedoroff.
2. Etiology, Therapy, and Prophylaxis of Bladder Stones. By Jos. Preindlsberger.
3. Origin, Treatment and Prevention of Bladder Stones. By Felix Schlagintweit.
4. The Röntgen-Ray Diagnosis of Ureter Stones. By Franz Weisz.
5. The Use of High Frequency Currents in Urology. By H. Wossidlo.
6. Results with Thermopenetration in Genito-urinary Diseases. By H. Lohnstein.
7. The Treatment of Papillomata of the Bladder by Intravesical Electrolysis. By Rudolf Oppenheimer.
8. Purpura Vesicæ and its Sequelæ (Ulcus Simplex Vesicæ Pepticum). By V. Blum.
9. Formation of a Valve in the Bladder for the Drainage of Ascitic Fluid. By Paul Rosenstein.
10. Congenital Diverticula of the Bladder. By H. Brongersma.
11. Prostatectomy Statistics. By Dr. Preindlsberger.
12. Demonstration of Bladder Diverticulum with Report of the Case. By Dr. Preindlsberger.

1. Bladder Stones, their Origin, Prevention and Treatment.

The diagnosis of bladder stone is made from the subjective and objective findings. Pain, dysuria, and bloody urine are the usual clinical manifestations of the condition. Objective investigation is generally begun with the metal sound. Cystoscopy is also of great value. One of the most exact methods is X-ray examination. This is especially helpful in children, in cases where the urethra is obstructed, in severe cystitis, in marked prostatic hypertrophy and in neurasthenic patients.

As regards the therapy of this condition Fedoroff comes to the following conclusions:

1. Litholapaxy is the operation of choice at all ages.

2. In those cases where litholapaxy is impossible or for any reason contraindicated, sectio alta must be attempted.

3. In doing the high section operation care must be taken to close the bladder completely with a suture of absorbable material (catgut).

4. When the bladder is hermetically sealed it is better to omit the permanent catheter in the post-operative stage.

5. The perineal route for stone-operation must be reserved for exceptional cases.

2. Etiology, Therapy, and Prophylaxis of Bladder Stones.

Preindlsberger takes up first the relation of the geology of the land to the frequency of lithiasis in the inhabitants residing in any given district. He mentions various observations based on soil and water analysis in this connection. He then discusses other factors in the etiology of lithiasis, such as the question of precipitation of the stone-building substances, supersaturation, the role of foreign bodies, the role of the organic framework found in calculi, etc., etc. He next takes up the question of uric acid infarcts in the young. He believes that the frequency of lithiasis in Bosnia and Herzegovina is due to the fact that the children are very poorly nourished, are kept on the breast until three and four years of age and that thus the regular flushing out of the kidney does not take place. In this manner congenital uric acid infarcts remain behind and become the starting points for calculus formation. In 587 cases 429 occurred under twenty years of age.

The remainder of the author's paper—which is rather extensive—is given over to a comparison of the two methods of operation: (abdominal) section, or stone-crushing. He discusses the indications for each procedure as determined by the age of the patient, size of the stone, etc., and quotes the opinions of various authors. The author finally gives his own results in the 377 bladder stone operations he performed up to December 31, 1912. He divides his material into four series for the purpose of presenting his cases in greater detail. In all he has performed 177 sections (abdominal) with a mortality of 11.3%, 100 perineal cystotomies with a mortality of 7%, 55 lithotripsies with one death, 5 lithotripsia perinealis and one sectio perinealis lateralis. Thirty-six cases of urethral stone all recovered.

Preindlsberger concludes that:

1. Lithotripsy is the operation of choice and gives the best results.

2. When lithotripsy is not applicable either sectio alta or cystotomia perinealis may be performed. The latter is especially valuable in children.

3. Origin, Treatment, and Prevention of Bladder Stones.

Schlagintweit presents a comprehensive study of the entire subject. Not only have surgeons been interested in the physical and mechanical aspects of stone formation, but biologists have been trying to solve the question of stone origin and stone growth and still others have been studying the broader subject of stone-distribution from the standpoint of climatology, geology, hygiene, ethnology, and sociology. The author concludes from such studies that in highly civilized countries there is no such thing as endemic stone occurrence, and that in such countries as Bosnia, Russia, India, and Egypt, where bladder stone is endemic, it is generally poorly nourished children, or riotously-living adults who are attacked. Furthermore, the factors which have been regarded as causes for stone-formation in stone countries, are not found to apply in individual cases in civilized lands. We are more and more inclined to the belief that the "endemic" frequency of stone is to be ascribed rather to primitive methods of hygiene, especially to poor nourishment in childhood. The sporadic occurrence of stone in individual cases should be ascribed rather to familial and hereditary diatheses.

In discussing the formation of urinary stones the author emphasizes the latest work done from the point of view of colloid chemistry. Thus Posner has called attention to the colloid framework existing in every calculus, and believes that the nubecula present in urine furnish the basis of the organic structure. Furthermore Lichtwitz has pointed out that the solubility of the stone-forming salts in the urine depends on the presence in the latter of a protective ("Schutz") colloid. [Both Posner's and Lichtwitz's papers have been abstracted in the December, 1913, number of this journal.—Ed.]

The chemical composition of a bladder stone is important inasmuch as it helps to explain the point of origin of the calculus, and the reason for its failure to pass out with the urinary current. Of the 326 cases of stone in the author's records the great majority were composed of urates, showing that these calculi usually originate in the kidney. Phosphate stones almost always originate secondarily in the bladder. The chief causes for the failure of the calculi to pass were prostatic hypertrophy, strictures, paralysis of the bladder, and poor contraction of the bladder, with urate cystitis. In about ten per cent. of the cases no cause was discoverable.

The diagnosis of the bladder stone may be made accidently by the passage of a soft instrument. The passage of the special stone sound or lithotriptor may be of value, especially when this is combined with auscultation of the bladder region. The cystoscope, is after all the most valuable instrument, especially as the beak may be used as a sound. Palpation through the vagina or rectum may be of help, especially in children. This is a very ancient method of diagnosis. Radiography is of course of great assistance especially in cases where the cystoscope cannot be introduced.

As regards the technic of stone operations, aspiration through an evacuation catheter or irrigation cystoscope should always be done if possible. Otherwise litholapaxy is easily the operation of choice. In this connection the author takes up the preliminary preparation of the bladder, points of asepsis, choice of anesthetic, technic (Guyon's) and difficulties and accidents encountered in the performance of the operation. Schlagintweit does not use the permanent catheter in the routine after-treatment of these cases. A comparison of the mortality statistics of lithotomy and lithotripsy is very much in favor of the latter, the former operation carrying a death rate of between 3.6 and 24.3%, and the latter one varying only between 1 and 4%, according to different authors.

Although lithotripsy is generally to be preferred to a sectio alta or perinealis, one of the latter may have to be resorted to under the following conditions: (1) when an instrument cannot be introduced through the urethra, (2) when the stones are too large, or too hard or too numerous, (3) when the stone is immovable, (4) when the stone is associated with a tumor, (5) when a permanent catheter is found insufficient for the drainage of a septic bladder or when a sectio alta is planned anyway for the removal of a tumor, (6) in the presence of certain foreign bodies which cannot for any reason be broken.

There is so far no way of preventing the formation of bladder stones. We may however avoid operation in many cases by repeated cystoscopies and removal of a beginning (early) calculous deposit by aspiration.

4. The Roentgen-Ray Diagnosis of Ureter Stones.

Weisz reports the case of a woman who suffered with attacks of severe abdominal pain with great tenderness in the right half of the abdomen most marked toward the bladder. There was dysuria with pain especially before urination. Cystoscopy revealed a normal left ureter opening, but the right was inflamed, edematous, and pouting. The right urine contained more pus than the left; no tubercle bacilli were found, and the urine injected into guinea pigs proved subsequently negative. An X-ray plate showed a shadow on the right side near the bladder. Ureteral catheterization of the right side met with no obstruction. On opening the abdomen the right ureter was isolated, opened and probed carefully in both directions. No stone was found. The wounds were closed and healed well but the patient died about a month later from cardiac failure. At autopsy there was found sclerosis of the coronary arteries. There was a fibrotic tuberculous kidney on the right side which did not appear in the X-ray plates on account of the adiposity of the patient. The shadow at the vesical orifice of the right ureter was probably caused by a similar mass of fibrotic or calcareous substance which was perhaps wiped away during the course of the operation.

5. The Use of High Frequency Currents in Urology.

The heat of resistance of the high frequency currents may be employed either to warm the body or one of its parts (general or local diathermy) or to destroy tissue (surgical diathermy). Local diathermy has given some fair results in chronic urethritis, but only when used in conjunction with dilatation. Better effects were obtained in posterior urethritis, in prostatitis and in chronic epididymitis and gonorrheal arthritis.

Surgical diathermy or electrocoagulation has given the best results in the treatment of bladder tumors. This method of treatment is easy of application, free from untoward effects, and painless. Very good effects have been obtained in papillomata (benign) of the bladder and of the posterior urethra.

6. **Results with Thermopenetration in Genito-Urinary Diseases.**

High frequency currents may be used either for the purpose of warming the body or for cauterization (cold cautery, fulguration). Clinically, the effect of diathermy is first to increase, then to diminish mucus secretion, to soften hard infiltrations in the urethra, prostate and testicle, and to relieve the pains of organic inflammation.

Lohnstein has treated 45 cases in 9 months by the so-called conservative diathermy. He varied the exact procedure according to the organ affected, the cause of the symptoms and the object of treatment. In general the cases selected were those which had remained unaffected by the ordinary methods of treatment. He reports favorable results in cases of chronic gonorrhea due to urethral infiltrations, in chronic prostatitis, in neurasthenia sexualis and in nervous impotence, in gonorrheal epididymitis, and in one case of chronic hemorrhagic nephritis.

The author has gained the impression, from his personal experience with the method, that diathermy is a valuable curative factor, that it often actually brings about or at least hastens a cure where other methods fail, but that in its present form (excluding the cold cautery) it can give no one a priori assurance of a more certain or more rapid cure than the other (older) methods of treatment.

7. **The Treatment of Papillomata of the Bladder by Intravesical Electrolysis.**

The patient's body is covered with moist towels and the anode is applied in the form of a medium sized platinum electrode. At the same time the cathode is introduced into the bladder. The cathode is a bougie-electrode provided with a metal tip 2 to 4 mm. in length, and is introduced through an ordinary ureteral cystoscope. The bladder is irrigated and distended and the electrode is introduced into the base of the tumor until the whole of the metal tip is buried in the growth. A current of 60 volts is then introduced slowly and applied, according to the patient's tolerance, in a strength of from 10 to 45 milliamperes. The current is allowed to act for about a minute, then discontinued, and reapplied in another place.

The advantages of intravesical electrolysis, according to the author, are the following:

1. The method is technically simpler than the use of snares.
2. Bleeding and pain are slight.
3. After the tumor is removed the base may be attacked intensively.
4. Electrolysis has the advantage over high frequency treatment of a simpler armamentarium and the slighter chance of bladder perforation.

The method has the disadvantages, first, of causing the appearance of gas bubbles thus clouding the operative field and necessitating frequent irrigations, and secondly of taking a long time and requiring many sittings for the complete removal of a given growth.

8. Purpura Vesicæ and its Sequelæ (Ulcus Simplex Vesicæ Pepticum).

Blum has made a special study of this subject and finds:

1. Acute hemorrhagic cystitis, characterized by the appearance of multiple solitary foci in the bladder mucosa, is similar to purpura hemorrhagica rheumatica, is a sequel of a general infection or intoxication, appears at definite seasons, and is therefore properly to be described as a purpura vesicæ.
2. The hemorrhages into the mucosa may be absorbed under favorable conditions. The clinical picture, in such cases, shows a rapid regression. As a rule however the bleeding goes on to a hemorrhagic erosion, and later to a superficial or deep ulceration, which may lead to a perforation of the bladder.
3. Every "spontaneous" perforation of the bladder is the result of a previous hemorrhagic lesion.
4. The formation of an ulcus simplex from an intramucous or submucous hemorrhage is explained by the peptic characteristics of the urine. There is a far-reaching analogy in the clinical symptoms, course, etiology, and pathogenesis between ulcers of the bladder and those of the stomach.
5. In addition to urinary disinfection and local treatment the therapy of cases of beginning ulcus vesicæ consists in a permanent alkalinization of the urine.
6. In order to prevent the formation of a peptic ulcer the urine should be rendered alkaline in every case of purpura of the bladder.

9. Formation of a Valve in the Bladder for the Drainage of Ascitic Fluid.

Rosenstein opened the abdomen and exposed the peritoneal aspect of the bladder. A metal ring, 3 cm. in diameter was then placed on the vertex and this portion of the bladder pushed through. The vertex was then incised and the cut surface of the serosa united to the serosa outside the ring in circular fashion. In order to prevent expulsion of the bladder contents into the peritoneum during contraction, a circular strip of serosa and muscularis about 4 cm. in width was excised outside the line of serosa suture. In this way the mucosa was exposed. The cut edges of muscularis and serosa were then united together causing the underlying mucosa to pucker and act as an effective valve during bladder contraction.

In the case reported the valve worked well although all the ascites was not gotten rid of by the method, supplementary paracenteses being necessary. The urine was cloudy and contained albumen, leucocytes and fat globules, originating from the ascitic fluid.

10. **Congenital Diverticula of the Bladder.**

Congenital diverticula are those in which all the elements making up the bladder wall are present and which do not contain a ureteral orifice.

The author presented four specimens which he had successfully removed extraperitoneally. The characteristic points in the anamnesis were the feeling of not having emptied the bladder after urination, and urination in two attempts. On irrigating such bladders the alternation between a clear and a cloudy return fluid is characteristic. Where no inflammation is present the same effect may be produced artificially by first introducing a collargol solution. The X-ray however is the best aid to diagnosis, and may be employed either in connection with an X-ray catheter or a collargol solution introduced into the diverticulum.

The prognosis in such cases is influenced by the pressure exerted by the diverticulum on one or both ureters with resulting stasis and by the occurrence of infection. The latter is a serious complication and, according to Englisch, involves a mortality of 83 per cent.

ANNALES DES MALADIES VENERIENNES.

Vol. IX, No. 4, April, 1914.

1. Neosalvarsan and Distilled Water. By Drs. A. Richaud and Gastaldi.
2. Two Cases of Cervical Vertebral Disease of Syphilitic Origin. By Drs. Gaucher and Bory.
3. Practical Considerations on Antigonococcic Serotherapy. By Giacomo Define.
4. Clinical Study of the Antigonococcic Vaccine of Nicolle and Blaisot. By André Weil.
5. Two Cases of Extragenital Chancre: Chancre of the Nares and of the Finger. By Dr. Payenneville.

1. **Neosalvarsan and Distilled Water.**

The majority of clinicians regard the untoward results following the new arsenical preparations as due either to the toxicity of these products or to a particular susceptibility on the part of certain individuals to these drugs. Other physicians have attributed these untoward effects to the presence of bacterial bodies in the distilled water used as the medium for the injection. Sicard has recently pointed out that some of the reactions resemble lead poisoning and might therefore be due to the presence of lead in the injected fluid, the lead arising from the glass of the distilling apparatus. The authors do not accept this theory and point out that the lead in the glass is in the insoluble form of silicate.

In order to prove definitely that the lead did not enter as a factor in the problem they performed the following experiments with the condenser used by Sicard in the preparation of the distilled water with which he got his so-called lead reactions: 1. The apparatus was thoroughly washed with sulfuric acid and distilled water and then connected with a distilling flask. Four liters of water were then distilled and evaporated to dryness. Although no residue was perceptible, the washings of the crucible were tested for lead and found negative. 2. The condenser was broken into small fragments and 30 grams of these were powdered and boiled in a reflux condenser for one hour. The liquid was then concentrated and examined for lead; none was found. Finally the authors examined several specimens of distilled water obtained from various Parisian druggists but could find no lead in any of them.

The authors are not inclined to accept Ehrlich's contention that the reactions may be due to catalases present in the distilled water. They point out, it seems with justice, that when a reaction follows an injection of pure water plus neosalvarsan, there is no a priori reason why the latter, other things being equal, should not play a part in causing such reaction. It may very well be, for example, that some individuals are susceptible to the particular action of this drug, or that some of the preparations of the drug may not be chemically perfect, or finally, that the simple aqueous solution of neosalvarsan does not constitute the ideal form for the intravenous introduction of this drug.

The authors conclude that it is not necessary to attach too much importance to the preparation of the distilled water and that the frequent changing of the distilling apparatus to prevent the solution of various substances from the glass, is, to say the least, quite superfluous.

2. Two Cases of Cervical Vertebral Disease of Syphilitic Origin.

The first case was that of a woman of 27, who had contracted syphilis seven years before. She had been insufficiently treated and at the time of examination presented a tumefaction under the skin involving the second, third, and fourth cervical vertebrae. The swelling was more prominent on the right side and seemed to consist of a gummatous osteo-periosteal infiltration enveloping the laminae and vertebral bodies. The mass was not tender on pressure, but induced some pain and stiffness on movement of the neck, and ultimately came to exert pressure on the cord causing a right spastic hemiplegia. Under mixed treatment the condition improved considerably.

The second case was that of a woman of 40 who contracted syphilis 8 years before, and developed gummata of the sternum and of the frontal bone. For the past year and a half a gibbus had been developing insidiously at the nape of the neck, but outside of causing a little stiffness it gave no other symptoms (such as those of compression of the cord). A radiograph clearly showed a sinking in of the bodies of the first two vertebrae. The Wassermann reaction was strongly positive.

In discussing the symptomatology of syphilitic disease of the vertebrae the authors point out the absolute clinical similarity of this condition to Pott's disease. Sudden death may also occur in the syphilitic process from dislocation of the odontoid process or from ascending paralysis. There are certain points of difference, however, between the two conditions. In the first place, vertebral disease when it begins in the adult and the general condition is good, is more likely to be specific than tuberculous. The past history of syphilis is of confirmatory value but too much importance should not be attached to this nor even to a positive Wassermann reaction unless there has been a previous tendency to involvement of the bony skeleton. On the other hand however syphilitic Pott's disease may be the only or the first lesion affecting the bones. In this case the diagnosis would be made only by the characteristic improvement under specific treatment.

An important point to bear in mind is that osseous syphilis in the adult is rarely accompanied by a change for the worse in the general condition, whereas when it occurs in youth, in the form of hereditary syphilis especially, it may very well be accompanied by a cachexia resembling closely that of tuberculous Pott's disease. It is therefore wise in every case of the latter condition to think of syphilis as a possible etiological factor.

3. **Antigonococcic Serotherapy.**

The real indication for antigonococcic serum is found in the complications of a urethritis due to the gonococcus or its toxins, for the serum has a definitely specific action. As to the effect on the urethral process itself, opinions differ. Some think that the serum may be of value inasmuch as it may aid the tissues in responding to the effect of local treatment. Others feel that this action is negligible or at least not proven as yet.

The action of antigonococcic serum is preëminently analgesic and resolvent. As regards administration, it is unnecessary to resort to the intravenous route. Injections are made daily into the subcutaneous connective tissue, are not painful, and are well borne by the patients. The number of injections varies according to the case. The author has given as many as sixteen. The best guide to the limitation of such treatment is the appearance and character of anaphylactic phenomena.

4. **Clinical Study of the Antigonococcic Vaccine of Nicolle and Blaisot.**

Through the kindness of Dr. Blaisot of Tunis, Weil was enabled to treat ten cases with the vaccine of Nicolle and Blaisot. In the series were 2 cases of chronic gonorrhea, one gonorrhea with prostatitis, 2 cases of gleet, 4 cases of acute urethritis, one vaginitis with urethritis.

The technic is simple. Two ampules are provided, one with distilled water, the other with the vaccine. A two c.c. syringe is used and first one-half c.c. of vaccine and then $1\frac{1}{2}$c.c. of water are aspirated and injected intramuscularly in the usual manner. From his experience with this method of treatment the author concludes as follows:

1. Intramuscular injections of the vaccine have always appeared harmless. Although slightly painful the injections have been well supported.

2. Only one attempt at intravenous injection was made. The patient had an intense reaction with severe general symptoms suggestive of septicemia.

3. Vaccine treatment alone seemed to have no great effect on the discharge. The course of the disease did not appear to be shortened.

4. There was clear analgesic effect in five out of six cases with pain.

5. On the other hand, the vaccine does not seem to prevent complications, for in two cases an orchitis developed in the actual course of treatment.

6. In short this treatment would appear to be of value only in painful manifestations where it exercises a very rapid sedative action. Otherwise the results appear to be inconstant.

5. **Two Cases of Extragenital Chancre.**

The first was that of a woman of 45, who noticed a slight erosion at the edge of the right nostril. The ulceration spread and became covered with a thick crust, the tip of the nose became red and swollen, and the submaxillary glands became enlarged on both sides. Contrary to the general rule with head chancres, the roseola appeared rather late,—somewhat more than two months after the discovery of the chancre. A series of neosalvarsan injections supplemented by active mercurial treatment brought about a rapid healing of the lesion. On questioning the woman it was found that her grandson, whom she was bringing up, had the full-blown lesions of congenital syphilis. The father of the child had a positive Wassermann and admitted having had a lesion of the penis several years back which "healed by itself." In this case the father had infected his mother and son and perhaps his wife as well.

The second case was that of a factory overseer who complained of an infected eczema of the hands. This cleared up under local treatment except for a periungual ulceration of the right middle finger. The finger itself was swollen and there was a large gland in the axilla. An ultramicroscopic examination of the secretion from the lesion was made but no spirochetæ were found. The Wassermann however was three plus and a characteristic roseola removed every element of doubt as to the nature of the process.

On interrogating the patient it was brought out that a month and a half before he had injured the finger while working in the factory. About ten days later he had a suspicious intercourse. The wound had never healed. The questions to be decided here were: (1) Was this a professional infection as a result of trauma? (2) Even if the venereal infection is conceded should not the previous traumation be regarded as a contributing factor facilitating the entrance of the infecting agent?

REVUE CLINIQUE D'UROLOGIE.

March, 1914.

1. So-called Prostatics Without a Prostate. By Nicola Carraro.
2. Notes on Nephrolithiasis. By Le Clerc-Dandoy.
3. A Case of Urethroplasty by Transplantation of a Piece of the Internal Saphenous Vein. By Dr. Cealic.
4. Pathology of the Seminal Vesicles (Continued). By M. Palazzoli.
5. Sexual Disorders of Psychic Nature (Continued). By A. Wizel.

1. So-called Prostatics Without a Prostate.

Carraro has made a special study of such cases. He describes the usual course with increasing difficulty in emptying the bladder, distention, and the supervention of terminal complications. He then reports four instances in which a diagnosis of prostatic adenoma was made cystoscopically, rectal palpation and other methods of examination failing to reveal an obstruction to the urinary current.

Cystoscopy is therefore of the first importance and enables us to size up accurately the anatomical condition of the neck of the bladder, revealing slight deformities produced by prostatic adenomas not palpahle per rectum. These adenomas are the cause of the great majority of cases of retention formerly attributed to "vesical prostatism."

The treatment of these cases is radical and the operation of

Freyer with complete enucleation of the nodules, is the procedure of choice. When successfully performed this permits of practically normal urination just as in the cases of prostatectomy for hypertrophied prostate. Microscopic and pathologic study of the removed growths shows conclusively that the nodules are arranged within the vesical sphincter, and that they do not originate within the prostate but in the submucous pericervical glands.

2. **Notes on Nephrolithiasis.**

The author reports nine cases of kidney stone with X-ray figures. Radiography is of the first importance in such studies not only for purposes of diagnosis but because in many instances it can help decide the operative procedure to be employed. Thus we are enabled to arrive at the decision as to whether a pyelotomy can be successfully undertaken. When the stone is very large, and the overlying renal cortex reduced to a thin shell, such a procedure or even a nephrotomy is out of the question.

The author agrees with Bazy in regarding pyelotomy as the operation of choice and nephrotomy the operation of necessity in removing kidney stones. Posterior pyelotomy is preferable to an anterior incision. Fistulæ are less common and the risk of hemorrhage is diminished. A pyelotomy wound cicatrizes very rapidly. In some cases it may be necessary to supplement a pyelotomy by a nephrotomy.

The chief symptoms of nephrolithiasis are pain and attacks of "congestive" nephritis. The pain extends over the entire loin and may be so severe as to prevent sleep for years. Very occasionally a calculous "friction" may be obtained on palpation. The author describes one such case. Cystoscopy is of importance. Fenwick has insisted that when the cystoscope reveals normal ureteral orifices a renal or ureteral lithiasis may be excluded; and that in cases of nephrolithiasis the ureteral orifice (corresponding side) is generally redder and more dilated than the other. This sign however is not absolute. What is of importance is that the cystoscope can establish the integrity of the bladder in the cases of unilateral renal suppuration.

4. **Pathology of the Seminal Vesicles. (Continued.)**

In this instalment Palazzoli first takes up the microscopic anatomy of the vesicles. He describes the various coats, fibrous, muscular, and fibro-elastic, and finally the epithelial lining. He then takes up the anatomy of the ejaculatory ducts and next goes into the development of the seminal vesicles. Among their anomalies he discusses: (1) Absence of the seminal vesicles, (2) Fusion of the vesicles, (3) Duplication, (4) Communication with the urethra, and (5) Atrophy. In this section especially full references are made to the literature.

Treatment of Gonorrhea with Santyl, the Salicylic Acid Ester of Santalol.

Dr. Antonio Acebo (Espana Medica, 1914, no. 107) has prescribed Santyl-(Knoll) during the last $2\frac{1}{2}$ years in numerous cases of gonorrhea. Disturbances so common during the administration of other balsams, such as gastric and intestinal disturbances, eructations or bad breath were not seen nor was there any record of renal pains or excretion of albumin.

Patients already treated without success with other balsams and complaining of pains in the renal region received daily 15-75 drops of Santyl. There always was an anesthetic effect, erections and hematurea disappeared, the urine cleared up and a definite cure was soon established. With combined treatment, other balsams were also tried but in the author's hands Santyl always proved to be the best internal remedy. Surprising results were also obtained in the urethrocystitis of women.

BOOK NOTICES

THE PATHOGENESIS OF SALVARSAN FATALITIES. By Sanitäts-Rat Dr. Wilhelm Wechselmann, Directing Physician of the Dermatological Department, Virchow Hospital in Berlin. Authorized translation by Clarence Martin, M.D. Fleming-Smith Co., St. Louis, Mo. Cloth, pp. 143, $1.50.

Whether one is an enthusiastic adherent of salvarsan or a bitter opponent he will do well to read this book by Wechselmann, who, while he cannot be considered a perfectly unbiased observer, has nevertheless had an enormous experience with the drug, and whatever he has to say must be taken into consideration. The volume before us is not a complete translation of Wechselmann's original work, many case reports having been omitted. It is sufficient, however, to give a complete idea of Wechselmann's standpoint. In conclusion of his volume the author gives certain precautions which may be reiterated here: These precautions are:

"1. The most exact technique. 2. A dose of the drug carefully adapted to the individual case. 3. Careful observation of the urinary secretion when employing salvarsan; resorting to the most exact chemical and microscopical examination of the urine. This holds good particularly when the combined treatment is employed. 4. The conjoint use of salvarsan with heavy mercurial treatment is dangerous. If one will use the combined treatment, then give mercury very carefully many days after the last salvarsan injection, but never reverse this rule. 5. Take into careful consideration every general reaction or rise of temperature, following the use of salvarsan, and make a full investigation of the causes of such effect."

DIE MODERNE THERAPIE DER GONORRHOE BEIM MANNE. Ein Leitfaden für Studierende und Artze. By Prof. Dr. Paul Asch.

Illustrated. Paper, bound. A. Marcus & E. Weber's Verlag, Bonn, Germany.

Although this little volume contains only eighty pages it presents a very satisfactory review of the modern treatment of gonorrhea in man. The author's presentation of the subject is very clear, and in spite of the number of volumes we have on the treatment of gonorrhea it is a welcome addition. The treatment of this refractory disease is still in such an unsatisfactory condition that no book presenting the personal opinions of an experienced specialist can be considered superfluous.

We read this volume with pleasure and we cheerfully recommend it to general practitioners interested in the treatment of gonorrhea. And even specialists might get a useful hint from its perusal here and there.

LE TRAITEMENT DE LA SYPHILIS EN CLIENTELE. By Prof. H. Gougerot. Pp. 492, with 75 illustrations and 19 colored plates. In paper covers, 10 francs; bound, 12 francs. A. Maloine, 25 due de l'Ecole de Medecine, Paris.

It affords us great pleasure to recommend this exceedingly practical volume which deals with what is indispensable to know in syphilography. Of course the latest developments in the treatment of the disease are considered in detail, and the author is not an extremist. The general practitioner will find in Prof. Gougerot's book a safe and reliable guide to the diagnosis and treatment of syphilis.

DEPARTMENT OF SEXUAL PSYCHOLOGY

NOTES ON THE PSYCHOLOGY OF SEX.

By Douglas C. McMurtrie, New York.

VII

A REMARKABLE OPINION ON PROSTITUTION.

There has recently been issued in Atlanta, Georgia, a most interesting volume [10] dealing with the prostitute and her profession. I have read the work and could comment upon it, but I should like to quote instead a very able review of the book which appeared [11] in the *New York Medical Journal.*

"This little work is in many respects a remarkable one. The writer apparently started on his investigations with the prejudices and the point of view of a country clergyman of the old school, an upholder of a cosmogony that includes the tower of Babel and the Noachian deluge, a thinker who looked upon the social evil as nothing more or less than a series of deliberate violations of a Mosaic law against adultery, unaware of the modern view that this law was directed solely against infractions of property rights and that nothing was further from the early Israelite mind than Christian ideas of purity. Apparently he intended to abolish the social evil by the methods of an old time revival and by personal exhortations. After visiting 3,000 brothels, however, and talking with over 15,000 prostitutes, the writer's views have undergone a complete reversal; he has learned that the great majority of people know nothing of the causes of prostitution; he has seen that there is no 'white slave' traffic and that the women in the business are there because their 'very being is permeated with a gross carelessness of good morals and high ideals. They are what might be termed low brows; possessing not one iota of courage to face the world bravely; devoid of womanly instinct, of character, and of principle. The motherhood instinct that lies in the average woman's heart and soul is missing in this class of women. . . . It is not their fault. They are in most instances doing the best they can, the best they know

[10] Albert W Elliott. *The cause of the social evil and the remedy.* Atlanta, Ga., 1914.

[11] *New York Medical Journal,* 1914, xcix, 658.

how. . . . They cannot understand why one should want good character. Possessing no high ideals themselves, the whole thing is simply foreign to them.'

"Mr. Elliott offered every prostitute he met a chance to reform; of the immense number fifty accepted or pretended to accept, and of the fifty a single one did really reform. Being convinced that once a prostitute always a prostitute, and that the prostitute is born so, the writer sees no remedy, but as a palliation insists upon segregation. Coming from the type of man that it does, this book deserves wide reading; we have given it space somewhat commensurate with its importance, despite its small size. The medical reader will smile at many naivetés in the work, for, outside of his views on the one subject, the author's philosophy has not broadened in the least and other vast problems of our civilization he still regards from the standpoint of the village pulpit."

I might add further that Mr. Elliott has sent me a copy of a journal which he edits, and in which appear commendations of the book referred to from people eminent in various lines.

HOMOSEXUAL INFATUATION BETWEEN WOMEN.

A recent report which has reached me from a middle-western city in this country seems to justify a diagnosis, on the basis of social relations alone, of sexually inverted infatuation.

Two young women, aged approximately twenty-eight and thirty-one years respectively, of good family standing and education, lived together in a luxurious house, the property of one of them who is very well-to-do. They employed several servants but none of these latter slept in the house, going home each night instead. The two ladies were never known to attend any social functions, but whenever they were seen, were invariably in each other's company, either driving, walking, or shopping.

The aggressive member of the pair was the elder, the one who had the money. She dressed in masculine fashion, wearing stiff collars and plain fedora hats. The second young woman exhibited feminine characteristics. Her appearance was comparatively weak.

AN ANTHROPOLOGICAL DATUM ON FEMININE INVERSION.

In a report to the Société d'Anthropologie of Paris, Roux

has reported [12] a case of sexually inverted practices by an old woman during a temporary period. The author considered the case interesting by reason of its rarity and because he was able to secure for presentation with his paper the artificial organs utilized by the female subject. The observation was made in 1900 on the Island of Maintirano, to the west of Madagascar.

Among the people of this island, the *sarimbavy*, a man dressed as a woman, having been already described in the scientific literature, Roux terms the woman regarding whom he reported a *sarindahy*, a woman with the figure, clothing and desires of a man. Its derivation is as follows: *sâry*, having the appearance of; *lāhy*, man.

"In 1900 Fatima was an old woman about sixty years of age who had been married but who had lost her husband in 1890. From this time on she shaved her head, assumed the native head-dress, and clothed herself in the great white robe, the garb of the male natives. She sought the favors of the Sakalave women, remunerating them handsomely. She made herself a male organ out of ebony. Through its base passed a cord which attached the article to her girdle. The testicles were represented by a bit of raffia. Means for adjustment were provided. Fatima, however, soon exhausted her pecuniary resources and she was deserted by her young women lovers. She then married and supported an aged woman in relation to whom she acted the male rôle but with diminished pleasure. She soon even abandoned male clothing and discontinued the practice of shaving her head. Finally in 1899 Fatima entirely ceased the vicious practices in which she formerly took pleasure. The majority of the people regarded her sexual misdeeds with indulgence, having a certain consideration for her age." Dr. Roux exhibited the artificial penis of Fatima at the time his paper was presented.

Zaborowski, in discussion, said [13] that the practices of this *Comorienne* were known to be widespread on the east coast of Africa, especially in Somaliland. In his opinion, it was from this region, always in communication with Madagascar, that the customs described were derived. Ivory instruments single or double were used by the women in mutual relations. In this region also, infibulation of women and girls was practiced.

[12] Roux. Note sur un cas d'inversion sexuelle chez une Comorienne. *Bulletins et Mémoirs de la Société d'Anthropologie.* Paris, 1905, 5th ser., vi, 218-219.

[13] *Ibid.*, p. 219.

DEFINITION OF THE SEXUAL INSTINCT.

One of the most important recent expressions concerning the sexual instinct is dealt with in a most interesting editorial in the *Medical Record.*[1] It ran as follows: "Many attempts have been made to define the sexual instinct but without success. Freud and his followers attribute to this instinct the production of many if not the majority of nervous disorders, but, as a rule, the English-speaking psychologists do not agree with the far-reaching views of the Freudian School. At a joint meeting of the Section of Psychiatry of the British Royal Medical Society and the British Psychological Society, on March 10, Dr. William McDougall read a paper on the 'Definition of the Sexual Instinct.' He said in part that the present attitude of both academic and medical psychologists on the nature and rôle of instinct in general, and the instinct of sex in particular, was chaotic; and it was only by coöperation of medical with other psychologists that a right understanding of sex instinct could be hoped for. The erroneous views could be classified into two groups: (1) Those which were unduly simple, representing the sex instinct as merely the tendency to respond to certain disagreeable sense-stimuli with movements which abolished the disagreeable and produced pleasurable sensations; and (2) Those which ascribed to the sex instinct a variety of mental and bodily processes which originated in other and distinct roots. The Freudian doctrine, in his opinion, comprised several errors. Against the view that the sex instinct arose from the desire for pleasurable gratification was the fact that in some cases the instinct continued after complete castration. The speaker strongly disagreed with Freud's contention that the sex instinct was normally present in infancy; it appeared to have its earliest beginnings at about the eighth year and progressed steadily to puberty. Though the sex instinct was admittedly complex, it should not be regarded as comprising two distinct impulses."

CASE OF EXHIBITIONISM IN THE STREET.

It is very seldom that a full clinical record of a case of exhibitionism can be secured, because such cases very seldom come professionally under the care of a physician. A good many more or less fragmentary reports, however, reach me from thoroughly

[1] The sex instinct. *Medical Record,* New York, 1914, lxxxv, 852.

reliable sources and they seem worth while recording, since the available data on this subject are few.

At six o'clock one Sunday morning, a man of respectable appearance, came to a corner diagonally opposite a large hospital where it would be known a number of trained nurses would be on duty. He stood there until he knew that he was observed; then unfastened his clothing and exposed his penis, at the same time performing manual masturbation. Having accomplished this, he went to early service in a church at the next corner. Coming out about half an hour later, he watched for a favorable opportunity and repeated his previous performance. At the time of orgasm he experienced a veritable frenzy, swaying from side to side and, according to my informant, "jumping all over the street." When his acts were completed he went quietly away.

THE EXTENT OF TRIBADISTIC PRACTICES.

The practice of tribadism, in the opinion [2] of Kisch, is more widely diffused than generally imagined. "I have often encountered instances of it in ladies of good position, who were past their first youth, and who would not, or could not marry, and who took extensive trips with a female 'companion' of similar age or perhaps a little younger. Their erotic needs, which could not be gratified in normal fashion, led to this sexual perversion—a tendency observable especially in persons with neuropathic predisposition, or with a liability to hysteria or to epilepsy. Sometimes such girls, even before puberty, show an inclination to wear boys' clothes, to avoid all feminine labor, and to examine and to handle the genital organs of their playmates. Even after puberty, such tribadists like to make a parade of masculine attitudes, they have their hair cut short, wear clothes of a masculine cut, smoke a great deal, and show in their conversation, and still more in their letters, great exaltation of the passions. It not infrequently happens that an elderly lady who has lived well in her day, and from youth upward has had much intercourse with men, comes at last to lament her worthlessness to men, and from this proceeds to the idea of obtaining sexual enjoyment by means of tribadism. The tribadistic union sometimes lasts for several years, but in most cases the alliances are quickly and frequently changed."

[2] E. HEINRICH KISCH. *Das Geschlechtsleben des Weibes.*, 2nd edit., Berlin and Vienna, 1907, p. 197.

THE AMERICAN JOURNAL OF UROLOGY, VENEREAL AND SEXUAL DISEASES

WILLIAM J. ROBINSON, M.D., EDITOR

VOL. X AUGUST, 1914. No. 8

PRESIDENTIAL ADDRESS TO THE SECTION ON UROLOGY OF THE XVIITH INTERNATIONAL MEDICAL CONGRESS IN LONDON.

By PROFESSOR E. HURRY FENWICK.

GENTLEMEN,—The note of cordial welcome which was sounded yesterday by Sir Edward Grey in open assembly is being echoed sympathetically this morning by every President, in every section. I count it as belonging to the privileges as well as to the pleasures of my office to be able, on behalf of my colleagues and myself, to say that that chorus evokes an especially vibrant harmonic note with us, for I feel that you are welcome here, not merely as visitors to the section, but as colleagues, as co-workers, and as friends.

Since a similar greeting was extended in this city to a similar Congress of medical men, over thirty years have elapsed; and those of us who were present then, in 1881, and enthused by the sight of those master minds, Pasteur, Koch, Virchow, Charcot, Huxley, Lister, Langenbeck, and Volkmann, and our much beloved leader of thought and teacher of men, Sir James Paget, may well feel proud of having continued the work which they initiated, whilst all of us may congratulate ourselves in having been instrumental in the production of the most wonderful wave of scientific progress which has ever been chronicled in the history of the healing art.

But what has this tidal wave brought us as a profession? Has it caused some lightening of our load of learning, some diminution in the responsibility which knowledge rightly entails upon the holder? Far from it. Both have increased beyond expression. The actual sum of knowledge of that complex science, medicine, which was then already great, has grown so vast, that it is now beyond the power of the average mental capacity to possess or hold it. The pressure of responsibility which a censorious public thrusts upon us is now so intolerable that men seek others to share the burden with them.

Hence divisions, re-divisions, then sub-divisions in the art and science of medicine, until, as was anticipated in 1881, and feared and as bitterly opposed, the appearance and rapid growth of special study, special learning, and special practice.

But specialism in medicine is no new feature. In the very dawn of history, in Egypt under the old Empire, sixty centuries ago, the science of medicine was already in the hands of special physicians, and later, forty centuries ago, each physician had to be a specialist. Moreover, if we glance down the arcades of time, we see appearing—where history flecks the pavement—men whose originality of mind and natural bent have forced them from the beaten track, to engage in the pursuit of special knowledge. But it may be acutely noticed that, when there has been no jealous opposition, no tyranny of tradition, of custom, or of prejudice to warp the worker's instincts, the special knowledge he has gained has returned to enrich the general fund—for the avid searcher after knowledge differs from the groper after gold—in that he is always anxious to share his gain with others.

The danger in specialism lies not in narrowness or in superficiality, as was urged in 1881, for the appetite for knowledge grows by what it feeds on. The danger lies in obstructing, and not directing wisely, the superabundant energy and originality of the workers; in ostracizing them, for this delays diffusion of knowledge; in isolating them, for this encourages selfish retention of experience gained.

The bureau of our International Congress of Medicine has realized these changes in the pressure and has noted the more generous policy of the profession, and has established, as the years went by, new sections for every new field of thought which showed fertility, so that when that field was harvested the gains could be garnered for the general good and universal progress. Our section—the Urological Section—is one of the later additions to the conclave of knowledge and is an adjunct to that of surgery—for expert urology without a mastery of surgery is inconceivable. But if urology is hopeless without surgery, it is helpless without many other of the sister arts and sciences of medicine. Medicine, gynecology, microscopy, bacteriology, radiology, and electro-therapeutics must all be utilized by the expert urologist and should be known to him, for he must always be responsible for their findings in his diagnosis and operative treatment. Can such a worker be called a "specialist"? Or is it possible to look at urology as a narrow superficial study? I contend that the term "specialism" applied to urology is a misnomer. I claim that the urologist is an expert surgeon with a bias to the study and treatment of one of the most difficult and lethal sections of surgery. Can this view be supported? Has urology justified the judgment of the bureau in making it a section? In answering, I feel an ample answer lies to hand—I have only to look round here and to remember others who are absent, but here in sympathy, and know that you all, working together, have created the art and science of urology.

When the genius of Nitze evolved the perfect cystoscope in 1887 an area of almost virgin soil was exposed. There had, of course, been toilers in that field before, and to the last of the great clinical masters, Guyon and Thompson, we are deeply indebted, but they all lacked in their research what Nitze and Röntgen gave us—*light*—and without *light*, urology is not.

So many earnest workers were attracted to the study of urinary disease, and facts accumulated so rapidly, that, within a decade, nearly every civilized nation had its society for discussion of the problems. France, America, and Germany had yearly congresses, and finally there was constituted that fusion of congresses and that reflection of their worth and dignity—the International Congress of Urology.

With so many ardent disciples of Nitze, the symptomatology of diseases of the lower urinary tract has been entirely reconstructed. Facts have replaced unstable supposition. Each phase in the life-history of each vesical disease has been studied by means of the cystoscope and so accurately described that there are now few bladder or prostatic complaints—if we except those of nerve origin, which are not recognizable to the expert, merely on an enumeration of their complexus of clinical features: but in most the final diagnosis is referred to the cystoscope for confirmation.

With all this precision there are flaws in the accuracy. The eye sometimes fails to distinguish between patches of infiltrating bacillary colicystitis and infiltrating tuberculous cystitis. Especially difficult also to differentiate are the advanced stages of either disease, and here bacteriology is our main stay. The correct clinical deduction of cystic changes in the glands of the mucous membrane has yet to be formulated.

Malignant changes in the base of luxuriant villous papillomata and the early stages of primary carcinoma of the median lobe of the prostate are most difficult to determine. These are some of our real difficulties of diagnosis. How about treatment?

With all the accuracy of diagnosis we possess, there remains, however, a diversity of opinion as to operative technique. For instance, many differ as to how to treat *malignant* growths of the bladder. Whether to remove the bladder in the earliest discovered stage or to leave the sufferer to succumb, for there are no half-measures, unless the growth attack the very apex. The removal of the entire bladder, if the stream of urine be first diverted, is neither difficult nor lethal. Good results are recorded, and I may mention here that one of my first patients operated on five years ago is still a manager of a large office in the city and is capable of heavy work.

Nor do we yet agree as to whether the preliminary urine drainage in excision of the bladder should be by bilateral nephrostomy or ureterostomy. I believe the latter is the simpler and the safer.

Whether the enlarged prostatic lobes have to be removed by the suprapubic or the perineal route will always remain a matter for the personal predilection of the surgeon. In suprapubic prostatectomy it is not as yet decided as to whether the lobes should be shelled out as McGill taught us in 1890, or the whole removed *en bloc*, as practiced by Freyer. This, I think, is a minor matter, for in both methods malignant disease has been known subsequently to attack the outer capsule. The next movement will be to early operation rather than to depend upon any fancied value in the route or capsular treatment. Probably the advance in the treatment of malignant prostates will be in more accurate diagnosis by rectal touch and by removing those prostates thus affected, by Young's method, at the very earliest opportunity. One of mine, thus treated five years ago, is still a farmer in active life and health.

Hence, although the diagnosis of disease of the lower urinary tract is, in the main, more precise than the operative interference, yet we can fairly claim that our operative technique, based on accurate diagnosis, has reduced the immediate mortality of nearly every vesico-prostatic disease to a minimum which does not exceed 5 per cent.

Perhaps the greatest triumphs and the greatest scope for future progress in urology will now be found in the diagnosis and treatment of diseases of the kidney. I can conceive of no greater triumph for the cystoscope, and of no greater advance in renal surgery than for the following sequence of events to take place. First, for *latent* tuberculous disease of one kidney to be detected merely by ureteric meatoscopy and confirmed by bacteriology of the urine; then for the entire kidney and its perirenal fat and upper ureter to be removed, without opening the renal pelvis; then for primary union, thus secured, to ensue, and then for that agonizing vesical distress consequent upon the scalding of the bladder neck by the caustic toxins of the disease, to be completely and permanently relieved. Yet this is now a matter of everyday experience.

To my mind there appears no triumph greater for a surgeon than to be able to assure a patient who has suffered renal torture for many years, that it is possible to cure him. To find that one is able by means of kinetic and postural radiography not only to detect the cause of pain to be due to a calculus of the kidney, but also to be able to take pen and pencil, and outline the kidney and the stone, indicating patches of disease in it, perhaps sketching a cyst in its substance due to closure of a calix or an obstructed papilla, maybe marking circles in the cyst to show that it contains one or many small stones; then to take caliper and rule and plan the line of the operative incision into the cortex, so that the disease can be reached and removed with a minimum of risk to the secreting structure of the gland; finally to operate before a critical group of experts and fulfill every statement made and every condition foretold—this indeed is a triumph both of science and of art. Such knowledge would have been worth a king's ransom ten years ago, and yet to-day it is a matter of not infrequent occurrence!

Or again, what can appeal more to one's surgical instincts than to say determinately and beyond refute in a given case that the suffering kidney must be left alone—that a smaller and better planned incision over the lower ureter will allow of the removal of a stone lodged there, and that the kidney will ultimately recover from the damage occasioned by the ureteric block? But this, a routine practice of to-day, is possible only for the last eight years, since the ureteric shadowgraph bougie and stereoscopic radiography have been utilized.

What can be a finer subject of congratulation to both patient and surgeon than the removal of a kidney detected so early in its invasion by cancer, by means of a ureteric meatoscopy, that the growth in the cortex is no larger than a monkey-nut? What can be more encouraging than to find by radiographic pyelography that years of indefinite abdominal pain are due to a dilated renal pelvis, and by the simple operation of cutting an aberrant leash of vessels to relieve the ureteric bend they have induced, and to save what still remains of the kidney, to restore it to functionization, and the patient in time to absolute health? But these are mere incidental procedures of our ordinary work.

Finally, gentlemen, consider for a moment that life-saving nephrectomy in unilateral hemic strepto-staphylococcic poisoning of the kidney, for this is on a plane with the life-saving operation for perforating gastric ulcer, for fulminating appendicitis, or for ruptured tubal gestation.

Is there anything more brilliant in urological surgery of to-day than to be confronted, as Emerson Brewer of New York was, with a patient suffering from a high grade of fever, abdominal pain, and the coma of profound bacterial poisoning; a patient whose scanty urine, containing bacterial casts, epithelia and blood, and whose rigid side were the only guides to an accurate diagnosis of bacterial invasion of the kidney, and then within a few hours after nephrectomy to see the same patient bright and alert and saved from impending death? But many, if not all of us, have followed in his footsteps, and secured the same success!

These are a few of the clearer and more sharply cut lines of diagnosis and operative treatment in disease of the kidney, bladder, and prostate, which serve to justify my contention that a true expert urologist is something more than a surgeon and that urology is worthy of special study.

But there are many failures to record in our work, much difficulty and doubt, many problems to solve, or we should not be here in section or in congress.

The uratic stones still baffle radiography—sluggish tuberculosis or septic wounds continue to destroy our surgical confidence in asepticity. Fatalities dog our attack on renal, vesical, and prostatic cancer.

Let us leave the subject and answer a question of ethics. Have we enriched the sister sciences by the study of urology? for the secret of true progress lies, though it is a platitude to say it, in the "give and take." We need not touch on surgery; we are one of its arms and have just proved it. The radiologist has gained from us a fair knowledge of false shadows of the pelvis. We can separate phleboliths from calculi by means of the shadowgraph bougie. By means of the elements of postural and kinetic radiography, which arose with us, we have taught him how to eliminate the false shadows of calcareous glands in the mesentery, and incidentally we have taught him, if he uses the same method, much that is useful in the radiography of the viscera.

The gynecologist also receives something from our study. He obtains a knowledge of those latent uterine pressures and subacute tubo-ovarian inflammations which cause so much bladder distress and renal danger. But it is especially to the physician that we pay a little of our indebtedness. In a single decade the urologist has limited the conception of the physician of what used to be termed Bright's disease to a more definite entity. The physician has secured through us the knowledge that many diseased conditions of the kidney and bladder resemble the nephritides very closely. Thus the bacilluric nephro-pyelitides of hemic origin, the albuminurias of irritation, such as that caused by a latent and embedded oxalate stone in the renal calix, the profuse "tension albuminuria" sometimes noticed in the enlarged prostate, and the slighter albuminuria found in the initial stage of vesical carcinoma, all these are revelations to the mind which once regarded albuminuria as due merely to renal degeneration with widespread cardio-vascular change. Finally, may I ask, does urology afford problems which, if solved, can exert far-reaching effects upon the practice of the healing art? Yes, they are numerous, and arresting. But I should hesitate to indicate even one, were I not able to take the simplest of all simple matters as a theme, the posture in sleep, and in defense remind you that the simplest matter may contain the germ of the most abstruse.

THE INFLUENCE OF SLEEP POSTURE UPON THE LOCALIZATION OF DISEASE.

It will be found that few healthy men lie supine in sleep. Fewer still, and they are women, sleep in the prone position. Most adopt one or other side.

It will be noticed that when one side is exclusively chosen for the eight hours' sleep, whether it be left or right, various results coincide with the side adopted. In acute hemic colibacilluria, in which we recognize the kidney as always being the first affected, that kidney is first attacked (for the symptoms are often unilateral to begin with) which belongs to the side habitually slept upon. One cannot avoid the inference that the passivity and position of that organ in sleep, by inducing hypostatic congestion, may depreciate resistance to disease, or that the hypostatic position of the gland for hours together favors deposition of the circulating microbe in the secreting structures. But these circumstances of position and incidence may be coincidental.

Take a step further—pass from the lowest grade of microbic invasion of the kidney to that of tuberculosis of the organ. The kidney first affected by urinary tuberculosis is generally that one upon which the patient habitually rests.

Take another step. If a vesical papilloma is found single and early in the bladder, it will be seen to arise from that side of the bladder on which the patient sleeps. It will be immediately behind and to the outer lip or side of the ureter of the sleep posture side. But this cannot be due to any alteration in the health of the vesical wall: it is due to some irritation arising from the urine of the kidney slept on. What possible changes, I ask you, can have occurred in the kidney slept on, to cause the urine it secretes to evoke growth by its mere contact with a healthy mucous membrane? That this correlation is not coincidental can be gathered from the cystoscopic examination of the bladder in early tubercle of the kidney. The side of the bladder corresponding to the sleep posture is seen to be eroded by the caustic action of the urine issuing from the ureter of the diseased kidney, and this occurs before any other part of the bladder is affected. In this I join issue with my friend Professor Rovsing. Now mark this, when this same patient has to rise more frequently at night because the urine irritates that side of the bladder upon which he has habitually rested, and when he turns for greater relief on to the other side to sleep, then that side of the bladder, on which he now lies, becomes in its turn eroded by the infiltrating toxins which gradually precipitate on to it. This side is now visibly infiltrated, although the adjacent ureteric orifice itself is absolutely normal.

Where are we carried to now in speculation—what lines of study open up to us? Do all the viscera obey some such law? Does tubercle of the lung, malignant disease of the stomach, and acute inflammatory trouble arise first on the side habitually slept on? If so, where is the clew to be found? It may be we possess it in the following incident, though its unraveling is beyond my power.

I removed a small papilloma from the bladder of a lady who had had her breast removed for cancer by Mr. Bryant of Guy's fifteen years before I operated. There had been no recurrence of the breast growth, but three years after she had been operated on by Mr. Bryant she had had intermittent hematuria, more or less severe, until she consulted me.

One year after I had checked this hemorrhage by removing the papilloma, the cancer returned in the breast scar and was so exuberant that it quickly closed the scene. Did the recurrent hematuria deplete the blood of some subtle pabulum which could feed a cancer? Had I, by removing the bleeding polypus, suppressed an outlet for the escape of that subtle pabulum which was able to feed a cancer, so that it remained, increased in amount, until it re-started the breast growth again? I feel sure I had. I contend that the next great step in the progress to the discovery of a cause and a cure for cancer is a greater knowledge of the *chemical* composition of that subtle fluid-medium—the blood. I further submit that the blood is altered in the act of sleep, and that hypostatically congested viscera are thus impaired. I venture to believe that the solution of the mystery of the incidence of cancer may be found in connection with the changes which occur in the tissues themselves during the torpor of sleep, and that the remedy will ultimately be discovered in chemio-therapy of the blood.

Gentlemen, I well remember the expectant mental hush of the last Congress here, when the discussions commenced. How eagerly each one waited for some startling theory to be propounded or some wonderful new power to be revealed by the workers of the Congress! There is the same hush of anticipation now. To whichever of our earnest workers falls the palm of the most brilliant discovery of this Congress, and to whichever section the credit will belong—though I hope it will be to ours—I can say this without fear of contradiction, that that man will be applauded by all of us, that the credit he will win for himself and section will be grudged by none, and that the benefit of his discovery will be shared by sufferer and scientist alike.

DIAGNOSIS AND TREATMENT OF HEMIC INFECTIONS OF THE URINARY TRACT[1]

By Frank Kidd, F.R.C.S., London.

TO obtain accurate results in the diagnosis and treatment of cases of hemic infection of the urinary tract it is necessary to apply an accurate method of examination to every case of febrile pyuria and to apply each method of treatment that it is desired to test to a consecutive series of cases so examined, and then to compare the results obtained with the results in a series of control cases left to take their course.

Scientific proof that a method of treatment does actually modify in favorable manner the natural course of a disease can only be attained if the following tests are satisfied:

1. In a series of cases adequately examined the method of treatment should show a far higher percentage of cures (adequately tested) than is found to occur in another series of control cases simply left to take their course.

2. The method of treatment should cure most, if not all, of the very chronic cases.

Practically the problem for solution is that of febrile pyuria. The first step then is to formulate an adequate method of examination in all cases of febrile pyuria.

During the last three years I have devised the following method, which I believe to be accurate, and have applied it to thirty-three cases of pyuria. The results obtained I wish to bring forward in this paper.

Method of examination. The patient is asked to pass water into two glasses. If the second glass is clear, the pus can only be coming from the urethra and its attached glands. The secretion of these glands is therefore obtained by massage, examined microscopically, and the diagnosis in this way rendered complete.

If, however, the second glass is hazy with pus, such pus may be coming from the bladder or the kidneys or both.

In such a case cystoscopy is performed if it is feasible, but some days later if there is high fever and great irritability of the

[1] Read at the International Medical Congress in London, Section on Urology. Infections by the tubercle bacillus are excluded from consideration in this paper.

bladder, that is to say, when these symptoms have somewhat abated.

The urethra in the male, or vagina in the female, is irrigated with 2 pints of oxycyanide of mercury (aqueous solution 1:4,000), a sterile catheter passed, and the bladder urine obtained for examination by means of film preparations and cultures. The bladder is thoroughly flushed out with oxycyanide of mercury solution and the interior is inspected with a cystoscope. The bladder is then emptied and flushed out several times with sterile salt solution. By this means all traces of antiseptic are removed from the bladder, as even the smallest trace of antiseptic was found by experience to interfere with the growth of bacteria from specimens of urine drawn off by ureteric catheters. The ureteric catheters and cystoscopes, which have been sterilized in formaline vapor, are washed out with sterile salt solution so as to remove the formaline, the ureters are then catheterized, and the lower ends of the catheters, having been flamed, are allowed to drip into sterile test-tubes. Cultures are taken from these specimens, which are then centrifugalized so that film preparations may be made and examined for the presence of pus cells and bacteria. By these steps it is possible to learn whether pus and bacteria are coming from the bladder alone, or from one or both kidneys.

To make the examination complete, skiagrams were taken to exclude stone, which is often the starting-point of bacterial infections of the kidney, and collargopyelo-radiograms were also applied when considered necessary to exclude strictures and kinks of the ureters. By the application of these methods to this series of cases I feel justified in laying down the following principles:

1. Pyuria, if accompanied by fever, means that the pus is coming either from the deep urethra or from the kidney. In males, therefore, a two-glass test is necessary to distinguish between these two origins, but in females febrile pyuria means that one or both kidneys are infected. (For general practice the detection of pus in the urine, the use of the thermometer, and the two-glass test will enable the main facts of the case to be immediately elicited.)

2. Spontaneous natural cure is the rule rather than the exception in hemic infections of the urinary tract. In nine cases of this series (27%) spontaneous cure occurred at the end of three to four weeks—the patient being kept quiet in bed till the

fever had disappeared and flooded with water and urotropin. Five further cases (15%) got well in from three to six months after living a quiet regular life and taking urotropin four times a day regularly. Forty-two per cent. or nearly half the cases, therefore, appeared to get well on very simple treatment. Seeing that the urologist is only called in for the difficult and defiant cases and is not asked to see the minor cases that get well quickly, I think it is fair to state that at least half the cases of pyelitis will get well within six months on the simple treatment outlined above. Advocates of special treatments ought, therefore, to be able to show a far higher percentage of cures within less than six months if they wish to prove that their remedy is helpful.

3. The kidneys may recover long before the bladder. This fact I was able to prove in six of the cases (18%). For instance, in the case of one woman I found pus and streptococci in the urine drawn off from each kidney. A week later, the fever having subsided, the bladder urine still contained pus and streptococci, but urine drawn off from each kidney was clear and sterile. During the ensuing fortnight I administered two bladder instillations of silver nitrate (5 gr. to the ounce of water), which sufficed to bring about a complete cure.

Three of these cases cleared up immediately after the prolonged lavage associated with cystoscopic examination, to the great gratification of the patients.

I will quote as the best example the wife of a doctor who developed left-sided pyelitis of pregnancy, which persisted for nine months after the birth of her child in spite of vaccine treatment. At that last stage I was called in and asked to cystoscope her, and though the mouth of the left ureter was swollen, the urine I drew off from the left ureter was clear and sterile. Three days later, without any further treatment, all the pus had disappeared from the urine, all the symptoms had vanished, and she has since remained perfectly well.

In the remaining three of these six cases the pyuria and the symptoms disappeared after two or three instillations into the bladder of 5 gr. to the ounce silver nitrate.

This fact explains why lavage of the bladder may alone suffice to clear up a chronic case of pyelitis; yet many authors appear to think that if a case clears up on bladder lavage, this is in itself a proof that the case has not been one of pyelitis. I am convinced that this is a mistaken notion.

4. Lavage of the renal pelvis cures most, if not all, of the very chronic cases.

I washed out the renal pelvis with 5% collargol in four cases which had resisted all other forms of treatment, and all four cases were cured after two or three washes.

I have found from my experience with collargo-radiography that collargol injected into the renal pelvis is absorbed into the lymphatics of the kidney and can be demonstrated in the lymphatic glands and in the perirenal fat. The kidney, therefore, is a sponge which can soak up a non-irritating antiseptic like collargol. It is thus possible to understand how renal lavage can rid the kidney of bacteria. That such a percentage of collargol does no harm I have proved by testing the urine drawn off from these kidneys after they are cured. It contains no albumin or casts, has a normal specific gravity and urea content. So impressed am I with renal lavage in the very chronic cases that in future I intend to employ it in all cases which do not recover naturally in three to four weeks.

5. Pyogenic bacteria may enter the urinary tract from the blood-stream by way of the prostate and not by the kidney. In this particular series two cases in males proved to be cases of hematogenous bacillus coli prostatitis and not pyelitis at all, and I have records of several further cases of this nature. This group of hematogenous infections of the prostate is of great interest and one to which not enough attention has been paid. Bacilli of the colon group tend to attack the prostate in those who ride to excess and who are run down from overwork. It can do so in complete absence of venereal history, and in two cases which do not enter into this series I have seen it attack not only the prostate but the testicle also and lead to testicular abscess.

Of the two cases in this series the first patient was a major in the army who for two years had been treated by the vaccinists without any effect, and had had his right kidney removed by another surgeon with the idea that it was the cause of the infection. He was having rigors every few weeks and life had become a burden to him. The two-glass tests showed the second urine quite clear and free from bacteria. Examination of the prostatic fluid showed a large amount of pus and a pure culture of the colon bacillus. After eight treatments, which consisted of prostatic massage and deep urethral instillations of silver nitrate, the patient was completely cured. This case serves to illustrate how important it is, in infections of the urinary tract, to search out the primary focus and treat that.

The second case was an army doctor who was very run down by examinations. He suffered from rigors and pyuria for two months; autogenous vaccines administered by the army doctors had had no effect. I was able to demonstrate that the primary source was a colon bacillus infection of the prostate. Three treatments applied to the prostate sufficed to cure the trouble completely.

6. Residual cases of the series. Two cases turned out to be cystitis only and were quickly cured by bladder lavage. In four more the results are not accurately known as they ceased to attend and have changed their addresses. I have every reason to think they were cured, but they did not attend for their final complete examination.

Only two cases remain (6%) which I know are not cured. The first is that of a young girl with bacillus coli pyelitis of the right kidney. She has attended the vaccine department for over two years without the slightest effect, and I am shortly going to try the effect of renal lavage under anesthesia, as she is too young for renal lavage in the ordinary way. The second is a man with congenital pouches of the bladder, and stones in his prostate gland. The bacillus coli in this case appears to have its primary seat in the prostate gland. He has attended the vaccine department for two and a half years and has had every variety of dose of autogenous vaccines without the slightest effect. These two cases serve to illustrate the persistence of the vaccinists and how slow they are to acknowledge failure.

7. Another principle which has come out very clearly, not only from my own cases but from an examination of the London Hospital records, is how very seldom the disease is fatal, at any rate in England, even though many patients appear to be at death's door during the early acute stages of the attack.

Only one of my thirty-three cases died (3%). This was a woman who had granular kidneys and who for six months had had symptoms of bacterial infection of the kidney. My examination showed staphylococcus aureus, pus, and granular casts coming from both kidneys. She died of uremia a few days after leaving the hospital.

At the London Hospital in 1911 there was only one death from hematogenous pyelitis—a child who came in moribund after a three weeks' illness and died in twelve hours. She had complete bacillus coli infarction of one kidney only.

In 1912 there were no deaths. In 1910 there was a little epidemic of five deaths, all in children under one year old who were suffering from summer diarrhea. In four out of five cases the disease was bilateral. Clearly there was not much chance here for operative interference.

It is extraordinary how ill the patients can appear to be and yet how quickly they recover. I have seen a woman with profuse hematuria and pyuria and a temperature of 108° get quite well in twenty-four hours. I do not think that American investigators have quite appreciated this fact, or else the cases met with in America must be of a far more virulent type.

Brewer frankly advocates nephrectomy for severe cases of unilateral pyelonephritis. I quite agree that the operation cures the cases, but can he feel quite sure that the cases might not have got well without operation? I have noted reports recently in the American journals of nephrectomies carried out on cases which, to judge from the case records, I cannot help feeling might have got well without operation.

I do not think it is justifiable to remove one kidney unless you feel morally certain the patient will die if you leave it alone. I think Brewer and his American followers will have to bring forward far stronger proofs of the danger to life in leaving these kidneys behind if they are to prove their case for nephrectomy.

The disease only appears to be fatal under the following conditions: if the patient is in very poor condition at the onset of the trouble, e.g. children with enteritis and marasmus; if there is gross infarction of practically the whole kidney caused by a very virulent germ; or if there is some cause of obstruction to the ureter by stone or abnormal vessel which remains unrelieved. For instance, one of my colleagues removed a kidney in a case of right-sided pyelitis as he thought the patient was going to die. He found that there was dilatation of the pelvis over an abnormal blood-vessel which had prevented free drainage and had therefore endangered life.

I wish to join issue very strongly on this question of nephrectomy and hold that nephrectomy should be reserved for two classes of cases only:

(1) For a few hyperacute cases, to pick which will require great surgical judgment.

(2) For a few unilateral chronic cases which resist all other treatment for eighteen months or more.

8. Lastly, I do not believe that vaccine treatment has any influence in effecting a cure. In some cases it appears to produce a sense of well-being and relieves the irritation for the time being, but it does not produce cures in any cases except in that class of case which gets quite well without it, whereas in the chronic cases it appears to be quite powerless. Yet these should be just the cases where it should be helpful, if vaccines act as they are said to act by stimulating the resistance of the tissues.

Out of my thirty-three cases eight had vaccine treatment, and of these two cleared up quickly—that is to say, only 25% less than the percentage of natural cures. In the other six it had no effect whatever, though three had had every kind of vaccine treatment for two years or more. Of these six I quickly cured four—two by finding the disease was in the prostate, and two by washing out the kidneys. Several of my cases wished to have vaccine treatment, but when the vaccinist tried to grow the urine he found that it had already become sterile, as a result of simple treatment. Yet if these patients had had only one dose of vaccine they would have been counted as cures by vaccine treatment.

As far as I am aware the results of vaccine treatment at the London Hospital for infections of the urinary tract have not been published, and I have reason to believe that they are poor. I notice also in the literature that men who some years ago were earnest advocates of this form of treatment are now stating that they are disappointed with it.

A large number of papers are published from time to time by men who treat a few cases with vaccines and state that such and such a percentage is "cured" and such and such a percentage is "improved," the treatment often having been persisted in for a year or eighteen months.

In my view these papers prove simply nothing and are in no way helpful to the elucidation of this question.

The results obtained need to be contrasted, as I said before, with results obtained in a series of cases not treated with vaccines. Till the question has been treated on a large scale in this manner I shall refuse to be convinced that vaccines effect anything in this complaint.

CONCLUSIONS.

The following line of diagnosis and treatment is what I would recommend in cases of acute pyelitis as a result of a careful study of this series of cases.

A patient suddenly seized with pyuria and fever should be put to bed and kept there until at least a week or ten days after the fever has disappeared. Over-exertion is the great predisposing cause of infection and reinfection, and nothing is more helpful than absolute rest in bed. Diuresis and diaphoresis are promoted by the usual methods. Potassium citrate is exhibited in large doses for two or three days until the fever shows signs of abating, when a change is made to urotropin in 5 to 10 grain doses four times a day. Meantime a catheter specimen of the urine is sent for bacteriological investigation. If the case were hyperacute and likely to prove fatal, nephrectomy certainly ought to be carried out after the trouble had been proved to be unilateral; but in the large majority of cases as soon as the fever abates skiagrams should be taken to exclude stone, bacteriological investigations be made of the urine drawn off from each kidney, and collargograms be taken if considered necessary. At the end of another week the ureters should again be catheterized, and if the kidney by this time has recovered, nothing is required except a few instillations of silver nitrate to the bladder itself. If on the other hand the kidney is still infected, either the catheter should be left *in situ* to drain the pelvis and enable the pelvis to be washed out for a few days twice a day with oxycyanide of mercury (1:4,000), or the ureters should be catheterized every fourth or fifth day and the pelvis be washed out with 5 c.c. of 5% collargol. Few cases will fail to yield to this treatment.

In the chronic cases that are left the general treatment of the patient is most important. These patients' tissues have a very unstable resistance to the bacillus coli.

Everything must therefore be done to increase the resistance of the tissues. The worst enemy to be feared is over-exertion. If they go to work at all the work must be taken very easily, no violent exercise must be indulged in, and there must be great moderation in sexual life. The greatest care must be taken to keep the alimentary canal in a natural condition.

The daily action of the bowels produced by a suitable diet and a good habit is the only way to keep the bacteria of the intestines in a state of balance so that the bacillus coli does not become too virulent. So-called intestinal antiseptics are of little use and the use of purgatives or laxatives is to be discouraged. Great care should be taken to see that all food eaten is fresh, there being a great risk of swallowing virulent colon bacilli in the food of large towns, such as milk or foreign meat, brought as it is from a long distance, at a great risk of contamination.

Urotropin should be prescribed in 5 gr. tabloids and the patient enjoined to take one regularly in plenty of water four times a day after meals without intermission for at least six months. The dose may be increased to 7½ or even 10 gr. if the pus does not disappear from the urine in a few weeks.

If the urotropin is left off when the patient appears to be cured relapses are common, but if the drug is continued long enough the tendency to relapse seems to die out.

It is no good prescribing urotropin in a fluid mixture as it decomposes almost at once. This may explain why some people have had disappointing results with urotropin.

By following out this line of treatment I find that a very small percentage (6%) is left uncured, and it is these cases for whom nephrectomy should be reserved when one has proved that the disease is unilateral and that the other kidney is adequate to carry out the renal functions.

Such then are my considered opinions after a review of the cases I have observed during the last four years.

An air of hopelessness had grown up around the chronic cases simply because they have not been rigorously examined and treated on true scientific principles. If, however, all these cases were sent to the urologist from the start for proper instrumental examination, which aims at searching out the primary focus of infection and treating it, I doubt if there is a single case which could not be cured along the lines of treatment I have sketched in this paper.

UNDESCENDED TESTICLE

By Charles Greene Cumston, M.D.

Privat-docent of the Faculty of Medicine,
University of Geneva, Switzerland.

PRIMARILY seated in the roof of the abdominal cavity, the testicles undergo a descent or migration which appears to begin at the end of the third month of intrauterine life. They come in contact with the internal opening of the inguinal canal at about the sixth month, enter into it, follow the canal and reach the bottom of the scrotum at the end of intrauterine life. If this descent is incomplete or in any way deviated from the normal, the result is an ectopic testicle. The anomaly may be single or bilateral.

Under the influence of causes as yet not fully understood, the spermatic gland may become lodged at any point along the course of its descent, in the lumbar region, iliac fossa or in the inguinal canal. It can also become deviated from its course and become fixed at some point quite a distance from its usual situation.

In this paper it is the writer's intention to consider only the surgical treatment of undescended testicle seated either in the inguinal canal (inguinal ectopia), or just behind and against the internal inguinal ring (retroperitoneal ectopia). Aberrant migrations are uncommon and far too variable in nature to permit one to lay down any fixed rules for surgical interference and technique. In deep seated abdominal ectopia, all conservative operations are out of the question on account of the serious destruction that is required in order to bring the gland down to the scrotum and also the entire performance is surrounded by uncertainty on account of the impossibility to locate the seat of the testicle before opening the abdomen. The anatomical result is ordinarily bad, the functional result very problematical, because the gland is greatly degenerated in these cases. Consequently, any such tentative is not to be considered, but removal of the gland is, in my opinion, decidedly indicated, as undescended testicles within the abdomen often undergo malignant transformation later in life and are, therefore, a source of danger to the individual.

On the other hand, when one is dealing with a case of inguinal ectopia, placing the testicle in its normal position is always a useful and often a necessary operation. Here again, let me point out the frequency of malignant change in testicles which have been allowed to remain within the inguinal canal.

It is at present generally admitted that the bringing down of the testicle into the scrotum has a favorable influence on its ulterior development and may improve the functional value of the gland. We are no longer in those days when castration was at once recommended, because from histological examination it was supposed that an ectopic testicle was a useless organ. Undoubtedly it is true that in the majority of cases the spermatozoids are absent, but on the other hand, there are several recorded cases of cryptorchids in which the spermatozoids were found, and many are the instances of cryptorchids giving issue to large families, which is proof positive of their fecundity.

At the Royal Academy of Medicine at Turin in January, 1910, Uffreduzzi declared that the frequency in ectopic testicles of tubules having complete spermatogenesis was greater than was commonly supposed, reaching probably about 10%, and this assertion he based upon the no mean experience of a study of ninety cases. In the *Comptes rendus de la Société de Biologie*, July 5, 1912, Kervily and Branca, having examined comparatively the two testicles of an infant, one being undescended, found little difference in the histologic make-up of the two glands.

And last but not least, the function of the testicle is not merely that of spermatogenesis. The internal secretion of the interstitial gland, whose importance has been demonstrated by the labors of Regaud, Ancel and Bouin, controls the development of the skeleton, the attributes of virility, the sexual characteristics, genital instinct and the aptitude for coitus. It also influences the general metabolism. Now, bringing down the testicle into the scrotum exercises a most happy effect on the development of the interstitial gland and a case recorded by Kirmisson is quite to the point in this respect. A fourteen-year-old crytorchid, very large for his age, with a high pitched voice, the pubis and axillæ hairless, a rudimentary penis and a marked adiposity, in short all the evidences of a diastematic insufficiency, was brought by his parents to Kirmisson for treatment. The latter decided to operate. Both seminal glands were about the size of a pea and were brought down as far as possible. Beyond all expectation, the testicles developed admirably and the boy underwent a complete transformation physically. From a eunuch he was made a man, owing to the fact that the nutrition of the seminal glands was improved by the surgical interference.

In inguinal ectopy, the coexistence of a hernia is almost always the rule and is a formal indication for operation, because the canal will have no tendency to close as long as it is occupied by the testicle, so that the walls will become weaker and weaker as time goes on. Even when there is no clinical evidence of hernia there is always, as has been pointed out by Berger, a commencement of a hernia.

The explanation may, perhaps, be given as follows: I am of the opinion that many cases of inguinal hernia are the undoubted result of a premature obliteration of the vaginoperitoneal canal. In place of an elastic peritoneal membrane, an inelastic fibrous band results, which opposes the descent of the gland. The muscles of the abdominal wall contract in order to force down the testicle, which acts as a foreign body in the inguinal canal, and the pedicle of the latter pulls upon the peritoneum so that a commencement of hernia results, which later on develops into a true hernia. Whatever may be the correctness of this pathogenic explanation, it is evident that an operation which radically cures the hernia and restores the canal and at the same time brings down the ectopic testicle is clearly indicated.

Although undescended testicle is usually indolent, some patients suffer from severe attacks of pain, to which the name of "testicular colic" can very properly be applied. These paroxysms may be considered as congestive attacks or compression of the gland resulting from contraction of the abdominal muscles or the presence of a hernia in the sac. However this may be, it is indicated to do away with the patient's suffering and to prevent the gland from undergoing strangulation or torsion of its pedicle.

As to the proper age at which to operate, it should be at once said that by the time of puberty the testicles should be in their proper place in the scrotum. Everyone is in accord on this point. But since an ectopic testicle is histologically normal during childhood it seems only rational that an operation should be resorted to before puberty. One should not wait to see if eventually migration of the gland may not take place and an active development of the ectopic organ should not be allowed to be prevented by the abnormal situation of the testicle.

During early childhood, up to the age of four years, orthopedic measures may be resorted to. By daily massage carefully and properly applied, one endeavors to mobilize the gland, break up the existing adhesions and bring the organ down to the external ring. I am utterly opposed to the use of any form of truss, as it never prevents the testicle from going back into the canal no matter how well made and fitted, and it is almost always the cause of testicular pain.

After the age of four years the question of operation may very properly be considered. Personally I prefer to operate between the ages of five to six years, because I am strongly of the opinion that the ectopic testicle is a hindrance to the occlusion of the inguinal canal and, therefore, creates a predisposition to hernia, if one does not already exist. Some prefer to wait until the thirteenth or fourteenth year before operating, and during this time continue the massage, a useless practice it seems to me, but when a hernia is present at the same time it is generally conceded that an operation is indicated without delay.

The selection of a proper technique is of greatest importance but I have found that devised by Walther of Paris to be, all things considered, the most satisfactory and it has certainly given me permanent results in those cases on which I have performed it. Therefore, I will give the technique in detail. I must confess that Colley's technique does not tempt me.

The skin incision should be made over the entire length of the inguinal canal and extend down the scrotum to the extent of at least four centimeters. The subcutaneous fat is at the same time incised in order to expose the aponeurosis of the great oblique and the spermatic cord. The external inguinal ring having been well exposed its borders are caught up with Kocher's hemostats and the anterior wall is incised sufficiently to expose the entire inguinal canal. The elements of the cord must be freed very high up and very completely, particularly at the peritoneal cul-de-sac, at which point the commencement of a hernia will be sure to be found when the ectopia is not accómpanied by a true hernia. In those difficult cases in which the cord is very short the dissection of the latter must be carried well up into the abdomen by detaching the peritoneum from the spermatic vessels and vas deferens. Sometimes one is obliged to free it down to its end in the pelvis.

When, as is usual, the ectopia is accompanied by a hernia

it is good practice to incise the vaginoperitoneal canal so as to retain at its lower part a pocket capable of covering the testicle. The shortness of the anterior vascular trunk, composed of the spermatic artery and veins, usually will still prevent bringing down the testicle but gentle traction and superficial incisions into the fibrous sheath surrounding these vessels will usually overcome this. These incisions should be made on the anterior, lateral and posterior aspects of the vascular trunk and should only include about one half of the circumference. Should this not be sufficient some of the most superficial veins must be sacrificed and thus the deeper vessels will elongate sufficiently to allow the testicle to be brought down.

The radical cure of the hernia, if it exists, or the starting point of the latter which is represented by the little cul-de-sac of peritoneum adhering to the cord at the internal inguinal ring, is accomplished according to the ordinary rules, and the sac ligated and resected is followed by the repair of the posterior wall of the canal after Bassini's method.

Next the cellular tissue of the bursa is broken down with the finger on the empty side of the scrotum as far down as possible and when the septum is cleaned and well exposed, it is incised low down in a vertical direction. This, I would say, is the most difficult part of the technique, because, the septum being composed of several layers, it is not always an easy matter to determine whether or not one has included the entire thickness and has entered the opposite cavity of the bursa. The best way to accomplish this is to seize the healthy testicle with the left hand and to put the septum on the stretch along with the seminal gland. Thus the testicle is held in a fixed position during the incision of the septum by the three last fingers of the left hand, which should not change its position during the making of the incision. If one allows the testicle to escape, if it should slip between the fingers, it may happen that the incision will slightly deviate and the knife be directed, not on the testicle, but on the envelope of the corpora cavernosa, whose aspect and consistency may cause confusion with the seminal gland. The healthy testicle and septum being firmly held on the stretch, the incision in the latter is made cautiously until the normal gland appears covered by a very thin membrane. At this point the right index finger is pushed through the incision and ascertains if the septum is incised through all its layers.

Once the incision completed, all the layers of the septum having been solidly caught up in hemostats, the finger freely enters the opposite cavity of the scrotum and at this moment the undescended gland can be brought down and placed in proper position. Then, drawing up the borders of the incision in the septum, the testicle is pushed through the buttonhole. Care must be taken to keep it in place, as it easily slips out, with the finger or hemostat, and sutures are quickly placed in the incision of the septum above and below the cord in order to close the former and retain the testicle in its new position. The opening left must be sufficiently close around the cord to prevent the testicle from slipping out, but the constriction of the cord must not be too great, otherwise the circulation would be interfered with. For greater security, it is well to insert one or two superficial sutures uniting that part of the septum which is in the neighborhood of the cord above the incision. These sutures also relieve the traction that the septum undergoes from the testicle. The skin incision is then sutured with a buried layer of catgut and superficially with silkworm gut or bronze and aluminium wire.

After the operation the scrotum appears to be deformed on account of the deviation of the raphé and the presence of two lumps on the healthy side of the scrotum, representing the two seminal glands now occupying one side of the scrotum. One lump is above, the other below, the latter being the ectopic testicle, which will always be seated below its fellow. This position is maintained, as examination months or years after the operation will show. Both glands will be found freely movable and the cord on both sides retains its suppleness.

54 Route de Frontenex.

COMPOSITION OF THE SEMINAL FLUID; DESQUAMATIVE BLENORRHAGIC ORCHITIS.*

By Prof. Zelenev,

THE normal seminal fluid emitted at intercourse contains not only the secretion of the testicles, that is, spermatozoa and a small quantity of albuminous fluid, but also other glandular products from the epididymis, the seminal vesicles, the prostate, Cowper's glands, and the urethral glands. Outside of spermatozoa, the seminal fluid contains the following morphological elements:

1. Large round testicle cells, nucleated, containing small round bodies.

2. Testicle cells without nuclei, probably protoplasm globules arising from the spermatozoa.

3. Lymphocytes.

4. Hyaline bodies resembling globules, a large number of fatty cells and albuminous and pigmented granules probably arising from proliferating cells.

5. Numerous small lecithin granules and relatively large amyloid corpuscles, arising from the prostate.

6. Waxy concretions from the seminal vesicles.

7. Cylindrical epithelial cells from the seminal vesicles and small pigmented globules which may be absent when the semen commences to cool and to dry up.

8. Spermatic crystals of various size and shape.

Zélenev has studied the pathological constituents of the semen. In the first place the presence of blood or pus is distinctly abnormal. Tubercle bacilli have been found, even where there were no lesions of the seminal vesicles. The author has found gonococci in the tail of spermatozoa. He is therefore convinced that the seminal cells undergo important changes in their characteristics under the influence of infectious products. He has had the opportunity of studying the seminal fluid from two cases of

* Journal Russe des Maladies Cutanées et Vénériennes, May, 1913.

chronic gonorrhea, in which he found that the testicle cells and spermatozoa had been distinctly affected by the gonorrheal process.

In taking up the cellular constituents of the semen in greater detail, the author points out that the chief ones are either round or polygonal. The round (or oval) cells vary greatly in size, sometimes show oval buds and may be in close relation to spermatozoa. The cytoplasm varies in amount; sometimes there are granules in the center, from which filaments spread to the periphery. In some of the cells crystalloid formations are seen. The author assumes from the above characteristics that these round cells must arise from the spermatozoa.

The polygonal cells are usually octagonal. Their protoplasm contains both small and large granulations. They do not correspond in their appearance either to spermatozones or to intermediary cells and are probably a special type not previously described.

Zélenev next goes into a detailed description of the crystalline formations he found present in the specimens of diseased semen and shows that the crystals differ radically from those described by Reinke, Lubarsch, Boettcher and Charcot, and Spangaro. The author believes that in general the different forms of spermatic crystals are governed by general principles modified by the time necessary for reaction and the various chemical changes taking place in the tissues in question. In view of the fact that the crystalline forms described by the author represent a distinct type of abnormal spermiohistogenesis as a result of gonorrheal infection and cause an exfoliation of testicular cells, Zélenev suggests for this affection the name orchitis desquamative gonorrhoica.

CASE REPORT OF A SEXUAL PERVERSION: DOG'S PENIS REMOVED FROM MALE HUMAN BLADDER

By Frederick R. Charlton, M.D., Indianapolis, Ind.

I BELIEVE the following case is unique.

C. K., male, 53. Admitted to Indianapolis City Hospital, March 10, 1914. History contradictory and unreliable. He stated that for many years he was a sheep herder in the West and that during this time he habitually had sexual intercourse with the sheep. About the middle of February, 1914,

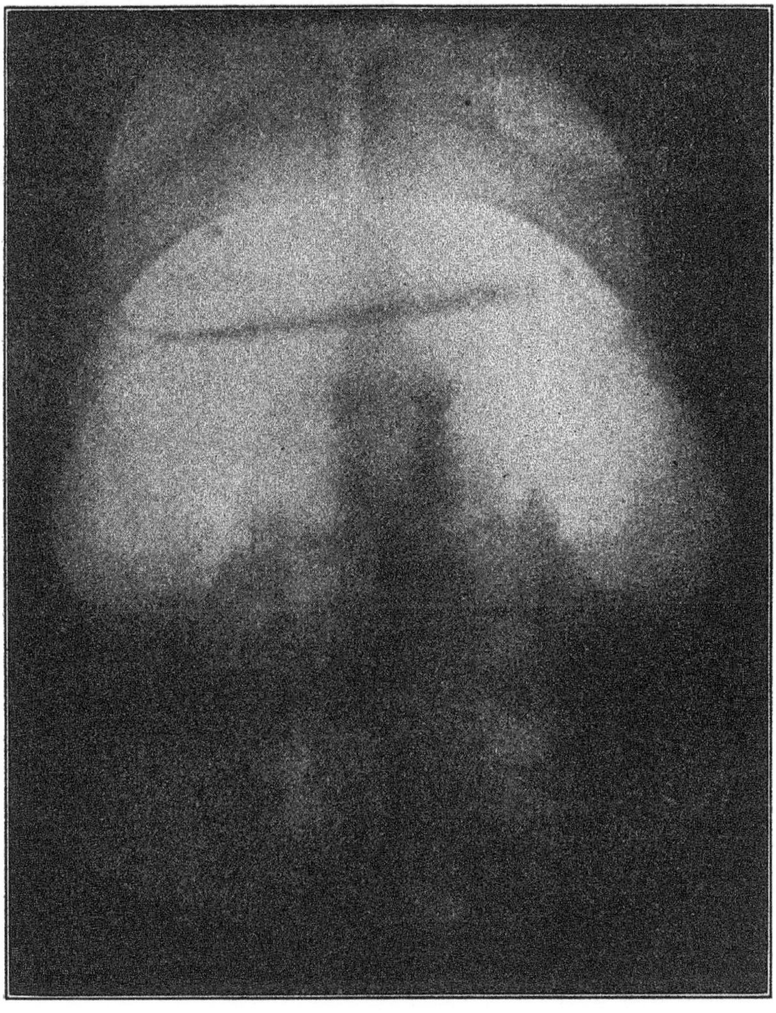

while intoxicated, he killed a large dog, cut out the entire penis, and pressed it into his own urethra, when it escaped and passed into the bladder. My impression was that the act was for purposes of intra-urethral masturbation. This he denied, and explained that he did it in order to get an erection (this power having failed him) and that he thought the bone in the dog's penis would hold the penis up so that he could "go with a woman." The entire dog's penis was used, fleshy parts as well as bone. (All of the dog and cat families are provided with the penile bone.) In explanation will say that the patient's penis was enormous (abnormal) and that a large hypospadias existed, either congenital or produced by some such practice as here reported.

The accompanying roentgenogram shows the shadow of bone lying transversely in the bladder. This bone measured 3½ inches in length, and still had partially decomposed flesh attached. The size of the bone was a surprise to those of us not conversant with comparative anatomy.

Operation was of course done, hastened by active hemorrhage and pain. (The ends of the bone had almost perforated the bladder on either side.) An interesting detail was that no deposit of urinary salts had taken place in spite of the bone having been over three weeks in the bladder. Recovery was uneventful and the patient was discharged.

The question immediately arises whether this man should have been liberated on the community?

Hume-Mansur Bldg.

REVIEW OF CURRENT UROLOGIC LITERATURE

ZEITSCHRIFT FUR UROLOGIE.

Third Supplementary Number

Proceedings of the Deutsche Gesellschaft für Urologic

Fourth Congress, Berlin, Wed., Oct. 1, 1913.

1. The Phenolsulfophthalein Test. By Max Roth.
2. The Influence of Peripheral Obstruction of the Urinary Current on the Function of the Kidneys. By Oswald Schwarz.
3. So-called Nervous Pollakiuria in Women. By Oswald Schwarz.
4. Clinical Manifestations of Nephroptosis. By Fr. Necker and Th. Lieben.
5. Pyelography. By Erich Wossidlo.
6. Diagnosis and Treatment of Kidney Infections. By Theodor Cohn.
7. The Employment of Biological Tests for the Early Demonstration of Tubercle Bacilli in Animal Inoculations. By N. Meyer.

A Case of Intravesical Seminal Vesicle. By Alfred Zinner.

9. Casts and Cylindroids. By C. Posner.
10. Arteriosclerosis of the Kidneys. By R. Th. Schwarzwald.
11. Anuria and Spontaneous Rupture of the Kidney. By Dr. Berg.
12. Secondary Coli Infection of the Kidney Pelvis. By A. Bloch.
13. A Biological Relationship Between the Prostate, Breast, and Sexual Glands. By Arthur Götzl.

The rest of the number is taken up by reports of demonstrations, as follows: Technic and Results of Endovesical Methods of Operation, by Dr. A. Levin; Carcinoma of the Kidney Pelvis, by Dr. Kielleuthner; Papilloma of the Kidney Pelvis, by Dr. Karl Lion; Pathology of Hypernephroma, by Dr. Wilhelm Israel; Chyluria Cured by Endovesical Operation, by Dr. A. Bloch; An Instrument for Mesothorium Treatment of Bladder Carcinoma, by Dr. H. Wossidlo; Contribution to the Pathological Anatomy of the Colliculus Seminalis, by Drs. Heller and Sprinz; Demonstration of Various Preserved Specimens, by Dr. Schwarzwald; The Distribution of Blood Vessels in the Vesical Mucosa, by Dr. Bachrach; Urethral Stone, by Dr. Konrad; A New Instrument for the Expression of Retention Foci of the Urethra Under Control of the Eye, by Dr. H. Lohnstein; A Case of Urethral Diverticulum Successfully Operated on by the Endourethral Route, by Dr. Lohnstein; Hyperemia Treatment in Inflammatory Infiltrations of the Urinary Tract, by Dr. Ernst R. W. Frank.

1. The Phenolsulfophthalein Test.

One cubic centimeter of the phenolsulfophthalein solution which comes in ampules is injected into the lumbar muscles. In 5 to 10 minutes the drug is excreted in the urine where its presence can be demonstrated by the addition of alkali. In the first hour thereafter at least 40%, and in the first two hours at least 60% of the drug injected should be normally excreted. In order to test the above values

Roth made 50 tests on normal humans and 23 tests on healthy dogs and found the figures as given by Rowntree and Geraghty to be confirmed in every instance. Many authors however have been unable to obtain these results and Roth explains their failure as due to some of the following causes: Some of the tests have been made on women shortly before labor or on those suffering from disease of the internal genitalia. In such cases the kidneys should not be regarded as normal because of the likelihood of pressure on the ureters with consequent obstruction to the urinary outflow. In other cases the bladder was not emptied by catheter and therefore not all of the urine was obtained for examination. Many of the authors have made use of a cheap local preparation instead of the more expensive American product. The author has shown that the former contains from 24% to 40% less coloring substance. A very important factor is the point of injection. All the authors who have obtained poor results have injected intragluteally where fat is abundant and the blood supply poor, whereas Rowntree and Geraghty have explicitly recommended the intralumbal injection because of the active circulation in this region.

In regard to the question, "Is every kidney which excretes the above values to be regarded as normal?" the author mentions that in 9 cases of chronic nephritis the excretion was practically normal. This is owing to the fact that the lesions were vascular and that the kidney cells proper, through which the coloring material is excreted, were unaffected. This is also in accord with the general sense of well-being shown for many years by chronic nephritics. In order to prove the above theory experimentally Roth produced a glomerular nephritis in dogs with cantharidin. He found that in a severe vascular nephritis of this nature the phenolsulfophthalein excretion was either normal or only slightly diminished. This shows that a good phthalein excretion does not necessarily mean an absence of nephritis. On the other hand Roth found that if the coloring matter appears later than in 10 minutes a pathological condition is always present and if later than in 20 minutes the case is a serious one.

Rowntree and Geraghty have reported cases in which the urinary and clinical manifestations of uremia were absent, yet in whom the phthalein excretion was very low and who died soon after the test, from kidney failure. In order to study this point Roth produced a tubular nephritis in dogs with potassium bichromate. He found that the phthalein excretion was depressed in exact proportion to the amount of poisoning. In one case in which the values had been very low the excretion increased as the animal recovered. The author concludes that if the excretion does not improve under treatment in any given case of nephritis the prognosis is bad.

The method has still another advantage, namely, that it can

help establish in cases of surgical kidney disease whether the process is bilateral or not. This is of special value when ureteral catheterization is impossible. If the phthalein excretion is considerably below normal disease of the other organ can be definitely assumed since a normal kidney can very soon make up the deficit due to unilateral involvement. On the other hand a normal excretion does not necessarily limit the disease to one kidney since certain tuberculous changes need not in the slightest disturb the kidney function.

Phenolsulfophthalein can be used for chromocystoscopy in the same manner as indigocarmine, only its use must be preceded by two hours by the ingestion of 5 to 10 grams of sodium bicarbonate in order to alkalinize the urine. As regards ureteral catheterization and separation of the kidney urines, the phenolsulfophthalein method can be used only with very large (No. 7 or 8) catheters, otherwise the urine will leak through alongside the thinner catheters and quantitative estimation of the separate output will be impossible.

In conclusion Roth takes up certain advantages as well as disadvantages of the new method over the older ones. He feels certain that the phthalein test has come to stay and will form one of our chief methods in the functional examination of the kidneys.

2. **The Influence of Peripheral Obstruction of the Urinary Current on the Function of the Kidneys.**

Schwartz has found that in many cases in which the free flow of urine was obstructed—as in cases of prostatic hypertrophy, stricture, and spinal cord lesion causing retention—the phenolsulfophthalein output was the same in both the first and second hours. When the obstruction is removed the normal excretory relationship is resumed. The peculiar type of secretion is regarded by the author as an expression of diminished ability to concentrate on the part of the kidney. In other words there is a functional deficiency of the tubules. In such cases the time of appearance of the coloring matter and the total amount excreted in two hours remains normal.

3. **So-called Nervous Pollakiuria in Women.**

The author has found that many women who suffer from pollakiuria are free from this symptom during their menstrual periods. He assumes that this is due to an overfunctioning of the ovary at this time and to a resultant diminution in the excitability of the sympathetic system governing the emptying of the bladder. When, on the other hand the ovary is quiescent, the sympathetic tonus is increased and as a result the bladder is emptied by subnormal stimuli. The practical value of this theory is that by the administration of ovarian extract the author has been able to control the pollakiuria in certain cases in the intermenstrual periods. The occurrence of pollakiuria after the menopause is explained by the author on the same basis.

4. Clinical Manifestations of Nephroptosis.

The authors have studied the simultaneous occurrence of movable kidney and disease of the biliary system. In Zuckerkandl's service there were performed, between 1904 and 1911, 600 laparotomies and 500 kidney operations. Among the former there were 44 operations on the biliary tract; of the latter operations only 6 were nephropexies, showing how rigorous were the indications for this operation. In 30% of the gall bladder operations there was a simultaneous occurrence of movable kidney whereas 2 of the 6 nephropexies had to have a simultaneous cholecystectomy done. The most common combination (8 cases, 5 operated) was the coincidence of hydrops of the gall bladder and movable kidney. In these cases the symptoms were not characteristic, but on palpation there could always be felt a large round smooth tumor in the upper right quadrant, the mass being ballotable, freely movable, and descending with respiration. If the mass was pushed over as far as possible to the left and the patient examined lying on the left side, the right kidney could be felt, low down, and displaced against the spinal column.

Another palpation phenomenon which is regarded as characteristic for hydrops of the gall bladder is the following: if the tumor is pushed down as far as possible and the patient told to breathe deep he will be seized with severe abdominal pains, often radiating to the shoulder. A movable kidney will not cause this response.

The authors report two cases of error in which the mass appeared clinically to be simply a kidney tumor but where there was in addition to a movable kidney a mass associated with the biliary tract. On the other hand various kidney conditions (cyst, carcinoma of the adrenal) have been mistaken for gall bladder disease chiefly because of a misleading history of icterus, characteristic pain radiating to the shoulder, etc. In such cases the usual kidney palpation findings are of no value, for not only ballottement and respiratory mobility but even typical renal configuration may be lacking, and in two cases, owing to the development of a mesonephron, the kidney actually overlay an inflated gut.

In diagnosing this group of cases functional renal tests are of no value when we are dealing with kidneys with normal parenchyma. Much more aid can be obtained from a pyelography which shows not only the form and position of the kidney pelvis, but which allows of a much more accurate definition of the entire kidney shadow.

5. Pyelography.

Wossidlo studied experimentally the effect of injecting collargol into the kidney beyond the capacity of the kidney pelvis. He found that as soon as the pelvis capacity was exceeded in normal kidneys the collargol crept into the interstitial connective tissue spaces between the uriniferous tubules causing the formation of rents and lacunæ by the tearing apart of the tissues and accumulating there. With very large doses the collargol passed through the walls of the kidney pelvis into the surrounding connective tissue.

The author also injected kidneys which had been previously injured by passing a needle through the pelvis into the kidney substance. The collargol was found to pass not only into the preformed hole but it spread out throughout the remaining parenchyma as well. That the drug did not diffuse through the vascular system was shown by sections demonstrating the integrity of the capillary lumina. The secretory duct system of the kidney was free except for slight traces of collargol in some of the collecting tubules.

Wossidlo also injected animals with tubular nephritis produced by uranium poisoning and found only very little collargol in the interstitial tissues. This he explains on the basis of an increased resistance of the kidney due to a heightened internal pressure resulting from a more compact arrangement of the tissues than in normal kidneys. In injecting hydronephrotic kidneys the author found that the collargol was practically always limited to the urinary tubules and that it did not enter the connective tissue spaces.

From these studies on animals the author concludes as follows: (1) We are never justified in injecting a human kidney beyond its normal pelvis capacity; (2) Whenever there is bleeding from a kidney pelvis, indicating a lesion in the pelvic mucosa disturbing or breaking its continuity, we are unjustified in injecting collargol whether for purposes of pyelography or of therapeusis; (3) Owing to the increased diffusibility of collargol through hydronephrotic kidney we are unjustified in injecting a greater quantity of the drug than corresponds to the residual urine; (4) The dangers of exceeding the pelvic capacity can be largely avoided by using a thin (No. 5) catheter which allows of the excess collargol escaping by its side into the bladder.

6. Diagnosis and Treatment of Kidney Infections.

Cohn has studied 109 cases of kidney infections of non-tuberculous nature and concludes as follows:

1. Non-tuberculous pyurias in which the urethra is intact prove on careful urological study to be of renal origin in the great majority of cases.

2. It is very difficult to prove the existence of a primary, idiopathic catarrh of the bladder, of a non-tuberculous nature.

3. Where there are no cystoscopic evidences of bladder involvement the treatment of cystitis should always be directed with a view toward combating the kidney condition. In such cases the author recommends his internal and general treatment as giving good results.

7. Employment of Biological Tests for the Early Demonstration of Tubercle Bacilli in Animal Inoculations.

In all operative urologic cases it is essential to establish definitely either the presence or the absence of tubercle bacilli in the urine in question. Several methods have been proposed for shortening the period of six weeks necessary for a report on a guinea pig inoculation. Thus Bloch has proposed the gland crushing method, but this has the disadvantage that bacteria other than the tubercle bacillus may produce an adenopathy and that a microscopic search is still necessary. Oppenheimer has suggested intrahepatic inoculation but as the animal must be killed early a slowly devoloping tuberculosis may not be discovered.

In 1910 the author and Martin Jacoby began the study of biological reactions in injected guinea pigs. They worked mostly with the subcutaneous injection of 0.5 c.c. old tuberculin. In animals which had developed tuberculosis or were sensitized there occurred a characteristic fall in temperature generally followed by death. The authors were able to obtain this characteristic anaphylactic reaction in 11 to 14 days in 88% of cases. They have recently compared their results by this method with the intracutaneous injection of 0.02 c.c. O.T. as recommended by Römer and come to the following conclusions:

1. The subcutaneous tuberculin injection forms a simple, reliable, and rapid method for diagnosing tuberculosis in guinea pigs.

2. The intracutaneous method is somewhat superior to the subcutaneous as regards the reaction time, i.e. the waiting interval is shorter. However its technic is not so simple nor the interpretation of its results so easy.

3. In actual practice it is recommended to combine both methods. In fact these two may very well be combined with the methods of Bloch and Oppenheimer, as all four procedures may be carried out on the same animal.

9. Casts and Cylindroids.

Posner has made studies of casts and cylindroids by the dark field illumination method. He concludes that cylindroids are of real pathognomonic importance. Thus they appear in large numbers at the onset, and during the recession, of an acute nephritis. They may also be numerous in the so-called pre-tuberculous albuminurias and deserve to be carefully watched for in this condition.

10. Arteriosclerosis of the Kidneys.

The author observed three cases characterized clinically by the syndrome of kidney colic and hematuria which showed pathologically arteriosclerosis of the kidneys. The arteries showed the changes typical of this condition and Henle's loops, the convoluted tubules, and to a less extent the collecting tubules were found to contain blood.

In the neighborhood, owing to the disturbed blood supply, there were found foci of tissue atrophy bearing the evidence of reactive inflammation.

This symptom complex seems to be analogous to certain dysbasias and dyspraxias described by Erb, Schnitzler, and Ortner, and Schwarzwald therefore suggests for it the name dyspraxia renis intermittens angiosclerotica.

11. **Anuria and Spontaneous Rupture of the Kidney.**

Berg reports the case of a four months' pregnant woman of 36 who came to the hospital with a history of three days' anuria and with colicky pains in the left kidney and outspoken uremic symptoms. At operation the left kidney was found to be ruptured in two places and surrounded by much clotted blood. The latter was removed, the kidney drained,—X-ray being negative for stone—and the patient for a time improved rapidly. She aborted on the day following the operation. Exitus was sudden over a month later from cardiac failure.

At autopsy the right kidney was found to be atrophied with a connective tissue or hyaline degeneration of all the glomeruli. The left kidney showed a small, perfectly movable stone in the upper part of the ureter. The kidney itself had undergone severe degeneration and necrosis and was found on section to be full of bacteria.

The author believes that the sequence of events in this case was the following: The pyelonephritic process prevented the kidney from compensating for its functionless fellow. A slight jar was sufficient to rupture the rotten organ and the resulting shock or hemorrhage caused the anuria. That the stone did not prevent the urine from flowing was evident from the post-operative course.

12. **Secondary Coli Infection of the Kidney Pelvis.**

From a study of 63 cases Bloch comes to the following conclusions:

1. Secondary coli pyelitis is a very common complication of gonorrhea.

2. We can distinguish a pyelitic, a nephrotic, and a pyelonephritic form of this disease.

3. The first two forms may appear in the acute stage without causing especial subjective symptoms so that the disease can only be diagnosed for the first time when it has gone over into a chronic stage.

4. Coli infection of the pelvis ascends from the bladder by the lymphatics or urinary passages.

5. Factors favoring ascent of the infection are a temporary increased pressure in the bladder such as may be caused by irrigations, a retardation of the urinary current from a slight obstruction in the ureters, and mechanical irritation superimposed upon a hyperemia of the urogenital system.

6. In the acute stage the pyelonephritic form is to be treated by internal medication, whereas the pyelitic and nephrotic forms are always to be treated locally.

7. Secondary colipyelitis, if recognized and treated early, is always curable.

8. In all cases of gonorrheal cystitis pyelitis must be thought of whenever special kidney symptoms are absent and the urine persists in being turbid despite appropriate treatment.

13. **A Biological Relationship Between the Prostate, Breast, and Sexual Glands.**

The author carried out a series of anaphylactic experiments in animals by injecting them with extracts of various glands of internal secretion. His conclusions follow:

1. The sexual glands (testicle, prostate, mamma) lack specificity as regards each other.

2. The organic specificity of the sexual glands applies to both sexes equally.

3. Both the prostate and mamma share in this organic specificity of the sexual glands.

4. Testicle, ovary, prostate, and mamma seem to possess a common albuminous sensitizing substance. With one of these organs we can sensitize against the other three.

5. Thymus, thyroid, adrenal, liver, and kidney do not seem to possess the above anaphylactogenous substance.

6. The latter named organs do not seem to possess a common anaphylactogenous substance.

ZEITSCHRIFT FUR UROLOGIE.

Vol. VIII, No. 3, 1914.

1. **The Practical Value of Urethroscopy.**

For the endourethral endoscopic treatment of the *anterior* urethra the author uses the Oberländer urethroscope and its set of operating instruments and the Schlenzka irrigation urethroscope with its endourethral armamentarium.

For the destruction of glands which may harbor germs in a chronic urethritis the author prefers to employ the galvanocautery through the air urethroscope, as this procedure is less painful to the patient, and a clearer view of the field is obtained than would be the case with the other methods. The author uses the same combination in the destruction of diseased lacunæ. For the destruction of bands or trabeculæ of the anterior urethra the galvanocautery may be used equally well through the air- or through the irrigation-urethroscope.

For the removal for examination of a piece of a wide-based papilloma the air-urethroscope is preferable. For the complete removal of such a growth curettage through the Oberländer urethroscope is the procedure of choice. Bleeding is readily controlled by hot irrigations and if necessary by the permanent catheter. Sessile papillomatee with long stems are best removed with the galvanocautery through the irrigation-urethroscope. In the treatment of strictures either form of urethroscope may occasionally be of value in the passage of filiform bougies.

The treatment of diverticula varies with their size and position. Small, narrow pockets are best destroyed with the electrolytic needle through the irrigation-urethroscope. Larger pockets may be broken up by destroying the septum separating them off from the urethra with the galvanocautery. Very large sacs are simply to be treated locally through the endoscope with very strong silver nitrate solutions.

For the endourethral endoscopic treatment of the *posterior* urethra we may use either the Goldschmidt, the Lohnstein, or the Wossidlo instruments. The author's instrument has the advantages that the optic (introduced through the irrigation-urethroscope tube of H. Wossidlo) is so placed as to allow free play for the operating instruments and that the latter may be interchanged ad libitum without removing the tube once in place. Of procedures in the posterior urethra one of the most common is the cauterization of a hypertrophied colliculus either with silver nitrate, lactic acid, or trichloracetic acid. When these simpler measures are unavailing recourse must be had to the galvanocautery. Other forms of inflammation of the posterior urethral mucosa which are benefited by intensive local treatment are bullous edemas and granulation tissue formations. Single polyps are best removed by the galvanocautery through the irrigation-urethroscope, especial attention being given to a thorough cauterization of their base. Polyps on the bladder side of the colliculus should be removed with the sharp snare forceps and their bases cauterized with silver nitrate.

The treatment of multiple polypi depends on their situation. If grouped at or about the colliculus they are best destroyed with the galvanocautery. If situated in the prostatic fossa the author employs the flat cautery and, if there is much bleeding, the sharp curet as well. Tuft-like polypi of the walls he always curets whereas multiple polypi of the sphincter internus he removes singly with the galvanocautery. The latter method he uses also for cysts.

Electrolysis is seldom used on account of the difficulties in its employment. On the other hand electrocoagulation is of value in large growths. As regards dosage the author recommends weaker currents than are used in the bladder. Strong currents may lead to crater-like necroses which may be followed by strictures. Coagulation gives the best results in large benign tumors of the posterior urethra. It is not right to use endoscopic methods for the treatment of prostatic hypertrophy, as the cutting through of the barrier with the galvanocautery and the temporary relief of the distention gives a false idea of improvement. Likewise, and for similar reasons, these methods should not be used for the treatment of tuberculous lesions. Polypi of the female urethra and sphincter vesicæ should be removed in the same way as outlined above.

As regards the indications for the employment of endourethral endoscopic methods, the author points out that they simply follow the diagnosis. However, in cases of colliculus swelling we should be especially careful how we proceed. Only then, says Wossidlo, are we justified in attacking the colliculus with nitrate and the cautery, when we have excluded every other basis for the symptoms. It is important also to let the parts rest after such treatment and not to excite them, so to speak, by pushing Yohimbin, etc. It must not be forgotten, finally, that atrophy of the colliculus may also be the cause of similar symptoms.

As regards the frequency of sittings and the interval between them, the author suggests that in the case of growths no more than five should be removed at one session. In general, moreover, endourethral manipulations should not be done more than once every ten to fourteen days, otherwise complications such as prostatic abscesses may ensue. The colliculus should not be cauterized more than two or three times.

In over 600 endourethral operations Wossidlo has seen but two cases of complicating cystitis, and two instances of continued hemorrhages. About 92% of the cases were cured, 6% improved for a period up to one year, 1¾% improved for a period up to 6 months, and ¼% were unimproved.

In conclusion the author cautions against the temptation—on account of the simplicity of the technique—of too much interference and too much cauterization. He strongly urges the necessity of giving the urethra periods of rest and of offering the system the opportunity of supplementing our local treatment.

2. The Local Treatment of Gonorrhea in the Male.

The objections to the ordinary hand injection treatment of gonorrhea are numerous. In the first place much of the antiseptic fluid is lost during the process of injection. Furthermore the patient has great difficulty in retaining the fluid for the prescribed length of time owing to the early cramping of the fingers compressing the meatus. The more complicated forms of treatment (such as irrigations) are open to the objection that they are only successful when carried out by the physician and hence are unavailable to those patients who for reasons of secrecy cannot be seen visiting the doctor's office.

Heinemann has been teaching his patients to use a simple apparatus described by Dr. H. Müller in the *Münchner Medizinische Wochenschrift*, No. 52, 1910. The apparatus consists of a glass bell shaped to fit over the glans penis and communicating with a suction chamber. The latter in turn opens at its side into a suction tube and at its end into an injection tube with air-tight fittings. The injection tube is furnished with a removable attachment which runs back through the suction chamber and for a short distance into the glass bell. The attachment is fitted with an olive tip for insertion into the meatus.

The apparatus ("Haftofer") is used by the patient in the folfowing manner. The injection tube is closed off with the stopcock, the suction tube is connected with the rubber bulb which comes with the apparatus, and the glass bell smeared with ointment. The patient then urinates, draws back the foreskin and grasps the penis and apparatus so that the shaft of the former lies on the small, ring, and middle fingers of one hand whereas the thumb and forefinger hold the suction chamber so that the instrument lies in line with the penis. The bulb is then compressed and the glass bell fitted over the glans. As the pressure is released the glans is sucked into the bell and the meatus comes to fit snugly about the olive-tipped prolongation above described. The suction tube stopcock is now closed and the rubber bulb removed. The special 10 c.c. syringe is now filled with 8-9 c.c. of the solution and is fitted to the injection tube. The stopcock is now opened and the piston of the syringe withdrawn to the full thus removing the air from the injection tube and collecting it in the form of a bubble on the top of the solution to be injected. The injection is now made with the syringe pointing downward and it is found that not a single drop is lost. The injection tube is now closed off, the syringe filled again and the injection repeated. By means of this apparatus the injection can be retained just as long as is desired. To remove the apparatus it is only necessary to open the injection tube and the suction tube in turn. The Haftofer can be sterilized by immersing the rubber parts in a carbolic acid solution and by boiling the glass attachments.

The first injection should consist of a ½% protargol or 1% lead acetate or zinc sulphate solution to be expelled immediately and followed by a second injection to be retained 5, a third to be retained 10, and a fourth to be retained 15 or 20 minutes. Three to five injections are to be given in 24 hours and 14 to 17 c.c. used at each injection. By this method the course of both acute and chronic gonorrheas is materially shortened. There can be no question that by this means the greatest distention of the urethra with the injected fluid can be produced and it is for this reason that the author regards weak solutions fully as efficacious as strong ones when employed according to the older methods. Moreover a "selective maceration" takes place, whereby, according to Müller, the weak solution during its long contact with the mucosa affects only the parts injured by the gonococci and spares the healthy tissue.

No evil results have been noticed and injection of the urethral discharge into the bladder is claimed to be impossible. Patients soon take to the apparatus, especially as soon as they begin to feel the benefits resulting from its use.

3. The Use of Yatren in Urology.

Yatren (formerly "Tryen") is an iodine benzol derivative. It is a yellowish powder readily soluble in water. It was first advocated as a desiccating agent in vaginal catarrh and owing to its highly bactericidal action has been used by gynecologists instead of iodoform in the shape of a 5-10% gauze.

The author has used a 10% solution made up in freshly distilled (warm) water. No striking results were obtained in gonorrheal urethritis in men but in women the drug seems to be very efficacious. A slight burning in the urethra is complained of for about a half hour after the application. In non-gonorrheal urethritis in the male excellent results have been obtained and the author has seen a chronic discharge disappear after a single injection. Intravesically Yatren is of value in chronic cystitis and in bladder tuberculosis. Citron injects 50 c.c. of the 10% solution without inflammatory or general toxic reactions.

4. The Operative Treatment of Prostatic Atrophy.

There are six different forms of prostatic atrophy according to its etiology: (1) inflammatory, (2) that caused by exhausting diseases, (3) that caused by compression, (4) senile, (5) congenital, (6) functional. The inflammatory, as a result of gonorrhea, and the senile, associated with arteriosclerosis, are the most common. Pathologically there is an atrophy of the glandular tissue either with a fatty degeneration of the fibromuscular structures and small celled infiltration, or with an indurative connective tissue proliferation. In men over 50 this condition occurs in from 6.7 to 31.3% of cases.

THE AMERICAN JOURNAL OF UROLOGY, VENEREAL AND SEXUAL DISEASES

WILLIAM J. ROBINSON, M.D., EDITOR

VOL. X SEPTEMBER, 1914. No. 9

TWO CASES OF EXTIRPATION OF THE VAS AND VESICLE FOR GENITOURINARY TUBERCULOSIS, WITH REMARKS.

By FRANCOIS JOUET, M.D., Toulouse, France.

CASE I. Patient, age 51 years, presented himself at the Hôtel-Dieu for a left-sided genital tumor, presenting all the characters of an acute tuberculous epididymitis. The skin covering the diseased side was red, edematous and adherent, which suggested an early perforation of the tail of the epididymis. Per rectum, the left seminal vesicle was found irregular and enlarged, with perivesicular infiltrate. It rested upon a voluminous prostate. The general health was excellent; auscultation of the thorax offered no evidence of pulmonary involvement. There was no evidence of renal nor vesical tuberculosis; the bladder was slightly intolerant but the urine was clear.

Operation by Prof. Mériel in March, 1911. Technique of Baudet and Duval. By subperitoneal laparotomy the left inguinal canal was opened completely. The vas deferens was next dissected off from the elements of the spermatic cord and the internal border of the wall was retracted, along with the peritoneum, inwardly. The vas deferens thus freed in almost its totality, nevertheless ruptured at a point near the vesicle. The lower portion of the cord was next taken from above downwards, and removed with the vesicle.

The wound was closed with drainage. The immediate results were good but one month later there still remained a fistula in the region of the external inguinal ring. The patient left the hospital at his own request, but promised to return, which he did the following June. At this time there was still a small fistula at the point above mentioned and it was suggested that a perineal operation, for the more complete removal of the vesicle, should be undertaken, but this the patient refused and was lost sight of.

Case II. The patient was an Italian workman, age 25 years, operated on Dec. 12, 1909. Two months previously he offered the symptoms of acute tuberculous orchi-epididymitis on the left side, which after subsiding left very deep seated lesions of the epididymis, which was enlarged, hard, irregular and softened in spots. The vas deferens was normal up to the inguinal ring, but rectal exploration revealed most distinctly in the left vesicular region an induration about the size of a filbert. The prostate, right testicle and seminal vesicle did not show any evidence of tuberculous infection. The general health was good.

The one-sided location of the lesions and their limited extent and the physical condition of the patient, who was not too fat, appeared favorable for extirpation of the testicle, vas deferens and vesicle by the inguinal route, and this operation was undertaken by Prof. J. Martin.

An incision was made in the axis of the inguinal canal and down along the scrotum. The exteriorization of the testicle and epididymis was an easy matter and then the dissection and section of the vascular elements of the cord up to the inguinal ring was accomplished, the testicle remaining suspended by only the vas deferens. The index finger was then introduced into the inguinal canal and directed towards the prostate by following the vas, which was kept slightly tense. The vesicle was by this means easily reached and digital examination showed that it would be possible to dissect it out and remove it.

An incision was next made in the aponeurosis of the great oblique as in radical cure of hernia, the upper border of the incision being retracted upwards, likewise the lower border of the small oblique and transversalis. It was then easy to dissect out the vas deferens down to and beyond the vesicle, after which a clamp was applied in healthy tissue and the vas was cut with the thermocautery at the level of the prostate. I purposely say the vas, but in reality at the time of the operation it was thought to be the tuberculous vesicle adherent to the vas that was being removed and it was only after examination of the removed specimen that it was found that the vas alone had been removed. The inguinal canal was then closed in the usual way.

On the following day rectal examination revealed no more induration in the vesicular region and, consequently, a complete ablation of the organ had been accomplished. The patient recovered rapidly and left the hospital three weeks later. Unfortunately, he at that time showed tuberculous nodules on the right side and in the prostate.

Examination of the specimen removed showed, in a section comprising the testicle and epididymis, a diffuse tuberculous infiltration of the testicle and an almost complete caseous degeneration of the epididymis. The vas deferens was free from lesions up to the terminal tumor; this was manifestly formed by the dilated terminal portion of the duct whose walls were thickened and fungous within the lumen, the cavity containing a few cubic centimeters of pus. The seminal vesicle, which was probably healthy, since it could not be felt per rectum after operation, had remained adherent to the prostate.

Up to the present time, vesiculectomy has retained a method of exception, reserved for those cases in which the lesions are too advanced to allow one to adopt a more conservative treatment. Excepting certain cases of Roux which did not present very extensive tuberculous processes, the others reported have had numerous fistulæ of the vas deferens with greatly enlarged vesicles.

It is a question whether or not one should reserve vesiculectomy for the particularly serious cases or whether the operation should, by more numerous indications, become more general. I do not believe that this will be the case and if regression of the lesions does not always take place, one can certainly look for it and defer an operation which is very troublesome and sometimes dangerous. The indications of necessity, so well put forth by Marion, appear to me to be the following.

1. *Urinary fistulæ* kept up by lesions of the vesicles, not only fistulæ but simple urinary disturbances of reflex origin; evacuation per urethram of pus coming from the vesicle seems to me to be one of the conditions in which operation is indicated. A careful examination of the patient should be made to better ascertain if the urinary disturbances are the result of renal lesions or due to tuberculous seminal vesicles.

2. *Rectal obstruction due to perivesiculitis.* Such was the case operated by Routier. It is evident that removal of the vesicles is the only means for avoiding a recurrence, which may occur if one is content to simply open up and drain the tissues compressing the rectum.

3. If the poor health of the patient depends upon the lesions of the genital organs, it is evident that the operation should not

be deferred. Lesions involving all portions of the genital apparatus with fistulæ and abscesses react on the general health and the only means to correct the latter is the suppression of all these sources of infection.

Such are the three conditions indicating the removal of the seminal vesicles. But there is a certain number of cases in which, after having performed a simple epididymectomy for lesions which did not retrocede, one should interfere. These cases are those where the vesicle continues to enlarge and threatens to suppurate. In these cases one should endeavor to prevent the formation of fistula and other urinary disturbances and it is better then to do the operation as soon as a distinct fluctuation can be made out.

According to Baudet, there exists a treatment of choice which is reserved for large vesicles which do not yield to more conservative treatment. It is evident that in dealing with particularly large vesicles one can count little on regression of the lesions, but even in these cases I advise temporizing, particularly if the lesions produce no disturbance. For that matter it is difficult to estimate at just what volume the vesicles must be, to be considered very large. For some, when the vesicle is twice its normal size it is considered very large. For others, it was six times, still others only found diffuse limits. Such indications are far from precise, and again I repeat that it is better to wait until the lesion tends to suppuration before deciding to remove the vesicle.

Marion also mentions cases in which both vesicles were diseased, with a single testicle involved. Under these circumstances it is equally indicated to remove them both to prevent possible infection of the healthy testicle. To sum up, it may be said that vesiculectomy is to be done in cases of (1) vesical disturbances and fistulæ due to vesicular lesions; (2) rectal obstruction from perivesiculitis; (3) large vesicles on the point of suppuration, but not until conservative measures have been tried in vain; (4) bad general health of the patient depending on the tuberculous lesions of the genital organs; (5) the presence of two diseased vesicles and one healthy testicle.

Other than the above conditions, it appears to me that in most cases it is wise to abstain and that just as good results can be obtained by simple epididymectomy, vasoepididymectomy and castration in some rare cases. But an operator should never be absolute; he should take into consideration the social condition of his patient. A general treatment, such as climate, may improve the patient in many instances, but if on account of the conditions in which he lives, such as the need to work, he cannot follow such a treatment, the surgeon will find it necessary to perform some operation to remove the lesions which prevent the patient from earning his daily bread.

The contra-indications have been well described by Marion as follows:

1. *Tuberculous lesions of the urinary tract.* In a case presenting very distinct lesions of the kidneys and bladder removal of the seminal vesicles is only a partial interference and the renal and vesical lesions demand a treatment which is of much more vital importance to the patient.

2. *Distinct pulmonary lesions.* When these exist, the operation is too long and serious and, as Baudet has pointed out, a simple and quickly performed operation is here necessary.

3. *A bad physical condition resulting from a cause other than the genital lesion.* In this case all operative consequences must be avoided as much as possible as they would fatally react on the general health. But if the general health is dependent upon the genital lesions alone one should, as has already been remarked, operate as soon as possible. Marion questions, if, when the tuberculous cystitis does not improve by classical treatment, it is not advisable to remove the vesicles, these being the seat of the trouble. It appears to me that in this case it is more prudent to abstain, unless one has an absolute proof that the cystitis is dependent directly upon the vesicular lesion.

Le Dentu also upheld that in cases of commencing suppuration or liquidation of tuberculous foci, an operation was absolutely contra-indicated. He advises abstention from fear of opening foci in the pelvic cellular tissue and thus give rise to septic complications or to an extension of the tuberculosis in the loose meshes of this tissue too well disposed for tuberculous infiltration. To this one may object that the vesicular suppuration, continuing to develop, may open those foci referred to by Le Dentu, which might have been prevented by operating. Even in these cases it seems to me preferable to operate, because the evolution of the lesions may end in similar results to the patient. However, every precaution must be taken to avoid such a complication.

If removal of the vesicles is not an operation to resort to in all cases of genital tuberculosis, there is a more conservative interference which respects the testicle and, consequently, avoids suppression of the internal secretion of this gland. It has also given good results. It is, in reality, epididymectomy accompanied by resection of the vas deferens. Marion has frequently performed this operation and in all cases he observed a regression of the lesions of the prostate and seminal vesicles. Marinesco, in the *Journal d'Urologie*, 1912, has well summed up the indications.

There exists a type with very rapid evolution, accompanied with fever and severe pain, in which castration is indicated. But other than in this particular case, all the types have a chronic evolution, with a symptomatology which does not alarm, with simple foci in the epididymis and a thickening of the vas, which should be treated by simple vaso-epididymectomy. Of forty cases where this operation was done, Marion had two deaths from pulmonary generalization, six required castration two months later and in twenty-three the ultimate results, both general and local, were excellent. Only two instances of appearance of the disease on the opposite side were noted. Seven patients, with very encouraging immediate results, were lost sight of.

Vaso-epididymectomy is consequently indicated in the majority of cases. Other than the few conditions above indicated in which removal of the vesicles is necessary, one may give health to a goodly number of patients and completely stop lesions which might continue to undergo their evolution. As to castration, it has some rare precise indications, such as an acute evolution of the tuberculosis, numerous fistulæ, or a testicle completely tuberculous.

CYSTOSCOPIC APPEARANCES OF RENAL AND VESICAL TUBERCULOSIS IN THE EARLY STAGES DEMONSTRATED BY THE PROJECTOSCOPE.[1]

By David Newman, M.D.

IT is now generally admitted that tuberculosis starts by attacking one kidney, that spontaneous cure of a tuberculous kidney does not occur, and that the only hope of saving the life of the patient rests upon an early recognition of the disease and a speedy removal of the infected organ.

Upon physical signs we must rely. It is in the application of physical methods to the inquiry that the urologist has advanced this department of the healing art, and even very early in the course of the disease he has rendered the diagnosis mathematically exact. Symptoms are only danger signals.

The subjective conditions which call for a minute physical examination are:

1. Polyuria and frequent micturition, at first without pain.
2. Persistent slight pyuria and albuminuria in acid urine, without tube-casts.
3. Occasional hematuria, with comma-shaped clots in the urine.
4. Remission of the above symptoms, for longer or shorter periods.

Later, pain is experienced in the loin over a small area, but is at first easily relieved by warm applications. There may be difficulty in micturition, meatal pain is complained of during the act, the urine is pale and of low specific gravity, and contains a slight deposit of mucus, pus, and tubercle bacilli.

The most characteristic feature of the symptoms is their tendency to remission. In this lies a serious danger: the patient and the medical attendant may be led astray by the hope that all is well. The patient gains in weight, appears in good health, the temperature is not disturbed, the polyuria and frequent micturition are no longer present, and no blood can be found in the urine. But this does not last long; they all return again with fresh vigor. When this happens an exhaustive examination is demanded. As I have said elsewhere, "In all cases of transient

[1] Read before the Section on Urology at the International Medical Congress in London.

and slight albuminuria, hematuria, and pyuria associated with acid reaction in the urine, occurring in young persons, a careful inquiry should at once be made to clearly demonstrate the cause of these symptoms. To allow time to pass in the hope that the warning may be neglected is folly. These are the distant danger-signals of renal tuberculosis; wait not till the home-signals are in full view; they may appear sooner than you expect; then it may be too late to avoid disaster."

The objective methods employed are:

1. Physical examination of the abdomen, and of the ureters *per rectum.*

2. Bacteriological examination of the urine; inoculation experiments, and ophthalmo-tuberculin reaction.

3. Segregation of the urine.

4. Cystoscopy.

All these methods come within the domain of the general practitioner with the exception of the last mentioned. It requires the experience and skill of the expert, from whom very precise information may be obtained, not only with reference to the presence of urinary tuberculosis, but also as to the extent and locality of the lesion.

While limited to the parenchyma of the kidney, on account of its insensitiveness to pain, the disease unfortunately does not give rise to any serious discomfort, and often the tenderness in the lumbar region on superficial and deep pressure is due to muscular rigidity or a cutaneous sensory reflex. It is when the mucous membrane of the pelvis becomes involved that pain is conspicuous. The absence of the great danger-signal, pain, is here a misfortune; less prominent symptoms are liable to be looked upon as not significant, and unless the medical attendant is on his guard the disease may be permitted to advance undiscovered. The premonitory symptoms of tuberculosis may appear long before the development of a gross renal lesion, such as gives rise to enough enlargement of the kidney to be detected by palpation.

It is during this stage, when surgical treatment can be most successfully employed, that cystoscopy steps in and offers a most valuable aid to diagnosis in both renal and vesical lesions, but more especially in the former.

Writing on this subject many years ago,[2] I observed, "It must be admitted that in many instances a considerable time is

[2] *Surgical Diseases of the Kidney,* Longmans, p. 298.

permitted to elapse between the primary renal tuberculosis and the invasion of other parts. It is by making an early diagnosis, and by taking advantage of this interval, that the surgeon can hope to save or prolong the life of his patient."

During the time that elapses between the onset of the disease in the kidney and the invasion of other parts the surgeon can interpose with advantage. The most favorable cases for operation are those in which, from the very circumstances of the case, the diagnosis is difficult and the prognosis uncertain. Surgical treatment is, therefore, often not asked for until the disease is advanced, or it is even postponed to a time when serious complications have set in.

Unfortunately, when a patient is not suffering much actual pain or serious inconvenience it is difficult to convince him of the seriousness of his condition, but in all cases of primary renal tuberculosis the problem must be seriously placed before him, and nephrectomy advised.

I. CYSTOSCOPIC APPEARANCES IN EARLY RENAL TUBERCULOSIS.

When a kidney is tuberculous the orifice of the corresponding ureter indicates clearly the nature of the lesion, and this happens in several ways: by changes in the color and contour of the lips of the orifice; by the size, frequency, and regularity of the "shoots"; and by the character of the urine which escapes.

From ocular inspection, if carefully carried out by an educated eye, exact conclusions may be drawn which cannot be arrived at by other means, and the course of treatment can be decided upon early in the course of the disease. By so employing this method most valuable time may be utilized, which would otherwise be wasted, waiting for other evidence to prove the nature of the renal lesion. Too often when we wait until the subjective symptoms are sufficiently significant to form a basis for diagnosis the disease has advanced beyond our power to remedy.

I agree with Fenwick and Meyer when they assert that the appearances of the ureteral orifices are so characteristic that they act as a reliable guide, not only as to the nature of the disease, but also as to the existence of tuberculosis of the kidney on the side on which they are found.

Experience has led me to the following conclusions in cases of primary renal tuberculosis: (1) when the orifice of the ureter is strictly normal no serious disease exists in the corresponding kidney; (2) when the kidney is normal the orifice of the ureter is also normal; (3) when there is evidence of tuberculosis at the orifice of the ureter there is always associated with it tuberculosis of the corresponding kidney; (4) in tuberculosis of the bladder the ureter does not become involved if the corresponding kidney is free from disease.

To state the position briefly from the clinical standpoint, I may say in respect to early renal tuberculosis: (*a*) when one ureteral orifice is altered while the other is normal, the renal lesion is on the side of the morbid ureter; (*b*) the deformity of the orifice and the lesions there indicate the nature of the renal disease; (*c*) the character of the urine escaping from the ureter denotes the morbid changes taking place in the corresponding kidney; (*d*) the frequency, size, and regularity of the "shoots" from the two orifices indicate the functional activity or the presence of undue irritation in the respective kidneys.

The first axiom is not yet sufficiently recognized, so that it is still necessary for me to say what I can to enforce it, now many years after I first called attention to the importance of studying the appearances of the orifices of the ureter in renal disease. At first little heed was given to the subject, but now urological surgeons are coming to appreciate the significance of this sign of disease. In 1902 I wrote: "When there is distinct evidence of irritation of the orifice of one ureter, while the other is normal in appearance, it may be safely inferred that the renal lesion is, if unilateral, on the side of the morbid ureter."[3] The more I have studied the subject the more convinced am I of the value of this observation.

In most of the following cases the "shoots" were different in size and frequency on the diseased side from what they were on the side of the normal kidney, and also the urine escaping contained either pus or blood.

In early tuberculosis the lesions at the orifices vary somewhat, but they always show some deformity or distortion of the mouth, and usually thickening or retraction of one or of both lips. The following illustrations show clearly the changes referred to, and all are taken from cases of primary renal tuberculosis without any involvement of the bladder, or tuberculous lesion elsewhere as far as could be discovered. Indeed, in several, it was

[3] *The Diagnosis of Diseases of the Kidney amenable to Surgical Treatment,* 1902, p. 26.

only by reason of the changes in the ureteral mouths that the renal lesion was in the first instance suspected.

SHORT EPITOME OF CASES, AND DESCRIPTION OF MORBID CYSTOSCOPIC APPEARANCES.

CASE I. Tuberculous focus in upper pole of left kidney. History of frequent micturition and polyuria for 18 months; twice hematuria, and transient albuminuria in acid urine; no pyuria; no shadow with X-rays, and no deposit in urine; no tubercle bacilli; no pain in either renal region, but some tenderness on pressure over the left kidney, and evidence of slight enlargement. The bladder was normal with the exception of the orifice of the left ureter (Fig. 1), which was crescent-shaped; the floor was of a bright red color, and the lips were thin and very sharp. From the left ureter the intervals of the "shoots" were from 13 to 22 seconds; the "shoots" were usually small but sometimes very frequent and rapid, and the urine which escaped was clear. From the right ureter the "shoots" escaped regularly every 25 seconds, and the flow occupied about two seconds.

Two months after the cystoscopic examination a third hematuria occurred, more copious than the former bleedings, and was followed by a slight pyuria. An inoculation made at this time caused death of the guinea-pig from tuberculosis in three weeks. Nephrectomy-cure. Well in January, 1908, four years after operation.

CASE II. Early tuberculosis of left kidney and pelvis in a female aged 27. Frequent micturition without pain for over eight months. The urine contained a trace of albumin, but no deposit. The frequency of micturition increased and was associated with marked discomfort, after which sudden improvement set in. No organisms could be discovered in the urine, and inoculations gave negative results. A cystoscopic examination (Fig. 2) showed the mucous membrane of the bladder in the neighborhood of the orifice of the left ureter to be congested and swollen, while the mouth was dilated and elongated, and the inner or right lip was occupied by a distinctly nodulated swelling. The nodules were small, pale in their most prominent parts, and looked like small caseous bodies covered with congested mucous membrane. At the lower angle of the orifice the hyperemia was very marked, otherwise the bladder was normal. The "shoots" were small and irregular, but the urine was clear from the left ureter; from the right the shoots were normal. No pyuria; no pain in renal region or tenderness on pressure, but slight increase in resistance over left kidney was made out. Pus was first noticed in small quantities later, and when inoculations were made two in five gave positive results. The X-rays gave no shadow. Exploration of the kidney was advised, but the operation was declined by the patient.

CASE III. Primary tuberculosis of left kidney in a male aged 27. Suffered from frequent micturition, polyuria, and hematuria; urine clear in color; specific gravity, 1008; acid, and did not throw down a deposit. He was tall, thin, anemic, and was very anxious about his condition since he first noticed the urine blood-stained. Micturition was not only frequent but also painful, so that he was very desirous to have relief. No pain in the renal region; very slight enlargement of the left kidney. The urine contained a trace of blood, and pus and tubercle bacilli.

Cystoscopic examination showed the bladder to be free from disease (Fig. 3), with the exception of the orifice of the left ureter which was unduly prominent, the opening being enlarged, while on both lips there were small pale nodular projections, but no ulceration was seen. The "shoots" from the left ureter were small in amount, but regular in rhythm, and were slightly purulent. From the right ureter the "shoots" were large, and the urine escaping was clear. There was no evidence of tuberculosis elsewhere. The conclusion come to was that the left kidney was tuberculous. It was excised, and found to contain three tuberculous foci. The patient made a good recovery and reported himself well two years after.

CASE IV. Tuberculosis of right kidney in early stage in a female aged 31. Sudden pyuria thought to be due to cystitis. The bladder found to be normal, but the right ureteral opening was distorted (Fig. 4) and gaping. The mouth presented a sigmoid form; the floor was deeply injected, and the lips had lost their sharp outline. The ridge of the trigone was unduly marked; the left ureter was normal. The "shoots" from the right ureter were purulent, small in amount and irregular in rhythm, the intervals sometimes being 15 seconds, at other times 80 or 90 seconds. The left ureteral opening was normal. Tubercle bacilli were found on inoculation, but not in the deposit, by the microscope. No enlargement of the kidney could be made out, or tuberculous lesions discovered elsewhere. The patient refused operation.

Tuberculin treatment was adopted, and carefully carried

out for $2\frac{1}{2}$ years. After 13 months' treatment no tubercle bacilli were found in the urine, the pyuria disappeared, and the vesical irritation ceased. But I fear we cannot claim this as a cure.

Case V. Primary tuberculosis of the right kidney in a female aged 19. A profuse hematuria thought to be due to a fall on a stair. The bleeding not accompanied by any pain in the renal regions or in the bladder; the urine contained no abnormal constituent beyond blood corpuscles. During a bleeding the blood was seen to flow from the right ureter only. No tubercle bacilli were present. No pain in the lumbar region, and no distinct swelling over the right kidney. A fourth bleeding from the right ureter and some erosion of the lips of the opening; the floor was deeply injected, and the mouth was enlarged and sickle-shaped, and both angles were very pointed (Fig. 5). The "shoots" were regular, the orifice remained fixed and did not dilate or contract; bladder normal. Later the right kidney was distinctly enlarged, and for the first time tubercle bacilli were found in the urine. There was no pyuria. The patient did not complain of any pain, but her general health was deteriorating rapidly. An exploration of the kidney was advised, but declined.

Case VI. Early tuberculosis of left kidney in a male aged 31. Sudden, frequent, and painful micturition and slight albuminuria which lasted for six weeks and returned ten months later, and associated with acid urine and slight pyuria, without tubercle bacilli; nothing abnormal in the bladder or orifices of the ureters. Lasted for ten days only. Third attack occurred three months later, and the quantity of pus was greater, but still small and variable in amount. Tubercle bacilli discovered for the first time, also pain over the left kidney, with slight enlargement. Bladder normal, with the exception that around the orifice of the left ureter (Fig. 6) the mucous membrane was congested, the opening elongated, slightly crescent-shaped, and the floor and outer lip eroded, while the inner lip was sharp and very clearly defined. The "shoots" were purulent and very frequent in number. The kidney was removed and was found to contain two moderate sized tuberculous foci. The patient made an excellent recovery.

II. THE CYSTOSCOPIC APPEARANCES IN EARLY VESICAL TUBERCULOSIS.

I have had the opportunity of watching the very early progress of tuberculosis disease from a time before any characteristic disease could be discovered in the bladder until ulceration set in.

The first feature was marked anemia of the mucous membrane, a change so often seen in the mucous membrane of other surfaces, for example in the larynx and pharnyx. In early vesical tuberculosis following the stage of simple anemia the vessels ramifying in the mucous membrane are often obscured, and the cystoscopic field is ill-defined, probably due to edema of the mucous membrane (Fig. 7). The surface may be unduly pale elsewhere than in the immediate neighborhood of the tuberculous infiltration.

The next change observed is hyperemia, due to dilatation of the arterioles supplying the floor and the neck of the bladder, followed by proliferation of connective tissue cells. This leads to the appearance of minute nodules, which are at first clear like boiled sago grains, beneath the epithelium of the mucous membrane (Fig. 8). These during the earlier stage are scattered, but they soon become confluent. At the same time, by becoming opaque, they evince signs of caseous degeneration, while the blood-vessels around the little nodules become more and more engorged, forming bright red rings enclosing pale, chalky-looking, elevated nodules (Fig. 9). The deposit may be in the form of short bands or in irregular patches, which are generally covered by thin pale flecks of mucus or shreds of necrosed mucous membrane. When these are removed by washing, an irregularly eroded surface is seen surrounded by a zone of hyperemia. Two or three ulcers are generally found in the same bladder when this stage is reached, and, adjacent to the ulcers, miliary tubercles are generally seen. Several small ulcers may occupy the floor of the bladder, situated within the area of the trigone, the surfaces being covered by yellow slough, while the margins are deeply injected (Fig. 10).

The ulcer may involve the submucosa, and completely expose the muscular coat, forming the "trabeculated ulcer" (Fig. 11).

Figs. 7, 8, 9, and 11 represent the same lesion at different stages in the same case, while Fig. 10 shows several small ulcers at the floor of the bladder covered by sloughs, and Fig. 12 shows several submucous caseous deposits, elongated oval in shape, on the right side of the trigone. The whole of the mucous membrane of the bladder was deeply injected.

The bladder offers considerable resistance to the attack of tubercle bacillus, even when the mucous membrane is injured, as

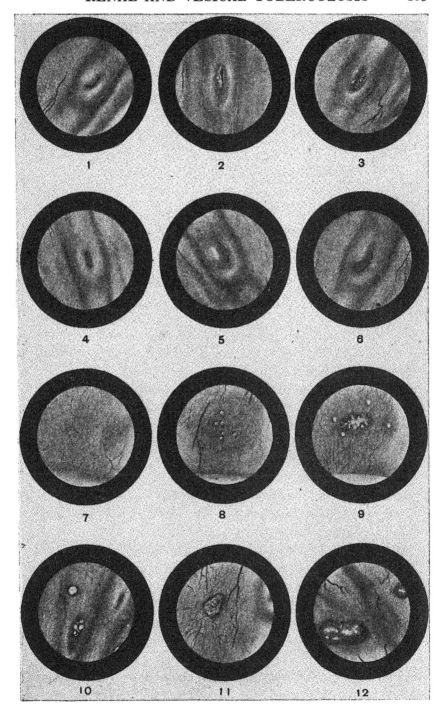

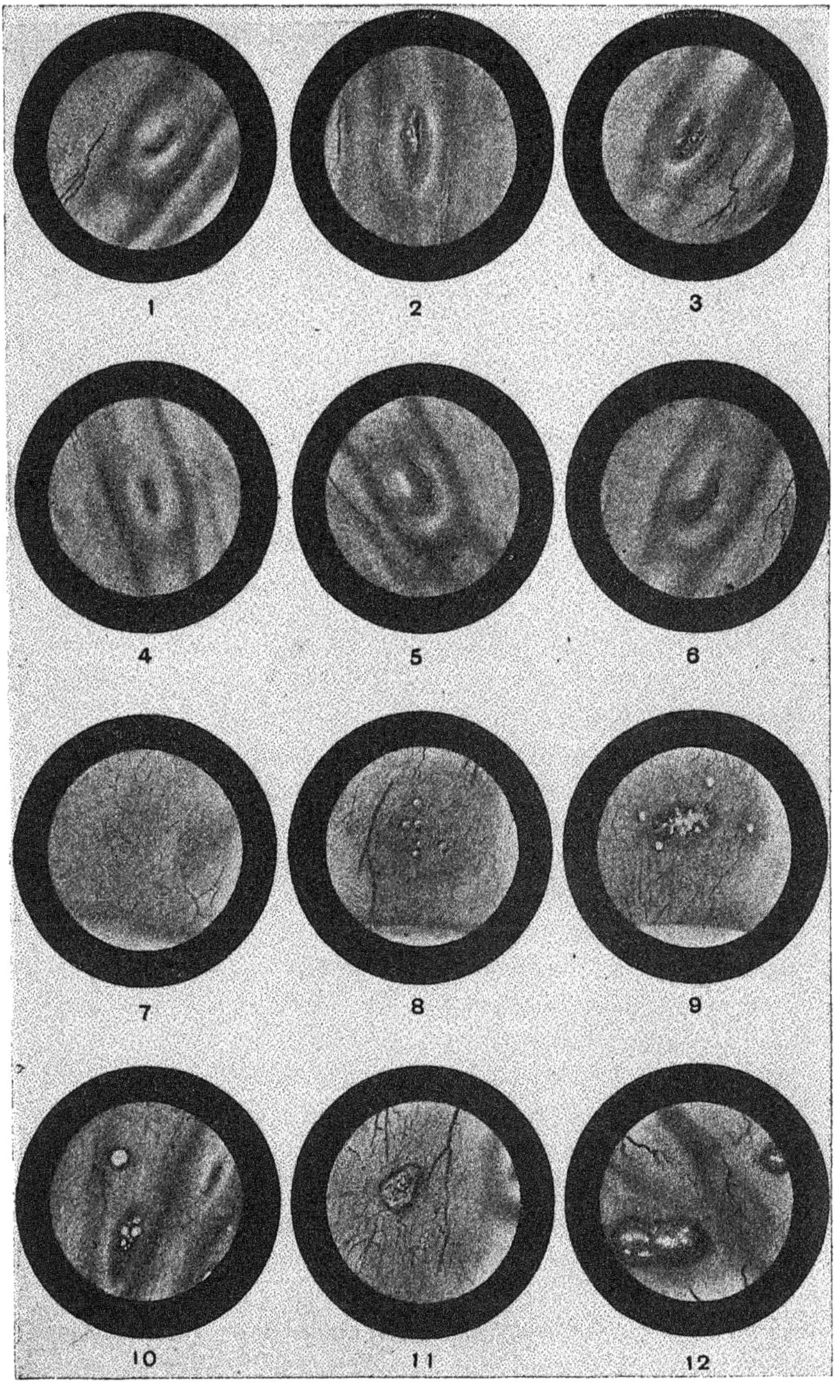

shown by experiments. Rovsing has demonstrated that tubercle bacilli, injected into the bladder and allowed to remain, often fail to produce a lesion. This explains how it is that in many cases of tuberculous nephritis the bladder remains healthy. But if other pyogenic organisms, and especially those which decompose urea, are present, the resisting power of the mucous membrane is greatly weakened, and secondary infection is almost certain to occur.

RESULTS OF MASTURBATION

By Victor Blum, M.D.
Assistant in Prof. von Frisch's Urological Department of the Vienna General Polyclinic

AUTHORIZED TRANSLATION. EDITED WITH NOTES AND ADDITIONS BY DR. W. J. ROBINSON

IN our intention of presenting masturbation as a disease sui generis, we meet the same difficulty, when we wish to consider its results, which we already encountered at the beginning of this division. The question again arises: Is masturbation a primary affection, or is it the result of a special neuropathic disposition?

The difficulty in answering this question lies in the fact that pathogenically masturbation presents no uniform clinical picture. Doubtless masturbation and its severe consequences for the whole organism are developed in quite healthy individuals by external influences. The way, however, in which the individual patients react to this injury of the sexual life is extremely variable. The more marked the abnormal, neuropathic constitution, the greater the effect of the abnormal sexual life upon the nervous system.

And then there arises the question: Is masturbation an "injury" at all; is it really an abnormality of the sexual life? It is denied by some authors that the act of masturbation is essentially different from the normal satisfaction of the sexual needs. Both arise from the same source, the human sexual instinct; both are physiologically and mechanically very similar actions; and yet clinical experience teaches that masturbation has an entirely different effect upon the nervous system from natural coitus. We have considered this question thoroughly elsewhere, and came to the conclusion, that habitual masturbation in some way represents an injury, in spite of the apparent identity of the two actions in their individual acts, because it is an abnormality of the sexual life.

The severe effects of masturbation, however, only occur when the injury affects an originally non-resistant nervous system, that is, when the unnatural sexual life is added as a specific agent to a nervous constitution.

When masturbation leads to severe nervous disorders in otherwise quite normally constituted men, we must suppose the cause of this to be the immoderate sexual activity in early youth, a time when the sensitive organism cannot bear without injury the repeated severe shocks to the nervous system resulting from the sexual acts and perhaps also from the frequent seminal losses.

The older authors refer especially to the latter circumstance with particular emphasis. Curschmann, however, rightly objects to the especial injuriousness of this loss of semen, that extremely precious body-fluid of such complex composition, which just as soon as it is deposited in the seminal passages, and so is out of the circulation, is already lost to the bodily economy. He says: "But if one objects, that with increasing frequency of sexual excesses it would be secreted in far larger amount than is normal, and so withdrawn from the body, yet the amount of material so used up is so small, that considerable disorders of nutrition could not in this way be even approximately explained."

[Here I decidedly disagree with both the author and Dr. Curschmann. It is my positive conviction that in some people the mere withdrawal of a certain amount of semen can have a disastrous effect on the economy. A consideration of the following *facts* should leave no doubts on the question. Certain confirmed masturbators have an ejaculation exceedingly rapidly; just a few manipulations and the act is over. There is no orgasm, no participation of the circulatory or respiratory system; no shock to the nervous system. It uses up about as much energy as the act of urination. And still this loss of semen is sufficient to give them a severe pain in the back of the head, or in the middle of the spine, a terrible nightmare when they go to bed; it is sufficient to cast them down in the utmost depths of depression, etc. Exactly the same is true of sexual weaklings who suffer with an extreme form of premature ejaculation: the normal sexual act with them is a matter of a moment; there is no orgasm, no shock to the nervous system, and still the effect of the withdrawal of the semen on the entire organism is what we might call staggering. Also the same is true of people who suffer from atonic pollutions, unaccompanied by any erotic dreams, or in fact by any dreams. There can be no question here about any "shock" to the nervous system—in cases of backward pollution the patient is even unaware of their occurrence—and still the effect of these pollutions is extremely weakening and depressing. The argument that the semen that is deposited in the seminal vesicles is lost to the economy anyhow is not a tenable one. For as soon as the seminal vesicles and the testicles are emptied of their reserve semen, the latter at once begin to elaborate new semen, and in the process of elaboration valuable vital material is withdrawn from the economy, material which evidently is of great importance to the brain and spinal cord—in short, to the entire nervous system. And we must assume that the injuriousness of sexual *abuse* lies both in the frequent irritation of the sexual centers and in the loss of extremely valuable vital fluid: which is the more injurious remains to be decided.—W. J. R.]

The principal injurious effect manifested is upon the nervous system, from the early suffered and frequently repeated severe shocks of the sexual act, and upon the general health, since in every sexual activity a coöperation of other organs is unavoidable. Thus we see disturbances occur in the circulatory and respiratory systems and in the functions of the visceral organs. The results of onanism upon the individual organs we have already reported in the chapter on sexual neurasthenia. The relations between masturbation and mental and psychic changes in the youthful masturbator have also been treated in that chapter.

As an example of the pathology and clinical symptoms of the masturbatory neurosis I will give here the clinical history of such an unfortunate, who made his confession in the form of a letter. The description of his disease and its origin seem to me interesting enough to justify giving it in detail:—

"I am now 20 years old, and lost my mother when I was seven. My mother died of encephalitis at the age of 52, my father of arteriosclerosis at the age of 70. Then of two sisters, one died of penumonia, the other of heart-failure.

"I was 8 years old when I first masturbated. Of course I knew nothing about the matter, for I was only a child. I gave myself up to my vice even at school, and got on poorly because of the accursed passion. I pressed my legs together and rubbed until I was tired and the semen poured out into my clothes. I did not trust myself to say anything, because I was afraid and ashamed, which I now regret bitterly. I continued this until the age of 11. Then I forgot it (!) for a year, until I was again reminded of this wretched idea by a comrade. I could not wean myself from it after that unlucky day, and have done it, alas! continually up to to-day, that is full eleven years.

"My education is the simplest imaginable. I passed through the elementary school, city school and business school successfully and attended to business. I have never had any particular interest in it. My wretched condition displayed itself especially through disinclination to occupation and to work. I could never stay long, because a strong impulse to wander seized me, yet all my employers were quite content with me. A longing after the unexpected had seized me, which after that never left me.

"I have not visited a prostitute for a year and a half, because each time I tried coitus, I failed, although formerly I had good erections. It sufficed me merely to seize, to touch, or even to look at the sexual parts in order to have an abundant ejaculation. I especially prefer women between 40 and 50 years of age, while I am very shy and helpless before younger ones, and must turn away my eyes, if such a one looks at me. I also have often a disgust for the female sex, which lasts for months.

"My present state is a sad one. Unfounded fears, quick

exhaustion of the entire body, especially of the hands and feet; poor memory, anger at the least trifle and especially pleasure in quarreling. I am fond of seeking lonely places, where I can sit all day and meditate on my lost happiness of youth. I should be happy to wander, if I could only go far, far away from Vienna.

"I get up in the morning more tired than when I went to bed, and have a morbid sleepiness so that I often sleep during my office hours. My complaints are: pain in urinating, pain in the feet and hands, then also in the hips and the head. The way in which I seek satisfaction is to rub the penis so long or to move to and fro so long on the bed until the pleasure comes, often in the reclining position, often in the standing during the day, three or four times and alas! oftener sometimes. The penis will not relax until the semen is emptied, which causes terrible pains. When the semen has been evacuated I am weak and cannot recover for twenty to thirty minutes, while the heart beats strongly and I have difficulty in breathing. Afterwards I can urinate only with difficulty, often with tears in my eyes.

"Pollutions occur quite often. Dreams in which women occur, but also dreams in which I cry out at night, when it seems to me as if I was pursued or murdered, are not rare with me. I have repeatedly dreamed that I lay before a bridge or before a train and was attacked from behind, so that I cried out aloud.

"To conclude, I fear that the end of these sad youthful errors will be madness; as the books all say at the end, there is no hope for me, and the madhouse threatens me. I have come to this supposition by reading the so-called popular—scientific books—thus incurable! Especially the book entitled 'Masturbation and its Terrible Results,' let no other thoughts arise in me than those of the madhouse."

REVIEW OF CURRENT UROLOGIC LITERATURE

ZEITSCHRIFT FUR UROLOGIE.

Vol. VIII, No. 4, 1914.

1. Closed Pyonephroses. By Robert Lichtenstern.
2. Hematuria Following Large Doses of Urotropin. By L. Simon.
3. The Significance of Diseases of the Pancreas for Surgery of the Urinary Tract. By Ernst R. W. Frank.

1. Closed Pyonephroses.

Zuckerkandl was the first to differentiate closed tuberculous pyonephroses. This condition is characterized clinically by a temperature curve of the type of a resorption fever, by progressive loss of weight, and by dysuria with often a clear urine. Cystoscopically there is closure of one ureter at the level of the kidney pelvis, and tuberculous cystitis, limited to the region of the affected ureter in early cases, widespread in severer forms. This form of kidney tuberculosis is very rare as only 25 cases have been collected from the literature.

Still more rare are closed pyonephroses of a non-tuberculous nature. The author has had the good fortune to observe three such cases. The first was that of a woman of 38 who had been running an occasional fever and chills for ten years. Clinical examination revealed no organic change. The urine was always microscopically and chemically normal. The patient had never had any abdominal pain. Finally cystoscopy was suggested and done. The bladder was quite normal, catheterization of the right ureter was normal but the left showed an obstruction at the level of the kidney pelvis. The indigocarmin test showed prompt excretion on the right side, none on the left. An X-ray plate showed a shadow, suspicions of calculus, in the left kidney region. At operation the left kidney was found embedded in adhesions, the ureter as thick as a finger. Pathologically, the organ was found to consist of a mass of pus sacs from which staphylococci were cultivated. No kidney tissue whatever was demonstrable on section, only sclerotic and inflammatory masses being present. The closure in this case may originally have been caused by a small stone which produced ulceration and scar tissue formation in the pelvis with subsequent cessation of the kidney function. Clinically, the absence of urinary symptoms could be explained by a rapid closure of the ureter which on the one hand prevented the occurrence of colic, and on the other blocked the passage of pus into the bladder. The rapid closure also prevented the formation of a large retention tumor.

The second patient complained of abdominal pains for some time.

They were worse during the past two years, became localized to the left hypochondrium, and were associated with fever. Examination revealed a movable tumor in the left upper quadrant. At cystoscopy exactly the same findings were obtained as in the previous case. X-ray examination was negative. At operation the left kidney was found to be bound down by adhesions, it was about four times the normal size, and with a pelvis dilated to the size of an orange. The preparation showed an enormous dilation of the pelvis with a corresponding atrophy of the parenchyma. The ureter could not be probed. The contents of the kidney was a thin, gray pus which was bacteriologically sterile. These findings can best be explained by assuming the kidney was at first a movable one. The ureter became kinked, a permanent obstruction resulted and a hydronephrosis was formed. This became infected by the hematogenous route and was changed to a pyonephrosis. Clinically, the original abdominal pains should be regarded as colic due to the hydronephrosis. The subsequent infection caused the fever and the distended pyonephrosis caused the recent continuous pain in the left hypochondrium.

The third case was that of an officer in the Bulgarian army who sustained a fall from his horse. The accident was followed by fever, emaciation, and the discovery of a hard, immovable tumor in the left hypochondrium. Cystoscopy revealed a condition quite similar to that of the other two cases. In view of the increasing cachexia, a diagnosis of malignant neoplasm of the left kidney was made. An X-ray of the skeleton failed to reveal metastases and so the kidney was explored. The large mass was found to consist chiefly of adhesions, exploratory aspiration of the kidney revealed pus, and the organ was finally removed after much difficulty. The kidney was found to consist of a series of thick-walled pus sacs from which staphylococcus albus was recovered. There was no trace of kidney tissue. In this case, although the original course could not he determined, the pyonephrosis was surely of long standing. It is also certain that the cessation of kidney function was sudden, for the patient observed no change in his urine and experienced no pain whatever. The fall from the horse had simply lighted up the quiescent process, thus showing that an encapsulated pus focus may not lose its virulence for years.

These three cases had as common features: (1) the absence of symptoms pointing to the urinary tract, (2) the characteristic cystoscopic findings. In two cases physical examination revealed a tumor in the kidney region. The removal of such organs is very difficult not only on account of the adhesions but of the shrinkage of the renal pedicle. This necessitates an intracapsular nephrectomy.

The author also reports two personal cases of closed tuberculous pyonephrosis.

2. **Hematuria Following Large Doses of Urotropin.**

Simon has observed the sudden appearance of hematuria in six cases which received large doses of urotropin. In these instances the drug had been given to combat meningitic symptoms and was ordered to be administered, one gram every two hours. The bleeding generally appeared on the third day after the urotropin was started and lasted in one case for 8 days after the stoppage of the drug. At autopsy the kidneys were generally intact but a severe hemorrhagic cystitis was observed in every case. The urine was found to smell very strongly of formalin.

The author succeeded in producing hematuria experimentally in rabbits. He increased the dose of urotropin until they received 8 grams daily. On the third day of this dosage the hematuria appeared.

Simon believes that if we keep urotropin in mind we may be able to explain an occasional case of hematuria of unknown origin.

3. **The Significance of Diseases of the Pancreas for Surgery of the Urinary Tract.**

Frank reports two cases of operation for prostatic hypertrophy followed by pancreatic symptoms. The first case was a man of 56 from whom the author removed an adenoma of the prostate. During the entire period of observation for this condition there were observed absolutely no symptoms from the gastro-intestinal tract. A few days after the operation the patient began suddenly to complain of nausea, constant eructations, and severe retching. There were colicky pains in the abdomen, the epigastrium was distended and rigid, and there was severe pain on swallowing. Next there appeared swelling of various joints and the urine became cloudy and was found to contain colon bacilli. The general condition became worse, the above symptoms became aggravated, the temperature began to rise, the patient developed a purpuric rash, and died on the fifth day. At autopsy there was found an acute hemorrhagic pancreatitis and healed and healing ulcers of the stomach.

The second case was a man of 71 in whom also prostatectomy was done for adenoma. A few days after the operation a small spot of gangrene was noticed at one of the stitch wounds. Following this the patient suddenly complained of feeling poorly and began to void large quantities of urine, which for the first time was found to contain sugar. This condition persisted, and diastase was found to be absent in the urine. Moreover the stools became copious, foul, and fatty. Nevertheless the patient soon began to improve under a very strict diet (tea, bouillon, cognac with eggs), his urine finally became sugar-free, and he developed a carbohydrate tolerance of 100 grams. He recovered completely.

Frank reports these cases for what they are worth. He does not claim to have been able to prove a causal relationship between the prostatectomies and the pancreatic symptoms.

JOURNAL D'UROLOGIE.

Vol. V, No. 2, Feb.-March, 1914.

1. Contribution to the Study of Hematuria in the Course of Various Forms of Appendicitis.

The authors conclude their exhaustive paper as follows:

1. Hematuria is little known as a complication of appendicitis yet it is of the greatest interest not so much from the prognostic standpoint as because of the confusion it may sometimes cause in the clinical picture.

2. Hematuria may be met with in every form of appendicitis, acute and chronic. In the acute forms the hematuria generally appears either simultaneously with or immediately after the cessation of the general symptoms of appendicular origin. Its appearance is sudden without premonitory symptoms. It is intermittent, of short duration, and variable in amount. In the chronic form the hematuria precedes the characteristic signs of appendicitis (cramps, fever, and localization of the pain to the appendix region). It appears in patients with a long history of varying abdominal complaints: gastralgia, with or without vomiting, constipation, meteorism, pains in the right iliac fossa. These hematurias always coexist with renal colics so that one is led to think of a renal or ureteral calculus. For this reason the differential diagnosis between appendicitis with hematuria and lithiasis becomes all the more difficult since these conditions may exist together. Even the most careful examination of the patient and a study of the leading symptoms will not clear up the diagnosis unless the urine is examined and cystoscopy employed. Even then the ureteral catheter may be arrested and the idea of calculus confirmed. Radiography may help but it must be born in mind that certain radiographic shadows in the pelvis are difficult of interpretation and that on the other hand appendix coproliths may be opaque.

3. These hematurias are in general benign. They develop

without rise of temperature or aggravation of the general condition and after their disappearance they ordinarily leave no urinary sequel.

4. Operative findings show that in cases of chronic appendicitis with hematuria, the appendix is often in a posterior position, adherent to the ureter and covering it. This explains the arrest of the ureteral sound during catheterization. In the acute forms as well the appendix is often in a posterior position, and in fatal cases autopsy reveals an intense congestion of the kidneys.

5. From the pathological point of view, hematuria in the course of appendicitis, outside of concomitant lesions of the urinary tract (lithiasis, tuberculosis) is due to: (1) General causes (nephritis); (2) local causes. In the latter case the theory which explains the majority of cases and which is most in accord with the peculiarities of the hematuria (sudden onset and cessation) and the absence of permanent lesions, is that of a *reflex renal congestion.* The condition would depend primarily on the inflamed appendix and would be propagated to the kidney by means of the abdominal sympathetics. Indeed, even if certain cases were to be explained readily by the anatomical relationship it must still be borne in mind that the appendix and the ureter possess a common innervation in the abdominal sympathetic system.

6. Strictly speaking, there is no treatment for hematuria of appendicular origin: (a) Because it is often only a warning sign of chronic appendicitis and as such indicates appendicectomy, after which it disappears. (b) Because in the acute forms it is a symptom which does not figure at all in the operative indications. (c) Because, finally, after appendicectomy, it is only a curious finding of convalescence.

None of the reported cases presented any important renal lesions which might affect the future of the patient.

2. Endoscopic Treatment of Vesical Tuberculosis with High Frequency Currents.

In a certain number of cases vesical symptoms persist after a nephrectomy for tuberculosis. These are generally due to a secondary cystitis and clear up under the usual forms of local treatment (lavages, etc.) Of these cases, there are a few, however, which are due to the abnormal persistence of tuberculous ulcerations, localized, and without much surrounding cystitis. It is such lesions as these that Heitz-Boyer successfully attacks with his high frequency sparking. According to him this method possesses the advantage over that of electrocoagulation that in attacking deep seated lesions, perforation of the bladder is less likely to occur. The technic of the sparking method has been described in full in the December number of the *Journal d'Urologie.* The author again emphasizes the necessity for destroying the surrounding tissue for at least one centimeter outside the lesion. The application, being painful, should be made under thorough local, or perhaps even general, anesthesia. The length of the treatment varies with the extent of the ulceration but it is essential to bear in mind that the wall of the bladder may be very thin.

The after effects are not troublesome and there is little pain. If cystoscopy is repeated it will be found that the ulcer has been replaced by an irregular projection formed of vegetations of unhealthy pale mucosa. These subsequently become detached and the involved area becomes covered by new epithelium. Complete cicatrization occurs in four weeks, with a coincident clearing of the urine and a subsidence of the pain. The author reports a case in detail. A colored plate and three black and white figures accompany the text.

3. The Demonstration of Tubercle Bacilli in Urine.

Gautier has made a special study of this subject and concludes as follows:

1. If the preparation is decolorized carefully with nitric acid, one-third strength, and absolute alcohol, the Ziehl-Neelsen method may be relied upon absolutely to demonstrate the presence of tubercle bacilli in the urine and to differentiate them from such less acid-fast bacteria as smegma bacilli.

2. The search for tubercle bacilli should be patiently carried out. A large quantity of urine should be centrifuged for a long time. The smears made with the sediment should be examined throughout their entire extent. If the first search is fruitless another specimen should be examined in a few days.

3. If in a specimen stained with methylene blue there are present red blood cells and degenerated polynuclears, even if no bacteria are seen, the presence of tubercle bacilli should be suspected.

4. Microscopic examination of the urine gives certain results and offers a rapid method of diagnosis in at least eighty per cent. of the cases.

4. Primary Vesical Lithiasis in Children and Adults in the Mussulmans of North Africa.

At the Sadiki Hospital in Tunis there were observed in the space of ten and a half years, 198 cases of bladder calculi. Of these 40 occurred in adults from 15 to 40 years of age and 50 occurred in children under fifteen. Although, therefore, vesical lithiasis was common, renal lithiasis was rare in these patients. Various factors have been invoked to explain the *etiology* of vesical lithiasis. Climate does not seem to play much of a rôle although vesical bilharziosis is said to be responsible for much of the disease among the Arabs of Egypt. All of the cases seen by the author occurred in the male sex. The most important etiological factor is alimentation. In the first place solid food is given too early in the life of these people. The diet is almost purely vegetable and too low in nitrogen, no meat being given. The enteritis so common in infants, is but an expression of such dietetic errors. In the second place the waters of this country are excessive in their content of calcium and magnesium.

The symptomatology of calculi in Arabs differs somewhat from that usually set forth. In children, pains on urination are complained of almost constantly. The penis and especially the glans in abnormally large. Hematuria is not important but prolapse of the rectum, when it occurs, is of significance. Incontinence of urine is seldom complained of but this is probably due to the slovenly habits of the poorer classes. The stream of urine is often interrupted.

In adolescents and adults the condition appears as a chronic cystitis with cloudy urine, frequent and painful micturition and terminal hematuria. When a patient complains of symptoms of stricture, of hernia, of prolapsus recti, or of hemorrhoids, it is wise to think of a stone obstructing the urethral orifice. The differential diagnosis is between vesical lithiasis and tumor or tuberculosis of the bladder. A positive diagnosis can be made by means of the sound, palpation by rectum (especially in children), cystoscopy, and radiography.

The treatment is either lithotrity or hypogastric section but as most of the author's cases came in the late stage with an accompanying cystitis, the latter operation was chosen.

Coudray gives the protocols of 90 cases with a mortality of 11%. In children the mortality was 6% of 50 cases; in adults 17.5% of 40 cases. The cause of death was usually an ascending renal infection due to a long neglected cystitis.

5. A Case of Vesical Exstrophy.

Cotte reports a case of exstrophy of the bladder which succumbed to infection of the kidneys. At autopsy there was found bilateral pyelonephritis, perinephritis, renal calculi (secondary) and dilatation of the ureters to the size of the index finger. Within the bladder the verumontanum, openings of the ejaculatory ducts and ureters were normal but the urethral orifice was missing. The generative organs were intact.

The author publishes this case to show the folly of attempting a plastic operation in such instances without first attempting in every possible way (radiography, catheterization of the ureters, determination of the coefficient of Ambard) to establish the functional activity of the kidneys.

6. Multiple Congenital Strictures of the Urethra

A sixteen-year-old boy was brought to Uteau complaining of inability to urinate. There was a tight phimosis and pin-hole meatus but neither circumcision nor meatotomy improved the condition. On exploring the urethra it was found that every instrument save a filiform was arrested in the balanic portion of the canal. An internal urethrotomy was then performed and two strictures cut, the first in the balanic, the second in the perineal portion of the urethra. A week later dilatations were commenced and successfully carried out. As post-operative complications there were fever and multiple arthritis.

In this case there was absolutely no past history of urethritis. From the very first the child had difficulty with urination, did not seem to know when he passed water and had both diurnal and nocturnal incontinence. After the operation, urination was normal, there was no more enuresis and the patient had gained weight.

7. **The Early Diagnosis of Syphilis.**

In the presence of a suspicious ulceration, especially a recent one, it is essential to establish the diagnosis of syphilis at the earliest possible moment when the Wassermann reaction is still negative. The diagnosis is often impossible or doubtful clinically. Recourse should always be had to an ultramicroscopic examination which permits of an early and positive diagnosis. In making the preparation a drop of distilled water is mixed on a slide with a drop of the secretion obtained from the ulcer with a platinum loop. The preparation is then covered with a slip so as to exclude the air and if the examination must be postponed the specimen is ringed with paraffin.

8. **A Simple New Apparatus for the Cystostomized.**

The apparatus consists of three parts. (1) An ordinary Nélaton catheter of a size corresponding to that of the suprapubic wound. To this is attached the third part. (2) A belt with perineal straps. The belt is 8-10 cm. in width, buttons at the side, and is provided with a reënforced opening for the catheter to pass through. (3) A round rubber disc, perforated and surmounted with a short tube. Through this tube and aperture the catheter is passed while on the stretch on a mandrin and is then allowed to slip into position at any given distance from its end. The catheter is introduced into the wound, is retained at the proper depth by the rubber guard, and the whole is kept in place by the overlying belt. The apparatus is simple and can be easily cleaned and sterilized.

JOURNAL D'UROLOGIE.

Vol. V, No. 3, March, 1914.

Extirpation; Vaginal Metastasis: Extirpation, Preservation of Excellent General Condition. By A. Grandjean.
7. A Case of Plastic Induration of the Corpora Cavernosa. By T. Pakowski.
8. Indications and Technic of the Transvesical Route for the Cure of Vesico-vaginal Fistulæ. By Jean Paris and F. Francey.
9. The Early Diagnosis of Syphilis. By Alfred Lévy-Bing.

1. **The Minute Histo-pathology of the Human Kidney.**

The authors have studied 53 fresh specimens removed at operation and fixed immediately thereafter. The larger bits of tissue were fixed and stained according to the method of Van Gehuchten-Sauer, the smaller pieces were fixed in J. de Laguesse's solution and stained by the Galeotti method.

The authors describe in detail the appearance of normal kidney cells and of the normal convoluted tubules. They then describe the cellular lesions of the human kidney and classify them as follows:

Acute lesions are characterized by protoplasmic cytolysis and homogenization. Chronic lesions also appear in two varieties: viz., tubular dilatation with transformation of the protoplasm and tubular atrophy.

The authors hope soon to be able to present a comparative study of the histological lesions of the kidney and its functional disturbances. The present article is accompanied by two excellent plates in colors.

2. **Sub-capsular Nephrectomy.**

Subcapsular nephrectomy is never an operation of choice but may at times become an operation of necessity owing to one or more of the following causes: large size of the kidney, extensive adhesions, abnormal vascularization. The ordinary or extra-capsular nephrectomy is especially dangerous in a secondary operation such as would follow a nephrotomy or nephrostomy for tuberculous or simple pyonephroses, renal lithiasis, fistulæ, or renal or perirenal suppurations and adhesions. Such adhesions unite the fatty capsule on the one hand to the capsule proper of the kidney, or on the other hand to the peritoneum on its anterior surface and to the nearest organs such as the liver or spleen, or to the renal pedicle. However even in some primary nephrectomies a long-standing septic process may produce inflammatory adhesions of such an extent that in order to free the kidney the latter must be detached from its capsule.

Mollá reports three cases in which the sub-capsular procedure was done. The first was a tuberculous pyonephrosis in which a nephrostomy was done in the first stage. At the subsequent operation a very large lumbo-abdominal incision and resection of the last rib were necessary to expose the inflamed organ which was found adherent to all the walls of the renal fossa. In removing the organ the pleura was opened, a pneumothorax formed, which was followed, despite immediate closure of the tear, by a septic pleurisy, and death from the infection. The second case was that of a woman in whom a primary sub-capsular resection was successfully done for a very large pyonephrotic sac. The third case was an enormous neoplasm which proved to be an endothelioma. Because of its size, this had to be removed sub-capsularly despite its adherence to the surrounding tissues.

3. Treatment of Tuberculous Cystitis with Vaporized Iodin.

Normand describes the apparatus he uses (that of Farnarier) and points out the value of vaporized iodin as a therapeutic agent. This treatment is especially indicated in tuberculous cystitis and in vesical tuberculosis after the ablation of a tuberculous kidney. Moreover it will give encouraging results where bilateral renal lesions or pulmonary or other involvement contra-indicate nephrectomy. The author has tried to remove errors in technic and to avoid the painful reactions which constitute the most serious objections raised against this method.

It is not claimed that vaporized iodin is a panacea against tuberculous cystitis or vesical tuberculosis, but it is probably the most valuable agent at our command in the treatment of these conditions. Even if cures are rare and it is still too early to assert that the cures are permanent we can at least point out that in general improvement and relief follow the iodin vapor treatment and that it gives rise to no unfavorable complications, if carefully administered. These claims are by no means insignificant if we bear in mind the terrible condition of these unfortunate patients whose existence is rendered almost insupportable by their frequent and painful urinations with the consequent loss of sleep and disturbed nervous system.

The vaporized iodin treatment is still in the experimental stage and will most likely undergo other advantageous modifications.

4. Inoperable Urethro-vaginal Cancer Cured by Radiumtherapy.

The case is that of a woman of twenty-six who in June, 1909, noticed a small tumor at the urethral orifice. She became steadily worse. By October, 1910, she was in a miserable state: pains were severe, urination was frequent and difficult and bloody, and the gentlest examination caused excruciating torture. By this time the whole upper part of the vulva was taken up by the cancer, which was ulcerating, bleeding, and hard. Three large masses fitted in the urethra, the induration involved the median part of both labia minora and extended up the course of the urethra to the cervix uteri. Biopsy showed that the growth was a carcinomatous epithelioma arising probably from the vaginal mucosa.

The first applications of radium were made externally with a flat apparatus containing 5 cg. of the metal. Six sittings of five hours each gave practically no result. On Oct. 31, a tube of 0.5 mm. thick, surrounded by three thicknesses of tarlatan and containing 5 cg. of radium was introduced into each of the lateral growths and allowed to remain 20 hours. In 20 days the masses had diminished in size, the bloody discharge was less, and there was less pain. On Nov. 23, 1910, a similar tube of radium but surrounded with only two layers of tarlatan, was introduced into the urethra for 22 hours. (It was replaced, when necessary, after urinating.) In two weeks or so the pains disappeared, as did the perivaginal tumors and the general condition had much improved. By February, however, there was a distinct recurrence at the urethra. On March 6, 1911, the urethral introduction of radium was repeated. By Oct., 1911, the general condition had become splendid; locally no tumor masses could be seen or felt, the urethra had been entirely destroyed and the neck of the bladder had opened into the vagina with a resulting incontinence of urine. The patient appeared absolutely cured.

In July, 1913, the patient insisting on relief of the incontinence, a double implantation of the ureters into the intestine was done which was followed in a week by death from peritonitis. At autopsy no trace of tumor was visible. Numerous sections through the vaginal mucosa, the remains of the urethro-vaginal septum, and the pelvic and inguinal glands, failed to reveal any trace of cancer.

5. Partial Exclusion of a Tuberculous Kidney with Clear Urine.

Heitz-Boyer has previously described what he calls the "segmental" development of renal tuberculosis and has reported specimens showing partial exclusion of tuberculous foci. The present case is one which he has had the opportunity of observing in the stage of pseudo-healing, that is, when the tuberculous focus is walled of, the urine being perfectly clear, and before the next renal segment has become infected.

The patient was a man with a fistulous tuberculous epididymo-orchitis, who eight years before had a pleurisy and some years later had renal crises in the right side. Examination of the urine and of the kidney regions gave negative results. Catheterization of the ureters gave perfectly clear urine on both sides free from tubercle bacilli. The right urine however came in greater amount and was of higher concentration as determined by functional tests. There seemed to be therefore a distinct compensatory hypertrophy of the left kidney. X-ray examination showed shadows characteristic of old calcareous tuberculous foci on the right side. A guinea pig inoculated with the right kidney urine showed a nodular spleen with distinct granulations of the liver and lung.

In view of the results of ureteral catheterization, functional tests, inoculations, and radiography, the author concludes that this was another case of partial exclusion of calcified lesions with integrity of the remaining kidney giving absolutely clear urine.

7. A Case of Plastic Induration of the Corpora Cavernosa.

The subject was a man of 59 who had a chronic urethritis with several strictures and a chronic prostatitis. Three months before he consulted the author he had noticed a nodule on the dorsum of the penis. The plaque was disposed along the long axis of the penis and seemed to invade both corpora cavernosa as well as to extend down by a sort of pedicle into the septum between them. The tumor had the consistency of a fibroma and was painful on pressure. During erection the penis was deformed, describing a curve with the concavity upward. This did not however prevent coitus.

Physical examination of the patient failed to reveal any of the etiological factors often invoked for this condition. There was no evidence of syphilis, of gout, of arteriosclerosis, of rheumatism, of eczema, of diabetes; there was no trauma.

As regards the symptomatology, the author points out that the induration was not in itself the cause of any difficulty in urination. On the other hand most of the other similar tumors reported in the literature were not painful on pressure. This induration was rather large—the size of a bean—but the resulting deformity was slight, which was in accord with the general observation that the deviation of the penis was not directly dependent on the size of the nodule.

As regards the pathogenesis of the condition the author does not believe it to be absolutely necessary to assume a previous chronic infectious cavernitis. He feels that the patient's urethritis, prostatitis and stricture acted as so many traumatisms and local irritants sufficient to bring about a plastic induration of the corpora cavernosa.

8. The Trans-vesical Route for the Cure of Vesico-vaginal Fistulæ.

The authors take up the indications and the technic of the operation and conclude that the transvesical route should be regarded as the best for repairing vesico-vaginal fistulæ which it is dangerous, difficult, or impossible to reach by the vagina. As a matter of fact the operation is easy when the bladder is well exposed. The method is rational because it gives a direct perpendicular access to the well-exposed fistula, because it offers the best opportunity for freshening and suturing the bladder walls without involving the ureters, and finally because it assures a perfect drainage of the bladder. Lastly, the method is efficacious as is shown by the cures obtained in the majority of cases and after a single intervention.

9. The Early Diagnosis of Syphilis.

The Wassermann reaction is always negative up to the fifteenth day after the appearance of the chancre. From the fifteenth to the twentieth day it is sometimes positive but it does not become regularly positive until at least the twenty-fifth day after the beginning of the lesion. During the first two weeks therefore the Wassermann test can give no information whatever and it is therefore necessary to resort to the ultramiscroscopic search for the spirochetæ.

There is one indication however for the employment of the Wassermann reaction at the beginning of syphilis, and that is when the chancre is cicatrized, whether as a result of local treatment or not, and secondary manifestations have not made their appearance. Here it is not quite justifiable to "freshen" the chancre because of the pain and the danger of contagion and one had best resort to a Wassermann test performed with a liver and cholesterin antigen.

JOURNAL D'UROLOGIE

Vol. V, No. 4, April, 1914.

1. Ultimate Results of Urethroplasty by Tunnelization and Dermo-epidermic Grafts in the Severe Forms of Hypospadias and Epispadias. By G. Nové-Josserand.
2. General Considerations on the Prostate and Prostatectomy. By Alberto Castano.
3. Abnormal Sub-urethral Canals. By Fernand Levy and Victor Planson.
4. Abortive Electrolytic Treatment of Gonorrhea. By G. Li Virghi.
5. Calcified Retro-vesical Hydatid Cyst Which Was Diagnosed. By M. Marion.
6. Reflux of Urine Through the Ureter after Nephrectomy with Report of a New Case. By M. Lévy-Weissmann.
7. Clinical Contribution to the Study of Experimental Polyuria. By E. Pirondini.
8. How to Collect Serum for the Wassermann Reaction. By Alfred Lévy-Bing.

1. Ultimate Results of Urethroplasty.

From a study of 21 urethroplasties which he had performed up to 2 years ago the author concludes that the dermo-epidermic graft has stood the test of time. Such new-formed urethræ have lasted six, seven, and up to twelve years and have successfully accomplished their double function. Some have increased in caliber by growth, others have remained stationary in size without causing functional disturbances even when their caliber has been below normal. Two cases have gone through an attack of gonorrhea.

Strictures were observed in four of the early cases and these were limited to the point of junction of the two urethræ and were due manifestly to a primary defective organization of the graft. The method of tunnelization with grafting seems therefore to be able to cure definitely extensive hypospadias and epispadias. The new canal opens on the glans, at the usual point, and resembles, as much as possible, a normal urethra. It is elastic enough not to interfere with erection and can attain a wide enough calibre, thanks to internal urethrotomy, so as not to interfere with normal urination. Fistulæ are exceptional, and otherwise the results, with good technic, are such that secondary operations are rarely necessary. The calibration of the urethra is the only difficult problem and demands careful attention but the difficulties in this respect are by no means insurmountable. The above method seems thus to be preferable to venous urethroplasty and to the other methods of transplantation.

2. **The Prostate and Prostatectomy.**

The author takes up various points which have been brought out in his experience. As regards choice of the anesthetic he warns against chloroform and ether as being dangerous to the kidneys and heart respectively and prefers ethyl chloride or bromide as giving a short and safe narcosis. In order to prevent pulmonary congestion patients should be sat up just as soon as possible after operation.

Castano insists strongly on rapidity of operation. He has accordingly reduced his technic to the simplest terms and has learned to perform an entire enucleation in less than a minute. He uses only a bistoury, requires no guide sutures for the bladder and does not sew up the bladder or abdominal wound on the principle that the entire field is rendered septic by the infected urine and primary union cannot be hoped for. Nevertheless his patients heal up entirely in most cases in three weeks' time. He introduces Freyer tubes modified by Marion at the time of operation, leaves them in place for 4 to 6 days, replaces them with simpler tubes for another week, and finally introduces a urethral sound for 4 to 6 days longer.

The author next takes up the question of urinary sepsis, describes the symptoms and outlines. the usual treatment. Before operating he gives calcium chloride in order to diminish the loss of blood. If the urine is found to contain less than 8 grams of urea in 24 hours he does not operate.

In discussing the nature of the prostatic tumor, the author accepts the work of Motz and Perearnau who believe that the mass is due to a hypertrophy of the periurethral glands but he also feels that in many cases it is the prostate itself which is involved.

Castano points out various technical difficulties in operating on certain cases and then goes into the physiology of the prostate. In the latter connection, he believes that the gland, in addition to an external secretion which gives vitality to the sperm, possesses an internal secretion, the rôle of which is to stimulate the sexual function. Chronic prostatitis is often a cause of sterility because the spermatozoa, instead of finding the secretion a favorable medium, lose their vitality when brought in contact with it.

3. **Abnormal Sub-urethral Canals.**

Under this head the authors describe abnormal passages opening at one extremity into the urethra and at the other upon the skin. Lévy and Planson are very careful to distinguish this condition from the "double" or "accessory" urethræ which have been described. After taking up in detail the anatomical pathology, structure, and pathogenesis of these canals, the authors discuss in detail the clinical features and methods of diagnosing this condition.

Treatment of this abnormality depends first of all upon whether the canal is infected or not. If it is not infected no treatment is necessary as a rule. If the canal is infected however it is necessary to destroy it, otherwise it is practically impossible to cure the urethritis either in the principal or in the accessory passage. To this end we may use either caustic injections, such as chloride of zinc, tincture of iodine, etc., or electrolysis, as has been used by Duhot. Neither of these methods however is as efficacious as surgical extirpation of the accessory canal, which is the most rational procedure and the one that should be used whenever possible.

4. Abortive Electrolytic Treatment of Gonorrhea.

This method is indicated in all cases in which the discharge is of less than eleven days' duration. The only contraindication is an exaggerated sensitiveness of the urethra due either to nervousness on the part of the subject or to a very severe infection. In the latter case it is best to wait a few days until the condition quiets down. The actual abortive treatment takes place in two stages.

First stage: The diagnosis of gonorrhea is established by microscopic examination. The patient urinates and the anterior urethra is irrigated with sterile water. Five cubic centimeters of a 2 per cent. cocaine solution are injected into the urethra, the lips pinched, and the canal massaged from before backward to insure good penetration of the anesthetic. The anesthetic fluid is then thoroughly expelled in order to prevent precipitation of the silver solution to follow. Next 5 c c. of protargol (strength not mentioned) are injected into the anterior urethra and retained there during the rest of the procedure. The positive electrode is now applied to the patient's body (left hip) and the negative electrode, consisting of a pliable insulated metal rod to the end of which is fixed a No. 13-14 Charrière bulb, is introduced into the urethra. The continuous current is then turned on and its intensity increased just below the point where a disagreeable sensation is felt under the positive (outside) electrode. At the same time the bulb is worked back and forth in the urethra and thus brought into contact with the protargol bathing the mucosa at all parts of the canal. It may be that electrargol is generated during this procedure. The application is continued from 3 to 4 minutes. This treatment is repeated the next day and on the third. The discharge is then again examined microscopically and if gonococci are present a fourth treatment is given. The result of this procedure is first to increase the discharge and to cause a burning sensation during urination. These symptoms soon disappear and in the great majority of cases, two or three electrolyses are sufficient to drive out the gonococcus.

Second stage: This consists in a daily lavage with boric acid solution or sterile water preceded, every second or third day, by a urethral massage on a straight sound. In addition, endoscopic applications of protargol or 4% silver nitrate should be made to the region of Guérin whenever indicated. The urethral discharge should be followed microscopically and if gonococci are still present a course of two electrolyses should be resorted to in order to insure the permanent disappearance of the organism. The case may be regarded as cured when there is no discharge for three days.

The author's results: Virghi has treated 92 cases in about two years. The duration of treatment varied according to the stage in which electrolysis was begun. In 57 cases in which the discharge dated one to three days, the average duration was 8 days. Twenty-four cases with a discharge of 4 to 6 days were cured in 12 days. Nine cases which had lasted from 7 to 10 days were cured within 25 days, and finally one case, which was first seen on the eleventh day, required 33 days to cure. The author concludes that, when rigorously carried out, the electrolytic method offers the best abortive treatment for gonorrhea.

5. Calcified Retro-vesical Hydatid Cyst.

The patient was a man of 54 who had had urinary trouble for ten years. At first there was pollakiuria which was only diurnal, then it became nocturnal as well and the patient began to have pain and difficulty on urination. Examination of the urethra revealed nothing abnormal. On palpation by rectum the prostate was found to be normal but just above it there was felt a rounded mass the size of a billiard ball, firm but movable, and giving a parchment-like crepitation on hard pressure. Cystoscopy revealed nothing but a bulging of the base of the bladder.

In view of the above findings the author made a diagnosis of a calcified cyst of the pelvis, most probably a hydatid cyst. X-ray examination revealed a large round shadow in the pelvis.

Laparotomy was done and the mass was readily stripped from the bladder and rectum. On incision, it was found to contain a brownish fluid with gelatinous débris, the evident remains of hydatid vesicles.

6. Reflux of Urine Through the Ureter After Nephrectomy.

A man of 32 began to complain of great frequency of urination and of pain in the right kidney region. Separate examination of the kidney urines showed that the right side excreted 3.78 parts of urea per mille whereas the left excreted 17.65 parts. Nephrostomy was done on the right side and this was followed a week later by nephrectomy. Advanced tuberculosis was found with conservation of but a single papilla. On the day following the operation there was a reflux of bladder urine through the dilated (cut) ureter and out of the lumbar wound. The amount of urine passed in this fashion reached a liter by the fourth day. Sitting the patient up stopped the reflux for a time but this recurred when the patient strained. Judging from the course of other similar cases the author hopes that the fistula will close spontaneously.

The author gives protocols of eight cases from the literature. He goes into the question of what causes the reflux in these cases. The consensus of opinion seems to be that there must be a dilatation of the ureter with a thinning of its walls. Moreover there is an increased irritability of the bladder as in tuberculosis in which the violence of the vesical contractions causes the sphincter to contract at the same time and the urine, not being able to pass out through the urethra, is forced toward the ureteral orifice. This, in turn, because of lesions at that point, or of gaping, offers a ready passage upward. In addition to the above we must assume a suspension of the physiologic contractions of the ureter which normally direct the urinary current downward into the bladder.

8. **How to Collect Serum for the Wassermann Reaction.**

The patient should be in the recumbent posture. A rubber tourniquet is applied at the upper arm. The arm at the elbow fold is disinfected with ether. A platinum Wassermann needle with a short sharp bevel point and rubber tube attached is held between the thumb and forefinger of one hand and a test tube containing the end of the rubber tube above mentioned is held in the remaining fingers of the same hand. The skin over the vein selected is stretched with the other hand and the vein thus immobilized. The needle, held almost parallel to, and in the direction of, the vein is now plunged into the lumen and the blood collected in the test-tube. When 10 or 20 c.c. are obtained the tourniquet is released and the test tube stoppered with cotton. Before use the needle and attached rubber tube are sterilized and dried, respectively, by passing through a flame and are then allowed to cool.

If the specimen must be sent any distance for examination it is much better to let the tube stand for a few hours in a slanting position. The serum is then found to separate out on the surface and can readily be transferred to another tube by pouring off or by pipetting with a sterile dropper.

DEPARTMENT OF SEXUAL PSYCHOLOGY

NOTES ON THE PSYCHOLOGY OF SEX.

By DOUGLAS C. MCMURTRIE, New York

LESBIAN ASSEMBLIES.

In the large cities, according to Hübner,[3] homosexual women have long assembled in clubs, literary circles, etc. Howard has expressed the opinion [4] that congenital sexual inversion is widespread in America, homosexual women being frequently found in societies and clubs.

HIRSCHFELD, CHAMPION OF HOMOSEXUALITY.

Speaking of a visit to Magnus Hirschfeld, Herts [5] remarks: "Our investigation started in the Doctor's office. We were introduced to two young 'ladies,' one apparently nineteen, the other several years older. There was nothing at all unusual in their appearance save that the younger was dressed in a somewhat mannish sailor suit. She was also exceedingly good-looking.

"The Doctor proceeded at once, and before them, to explain that the older was actually a man, fully formed and normal in all physical attributes. He had simply been able to secure from the government permission to wear feminine attire. This, moreover, had been granted because it was believed that he was more conspicuous in the clothes of his own sex than otherwise. The other young lady herself explained that she had been trying to get permission to dress as a man. She felt as a man and loved only women, she told us quite simply." The pair had been to Dr. Hirschfeld in the first place to see if by an operation they could change places sexually.

THE BIBLE AND FEMININE INVERSION.

There is mention in the Bible of inverted practices between women. The most specific instance is when Paul is describing [6] to the Romans the anger of God at certain types of sin. "Where-

[3] A. H. HUBNER, *Lehrbuch der forensischen Psychiatrie.* Bonn, 1914, p. 1008.

[4] WILLIAM LEE HOWARD. Sexual perversion in America. *American Journal of Dermatology and Genito-Urinary Diseases,* St. Louis, 1904, viii, 9-14.

[5] B. RUSSELL HERTS. Visits to three scientists. Haeckel the monist; Bloch the syphilologist; Hirschfeld, defender of homosexuality; *Medical Review of Reviews,* New York, 1913, xix, 490-496.

[6] Romans i, 24-27.

fore God also gave them up to uncleanness through the lusts of their own hearts, to dishonour their own bodies between themselves. Who changed the truth of God into a lie, and worshipped and served the creature more than the Creator, who is blessed for ever. Amen. For this cause, God gave them up unto vile affections: for even their women did change the natural use into that which is against nature. And likewise also the men, leaving the natural use of the woman, burned in their lust one toward another; men with men working that which is unseemly. . . ." The reference here is specific. In the Old Testament, while there are many references to abnormal sexual practices there is no definite mention of inversion among women, though in view of the many sins with which the Israelites were tempted and afflicted, it is probable that this particular anomaly existed among them. Chevalier after citing several passages[7] in the sacred books directed against unnatural practices between men, mentions[8] in a spirit of evident surprise that Moses took no account of analogous excesses among women.

A CRIME OF LESBIAN LOVE.

One of the most widely known cases of violent crimes due to sexual inversion in the female occurred in Memphis, Tenn., approximately in 1891, though the exact date is unknown to me. The facts were typical of sexually inverted affection and are of considerable interest. They have been reported[9] by Comstock.

"The facts were that there was an unnatural affection existing between Alice Mitchell and Freda Ward. Alice Mitchell seems to have been the ardent one. The love they had for each other, to the public, seems something hard to conceive or explain, but to experts in insanity it is nothing unusual. Alice exhibited in her passion for Freda Ward all the impulses of the male sex for a female. She was to have been dressed as a man and take the bridegroom's part in the marriage ceremony. She had already even arranged with a clergyman to perform the services, but Miss Ward's friends interfered and they were separated. This

[7] *E.g.* Genesis xx, 13; Leviticus xviii, 22, 29; Deuteronomy xvii, 28.

[8] JULIEN CHEVALIER. *De l'inversion de l'instinct sexuel au point de vue médico-légal.* Paris, 1885. p. 30.

[9] T. GRISWOLD COMSTOCK. Alice Mitchell of Memphis. A case of sexual perversion or "urning" (a paranoiac). *New York Medical Times,* 1892-1893, xx, 170-173.

disturbed Alice. When riding out with a friend, she meets Miss Ward. She suddenly stops and alights from the carriage, and overtaking Miss Ward deliberately cuts her throat with a razor which she carried for the purpose. She jumps into her buggy and drives rapidly home. She was arrested. She confessed the dreadful deed. She said she murdered her best friend because she loved her. For six months while in prison she did not exhibit any remorse or regret, but showed great devotion for the photograph of Miss Ward. And during the trial, and while the verdict was being rendered, her conduct was scarcely altered."

In accounting for the deed, Comstock, while diagnosing Alice Mitchell as a sexual "pervert," considers her insane. It appears that her mother in her first confinement had child-bed fever and puerperal insanity, and was confined in an asylum, and that before the birth of Alice she was deranged, and this aberration continued until some time after labor. Although no actual determination was made of Alice's mental state it was decided she was insane.

This may have been the case. In the light of present knowledge regarding this sexual anomaly, however, it may be said that no more insanity might have been involved in this crime of homosexual jealousy than is involved in analogous crimes of heterosexual jealousy which come constantly before the courts.

A full account of the case of Alice Mitchell giving the facts as proved in court and the various testimony of the medical witnesses is given [10] in the *Memphis Medical Monthly*. The article also contains a report of the direct examination of the defendant. It is noteworthy that in none of the medical evidence was there any mention of there having been a sexual condition chiefly accountable for the crime.

CASE OF PERVERTED SEXUAL TASTES.

Howard has reported [11] the following case. A woman of thirty-nine, a chronic masturbator, had practiced Lesbian love at boarding school. She married a strong healthy man when she was twenty years old, but derived no pleasure from normal intercourse. She greatly enjoyed masturbation directly after coitus, however.

[10] Forensic psychiatry; Alice Mitchell adjudged insane. *Memphis Medical Monthly,* 1892, xii, 377-428.

[11] WILLIAM LEE HOWARD. Sexual perversion. *Alienist and Neurologist,* St. Louis, 1896, xvii, 1-6.

Later she ceased sexual intercourse and forced her husband to mutual self-abuse. She no longer desired Lesbian relations, but endeavored to have a man expose himself and then she retired to masturbate herself. Any man would excite her thus but once, never a second time.

CONGRESSIONAL REGULATION OF PREVENTION OF CONCEPTION.

In a congressional debate on the authority of congress in the regulation of interstate and federal affairs, the power affecting "articles preventing conception (U. S. vs. Popper, 98 Fed., 423)" was cited.[12]

THE BERDACHE AMONG THE ILLINOIS.

Referring to the Illinois, Parkman[13] observes: "In their manners, they were more licentious than many of their neighbors, and addicted to practices which are sometimes supposed to be the result of a perverted civilization. Young men enacting the part of women were frequently to be seen among them. These were held in great contempt. Some of the early travelers, both among the Illinois and among other tribes, where the same practice prevailed, mistook them for hermaphrodites. According to Charlevoix (*Journal Historique*, 303) this abuse was due in part to a superstition."

According to Membré, hermaphrodites were numerous among the Illinois.[14] Regarding the male members of this tribe, Membré states as follows:

"They have many wives, and often take several sisters that they may agree better; and yet they are so jealous that they cut off their noses on the slightest suspicion. They are lewd, and even unnaturally so, having boys dressed as women, destined for infamous purposes. These boys are employed only in women's work, without taking part in the chase or war." [15]

[12] *Congressional Record*, Washington, March 11, 1914, li, 4989.

[13] FRANCIS PARKMAN. *La Salle and the discovery of the great west.* 11th edit., rev., Boston, 1879. p. 207.

[14] FATHER ZENOBIUS MEMBRÉ. *Narrative of the adventures of La Salle's party at Fort Crevecoeur, in Ilinois, from February, 1680, to June, 1681.* In: JOHN GILMARY SHEA. *Discovery and exploration of the Mississippi Valley: with the original narratives of Marquette, Allouez, Membré, Hennepin, and Anastase Douay.* Redfield, Clinton Hall, New York, 1852, p. 151.

[15] *Ibid.*, p. 151.

MORAL CONDITIONS AMONG SEAMEN.

In a recent conversation with a gentleman exceptionally conversant with all phases of the seaman's life, I was told that homosexual practices among sailors had decreased in recent years to a notable extent. This he considered to be due to several causes, the most important being the passing of long voyages, such as used to be taken in the old sailing ships, not touching land, in some instances, for six months at a time. The majority of trips at the present time are in fast steam vessels having a maximum period of two weeks between ports. Another reason for the decrease of the practice in question was the rise of public sentiment, condemning it, among the men. This would operate, of course, to put a check on the conduct of individuals.

THE KAMA SUTRA.

One of the most famous treatises in the world on sexual affairs is the Kama Sutra of Vatsyayana.[16] Without going into details, it may be noted that the work, written in Sanskrit, dates from some time between the first and the sixth centuries A. D. The work deals with various phases of the sexual life, methods of sexual congress, principles of courtship, marital relations, and the practices of courtesans.

The author's own statement regarding his work is most illuminating. "After reading and considering the works of Babhravya and other ancient authors, and thinking over the meaning of the rules given by them, this treatise was composed, according to the precepts of the Holy Writ, for the benefit of the world, by Vatsyayana, while leading the life of a religious student at Benares, and wholly engaged in the contemplation of the Deity. This work is not to be used merely as an instrument for satisfying our desires. A person acquainted with the true principles of this science, who preserves his Dharma (virtue or religious merit), his Artha (worldly wealth), and his Kama (pleasure or sensual gratification), and who has regard to the customs of the people, is sure to obtain the mastery over his senses. In short, an intelligent and knowing person, attending to Dharma and Artha and also to Kama, without becoming the slave of his passions, will obtain success in everything that he may do."

[16] *The Kama Sutra of Vatsyayana. Translated from the Sanskrit. In seven parts, with preface, introduction, and concluding remarks.* Reprint: Cosmopoli, MDCCCLXXXIII [1883]: for the Kama Shastra Society of London and Benares, and for private circulation only.

THE AMERICAN JOURNAL OF UROLOGY, VENEREAL AND SEXUAL DISEASES

William J. Robinson, M.D., Editor

Vol. X OCTOBER, 1914. No. 10

SOME POINTS IN THE TECHNIQUE OF PROSTATIC ADENOMECTOMY FOR ADENOMATOSIS OF THE PROSTATE [1]

By William M. Spitzer, M.D., Denver, Colo.

WITHIN the last few years there has been instituted a rather vigorous propaganda against the term "hypertrophy of the prostate." Unfortunately it has not met with very great success, for the reason that no substitute was offered for the old convenient term. I would therefore modestly suggest "adenomatosis of the prostate" to connote the pathological entity understood by the old expression. As we really do not perform a prostatectomy, and as the use of the name is still productive of radical surgery, I would also suggest, until a better name is proposed, the term "prostatic adenomectomy" which, as the name implies, is all that should be accomplished under the operation.

Many a one who operates for the above condition without having had considerable previous experience, is under the impression that he must "enucleate" the prostate gland, and as a result, he often removes much more than is necessary.

Of all the old men who come to us with obstruction of the urinary outflow, a large proportion are found to have adenomata in the prostate. Even in those where carcinoma is found, the malignant tumor may have been the outgrowth of an adenoma.

It is practically impossible to remove the prostate gland, because the recto-vesical fascia is so closely interwoven with the lower end of the bladder, the prostate gland, the anterior wall of the rectum and the seminal vesicles, that it cannot be torn away from any of these organs without dissecting the prostate itself. Moreover, this fascia, or one of its layers, extends into

[1] Read at the annual meeting of The American Urological Association.

the gland proper, accompanying the ejaculatory ducts, and dividing the prostate into two portions, the posterior one having no connection whatsoever with the anterior. The function of the former, if it have any, is not known, and as far as the operative work is concerned is of no importance. The anterior portion has running through it the urethra, below and to the sides of which lie the glands which give the name to this organ. Anterior to the urethra only muscular and fibrous tissue are found, and if a gland be seated here it is due to congenital misplacement.

The prostate has no capsule and no lobes, unless one chooses to call the anterior portion and the posterior portion, respectively, the anterior and the posterior lobes. Superior and inferior may be substituted for anterior and posterior with perfect propriety because the important portion or lobe of the organ lies both superiorly and anteriorly to the posterior when in the upright position.

The superior of the three layers of the recto-vesical fascia runs in front of the prostate, to which, as previously mentioned, it is firmly attached, and then continues forward and upward on each side to the pubes, forming the pubo-prostatic or pubo-vesical ligaments. The middle layer of the recto-vesical fascia, together with the inferior layer, covers the seminal vesicles posteriorly or inferiorly, and a projection of it accompanies the ejaculatory ducts to within a few millimeters of their entrance into the urethra, making a perfect fascial plate completely separating the anterior portion of the prostate from the posterior. This fascia is also inseparable from the organ. The inferior layer of the recto-vesical fascia blended with the middle layer, and known as the "fascia of Dénonvilliers," lies between the extreme inferior wall of the prostate and the rectum, and is also so attached to both of these organs that if an attempt were made to tear away either one or the other, a portion of the organ to be left would undoubtedly come away. All three of these layers comprise the anatomic capsule of the prostate, if capsule it be called, completely enclosing the organ. It is also not to be forgotten that the fibro-muscular structure of the prostate insensibly penetrates the deep layer of the triangular ligament, and intertwines with the fibers of the transversus perinei profundus, as it does with those muscular fibers of the bladder known as the internal sphincter. From the above it is clearly evident that it is absolutely impossible to remove the entire organ without seriously injuring the adnexa.

The object of the various operations which we employ to restore the impaired urinary outflow is to remove the obstruction. This is effected by restoring the internal opening of the urethra to the lowest point of the bladder which necessarily diminishes its length and brings the curve of the urethra back to its original status. This is very nicely accomplished by removing the adenomata which are located in that portion of the prostate lying between the urethra and the fascial plate. As there is no gland tissue anywhere else but at this site, there can be no other adenomata. With the removal of the tumors the operation is completed.

Dr. Wishard makes an incision on each side of the urethra and then proceeds to enucleate all the adenomata with which his finger comes in contact, after which he explores the bladder and finishes the operation by establishing good drainage and packing around it. He does this by way of the perineum, which it is true has certain advantages; but at the same time it also has its disadvantages. While his mortality is lower than that of those who operate by the suprapubic route, it is not free from the unfortunate accidents which occasionally occur when entry is gained through the perineum, such as incontinence of urine, perineal fistula, overlooking a stone in the bladder, or failure to cure the condition for which operation was performed. There is another accident which happens not infrequently, that a small adenoma which has been dug out slips into the bladder and becomes a nucleus for a stone. I therefore prefer to follow the supra-pubic route, as the operative results are perfect from every standpoint, the wound completely closes sooner or later as the case may be, and there are no sequela to bother the surgeon or the patient. In other words, only one of two conditions follow: either complete cure or death. While the mortality is higher than in operation by way of the perineum, I think we are justified in following the supra-pubic route rather than have the incomplete results that are so often a source of torture to the patient.

As to the technique of the operation after the bladder has been opened and the field inspected, an incision is made in the mucous membrane of the urethra on each side, one inch in length, with a small knife, or with the instrument that I beg leave to demonstrate. It is a pair of dressing forceps having a small knife on the outer side of the end of each blade. It is inserted into the urethra, opened, and then withdrawn, slight pressure being made to hold it open during the withdrawal. The blade is just large enough to make an incision of such a depth that the lines of cleavage are easily found. The finger is then inserted and passed through one of the incisions in the mucous membrane, the line of cleavage found, and the tumor enucleated, the finger again inserted into the same opening, and if another tumor be detected it is likewise removed, this operation being repeated until no more tumors are to be found on that side. The same operation is repeated on the other side. It is important to hug the tumors closely, so that no other tissue be removed and as little damage as possible be done to the true prostatic structure. The best results and the least bleeding are obtained in those cases in which each tumor is removed separately. This work, which is identical with the method of Wishard, excepting the change of route, should be done preferably with the gloved hand, the bladder walls being meanwhile carefully retracted. I am convinced that the shock is less in those cases where least trauma to the bladder wall occurs. Where the vesical walls are not well retracted the mucous membrane is injured very much by the constant passing in and pulling out of the ungloved hand and sharp finger nails. In those cases in which the prostate can be pushed up into the abdominal wound, there is less injury to the bladder wall, and consequently less absorption from infected bladder contents through a raw mucous membrane. The reason for making the incision in the lateral walls of the urethra is that they do not bleed as freely as the floor or the trigone of the bladder, for the venous plexuses are not in the vicinity of these incisions nor is the field of enucleation near these plexuses. While there is a rather sharp hemorrhage during the enucleation, it ceases immediately when the prostate is dropped back, and before the bladder wall is closed it will be seen that it has practically stopped. Another advantage of the lateral incision over that of the trigone, is that one is nearer the field of operation by the former route.

The entire operation is confined to that portion of the prostate which lies between the before-mentioned prolongation of the fascia of Dénonvilliers posteriorly and the urethra anteriorly. The urethra itself is not torn away or injured except when an adenoma cannot be separated from one of the small ducts which empty into the prostatic urethra. This may be avoided by snipping the duct with scissors when the tumor is enucleated.

Much has been said of the advantages of spinal anesthesia for prostatic adenomectomy, which it would be superfluous to detail in this paper, although I am in hearty accord with the opinion that it is the ideal anesthetic for this operation, particularly because of the relaxation of the abdominal muscles, and more especially of the levator ani, so that with a proper retraction of the wound and two fingers in the rectum one may in practically every case elevate the prostate into the abdominal wound and see the field clearly. This is of aid in avoiding shock, by eliminating injury to the bladder wall.

When is the operation completed? When there is no longer a projection of the prostate into the bladder; when the internal sphincter is at the lowest point of the viscus; when the finger no longer meets resistant rounded masses of tissue on being introduced into the urethra; and when a Van Buren sound whose curve is the arc of a very large circle can be introduced with ease into the bladder, not more than six and one-half to seven inches of sound being necessary to traverse the distance between the external urinary meatus and the bladder. This sound should be of large size.

Drainage can be as perfect through a suprapubic wound as through the perineum or the urethra if the bladder be closed very tightly about the drainage tube with a purse string, and if the abdominal wall be just as tightly closed around this soft rubber tube. The latter should not extend more than one or two centimeters inside the bladder wall, and should be tested by running water in and out of it before the patient is dressed. There should be no leakage around it. On putting the patient to bed syphonage can at once be established by attaching a soft rubber tube, previously filled with water, on one end to the tube left in the abdominal wound, the other end being inserted in a jar on the floor containing a measured quantity of antiseptic fluid. Syphonage will immediately be started and continue for the ensuing four or five days. The dressings on the abdomen by this procedure will be just as dry and clean as after a laparotomy.

I have been fortunate in obtaining post mortem examinations in most of my cases which terminated fatally, and have been able to demonstrate that the urethra was uninjured, that the prostate was left in situ, the ejaculatory ducts were intact, and the cavities remaining after enucleation of large adenomata were very small indeed. I have also found in some cases traces of small adenomata that had not been enucleated, evidently too minute to have been felt by the finger. This, however, is a negligible circumstance, as the growth of these tumors is so slight that years pass before they attain such size as to again obstruct the urinary outflow. Usually this does not come to pass, as the patient is of such an age when operated upon that he dies of an intercurrent affection long before there is a recurrence of his prostatic trouble. Personally I have never yet had a patient with a recurrence sufficient to worry him, although my oldest living patient had his adenomectomy performed by this method about nine years ago.

While the main objects of my remarks were to elucidate some points in the technique, I desire once more, in conclusion, to make an earnest plea for the substitution of the term "adenomatosis of the prostate" and "prostatic adenomectomy" for the present inappropriate terminology.

METROPOLITAN BLDG.

THE ANATOMICAL CONFIGURATION OF THE HUMAN VESICULA SEMINALIS IN RELATION TO THE CLINICAL FEATURES OF SPERMACYSTITIS.[1]

By Dr. R. Picker, Budapest, Hungary.

IN the evolution of the pathological conception and the treatment of infectious diseases of the *lower part of the male genito-urinary organs* in general two assumptions are to be distinguished.

The first lays the leading idea upon the disease of the bladder and finds the explanation for the so-called "bladder ailments" in the vesical retention, in the retention of infected urine and the urine-poisoning. The second seeks the explanation of those appearances, which do not depend upon vesical retention, rather in the "urethritis posterior" and urethrocystitis.

The discoveries of bacteriology, which seemed to throw at once a light upon the numerous unknown facts in infectious diseases, have in fact not forwarded the matter so much as we might have expected. The war against bacteria was carried on with fire and sword, because they were considered to be the *single motive power* in diseases.

Upon this conception was based the treatment of bladder and urethra posterior by means of very strong antibacteric medicaments, and the results, often only symptomatical ones, obtained by this procedure seemed to justify the assumption.

The important part played by the connexion between the glandular adnexa and urethra and bladder in the infectious diseases of these organs was overlooked, especially as regards invalids of younger age, while in the case of men of more advanced age suffering from prostatic enlargement, as already mentioned, the vesical retention and the prostatic obstruction became the essence of pathology and therapy.

Having occupied myself for more than 15 years with the clinical, i. e. *applied bacteriology*, and the *systematical treatment* of the infectious diseases of the lower part of the genito-urinary organs, I have been led (by the most exact examination of *every case* coming within my practice) more and more to attribute the greatest importance to the mechanical moments present in the anatomical texture and physiological behavior of the greater and smaller glandular adnexa of the male urethra.

Concerning the pathology of pyelitis, the French School,

[1] Read before the Section on Urology at the International Medical Congress in London.

with Albarran at its head, early discovered by means of exact anatomical studies the importance of the mechanical moment of retention in the pathology of infectious diseases of that organ being present in dilatations and malformations of the kidney pelvis, the fundamental anatomical work of Hyrtl (1872) having been almost forgotten.

With respect to the lower part of the urine passage and its diseases, the rôle of the prostate gland was early known and thoroughly studied, as may be seen from numerous textbooks and manuals (English, German, French), while the vesiculæ seminales and their diseases have been in the greater part superficially treated or clearly neglected. In America a good deal of work has been done concerning this matter in the past few years.

Lloyd and Fuller were almost the only ones who have *long* recognized the importance of the vesiculæ seminales in the clinic of infectious diseases of the lower urinary tract, and by their operative successes have proved the connexion, on the one hand, of these organs with chronic bladder ailments, and on the other hand with septic, metastatic, and arthritic appearances.

The experiences which I have had during fifteen years of practice in the treatment of infectious diseases of the genito-urinary organs have led me to a detailed study of the anatomy of the vesiculæ seminales, these being the most important glandular adnexa of the urethra.

I have examined about 150 seminal vesicles by filling them through the vas deferens with Beck's bismuth-paste to the maximum capacity ("surgical fullness"), after which I endeavored to disentangle the tube system. Thus I am in possession of 72 specimens, 56 normal and 16 pathological, the classification of which is to be seen from the following table:

TABLE OF SPECIMENS

		Pieces.	*Per cent.*
A.	Simple straight tubes	2	4
B.	Thick twisted tubes with or without diverticula	8	15
C.	Thin twisted tubes with or without diverticula	8	15
D.	Main tube straight or twisted, with larger grape-like arranged diverticula	19	33
E.	Short main tube with large irregular ramified branches.	19	33
		56	100

F. Varia.

1. Embryological abnormities:
   Reduplication of vesic. seminalis ....piece A. 1.

Rudimentary seminal ves.	piece 59
Ductus Mulleri persistens	piece B. 17
Vesicula seminalis covering ampulla....	piece 50
Ductus ejaculatorii in the posterior wall of prostate	piece 44

These all belong to otherwise anatomical pieces.

2. Pathological conditions:

Inflammatory cicatricial adhesions not to be disentangled, cicatricial occlusion of both ducti deferentes, &c.	15
Carcinoma vesicæ seminalis	1
General total	72

The complete collection of specimens (Röntgen-ray photographs and a set of 50 stereo-diapositives arranged in a desk) was shown by me in Vienna at the Third Congress of the German Urological Society (September, 1911). A part of the figures and the German paper I placed at the disposal of Professor Voelcker (Heidelberg) in the autumn of 1911; ten figures (Nos. 2, 8, 9, 10, 11, 12, 13; and 26, 27, 28) of his book, *Chirurgie der Samenblasen* (1912), are my preparations, and the text, pp. 16-22, and pp. 50-52, is reproduced from my paper. 26 specimens, 28 X-ray plates, and the arrangement of stereo-diapositives I have shown also in the museum of this Congress, cf. Catalogue, Nos. 2239-79.

SEMINAL VESICLES.

GROUP A. *Simple straight tubes*, 2 preparations, being about 4 per cent. of my anatomical material. These are of insignificant length (6 cm.) and volume 3 c.c. It is the rarest and embryologically simplest form of seminal vesicle, which is, so to say, only a diverticulum of the ampulla, i. e. of the vas deferens. Type of this group is piece A 1, showing on its right side the thorough reduplication of the seminal vesicle, each tube arising separately from the ampulla. On the left side of the tube bends laterally at its end; thus arises the form of vesicula seminalis named "shepherd's-crook," and described by anatomists as a typical form of this organ.

I may here mention the rudimentary form of seminal vesicle as shown in piece 59, presenting itself as a short stump about 2 cm. in length, arising under a very strongly developed ampulla.

GROUP B. *Thick twisted tubes*, with or without diverticula, 8 pieces, i. e. 15 per cent. of my collection.

This form is distinguished by its enormous volume (11.5 c.c.) and by the as yet undescribed considerable length (23 cm.) of the large tube which runs from the basis prostatæ towards the rectum, screw-like in form without any sharp bend and tanglement.

The tubes become towards their cranial end more and more thickened, showing there, in the greatest pieces, a transverse diameter measuring more than 1 cm.

Diverticula are rarely seen, ampullæ are often very strongly developed.

Group C. *Thin twisted tubes with or without diverticula,* 8 examples, i. e. 15 per cent. of my collection. Their volume varies between 2 and 7 c.c., their length between 8 and 11 cm. Type of this group is preparation No. 11. The thin tubes (o.3 cm. diameter), which run in narrow regular spiral convolutions without any bend, are arranged quite symmetrically. Their length in relation to their volume is very significant. In a part of the preparations there is to be observed a lateral bend, formed by the cranial extremity of this tube-system which is said to be typical by the anatomists. In some cases the diverticula are present in considerable number and high development.

As characteristic for group B and C, in disentangling the filled vesiculæ, I have met but seldom with any adhesions formed by coarse and dense connective tissue between the tubes and tubuli. On the contrary the intertubular connective tissue has in every case been found to be easily divisible.

Group D. *Main tube straight or twisted with larger "grape-like" arranged diverticula,* 19 examples, i. e. about 33 per cent. of my collection. The volume of the ducts varies between 2 and 6 cc., length between 4½ and 19 cm. The largest piece is No. 27, the volume of each tube being 5 c.c., lengths 11 and 19 cm. Both tubes bend round laterally and so recede to the base of prostate gland. The smallest preparation is No. 34, with 4 and 5 cm. length and 2 c.c. capacity for each branch.

In No. 19, the prototype of this group, I am sorry I could only work out one tube. This is a short straight duct covered with broad-based diverticula, varying in size from a pea to a hazel-nut, without which it would be a type of group A. I must also call attention to No. 24 on account of the very remarkable difference of length of the two branches, the left being 3½, the right 12 cm. long and ending in a T. No. 31 is typical on both sides, in spite of the total dissymmetry of the whole system.

The examples of this group mostly possess many diverticula (4-14), the ampullæ being mostly very rich, and thickened, so as to appear knotted.

GROUP E. *Short main duct with large irregular ramified branches,* 19 pieces, i. e. 33 per cent. of my anatomical material. In this group again are found very large vesicles, which attain a volume of 10 c.c. and a length of 14 cm. The average length is about 10 cm., even the smallest specimens being 6-8 cm. The relative small length with relatively large volumes is to be explained from the extensive surface of the branches so abundantly present. The numerous diverticula arise with narrow bases from the tubes. The main duct very often cannot be followed to the end, but is lost in a row of more or less similar large secondary ducts. In every case these secondary ducts dominate the field and give to each preparation its characteristic appearance, which is very difficult or impossible to describe.

The larger branches mostly bend laterally backwards (Prep. No. 41); but yet we more rarely find them bending in the medial direction. If two such branches, one lateral and one medial, meet at their extremity, then there appears to be formed the figure of a perfect circle (Prep. 45). This is, however, a false appearance, since in delicate and careful preparation the ends of the branches may be divided from each other. In observing the mechanism of the filling of these diverticula by means of Beck's paste, I have often seen the same fill themselves separately, and as the filling proceeds the blunt end of each diverticulum becomes more and more strongly marked. The perfect circle, which is visible in the figures of Pallin, might owe its origin to a mistake in the reconstruction by means of the "Plattenmodellmethode." (It is probable that those slices which contained the very thin walls of the adjacent blunt ends have fallen out in the reconstruction.)

I would specially call attention to preparation No. 44, both sides of which are quite asymmetric and irregular; on the right side the main tube shows at its end a large laterally-placed cyst.

In general the more richly developed pieces of this group are very difficult of description and may only be depicted by stereoscopic photographs. It is only in this way possible to demonstrate the space-relation of the numerous branches, running partly in front, partly behind, partly crossing each other and showing great differences in size.

Group F.. *Varia*, 16 cases. From these in 7 cases I have found strong cicatricial adhesions owing to the dense connective tissue which cannot be disentangled. In one case the vasa deferentia has been found obliterated high above the ampullæ; the filling of ampullæ and vesicles was only possible by stitching with the needle in the ampulla (collargol preparation No. 57). Besides this there were present in these specimens: pyelitis, callosities, and cicatrices in the epididymis; thickening of Cowper's gland, leucocytes in the prostatic and vesical secretions, and, so to say, in each case the dense cicatricial induration of the surrounding fat-tissue, particularly around the top of the vesicula.

AMPULLA OF VAS DEFERENS AND BASIS-DIVERTICULA.

The *ampulla* shows itself, when simply developed, as a straight narrow tube; its diameter widens slightly in relation to the caliber of the vas deferens. We also find ampullæ of simple form in which the vas deferens is twisted, thus resulting in slight thickening.

The construction given as a type of ampullæ by descriptive anatomy is to be seen in the next group: slightly swollen and thickened ampullæ with fairly numerous, small bud-like diverticula.

If the diverticula develop more strongly the symmetrical arrangement of the same gives to the ampullæ a feathery appearance.

The symmetrically arranged diverticula again show differences of the finer structure, partly being developed in form of cauliflower-like papillomata, and partly the diverticula get a downy appearance through the very fine and abundant ramifications.

The most complicated developments are shown by those ampullæ on which we recognize a separately-formed "corpus diverticulare" to be well distinguished from the main duct, which itself again shows varieties similar to the above-mentioned.

All these features are very difficult to describe. Their exact study is only possible by the analysis of Röntgen-ray photographs of the infected ampulla.

I have given the name of "basis-diverticula" to those outgrowths which, reaching a length of 1 cm. or more, are found lying in the corner between the seminal vesicle and the ampulla on the posterior surface of the "collum vesicæ seminalis."

In treating in a systematic way the cases of spermatocystitis I have met with the following classes of cases.

1. *Mild cases*, taking their course without any local symptoms, in which, in the absence of any morbid change to be felt on rectal examination, the correct diagnosis can only be made by the most exact topical diagnosis and thorough bacteriological examination of the pathological secretions got by means of rectal palpation and expression. The cure can often be quickly obtained.

2. *Serious cases*, accompanied by high fever and very marked clinical symptoms: bladder and rectal complications and metastases in the highest stage of the disease, i. e., in the course of the second or third week after the infection.

(*a*) *One part* of them *is healed quickly* and completely by the spontaneous discharge of considerable quantities of pus, accompanied often by violent colics, said to be in general cystitis, or by the draining off of the retained pus by means of rectal massage within a period of four to six weeks.

(*b*) *Another part*, in spite of the serious initial symptoms, the suppuration and spontaneous pus leakage, quite similar to cases described under (*a*), *takes a chronic course* and requires systematic expression treatment by means of digital massage through many (3-4-5) months. Often these cases are only definitely cured after several relapses of the fever and suppuration. The discharge drained off by the massage is of pus-like character only in the beginning; later on there is emptied a greyish, thin prostatic secretion intermingled with casts originating in the seminal vesicle, being partly totally normal (sago-like), partly showing slight inflammatory changes, and partly pus-like in appearance.

3. *Ordinary cases*, with feverish symptoms of more significant or abortive character, with very slight urinary troubles passing very quickly, causing scarcely any inconvenience to the patients and only to be remarked by thorough examination, the disease notwithstanding lasting often many months. In some of these cases I have observed the formation of great anatomical infiltrations, but very rarely is there present a well-marked diffused suppuration. In the treatment of these cases by massage one seldom succeeds in draining off greater quantities of pus, but in the large majority of cases there are emptied through a long period pus-plugs of all sizes in combination with seminal

casts of a normal or fairly normal aspect, containing little spots of abnormal appearance, which, taken apart and prepared for the microscope, are shown to be small pus-plugs, formed in the diverticula of the seminal tube, containing leucocytes and bacteria.

4. *Cases with recurrent epididymitis,* in which the ampulla of the vas deferens is found also to be affected, and in the course of massage treatment relapses of the epididymitis may occur once, or even more often.

It may be seen from the preceding that *great differences are observable in the course and final cure* of the acute forms of spermatocystitis. Bringing these clinical features in relation with the above-described anatomical forms of this organ, I have been led to the following conclusions.

When infected, *the straight, single tubes of group* A might not give rise to many complications, because the uniformly wide and straight tube possessing no diverticula offers no predisposition to the retention of inflammatory secretions.

The infection of form B, characterized by *thick, long screw-like twisted tubes with or without diverticula,* might in case of acute inflammation be accompanied by abundant pus-formation and high fever, lasting while the pus is formed and retained in the tube-system through the inflammatory swelling of the common ejaculatory duct. In these cases I have further remarked a very large inflammatory tumor extending to the ampulla of the rectum, as well as strong subjective inconveniences originating from the bladder and the rectum. In the given case I have in mind that with a disease of a vesicula seminalis of that configuration, after disappearance of the alarming and acute symptoms, the final cure of the serious disease takes place within an unexpectedly short time (3-6 weeks) by means of the complete evacuation of pus either in a natural way or through the massage treatment. The difficulties arising from the bladder consist principally in frequent and painful micturition, which symptom is usually taken for subacute cystitis, but in my experience is really caused by colics of the overfilled seminal duct. *The colic of the seminal vesicle* is characterized, as mentioned above, by very frequent and painful micturition without the patients being always able to urinate, but they frequently complain of a feeling as if secretions were entering into the posterior urethra.

In other cases where the inflammatory swelling extends more towards the rectum, patients complain also of frequent rectal "tenesmi," emptying only some mucus without any relief to their pains; under these conditions they also often have the feeling as if the rectum were full and are not able to sit. The fundus vesicæ being also involved in the inflammatory swelling, there results often an incomplete, more rarely a complete, retention of urine with clear or cloudy residuum, the amount of which varies between 80 to 300 grams. The capacity of the bladder is, in spite of the symptoms of "subacute cystitis," found to be almost normal.

The occurrence of the colics is clearly to be explained by the anatomical configuration of the long and large twisted tubes, when these are filled to a maximum by the products of the inflammation. The best proof of the correctness of my conception is given by *the immediate disappearance of the colics,* felt as a pressing desire to urinate, through the *evacuation of the pus,* the colic reappearing immediately after the tube system has been filled again to the maximum.

It is not even necessary to drain off the whole of the pus in order to make the colics cease; it is sufficient to lead off a little more than the overbrimming quantity of pus upon the urinary passage. This is the ordinary way in which "nature by itself effects the cure" ("Naturheilung"). The spermatic colics may be of such violence, that even great doses of morphia, administered in the subcutaneous form or in suppositories, may remain without any effect. I have observed this in many of my patients: the cramps appeared regularly after intervals of 3–5–10 minutes; the morphia was, at the most, only able to deaden in some measure the pains, but could not make the colics cease. However, the colics together with the pains disappeared *immediately*—at first only for 2 to 3 hours, later even for 6 to 8, and finally for 12 to 24 hours—*upon my draining off the secretion by means of massage.* When the colics, after the above-mentioned periods of relief, reappeared, they did so in the beginning at intervals of perhaps half an hour, and then became more and more frequent till they reached the maximal frequency, only being again stopped by the repetition of my massage treatment. Following this process and administering this evacuation treatment as often as necessary (even 3 and 4 times daily), I have been able to definitely free the patients from the colics, usually within one week, emptying *at one sitting* very frequently quantities of pus from 5–8 c.c., and in one of my most remarkable cases so much as 15 c.c., *of thick yellow pus.* The definite cure, i. e., the complete elimination of bacteria, takes place after this period of colic often in a very short space of time, which may in fortunate cases *not be more than 3 or 4 weeks.*

This *favorable end* of such a serious disease is to be explained simply through the structure of the seminal vesicles belonging to this group, the tube system of which—diverticula being almost completely absent—puts no obstacle in the way of the quick and definite draining off of the pus, but even *promotes* the same by the assistance of the colics. This is explained by the powerful muscular coat of the great and wide duct. In such cases the fundus of the bladder, as mentioned, being involved also in the great inflammatory swelling, the bladder must (under these conditions) be examined by introducing a thin Jacques-patent catheter (about No. 5 or 6 English scale) to find out if there be a vesical retention. A greater retention, which setting in in an acute form causes an augmentation of the frequency of micturition, gives rise in combination with the spermatic colics to such inconveniences that the patient's lot, sufficiently unenviable as it is, may become absolutely unbearable through these easily removable disturbances.

These cases connected with such an abundant suppuration might also be those in which, by shutting off the draining of pus or by insufficient evacuation of the retention, the morbid secretion makes for itself a path in the *neighborhood* of the vesicle and breaks down into the perivesicular and perirectal cellular tissue, into the peritoneum (Douglas's fold), or even into the rectum. The anatomical predisposition for these events is present at the entrance-point of the vessels, where there exist physiological clefts (dehiscences) of tunica fibrosa and muscularis, and also at those points where greater and smaller diverticula grow out (Petersen, Oberndorfer).

In my practice of fifteen years I have only had *one case coming to me with rectal gonorrhea* caused by *spermatocystitis,* in which I could prove the communication of the rectum with seminal vesicle in the form of a papillomatous growth felt on the top of the right vesicula; this disappeared and the fistula closed after ten days of forcible massage treatment, while the remaining spermatocystitis had to be treated further.

I have never yet observed the formation *of perispermatocystitic phlegmon* in cases of fresh infection conducted by me.

If in the course of an inflammation there takes place a cicatricial fixation of a badly-drained section of the tube-system (e. g., a greater secondary duct, cystically widened end of main duct), so there may arise, after spontaneous healing of a typical infectious disease, *empyema falsum*, liable to be attacked by any hematic or ascending secondary infection with all the sequelæ of general or local nature. The empyema falsum may last—after the fundamental gonorrhea has passed away for 10–20, even 30 years—the center of the most various forms of saprophytic urethritis and cystitis, of feverish conditions showing the clinical features of influenza, and finally giving rise to otherwise inexplicable rheumatic and septic diseases. These latter may in the form of cryptogenetic sepsis, with the most various symptoms belonging to the heart, joints, kidneys, etc., sooner or later cause the death of the patient, without the doctor having any idea that the manifold successive diseases are all attributable to a latent infection of the seminal vesicle.

C. Thin twisted tubes with or without small diverticula. I have until now not been able to separate amongst the various cases of spermatocystitis any cases presenting features characteristic of that anatomical configuration. In any case, however, theoretically the spontaneous uninterrupted cure of an infectious disease is more to be expected for the simply constructed organs than for the larger ones fitted with many diverticula.

D. Main tube; straight or twisted, with larger grape-like arranged diverticula. The many diverticula and windings predispose in the case of an infection, surely, to retention. The conditions of drainage are in general bad, apart from the vesicles with straight main tube. The great number of diverticula characteristic of that group may be looked upon as an obstacle to a definite spontaneous evacuation. The sharp bend of the main tube, which is found in very many pieces of this group lying in the top of the undisentangled organ, represents a physiological condition of poor drainage, which becomes more accentuated under pathological changes, especially when there exists a greater inflammatory swelling. In the course of massage treatment at these points I have observed the most resistent infiltrations. In chronic cases I have often met at this point with an isolated hardness sensitive to pressure, requiring in many cases a very intense treatment.

Group E. (Short main duct with large ramified irregular secondary branches.) I should in a given case consider that I was dealing with a seminal vesicle belonging to this group, when after the quieting down of the acute initial appearances and the abatement of fever, there is to be remarked an abundant draining off of pus similar to group B, but the final evacuation of the large and swollen seminal vesicle is only to be obtained after a systematic massage treatment extending over several months. Till the end of this treatment there are emptied, together with normal sago-formed seminal secretions, numerous long and thick pus-threads and plugs, which in shape quite resemble the normal sago-like secretions, and which are formed of leucocytes, partly containing those bacteria which produce, on interrupting the treatment, again and again the recurrences of urethral discharge and cystitis so often observed in the course of chronic urogenital ailments.

When not treated by massage, the examples of group E, as well as the complicated ones of group D, may represent those cases in which we meet with several attacks of cystitis combined with irregular fever and even with complete or incomplete retention. In these cases a feverish condition of long standing and irregular character with absence of urogenital symptoms may lead the physician to think that he has to do with a case of typhoid, especially when the fundamental acute infection has long passed away (10–20, even 30 years) and the symptoms of disease belong more to the organs of the digestive system.

It is very easy to imagine that in seminal vesicles of this structure, in case of infection (e. g., gonorrheal), an apparent cure of the symptoms belonging to the urinary passages may take place by inflammatory swelling and obstruction of a greater secondary duct, the inflammatory processes therein gradually quieting down.

In case of forced coitus there appear those unexpected, even heavy recurrences of urethral discharges, with which we have to deal so often after insufficient healing of a heavy gonorrheal infection. How to differentiate such old infections, often showing more acute symptoms than fresh cases, from the latter, I have in detail described in my *Studien zur Pathologie der infektiösen Erkrankungen der Harnorgane*, and in the "Gonorrheal cases in men treated without antiseptic."

In the course of the treatment these cases, which often show —when conducted in the ordinary way *without massage*—an apparently short cure, are characterized by the following features: when treated by means of strong massages indicated by more resistant infiltrates, there often arises, even in an advanced stage of treatment after a period of marked improvement, a typical "focus" reaction, showing itself in a feverish condition, fresh inflammation and exudation in the resistant infiltrated parts, bladder disturbances, and in some cases even through metastases. In chronic cases we meet with those appearances very frequently in the beginning of the treatment. Only after these symptoms, proving the correctness of my diagnosis, have vanished or quieted down, definite cure will be obtained by regular continuation of the massage treatment, emptying completely the focus of bacterial retention. Hand in hand with this there also disappear the metastases, in so far as they have not receded spontaneously with the other symptoms of the above-mentioned focus reaction.

The seminal vesicles belonging to this group are probably those which, after a gonorrheal infection of longer standing and "self-cured," form for the invasion and development of any secondary bacterial infection an apt soil on the base of the remaining and continuous post gonorrheal inflammatory changes, and so become the focus of many chronic urethral and bladder ailments, rheumatic affections, and cryptogenetic sepsis.

The pathogenesis of recurrent epididymitis may be clearly explained by the anatomical structure of the ampullæ. There is to be remarked in these cases on rectal palpation a marked sensitiveness more to the medial side of the infiltration involving the seminal vesicle. Recurrences of the epididymitis occurring in the course of treatment prove only the correctness of my diagnosis.

If we take in consideration that the first three groups (A, B, C), forming together 34 per cent. of my material, show good or relatively good draining conditions, and that group D and E, forming 66 per cent. of my material, show unfavorable draining conditions, it is evident that there must be many more cases of spermatocystitis which will heal badly and show an inclination to pass into a chronic stage, than such as possess favorable chances for a spontaneous cure. And in fact, my experiences teach me that it must be looked upon as a rarity when an infection of this organ is cured spontaneously, without any anatomical, i.e., inflammatory, residuum.

This is also proved by the pieces of group F, which show the advanced inflammatory and cicatricial changes and which have been all taken from persons over 30 years of age, some of whom have died in consequence of well-marked infectious urogenital disease.

In that view the most remarkable piece is No. 17, showing very extended inflammatory changes round the top of the right vesicle, extending along the vas deferens and the ureter of this side, there having been found a large abscess breaking into the peritoneum and giving rise to the diagnosis of pericecal abscess for which laparotomy was performed.

CONCLUSIONS.

The seminal vesicle possesses among the glandular adnexa of the male urethra by far the most extensive secreting surface, in combination however with the worst drainage conditions. This tube-system stands from my experience at the *center point of bacterial infectious diseases* of the lower urine passage, most of the appearances of which may be explained by direct reference to, or as a subsequent symptom of, a disease of this organ.

From my clinical and anatomical studies which I have here reported *en résumé,* it is clear that the symptoms of vesical pyuria going with fever, with or without increase of frequency of micturition, with or without residual urine, are due to spermatocystitis if we can exclude pyelitis and prostatitis.

Epididymitis, if arising spontaneously, or by catheterism, or by massage or any other damage, is for me, with respect to what I have already said, the strict proof of the diseased condition of the ampulla of the seminal vesicle.

Metastatic symptoms, whether they be of rheumatic and arthritic or of pure septic character, going with an infectious disease of the lower part of the urine tract, have in the majority of cases their origin in the infected but clinically latent state of the seminal vesicle. There a great part is also played by secondary infections which have established themselves on the soil of the changes produced by a typical acute gonorrheal infection long passed away, as I have mentioned in different places.

In *conducting* in the *rational way,* pointed out by my experiences, the *therapy* of infectious diseases of the lower part of the urinary tract, special attention must be paid to the *treatment* of the *adnexa* and to the *relieving* of the patients from their *complaints* arising from the diseased state of the *draining mucous surfaces.* The former is done by the evacuation of the glandular adnexa, the latter by cleansing the urine passage by means of mild antiseptic treatment.

In this evacuation-therapy there compete:

A. The evacuation in a natural way—

(1) by spontaneous cure,

(2) by massage therapy,

(3) by washing out the seminal vesicle through the vas deferens (Belfield's operation).

B. The operations which open the vesicles from outside—

(4) by vesiculotomy (Fuller, Lloyd),

(5) by vesiculectomy (Bransford Lewis).

My anatomical studies explain to me what I have experienced in practice:

A. (1) Why spontaneous cure can relatively rarely be expected in a short time.

(2) Why the systematic evacuation treatment by means of digital expression furnishes the best results in the great majority of acute and chronic cases, and why the vaccination treatment cannot act in the causal way of evacuation.

(3) Why I had no complete success with Belfield's operation alone; but combined with cutting abscesses in the epididymis I was able to shorten in many cases the duration of massage treatment.

B. (4) Concerning Fuller's operation, my studies explain the fairly large percentage of recurrences observed in the cases operated for arthritic and bladder complaints, because there are among the seminal vesicles, especially appertaining to groups D and E, such forms as cannot be completely opened and drained by the knife. In the given case I should for vesiculotomy prefer Voelcker's operation, giving as it does a better survey.

(5) The vesiculectomy is the most radical form of treatment, with which in the grave cases no other proceeding can compete.

The effect of antiseptic treatment of the surfaces of the urine passages is only symptomatic in the treatment of urogenital ailments, except pyelitis, where it acts directly, and in the causal indication.

I have proved this by the cure of gonorrhea without antiseptics, by the cure of bacterial and other post-gonorrheal saprophytic infections (urethritis, cystitis), and of various mild and serious cases of metastatic diseases originating in the infected state of the seminal vesicle, only by way of massage.

In cases of grave sepsis, where the systematic massage treatment remains without result after a certain period (say 2–3 months maxima), I should find the indication for vesiculectomy.

LITERATURE

Albarran.—*Operative Chirurgie der Harnwege,* Gustav Fischer, Jena, 1910.

Hyrtl, T.—"Das Nierenbecken der Saugethiere und des Menschen," *Denkschrift d. kais. Akademie,* Wien, 1872, Bd. xxxi.

Fuller.—"Seminal Vesiculitis," *Journal of Cutaneous and Genito-urinary Diseases,* September, 1893.

—— "Persistent Urethral Discharge dependent on Subacute or Chronic Vesiculitis," *Journal of Cutaneous and Genito-urinary Diseases,* June, 1894.

—— "Operative Interference in Aggravated Instances of Seminal Vesiculitis," *Journal of Cutaneous and Genito-urinary Diseases,* September, 1896.

—— "Relief of Urinary and Genital Conditions through Surgery of Seminal Vesicles," *Med. Record,* October, 1909.

Lloyd, T.—"On Inflammatory Disease of the Seminal Vesicles," *Brit. Med. Journ.,* April, 1889.

Picker.—"Studien über das Gangsystem der menschlichen Samenblase" (Referat), *Verhandlungen des III. Kongr. des Deutschen Ges. für Urologie,* pp. 9-302, O. Coblentz & G. Thieme, Berlin, Leipzig, 1912.

Voelcker.—*Chirurgie der Samenblasen,* F. Euke, Stuttgart, 1912.

Picker.—*Topische Diagnose der chronischen Gonorrhoe und der anderen bakteriellen Infektionen in den Harn- und Geschlechtsorganen des Mannes, O. Coblentz,* Berlin, 1909.

Pallin.—"Beitrage zur Anatomie der Prostata und Samenblasen," *Archiv. für Anatomie,* 1901.

Obendorfer.—"Beitrage zur Anatomie und Pathologie der Samenblase," *Ziegler's Beiträge,* Bd. xxxi.

Petersen.—"Beiträge zur mikroskop. Anatomie der Samenblase," *Anatomische Hefte,* Wiesbaden, 1907, Bd. xxxvii.

Picker.—"Der Symptomenkomplex der rezidivierenden Epididymitis," *Verhandlungen des II. Kongr. der Deutschen Ges. f. Urologie,* 1909.

—— "Studien zur Pathologie der infektiösen Erkrankungen der Harnorgane," *Verhandlungen des II. Kongr. der Deutschen Ges. f. Urologie,* 1909.

—— "Gonorrheal Cases in Men treated without Antiseptics," *Urologic and Cutaneous Review,* Tech. Suppl., January, 1913.

Belfield, W.—"Pus Tubes in the Male."*Med. Record,* May, 1907.

—— "Irrigation and Drainage of the Seminal Vesicle through the Vas Deferens," *St. Louis Medical Review,* February, 1907.

Picker.—"Ein Fall von geheilter kryptogenetischer Sepsis," *Medizin. Klinik,* 1911, No. 48.

TEN TESTS BY WHICH THE PHYSICIAN MAY DETERMINE WHEN A PATIENT IS CURED OF GONORRHEA. A STUDY OF 1260 TESTS BY CULTURE AND SLIDE OF THE EXPRESSED PROSTATIC AND VESICULAR SECRETIONS.[1]

By CHARLES M. WHITNEY, M.D., Boston,

Professor of Genito-urinary Diseases, Tufts College Medical School; Surgeon to the Genito-Urinary Department, Mt. Sinai Hospital.

THAT gonorrhea is a most serious and dangerous disease, is admitted by every physician who has observed its disastrous effects. It is responsible for one-fourth of all the blindness in the world, for thousands of deaths from secondary kidney disease following stricture, for many fatal cases of gonorrheal salpingitis and secondary peritonitis, and for metastatic gonorrhea (the so-called gonorrheal rheumatism) which results in temporary or permanent loss of function in one or many joints.

It is stated by specialists in that line that gonorrhea is the cause of 60-80% of all gynecological operations. We should add to our list of disasters sterility in both men and women.

From this brief review of the subject it is clear that all preventive measures which tend to lessen the spread of this disease should receive the thoughtful attention of every physician.

This paper will not discuss the ordinary clinical symptoms and treatment of this ailment, for it is wholly concerned in answering these very important questions, when is gonorrhea cured? How may we assure a patient who has had it that he may marry without danger of infecting his wife? It would seem at first sight that the answer was easy, that when the discharge stopped, and the urine was clear, and there was no return of the symptoms, that the case was well. This is usually the patients' view and because of this many serious and unfortunate results are observed. In spite of a clear urine and no discharge for months, gonorrhea may exist in an active and dangerous form. The explanation of this is found in the peculiar and complex structure of the urogenital organs. The urethra, in which the infection first occurs, is divided into the anterior and posterior portions by the compressor urethrae muscle. In the anterior portion there are along the

[1] Read before the Somerville Medical Society.—*Boston Medical and Surgical Journal.*

urethra, the lacuna magna, and the follicles of Littrè and Morgagni, in all of which the gonococci may be concealed and give no symptoms.

In the bulbous urethra upon the floor are the two openings of Cowper's glands, the ducts of which are nearly two inches in length and end in small glands which are situated between the layers of the triangular ligament. Along this duct the infection may extend, giving rise to no symptoms until some cause starts it into activity, when it may infect the urethra and cause a profuse discharge. When we pass the compressor urethrae muscle we enter a portion of the urethra which has many and important structures leading from it.

In the median line is the veru montanum, with the colliculus at its apex, on the walls of which the ejaculatory ducts are to be found. Along the floor are the prostatic sinuses, from which many glands lead into the prostate.

Connected by the ejaculatory ducts are the seminal vesicles, composed of tubules and blind cul-de-sacs.

It is possible for the gonococcus to enter these ducts and organs and remain latent many months or years. If the disease did not extend beyond the compressor urethrae muscle the danger of latency would not be as great, for probably 90% of relapsing cases are due to the prostate and vesicles, but the unfortunate fact is that from 60% to 80% of cases do progress beyond this muscle and become posterior, either with or without subjective symptoms. Hence it is obvious that before deciding upon a cure these organs should be carefully examined to determine that no organisms are present.

Assuming then, that a patient presents himself for examination as to whether he is cured and in proper condition to be married or to resume marital relation if already married, what steps should we take to assure him that the disease is no longer present?

Two classes of cases are seen: first, those in which the disease has been a first infection and has been acute and uncomplicated, and second, the chronic and protracted cases which have resisted treatment, are usually not primary infections and have resulted in some organic change in the anatomic structures.

In the first class there is less danger of latency than in the second.

1. *Discharge.* Regardless of which class the case belongs to, we should begin our examination by an inspection of the patient's

urethra to find out whether any discharge is visible at the meatus and if not, the urethra should be gently stripped.

If present it should be looked at with suspicion and carefully examined for gonococci. If it contains only mucus, epithelium and an occasional pus cell it may be harmless, but a culture of it should be made to prevent any possibility of error. If no discharge is present inquiry should be made as to how long a time has elapsed since urination, and the patient should be told to carefully examine the meatus in the morning before urination and if discharge is present it should be placed on a slide for examination.

2. *Urine.* If no discharge is found we should now examine the urine as to its clearness and freedom from shreds. A turbid urine which does not clear upon the addition of acetic acid, shows a chronic inflammation, and the examination need proceed no further for it is obvious that the disease is still present. If clear and shreds are present, their size and action in the urine should be noted. If they are large and sink quickly they contain a large amount of pus and indicate an inflammatory area somewhere along the urinary tract which must be located and treated. If small, or light and flocculent, they are chiefly mucus and epithelium and are not usually of diagnostic value, merely indicating a mild urethral catarrh.

Not a great deal of information is gained from the microscopical examination of these large shreds. Some years ago the writer investigated them by preparing over a hundred slides and several hundred fields were gone over with the result that gonococci were found in only two large shreds.

Therefore other means will tell us more quickly and accurately whether the disease is present.

3. *Instrumental Examination of the Urethra.* By the bougie-a-boule we should examine the urethra for stricture and for tender areas. If the meatus is small it should be divided to permit the passage of instruments.

If a 28 or 30 bougie-a-boule passes freely to the bulb and shows no stricture or tender spot, and if a 28 sound passes to the bladder easily and without causing bleeding we may feel fairly well assured that no stricture exists in the urethra which might cause a relapsing discharge.

4. *Urethroscopic Examination.* By this we can ascertain the condition of the urethral mucous membrane and can occasionally see the minute openings of inflamed follicles.

If localized congestions or erosions are present they should be placed under treatment by local application of silver nitrate, which will provoke a discharge which should be examined.

5. *Examination of the Prostate and Vesicles.* With the bladder partially filled with urine or boracic acid solution, the prostate and vesicles should be examined and their size, consistency and sensitiveness should be noted. If boggy, enlarged or tender, it indicates the need of treatment, at any rate, and the possibility of latent disease in these organs.

Whatever the condition found may be, gentle massage should be done and the vesicles stripped. The discharge appearing at the meatus should be saved on a slide, or Petri glass, and examined later.

The urine or solution should now be passed and if many "snowflake" masses are present they should be examined microscopically. They almost surely mean vesiculitis, and a patient having this cannot be called cured.

The very important and vital examinations of this expressed secretion by culture and slide will be later referred to at length.

6. *Test by Alcohol.* If the patient has successfully passed the foregoing tests he should now be permitted to take malt liquors (the so-called "beer test") or spirits.

The results should be carefully noted and also the character of any discharge produced by them.

7. *Coitus.* This test cannot properly be included among those which should be used, because no physician would permit a patient to risk infecting anyone else. Nevertheless, there are patients who have no sense of moral responsibility and from their errors certain conclusions can be formed, provided a protective covering is used. In case the discharge returns we know it was a relapse and not a new infection.

8. *Discharge Induced by Irritating Antiseptics.* This so-called provocative method consists in irrigating the urethra with some irritating chemical substance producing a urethritis, and the resulting discharge may show gonococci in the pus cells which have come from the deeper layers of the urethra. Nitrate of silver is the best antiseptic for this purpose and should be used as an anterior injection in the strength of 1-4000 and also as a deep urethral irrigation in the strength of 1% in a Keyes-Ultzmann syringe.

I am in the habit of passing a full sized sound before using the injections to dilate the urethra and to express from the follicles any retained contents.

9. *Bacteriological Examination of the Expressed Vesicular and Prostatic Secretion by Culture and Slide.* It is very interesting to note that in 1878, one year prior to the discovery of the specific organism of gonorrhea, the attention of the medical profession was called to the possibilities of its latency by Emil Noeggerath of New York. At that time his conclusions were ridiculed but to-day it is generally admitted that this disease may remain latent for months or years. The discovery of the gonococcus by Neisser in 1879 and its growth in a culture medium by Bumm in 1887 were the beginnings of better days, for it is no longer necessary to grope blindly in the darkness of ignorance for the causative factor of the disease, but its presence or absence may be seen in the clear daylight of scientific accuracy. The work so ably started by these pioneers has been the means of helping us to recognize many obscure conditions due to this organism.

The cases here reported which have been studied by my colleague, Dr. A. C. Pearce, and myself, have made us realize more than ever the responsibility placed upon the physician who is called upon to determine whether or not a man may safely marry.

In order to answer this question intelligently it is absolutely necessary that the patient should be under observation a sufficient length of time to allow various tests to be made, which require at least three weeks. We have been repeatedly called upon to determine whether or not a man is cured of his ailment and been told by him that he has made all arrangements for marriage in a week or ten days. He would certainly be placed in a very unpleasant position in case our examination showed the presence of gonococci. The insidious character of latent gonorrhea has repeatedly manifested itself in our series of cases. Time and again a patient has been examined who has a clear urine, no visible discharge at any time, with few if any shreds, and upon stripping the seminal vesicles we have found them loaded with pus. Whether or not we find the gonococcus in the expressed secretion we consider this man a menace to the community and he should not be allowed to marry until we have improved his condition. The presence or absence of chronic seminal vesiculitis cannot always be made by rectal palpation alone. It can only be made in some cases by a physical and microscopical examination of the expressed vesicular secretion, because the vesicles are not always enlarged to touch.

Manifestly, then, such an examination is indispensable in ascertaining the presence of a latent form of gonorrhea. In considering the prostate as a harboring place for these organisms we believe that too much importance has been given to it. We know that the disease does infect the glands leading from the sinuses, the colliculus, and may enter the tissues of the gland itself, but these are reached by treatment through the urethra, while the seminal vesicles, with their honey-comb structure so ideal as culture media for organisms, can only be indirectly treated by stripping and in intractable cases by incision or excision of these organs. This means a severe and mutilating surgical operation, which may be dangerous to life. While this is rarely necessary, there are cases which will yield to no other means. The fact that so few patients who have a low grade chronic prostatitis are sterile would lead us to believe that its secretory action is not markedly disturbed, but it may still excite the motility of the spermatozoa and may also stimulate the testes in the formation of them.

The patient is instructed to report with a full bladder. Any secretion appearing at the meatus is obtained on a slide and reserved for future examination. The anterior urethra is cleansed with normal salt solution, which will not affect the growth of the gonococcus, and the glans penis is cleansed with alcohol, which causes a temporary burning sensation if it enters the meatus or comes in contact with the scrotum. The patient then assumes a crouching position with the knees slightly bent and the back parallel with the floor. The vesicles are then vigorously massaged and the strippings allowed to drop into a tube containing the culture medium. A series of slides is made and then the patient passes his urine into a clear glass. This is later centrifuged and examined for pus and cocci.

The culture tube is incubated for 24 to 48 hours. The slide gently fixed with heat and placed in a solution of equal parts of ether and alcohol, to be stained later by the Gram method. The examination of the unstained slide is done immediately and the addition of a weak solution of acetic acid aids in detecting the pus corpuscles.

As the culture media we have chiefly used the nutrient blood agar in the proportion of one part blood to two parts nutrient agar. The latter is prepared by extracting one pound lean beef by immersion in 500 c.c. cold water for twenty-four hours, and then bringing it to a boil and skimming the surface. Then we add 40 grams of agar, 10 grams sodium chloride and 1 liter of water. The growth of gonococcus outside of the body in even the most carefully prepared media is uncertain because of its low vitality. One or two degrees of temperature above or below 38° Centigrade is sufficient to make the test valueless. It is therefore necessary to have the patient examined near to the thermostat in which the culture tube is to be placed because it cannot be transported from a distance in the varying temperatures which occur in this climate.

Another difficulty is the frequent and rapid growth of other organisms than the gonococci, for it is rare to get a pure uncontaminated culture.

The series here presented consists of 1260 examinations by culture and slide.

To properly understand the importance of the results obtained it is essential to state that nearly all these cases had been treated thoroughly by all modern means before they were subjected to these tests. In acute cases the vesicles were massaged after apparent recovery and the urethra examined, and in the chronic ones where the disease when first seen had existed from six months to eight years they had been treated for months by urethral dilatation and local urethroscopic applications, as well as by thorough and repeated prostatic massage and vesicular stripping, with the usual antiseptic irrigations and instillations. Further, the majority of these cases were private patients of the writer, others were sent by their physician for these tests, and a very small proportion were from the clinic, where they had been subjected to thorough and careful treatment.

Let us see what the examination of these well watched, carefully treated and apparently cured patients showed. Gonococci were found as follows: By slide alone, 63, or 5% ; by culture and slide, 44 positive, or 3½% ; by culture alone, 26 positive, or 2%. In other words, from two to five men in every hundred who were clinically well harbored active and dangerous gonococci. It is sad to think of what the effect of marriage upon innocent wives and future children would have been. No patient who has had gonorrhea even in the distant past should neglect the precaution of these careful examinations to protect his health and that of those who will be near and dear to him in future. None of these cases had less than three examinations and we should insist on that number of cultural examinations at least, and more if the slide contains much pus. Some of our positive results were obtained on the first examination, while in others they did not appear till the second or third one.

It is needless to say that everyone showing positive results was again subjected to treatment which was continued until we obtained three negative results, and up to the present not one of these men who have been married have had any return of their discharge nor have their wives been infected.

Many interesting results have been obtained from the bacteriological study of these cases as to the other pathogenic organisms which follow the gonococcus and serve to keep up a urethral discharge in some cases, but the limits of this paper do not permit a description of them. With new culture media the more accurate will be our results and the greater our assurance that physicians may do a beneficent work in the community by educating their patients to have these tests made.

10. *The Complement-Fixation Test.* This new and apparently valuable addition to our methods of determining the presence of gonococci or their toxins was first brought into notice by Schwarz and McNeil in an article published in the *Journal of the Medical Sciences* for May, 1911. Prior to that work along this line had been done by Mueller and Oppenheim, but it was not sufficiently conclusive to attract the attention of the scientific world.

This is similar to the Wassermann test for syphilis and follows essentially the same technic. It has been found necessary to use a polyvalent antigen, that is, one made from several strains (usually twelve) of gonococci. By this we determine the presence in the blood of an antibody produced by the gonorrheal organisms in the blood current or in the tissues of some organ, like the prostate, vesicles, or the joints. In an acute case it is not found before four weeks, and apparently remains long after the disease has clinically disappeared. It has been found after all microscopical and cultural tests have proved negative. These facts are most startling and point to the possibility that gonorrhea is not so local a disease as we have supposed it to be.

Not enough evidence has yet been produced for us to say that a positive result shows the presence of living gonococci somewhere in the tissues of the body, nor have we any way of knowing how long the antibodies may persist after cure. This is a most important fact to find out as otherwise we cannot wisely advise those patients whose test has proved positive. The test is exceedingly delicate and can only be done in a well equipped laboratory, and even there strange variations in the results are obtained. A clinically clear case of gonorrhea may show negative results, while one which is well by other and better tests may show positive results. The time has not yet arrived when we can depend upon this test alone and we must therefore place our faith in the tests which are of proven value and which will assure safety to our patients.

These tests which have been described are those which the physician should recommend to his patient, and by so doing he may lessen the peril of latent gonorrhea. He will do more than that for he will awaken in the public mind a realization of the fact that an apparently cured patient is not surely well, but that the consequences of his folly and misfortune may follow him all his life unless he receives competent and skillful treatment from his physician until he is cured, clinically and bacteriologically.

With the treatment of gonorrhea thus placed upon a plane as high as other diseases of far less importance we will hear less silly talk of the physician prolonging a case for financial reasons, we shall see fewer and fewer patients applying to druggists for nostrums promising a quick cure, and we will soon find that men having gonorrhea will aid their physician in their conscientious efforts to rid them of this dangerous malady.

[Very well. But what percentage of gonorrheal patients can afford the financial cost of a really thorough scientific treatment; and of repeated thorough diagnostic tests? Dispensaries? They are almost useless.—Ed.]

ZEITSCHRIFT FUR UROLOGIE

Vol. VIII, No. 5, 1914

1. **Modern Methods for Determination of the Kidney Function.**

The authors have employed the methods of Schlayer-Monakow, Ambard, and Strauss. The first of the three methods provides for the determination of the rate of output of chlorides; iodine, water, lactose, and nitrogen. It has been shown, for example, that a delayed output of chlorides and iodides indicates disease of the kidney tubules whereas a delayed excretion of water or of lactose or of nitrogen points to the existence of glomerular lesions. The authors have been able to find by the application of this method to orthostatic albuminuria cases that the latter condition is not always necessarily harmless but may be associated with a disturbance of the kidney function which may in turn lead to a disturbance of the general metabolism in the sense of a latent uremia.

Ambard's method was used for the determination both of the ureosecretory coefficient and of the chloridesecretory coefficient. The rest-nitrogen was determined by the method of Strauss. After studying their methods separately and comparing the results together the authors conclude that by the investigation of renal function in this manner the clinician can obtain results that will be of the greatest practical as well as theoretical value.

ANNALES DES MALADIES VÉNÉRIENNES

Vol. IX, No. 5, May, 1914

1. **Angina Pectoris of Syphilitic Origin.**

There are two kinds of angina pectoris: 1. In which the angina is associated with narrowing of the coronary arteries, always of syphilitic origin. 2. In which the angina is associated with neuritis or neuralgia of the cardiac plexus which may be due to various causes, rheumatism especially, syphilis occasionally, or to angiospasm. In the former class of cases, to the description of which this article is limited, the most common pathological lesions are: 1. A subacute diffuse aortitis going on to sclerosis. 2. A stenosing arteritis, or less commonly multiple aneurysms of the great coronary trunks. 3. Secondary changes in the smaller branches and in the myocardium.

Etiology — The spirocheta pallida has been demonstrated in the lesions. The disease may occur as a secondary manifestation of syphilis but it is more usual in the tertiary stage.

Symptomatology — The authors divide this into three classes: 1. Simple angina pectoris. 2. Latent syphilis and angina pectoris. 3. Syphilitic angina pectoris in an aortic. The attack may occur without warning in sleep, or it may be preceded by an aura such as yawning, or painful sensations in the limbs. Usually, however, as is well known, the attack is brought on by some exertion or sudden excitement. The pain, of course, is the most striking phenomenon. Its location is retrosternal. It is not increased by pressure. The radiations are centrifugal and are referred along the left upper extremity, less often up the neck or down the right arm or down the lower limbs. According to Friedreich these referred pains are increased by pressure. The heart action is generally normal during an attack. Occasionally the attacks show a tendency to be repeated at more and more frequent intervals, but even in untreated cases they may not recur for many years.

Diagnosis — Brachio-thoracic and intercostal neuralgias are distinguished from angina pectoris by the occurrence in the former of superficial, non-agonizing pain which is permanent with exacerbations and is localized to the emergence of the intercostal nerves. Diaphragmatic pleurisy (left-sided) is associated with fever, dyspnea, and the characteristic auscultatory phenomena. Acute pericarditis is not associated with severe pain. Acute aortitis may resemble angina pectoris but the crises are not separated by long periods of rest, the pain is almost incessant, and there are dyspnea, cough, digestive disorders, and a marked arterial hypertension. The diagnosis from aneurysm of the aorta or from paroxysms of bronchial asthma does not offer much difficulty. With the aid of the Wassermann reaction we have learned that angina pectoris is as often syphilitic as is tabes or general paresis.

Prognosis — This depends entirely on the establishment of specific treatment and the association with the angina of cardiac or aortic lesions. As a rule pure cases of angina are much improved or cured by treatment. The physical signs of aortitis of course persist unchanged.

Treatment — Mixed treatment should be instituted as soon as possible. Mercury cyanide should be given intravenously in 1 cg. doses at the same time that a similar dose of benzoate of mercury is given intramuscularly. This should be combined with 2 to 4 grams of potassium iodide daily by mouth, and if this is ill-borne the sodium salt may be substituted. After the attacks have ceased a less intense mixed treatment should be kept up indefinitely. The ultimate dosage should be controlled by auscultation, by the study of the arterial tension, the symptoms, by the age of the patient and the amount of previous treatment received by the patient.

2. A Case of Syphilitic Plantar Keratodermia.

In addition to palmar and plantar keratoses, congenital in origin, or appearing in childhood, which are ordinarily symmetrical, hereditary, and familial, there exist a certain number of acquired keratoses which occur in the adult and are always unilateral. Certain of these are toxic in origin, e.g., arsenical, the others come from various infections. Recently attention has been called to keratodermias of blenorrhagic origin. Gaucher, also, has shown that syphilis may give rise to keratotic vegetations. The authors report a case of this nature.

The patient was a woman of 53, who had had for the past year a lesion of the sole of the left foot. The posterior three quarters of the sole were covered with a horny layer from ½ to 1 cm. in thickness, which extended up on the sides of the feet. In addition there was a horny "island" on the dorsum about the size of a five franc piece. The keratotic layer was of a yellow color, fissured, and desquamating in sheets, and separated from the healthy skin by a reddish area of 1 cm. thickness. Pressure on the hypertrophied skin was tender, but the patient was not prevented from walking. The right foot and the hands were normal.

As regards the past history, there was a still-birth 25 years before, but no miscarriages. Within the past 6 years there were several attacks of gummatous ulcerations which cleared up under specific treatment, leaving numerous whitish scars especially on the lower extremities. There was no history of primary lesion. On the other hand there were some stigmata of heredo-syphilis — high-arched palate, faulty dentition, and maldevelopment of a metacarpal bone. In order to prove therefore, if possible, whether the plantar keratosis was due to an acquired or hereditary syphilis a Wassermann test was performed both with the Desmoulière and with the ordinary antigen. Both reactions proved absolutely positive which was in favor of an acquired syphilis since a patient with hereditary syphilis would hardly at the age of 53 give a positive Wassermann with the ordinary antigen.

3. Hemorrhagic Nephritis and Cystitis Following Neosalvarsan.

Nanta reports two cases which seem to prove conclusively that neosalvarsan may cause an intense congestion of the urinary passages, extending from the kidney (cylindruria) to the urethra (pain on micturition), and that it may provoke a real hemorrhagic nephritis and cystitis. However, these symptoms, it should be noted, were very mild in both cases and cleared up in four or five days on rest in bed and milk diet.

The first case — that of an old hemoglobinuric following malarial infection — was of additional interest in that the intravenous injection of the 250 cc. of 0.45% saline solution which contained the neosalvarsan brought about an attack of hemoglobinuria which was not reproduced by a subsequent injection with a small quantity (8 cc.) of distilled water.

It is of interest to point out that both patients presented marked hematologic or serologic abnormalities. In the first case the author determined a marked retardation of the coagulation time, corpuscular fragility, and a history of paroxysmal hemoglobinuria. In the second patient there was a distinct anemia. It seems noteworthy moreover that the hemorrhagic effect of the arsenic is independent of the previous condition of the kidney, for this effect has been observed in persons who never presented any previous renal symptoms, nor even albuminuria. In the other hand, in two children (reported by Prof. Audry) suffering from hemorrhagic nephritis of hereditary syphilis the renal symptoms cleared up after the use of salvarsan, whereas the previous employment of mercury and iodides had been absolutely non-effectual.

4. Pernicious Anemia and Syphilis.

Nathan reports a case of pernicious anemia which ran a very insidious and paradoxical course. The patient was a woman of about 40 who complained of vague dyspeptic symptoms. A fibroid of the uterus was found on physical examination. The organ was removed and the post-operative course was uneventful until the twelfth day when the patient had a profuse hemorrhage from the bowels. The diagnosis of gastric or intestinal neoplasm was made. There was complete intolerance of the stomach to food, extreme emaciation, yellowish pallor, weak voice, and a small and thready pulse. The hemorrhages were repeated either in the form of melena or as occult blood found chemically in the feces. There were no cutaneous or visceral hemorrhages. There was no icterus, nor diarrhea, no hypothermia as occurs in grave post-operative jaundice. The blood count showed a severe anemia, color index greater than 1, white blood cells 17,000 with excess of polynuclears; myelocytes were present. A Wassermann test proved completely positive. A dose of 0.3 gm. salvarsan was administered but the patient died nevertheless three days later. The author assumes that the anemia was probably specific.

The author discusses similar cases reported in the literature and concludes that pernicious anemias of syphilitic nature occur more often than we suppose. We must therefore from the beginning suspect syphilis when the etiology of an anemia remains obscure, but it would be dangerous to overestimate the frequency of this condition, for after all, despite the excellent means at present at our command for the discovery of syphilis recent studies have revealed but a very few proven cases of syphilitic pernicious anemia.

5. A Syphilide Superimposed on a Keloid.

The patient was a man of 31, who denied having had syphilis.

Three years ago, following a trauma, he developed a wound of the inner aspect of the right leg. This wound healed without internal treatment, leaving a pigmented area like those of varicose ulcers. About a year ago, without definite cause, he had a phlegmon of the left popliteal region which was incised. Cicatrization was slow and incomplete and hindered by the patient's occupation (ploughman) which he continued following.

The cicatrix became thicker and thicker and developed into a large, hard, painful, typical keloid. At the center of the keloid there was a round ulceration the size of a franc piece, the walls were punched out, the base yellowish red. Below the keloid are the lesions of dry, chronic eczema.

The wound at the center was diagnosed a simple ulcer by many. As a matter of fact it was a gumma, as was evident from the clinical aspect, the positive sero-reaction, and the rapid cure under mercurial treatment. The keloid was not modified by the specific therapy. In discussing the pathogenesis of this case the author offers two possible explanations: 1. The "phlegmon" was in reality a gumma which was incised by mistake and healed slowly leaving a keloid. Syphilis may therefore, like tuberculosis, be a cause of keloid. 2. The "phlegmon" was in reality a pyogenic suppuration. Its healing was followed by a keloid as after any simple wound, but this wound acted as a localizing point of least resistance for the manifestation of a hitherto latent syphilis.

The author concludes that because of the rarity of keloids in the course of syphilis the conditions for the development of these lesions must be very rarely realized.

REVUE CLINIQUE D' UROLOGIE

May, 1914

1. The Forms of Chronic Renal Tuberculosis. By Noël Hallé.
2. Syphilitic Chancre of the Urethra and Gonorrhea. By J. Brault and J. Montpellier.
3. The Rôle of the Reserve Power of the Kidney after Nephrectomy. By N. A. Mikaïlow.
4. The Possible Importance of Diseases of the Pancreas for Surgery of the Urinary Tract. By Ernst Frank.
5. Some Interesting Cases of Gonorrheal Complications Successfully Treated with Anti-meningococcus Serum. By M. Cealic.
6. Vesico-prostato-perineal Fistula Treated by Bilateral Ureteral Catheterization as a Means of Deviation of the Urinary Current. By P. Cifuentes.
7. Sexual Disorders of Psychic Nature. By A. Wizel.

1. **The Forms of Chronic Renal Tuberculosis.**

According to Hallé there are two main forms of tuberculosis of the kidneys: 1. A primary, closed, parenchymatous tuberculosis, which is hematogenous in its origin, slow in development, and spontaneously curable. 2. An open primary tuberculosis of the pelvis, lymphogenous in origin, acute in its manifestations, and hardly if ever curable spontaneously. These forms may follow each other or be combined in various ways.

Other points of pathological interest brought out by the author are:

1. The initial location on the calyces of the lesions involving the pelvis.

2. The constant accompanying obliteration of the excretory passages in complete lobar parenchymatous tuberculosis.

3. The mode of progress of intra-renal tuberculosis in lesions of the pelvis, viz., the disease ascends along the perivascular interlobar lymphatic channels.

4. The differences in histologic structure which separate tuberculous lesions into two groups, lesions of the pelvis being active and progressive, lesions of the parenchyma being extinct and regressive.

5. The existence of fibrous scars and healed lesions in different forms in tuberculous kidneys.

6. The diversity and complexity of simple secondary lesions which complicate tuberculosis of the kidneys.

Four plates with figures in black and white accompany the paper.

2. Syphilitic Chancre of the Urethra and Gonorrhea.

The authors report the case of a man of 25 who had had a profuse urethral discharge for about one month and a half. Two weeks after the onset of the condition there appeared three ulcerations on the penis, the sores being of the soft variety. There was a thick, purulent, urethral discharge; the inguinal glands were swollen and large on the right side, small and hard on the left. There were no general symptoms, and no rash on the body.

Bacteriological examination of the pus from the ulcerations revealed the presence of Ducrey bacilli in large numbers, but the same discharge failed to show the presence of treponema pallida. The urethral discharge on the other hand, contained not only gonococci but treponemata as well. After the patient had been a week under observation a slight ulceration appeared at the meatus giving the impression of a chancre of the urethra which was becoming exteriorized. At the same time there appeared a slight induration of the extremity of the urethra. Unfortunately, the patient at this stage insisted on leaving the hospital. This was therefore a case, the serious nature of which would not have been recognized, had not the microscopic examination revealed the existence of a double infection of the urethra.

3. The Role of the Reserve Power of the Kidney After Nephrectomy.

Mikhailow has studied 62 cases of nephrectomy (9 personal and 53 cited by Kapsammer in his treatise on "Nierenchirurgie"). In general, in man, the remaining kidney produces less urine in the first 24 hours following operation than before the nephrectomy but the specific gravity and molecular diuresis are both increased. Later in the post-operative period the remaining kidney varies in its function according to the disease which originally necessitated the intervention and according to its own reserve power. The author has been able to distinguish three types of diuresis following nephrectomy.

In the first type the remaining kidney puts out a steadily increasing amount of urine up to the eighth or ninth day following the operation at which point the diuresis remains about constant. In this group of cases the previous examination (before nephrectomy) of the remaining kidney (indigo-carmine, phloridzin, experimental polyuria) warrants our regarding it as normal or almost normal.

The second type of diuresis is seen most often after nephrectomies for neoplasm or tuberculosis. The reserve force of the kidney develops in an irregular fashion, by spurts, as it were. In such cases the previous examination of the remaining kidney reveals the fact that it reacted poorly with indigo-carmine or with phloridzin, that is to say that it was affected by pyelitis or pyelonephritis.

The third type of diuresis is characterized by insufficiency and rapid exhaustion of the reserve force of the remaining kidney, a point of grave prognostic significance. As far as can be determined from the material at our disposal the last type is met with in cases of long standing and pronounced compensatory hypertrophy of the remaining kidney, characterized (already before operation) by enlargement in the size of the organ, by polyuria (the ureteral catheter collecting 90-120 cc. of urine in ½-hour instead of the normal 30-60 cc), by the accelerated appearance of test dyes, and by the negative outcome of the experimental polyuria test. The presence of these clinical phenomena is a formal contraindication to nephrectomy.

The author concludes that a careful examination of the kidney to remain should be made before proposing a nephrectomy and that we may in this way gain important information on the function and reserve power of the kidney in question and will thus avoid operations which would compromise renal surgery.

4. The Possible Importance of Diseases of the Pancreas for Surgery of the Urinary Tract.

Frank's paper appeared originally in the "Zeitschrift für Urologie," Vol. VIII, No. 4, 1914, and has already been abstracted in this Journal.

5. Some Interesting Cases of Gonorrheal Complications Successfully Treated with Anti-meningococcus Serum.

The author reports four more cases. The first was that of a

double metastatic conjunctivitis, arthritis of the knee and instep, and myositis. The first complication especially, although treated for a long time in the ophthalmologic service immediately improved after the first injections of serum.

The second case was that of a gonorrheal sciatic who had tried many forms of treatment before admission to the hospital, but without relief. Three injections of serum cured this patient in twelve days.

The third case was a rather intense arthritis of the hip which confined the patient to bed. He also was completely cured by this treatment.

The fourth case was the most interesting. At first the gonorrheal infection assumed the aspect of a septicemia for not only were the testicle and epididymis and cord inflamed, but the hip and the knee were also involved, the general condition was poor, the temperature 104, the pulse 160, irregular and of poor quality. At the same time there was vomiting and diarrhea, cold sweats and great prostration. Two serum injections caused complete cure. The case was also of interest in showing severe anaphylactic reactions following the injections.

6. **Vesico-prostato-perineal Fistula Treated by Bilateral Ureteral Catheterization.**

The patient was a boy of 15, who was admitted to the hospital suffering from a perineal fistula, the result of an old perineal section for bladder stone. Urethral catheterization revealed no obstruction in the prostatic region. The external orifice of the fistula was situated a little in front of the anus. The tract could not be catheterized with a small filiform. When the patient was standing urine was continually escaping from the fissure, but when the patient was in the recumbent posture urine was passed only during micturition.

The first operation consisted in a transvesical attempt to resect and close the internal orifice of the fistula, and a perineal incision for the extirpation of the rest of the fistulous tract. Suprapubic drainage was instituted for twelve days and then a permanent urethral sound was introduced. When the latter was removed urine again flowed from the perineal wound, the attempt had failed and it was evident that deviation of the urine by suprapubic drainage was insufficient in that case and that contamination with urine had prevented cicatrization.

It was then thought that deflection of the urinary stream at a higher point — as by nephrostomy — might be necessary, but before this was attempted a bilateral ureteral catheterization was tried. This was successful and was accomplished by introducing a No. 8 Charrière catheter into each ureter and leaving a No. 15 in the bladder. The fistulous tract was then again excised by the perineal route and the wound sutured in part and packed with gauze. The ureteral catheters were retained in place for nine days, during which period they functionated well, being irrigated with weak silver nitrate solution twice every other day. After the ureteral catheters were removed a urethral catheter was introduced and renewed every other day for a week. The perineal wound healed rapidly, urination was normal, and two months after the operation the patient was entirely cured.

In summing up the case the authors point out that in order for the ureteral catheterization to be effectual it should be carried out with large catheters. Even under these precautions however there may be leakage into the bladder but this can readily be nullified by the use of a permanent urethral catheter.

MISCELLANEOUS ABSTRACTS

Non-gonorrheal Granular Urethritis.

From the many forms of non-gonorrheal urethritis Waelsch has recently separated a group most refractory to treatment. He states that complete recovery never occurs, but this is not A. Glingar's experience (*Wien. Med. Woch.*, Mar. 28). Various cocci and bacilli have been found but none is characteristic, and it is doubtful whether the etiology is invariably the same. In this chronic type of urethritis the writer includes only those primary cases in which the patients have never had gonorrhea. There is a long incubation period and only slight subjective and objective symptoms. In 18 cases, seen within 3 years, the writer used the endoscope. In 11 cases the appearance of the mucous membrane of the anterior portion of the urethra was similar. There was diffuse or circumscribed inflammation of the type described by Oberländer as soft infiltration. In the infiltrated mucosa; gray, or grayish-yellow, slightly raised granules of the size of a millet seed or pin's head were scattered either in groups or in confluent patches which involved the whole circumference of the urethra. These nodules closely resembled the granules of conjunctival trachoma. The two chief conditions from which they are to be distinguished are tubercles and the follicles present in chronic follicular urethritis (Oberländer). Compared with tubercles the nodules are more transparent. Tubercles are whiter and more opaque. But the diagnosis may be difficult. From follicular urethritis the chief distinction in recent cases is the absence of hard infiltration. But as in old cases of chronic non-gonorrheal urethritis infiltration may occur, other points of difference must be noted. The nodules of non-gonorrheal urethritis are smaller than the follicles in follicular urethritis and are more constant in size. If the follicles are pricked the liquid contents escape and the structure collapses. The nodules of non-gonorrheal urethritis bleed if pricked but do not collapse. In the latter the urethra is moist owing to a more or less profuse secretion; in the former the mucosa is of dry appearance. The number of nodules varies greatly and is in no relation to the quantity of discharge and the turbidity of the urine. The discharge is thin and more serous than purulent — at least in the earlier stages of the disease.

The writer is undecided whether any clinical or etiological difference exists between the cases with nodules and those without. In general the former appeared to be more refractory to treatment and more likely to give rise to complications. One patient had enlarged and painful inguinal glands, which disappeared after 3 months' syphilis was excluded. It is of interest that in one of the cases with nodules the patient during the sixth month of the urethritis acquired acute gonorrhea. On recovery from gonorrhea the urethritis and nodules had disappeared.

In chronic non-gonorrheal urethritis endoscopy has usually been performed to exclude other diseases — especially soft chancres, syphilis, tuberculosis, and gonorrhea. Characteristic appearances in chronic non-gonorrheal urethritis have never previously been described. Indeed both Königstein and Waelsch expressly state that no certain differences between the endoscopic appearances of gonorrheal and non-gonorrheal urethritis exist. The writer is convinced that the nodules described are characteristic of one of the forms of chronic nonrheal urethritis, though whether all cases have the same etiology cannot be stated. If the history points to a non-gonorrheal disease the presence of urethral nodules tends to confirm it. In oldstanding cases the presence of nodules does not exclude the possibility that both infections — gonorrhea and non-gonorrheal urethritis — may co-exist. In some cases of post-gonorrheal catarrh similar nodules were present and possibly accounted for the refractory character of the disease. The nodules do not appear to predispose to stricture.

Inoculation of the conjunctive of a monkey with the secretion of non-gonorrheal urethritis was without result and did not produce trachoma. The nodules have not been found in the female urethra.

There is no specific treatment. The nodules should be treated with caustics under guidance of the endoscope. The prognosis is then not unfavorable.

Torsion of the Testicle: Reduction by Manipulation.

Lieut. C. M. Finny (*Journ. Royal Army Med. Corps,* Feb., p. 201). — A lieutenant while at mess was seized with a violent pain in his left testicle. He went to his tent, where he vomited several times, while the pain continued to increase. As a boy he had suffered from an undescended testicle on the left side, which, however, had eventually found its way into the scrotum. On two previous occasions he had suffered from attacks similar to the present one, but they had ceased spontaneously in a few hours.

The left testicle and cord were much swollen and tender, so that it was impossible to distinguish the epididymis from the rest of the organ. The temperature was subnormal, pulse 100, and there was no abdominal rigidity.

Thanks to the history there was little difficulty in arriving at a diagnosis of torsion of the testicle, but in view of the spontaneous recovery in the two previous attacks palliative measures were first tried. These proved of no avail; the patient continued to vomit repeatedly and the pain was unrelieved. Before sending him to hospital — distance of 7 miles — the writer decided to try manipulation. Twisting the testicle inwards was found to increase the pain. It was therefore rotated outwards firmly. After passing through half a circle a sensation similar to that experienced on reducing a dislocation was felt as the organ suddenly resumed its normal position. The pain immediately abated, the patient went to sleep, and next morning felt quite well. The swelling had gone and merely a small effusion into the tunica vaginalis remained, which disappeared in a few days.

Two features are of interest. The first is that the torsion occurred while the patient was seated at table. The second is that, though the treatment is doubtless not original, the writer has not been able to find in surgical literature any other treatment than immediate operation. This case is submitted as a plea for giving less radical measures a trial.

THE AMERICAN JOURNAL OF UROLOGY, VENEREAL AND SEXUAL DISEASES

WILLIAM J. ROBINSON, M.D., EDITOR

VOL. X NOVEMBER, 1914 No. 11

THE TREATMENT OF PYOVESICAL FISTULÆ, WITH THE REPORT OF A CASE

By JEAN L. AUBOUIN, M.D., Bordeaux, France

SPONTANEOUS opening of suppurating collections into the bladder takes place in various ways and gives rise to various symptoms. Pollosson, quoted by Patel (*Revue de Gynécologie,* Aug., 1912), says: "The salpingitic or perisalpingitic collections of pus, when left alone, empty into the neighboring organs. The communication with the bladder is either direct by way of the Fallopian tube, or indirectly, resulting from rupture of a perisalpingitic abscess into the bladder. The operation will reveal the site of the fistula, usually on the posterior surface. A pyosalpinx will not give rise, when it empties itself, to the same phenomena as will an appendicitis, although frequently the case can be summed up in a few words: the ordinary signs of an encysted suppuration in the pelvis or lower abdomen, a sudden cessation with pyuria, this symptom preceded by more or less marked vesical disturbances. The presence of pus in the urine, persistent or not, sometimes becomes intermittent, and, later on, complications may arise unless an operation is considered opportune. Things may still pass in a different way. The evacuation, although abundant, does not bring about a complete calm. The physical and functional signs of pelvic abscess persist, the pyuria little marked, but persistent. The patient has hectic fever which undermines his health." Pozzi says: "An uncontrollable anorexia is one of the most striking characters of this condition. There are women who can take no food, who vomit everything, and literally die from inanition."

Sometimes the majority of functional symptoms are wanting; the pus collects without any clinical evidence, the vesical perforation occurs without pain, and the pyuria is the only symptom by which the trouble manifests itself. These patients die quickly. Then again, the pelvic lesion is of long standing; the patient is worn out, in complete cachexia, when the perforation takes place. Improvement is immediate but of short duration, until a new evacuation takes place. And so it goes on until death finally occurs.

The symptomatology will also vary if a communication between the intestine and bladder exists, between an ovarian cyst and the vesical cavity or between a suppurative lesion in the bones and the urinary reservoir. However, the most interesting is the general study of the evolution of a pyovesical fistula. "Peritonitis, generalized infection, progressive loss of strength and renal infection are the most common ways of death" (Gras, Thesis, Paris, 1905). In opposition to this opinion, I believe from the study of many reported cases of this condition that usually these patients recover.

If we compare the rupture of suppurating genital lesions into the rectum—which used to have such a bad prognosis and are now considered of little importance—with pyovesical fistula, there is just as much chance of recovery in one as in the other. When no meddlesome treatment is attempted, with rest and medical care, the intravesical opening has a natural tendency to close. And I believe that the prognosis depends more upon the degree of perivesical inflammation than on the size of the fistula or its origin. In cases of tuberculous fistula the same cannot be said, as the lesions progress more or less rapidly and continuously. And lastly, patients presenting a pyuria of extravesical origin should always be followed by the surgeon, who will judge if an operation is necessary.

Case Report. I am obliged to Dr. E. Monod, honorary surgeon to the Hospitals of Bordeaux, for the privilege of reporting this case, which has not been published.

Mrs. X, of good constitution and without hereditary or personal pathological antecedents. Menstruation at the age of eleven and always irregular, often with an interval of two, three or even six months. The menses are usually abundant and last eight to ten days.

Married in 1905. No change in the menstrual irregularity. A year after marriage, after a delay of two and a half months, the patient had a fall, which was followed by a severe loss of blood with clots and pain. It was thought that she had had a miscarriage, but this was not medically confirmed.

In December, 1907, after a voyage, she had what was supposed to be an attack of appendicitis, but the symptoms have not since returned. The menses continued to be irregular and profuse and a pink colored discharge made its appearance during the interval. A diagnosis of hemorrhagic metritis was made and the patient was treated by rest, antiseptic irrigations and medicated ovules, which resulted in a decrease of the discharge. It was at this time that a physician first noted the existence on the right side of the uterus of an enlargement the size of an almond, which increased in size during the menses and afterwards decreased.

In the month of September, 1908, another physician suspected the possibility of pregnancy, an hypothesis which was abandoned two months later, and the patient was subjected to a thyroid treatment with object of reducing her weight. She lost 9 kilogrammes in two months.

In May, 1910, after considerable fatigue, a free discharge with clots took place and this was followed by an attack of enteritis and vomiting. At this time the patient consulted a specialist for diseases of the digestive system, who placed her on a strict diet. Greatly improved by this treatment she remained in the country for three months in excellent health and without any discharge or menstruation. The latter did not recur until October and again in December. After a trip to Paris about Christmas time the digestive disturbances returned.

Towards the end of January, 1911, she had a severe attack of enteritis with peritonitis, cystitis and fever, which lasted three weeks. Absolute rest for a month. The uterus at this time was found enlarged and the possibility of pregnancy was considered, but after a very severe flow, with clots, the uterus considerably diminished in size.

At this time (the end of March, 1911) Dr. Monod first saw the patient. A treatment of saline baths at Briscous was ordered during April and after the seventh bath the menstruation appeared and was normal. During June an electrical treatment was tried, but each séance brought on a discharge lasting eight days so the treatment was stopped. Normal menses until November, after which they did not appear for three months.

At the beginning of 1912, the discharge returned with more or less intermittence. Second cure at Briscous in August.

Dr. Monod again saw the patient in May, 1913, and found the following condition: she was pale, thin and so weak that she could not leave her bed. Food was badly tolerated. Some vomiting. Chronic constipation. The temperature, which kept at about 38° C., showed intermittent rises to 39.5° C. The urine was cloudy and a manifestly purulent deposit fell to the bottom of the glass. A distinct swelling could be detected in the right iliac fossa and combined palpation revealed fluctuation. There was now no longer any doubt that there was a collection of pus, in all probability salpingitic in origin, which had opened spontaneously into the bladder, and after consultation with Prof. Vénot surgical interference was decided upon.

On June 25 a free posterior colpotomy was done, which gave issue to about 1500 c.c. of well mixed and odorless pus. Two large drainage tubes were inserted into the pocket and the vagina packed with sterile gauze.

After this the general health rapidly improved; the temperature fell and the appetite returned. Irrigation of the pus pocket with oxygenated water. One drain was removed in two weeks and the remaining tube was changed for others of smaller caliber as the vaginal incision decreased in size, and finally after three weeks the last tube was expelled spontaneously. During all this time the bladder was regularly irrigated with a solution of silver nitrate. The large amount of pus at first contained in the urine little by little diminished, but distinct traces were still present (end of August, 1913) at the time the patient left the private clinic.

She was last seen on Nov. 18, 1913, at which time her general health was good and she had gained in weight. Bimanual examination revealed in the right iliac fossa a hard tumor, the size of a large walnut and painless, the remains of the old pus focus which was undergoing progressive retraction. After standing in a glass the urine deposits a slight layer of pus so that it may be assumed that the fistulous tract connecting the salpingitic focus with the vesical cavity has not as yet completely closed.

Opinions most varied have been put forth as to the treatment of pyovesical fistulæ, but the majority seem in favor of abstention, unless complications should occur, and while cicatrization of the vesical opening is going on the bladder should be washed out with proper disinfecting solutions daily. After a time, should new symptoms appear, which would prove the presence of relapsing suppuration, operation is indicated.

In appendix abscess particularly it is, according to Bazy, not only useless but unsafe to interfere surgically when the process opens into the bladder. However, should the septic accidents persist a paravesical opening can be made at the lowest point which will give easy issue to the pus. Appendiculo-vesical fistulæ following acute appendicitis may heal spontaneously and one should not hasten to resort to laparotomy unless special indications exist. The treatment should at first be limited to frequent vesical irrigation and, if necessary, the use of the permanent catheter. Bazy is of the opinion that operation is, however, indicated in cases where the fistula persists.

Terrillon expresses a similar idea in cases of pelvic abscess which has opened into the bladder: "In some cases one should be in no hurry to interfere, because it is well known that these fistulæ are sometimes a mode of cure." Von Warker has quite the contrary opinion for he says: "The evacuation of pus by the bladder is not a real exit; there remains a suppurating cavity which cannot empty itself and sooner or later it becomes necessary to incise and completely empty it, in order to produce a cure." Ramon Y. Cajal (Clinica moderna, 1912) believes that suppurative lesions of the uterine adnexa and parametrium which have opened into the bladder is always a serious condition, which exposes the patient to septic complications of the urinary apparatus and septicemic manifestations which are often the cause of death, and reports cases to this effect.

It is probable that, in spite of these apparent divergencies of opinion, surgeons are almost of the same idea, holding themselves in readiness to operate if the evacuation of the pus is incomplete, if the general health does not improve and, above all, if symptoms appear which indicate an approaching cachexia or a tendency to the formation of a new collection.

The cases that I have been able to collect in the literature seem to show that operation must be undertaken in cases of chronic suppuration, because the condition of these patients becomes each day more serious and to defer operating may very well increase the gravity of the prognosis in spite of treacherous periods of seeming improvement.

The local and general conditions lead one to decide to interfere according to the ordinary rules of general surgery. The pyovesical fistula will have little tendency to heal, if two or three months have elapsed since its formation without any evidence of amelioration. Fever, progressive loss of flesh and the anorexia referred to by Pozzi also indicate that the cause of the pyuria persists without regression. It is also evident that it would not be prudent to wait for infection of the uropoietic system, although this may be late in taking place.

Consequently, although an operation at the beginning is only exceptionally required, on account of the technical difficulties and the resulting danger to the patient, it should be resorted to later on and with not too great delay.

The operations performed for the cure of pyovesical fistulæ are various and I shall not consider them in detail, as they are treated in most text-books. The vesical route, alone possible in the female, is a procedure of exception, the urethra allowing an exploration to be made but not an operation. Simon resorted to a vaginal incision into the bladder through which the bladder cavity is turned out and is thus easily explored and the fistula closed. For rectovesical fistulæ resulting from abscess, Tuffier and Chavannaz utilize the perineal route, passing between the urethra and prostate in front and the rectum behind. This route is useful and simple. In some few cases the anterior or posterior transpelvic routes may possibly be indicated.

In 1894 Prof. Pousson formulated rules for a simple technique allowing the bladder to be directly reached by its anterior face, namely, the transvesical technique. A little later the transperitoneal route was proposed and many successful cases have been reported. Colpotomy with drainage is indicated in some cases like the one here reported, but it is not always possible and in many cases is quite insufficient. Péau was greatly in favor of vaginal hysterectomy in cases of pelvic suppurations complicated by rectal, vesical and hypogastric fistulæ and this seems still applicable in selected cases. Simple abdominal incision has also its field of usefulness.

Laparotomy has, over all the other procedures, an undoubted superiority as it gives a full view of the lesions and offers plenty of room for any technique required for their cure. Likewise, by laparotomy drainage is easily established, combined or not with vaginal drainage. It is particularly indicated when one operates after the acute symptoms have calmed down.

The operative procedures applicable to pelvic suppurative processes which have opened into the bladder are numerous and have their particular indications. Two are to be particularly distinguished: (1) The urgent interference consists in a vaginal or abdominal incision, either alone or combined as the conditions indicate; (2) this applies to chronic suppurative processes, usually two or three months after fistulization, and laparotomy is the procedure of choice.

By this method, applicable to the majority of cases, the operator can break down the adhesions between the bladder, intestine or genital organs, free the latter, find the openings of communication, resect the diseased structures and suture the fistulæ.

It may happen that the vesical fistula is with difficulty discovered, the pyuria being kept up more especially by a pericystitis itself depending upon an active pelvic suppurating lesion. The suppression of the cause, be it appendicitis or pyosalpinx, and the closure of the opening into the bladder will bring about a rapid recovery, but this must be followed by careful local treatment of the vesical cavity.

Medical treatment must not be overlooked in all stages of the trouble, and to sum up what has been said we must expect, when in presence of a suppurating lesion which has ruptured into the bladder, that a spontaneous cure will ensue. If the accidents become serious and the local phenomena increase in intensity, an abdominal or vaginal incision will often suffice. Should waiting be permissible, the fistula being well established, a radical operation can be done and abdominal incision is the method to be selected, so that a thorough removal of all diseased tissue, with closure of the fistula, can be effected.

CONGENITAL DIVERTICULA OF THE BLADDER

By J. Swift Joly, F.R.C.S., London.

UNTIL recently diverticula of the bladder did not attract much attention clinically, except in those cases in which calculi were impacted or encysted in them. Even in these cases the energies of the surgeon were directed more towards the removal of the stone than towards the treatment of the cavity in which it lay. During this period we find scattered up and down throughout the medical literature records of cases who suffered from obscure urinary symptoms, which persisted in spite of treatment, and which were shown on the post-mortem table to be due to a diverticulum.

A second period in the history of this condition was ushered in by the introduction of the cystoscope. By means of this instrument the diagnosis of vesical diverticula was made easy, but even then most surgeons looked on them as interesting findings of no great pathological import, and the cystoscopic picture of a diverticulum was considered one that should be demonstrated to students chiefly as showing how easily the cavity might serve as a trap for calculi.

The third and last period commenced when it was found that not only were these pouches a source of great danger to the patient, but also that they came within the scope of surgical treatment.

Congenital vesical diverticula are of all sizes, from a tiny cavity which is contained in the thickness of the bladder-wall and does not form any projection on its outer surface, to an enormous sac which fills up the whole abdomen and contains a gallon of urine. This extraordinary condition was recorded by Warren Greene,[1] and occurred in an old man who died of retention of urine. At the autopsy an enormous diverticulum was found filling the left half of the abdomen, and pressing the stomach and intestines into the cavity of the diaphragm. The opening between the bladder and the diverticulum was about $1\frac{1}{2}$ cm. in diameter and was situated on the left side of the bladder about 4 cm. from the urethral orifice. During life the tumor was thought to be an ascites.

The time at my disposal only permits me to touch on two

[1] Read at the Section on Urology of the last International Medical Congress in London.

points in connexion with these diverticula, namely treatment and etiology.

TREATMENT.

Large vesical diverticula if left to themselves tend directly or indirectly to cause the death of the patient. This is due as a rule either to infection of the sac itself, or to infection of the whole urinary tree. In the former case the patient dies either of septic absorption, or as a result of perforation with either general peritonitis or pelvic cellulitis, in the latter of septic pyelonephritis. Besides this, even in the non-infected cases, there is a tendency to cause back-pressure on the kidneys by compressing or stretching one or both ureters. This of course paves the way for subsequent infection.

Once the gravity of the condition is recognized, the question of treatment becomes one of paramount importance. This may be palliative or radical. Among the methods of palliative treatment attempted in the past are—(1) catheterization and lavage; (2) drainage either of the bladder or of the diverticulum on to the surface of the body. This may be called "external drainage." (3) Operations devised to facilitate the drainage of the diverticulum into the bladder. These consist of dilatation of the orifice of communication between the two cavities, destruction of the wall between them, or the formation of a new opening between them at a more dependent part of the diverticulum. All these operations may be classed under the term "internal drainage."

Catheterization and lavage. The mere introduction of the catheter into the bladder and irrigation of that organ does very little to cleanse or disinfect the diverticulum. I doubt if the contents of a large sacculus are ever evacuated by mere catheterization; therefore the apparent residual urine (i. e., that withdrawn by the catheter) is less than the total amount left behind after micturition. Evidence in favor of this will be given later on. Even if the catheter can be insinuated into the cavity of the diverticulum, I doubt if it is thoroughly flushed out. The catheter cannot be passed far down into the sac, therefore only the part near the orifice receives much benefit from this procedure. I feel that lavage is of use only as a preliminary to some more radical operation, and that for this purpose it is inferior to a temporary cystotomy.

External drainage. This procedure is of the greatest benefit as a preliminary to excision of the diverticulum, and ought to be used in all badly infected cases. It enables the surgeon to do much to clean the bladder and the cavity of the sacculus, it relieves the patient from septic absorption, and enables him to regain strength to undergo the severe radical operation. Permanent external drainage has, however, little to recommend it. It may prolong the patient's life, but it will render him miserable from being constantly soaked in foul purulent urine, which excoriates the skin, and which on account of its odor prevents all social pleasures.

Internal drainage. At first sight this type of operation has much in its favor. It is simple, it does not put much strain on the patient, and it apparently gives free drainage by gravity from the diverticulum to the bladder. However, drainage into a contractile cavity like the bladder, in which the pressure is always raised, is very different from drainage on to the skin, and does not as a rule tend to bring about much diminution in the size of the diverticulum. The reason of this is that every attempt on the patient's part to empty his bladder results in the urine being driven in two directions: part of it is forced through the urethra, while the remainder is pressed back into the sacculus. Thus only an imperfect evacuation of the bladder results. Besides this, the tumor which is formed by the diverticulum remains, and may continue to exert a harmful pressure on the ureters or on other organs. If much advantage was to be gained from internal drainage, one would naturally expect that those diverticula that communicated with the bladder through a large opening should present fewer symptoms than those in which the orifice of communication is small. Yet we do not find this to be the case. In addition to these theoretical arguments we have the practical experience that in many cases very little good has resulted from these operations.

The radical treatment of these large diverticula is excision. Although the operation is in all cases severe, it is the one that should be proposed to all patients who have a reasonable chance of surviving it. It may be objected that in many cases the results of excision are not all that one could desire. I admit that this is so, but from a critical examination of the reported cases I came to the conclusion that where the infection was severe and of long duration the results were unsatisfactory; and as the severity of infection previous to operation diminished, so did the results of excision improve. After all, one can hardly expect a perfect result in a case where a severe infection of the bladder was present for periods extending up to ten years, and where the diverticulum and even the bladder itself became fixed and deformed by adhesions. I feel convinced that if the condition is attacked and a complete excision performed before infection has set in, the end results will leave nothing to be desired.

Another point is that some of the cases have been reported too early. I have seen slow but steady improvement continue for about two years after the operation. If such a case was reported early, the result of the operation would have appeared to be much worse than it really was.

I have operated on two cases which I wish to bring to your notice.

Case 1. Male, aet. 51, admitted to St. Peter's Hospital, January 11, 1910.

History. (Patient's own words.) "As long as I can remember I never had a strong flow of water, always taking longer to pass it than other people. In 1901 I first felt pain in my side, just above the left groin. I went to a doctor about it, and after passing a catheter he told me that I had an enlarged prostate gland, but did not advise an operation as it was not a very bad case. Up till this time my water had been quite clear, but about a week afterwards when passing water I felt a pricking sensation, and passed some white matter. This gradually got worse. This went on for several years, during which time I was attended by several doctors. They generally treated me for inflammation of the bladder."

The patient has had four or five attacks of hematuria during the last 18 months. During these attacks his pain (in the groin), scalding, and frequency of micturition were always much worse. He also suffered from backache, headache, and night-sweats during these attacks, but in the intervals between them he was fairly comfortable. He has lost weight. Denies syphilis and gonorrhea. Frequency of micturition from one to two hours both by day and by night. This has been getting worse for the last year, but all his life patient has had to get up once at night to pass water. Difficulty in micturition, stream slow and weak, straining. No after-dribbling, never had complete retention. Scalding in the penis and perineum during micturition: this has been present since 1901.

Urethra admits No. 18 Coudé catheter easily. Residual urine 13 ounces.

Abdomen. The bladder can be felt even when apparently empty, that is, when no urine flows through the catheter, as a tumor rising just above the pubis under the right rectus. The displacement to the right becomes more marked when it is distended. When empty it can be felt to become hard and soft like the uterus in the third stage of labor. The lower pole of the right kidney is just palpable.

Per rectum. The prostate is normal. Above it the bladder can be felt bulging into the rectum, but it is not indurated in any part, and does not bulge more on one side than on the other.

The other organs are normal.

Urine. Sp. gr. 1018, acid, albumin present, no sugar, urea 1%, deposit pus and blood.

Cystoscopy. Several attempts were made to wash the bladder clear enough for cystoscopy, but it was only after a long course of daily irrigations that it was possible to do so. The patient had a considerable amount of urethral spasm that rendered catheterization difficult. Finally a good view was obtained. Bladder distension 24 ounces. The right ureter was displaced towards the right, and the left almost to the middle line. The opening of a large diverticulum was seen above and to the left of the left ureter; the opening was round and appeared to be about the size of a cedar pencil. Surrounding this opening, except at its lower part, was a polypoid mass which proved to consist of edematous mucous membrane. The left ureter projected into the bladder and was somewhat dilated.

Operation, January 19, 1910. Anesthetic, chloroform and ether. Trendelenburg position. A vertical median incision was made extending from the pubis almost to the umbilicus, and a transverse one across the left rectus 1½ inch above the pubis. The operation was entirely extraperitoneal. The diverticulum was about half as large again as the bladder; it completely filled the left half of the pelvis, and extended to the right of the middle line, pushing the bladder before it. It was large enough to hold a large orange. The peritoneum was stripped upwards and the tissues peeled off the left side of the bladder, and off the upper surface of the diverticule. This process was continued down the left side of the sacculus between it and the pelvic wall. The vas deferens was here met with running in a groove in the lateral wall of the diverticulum. It was divided between ligatures. The dissection was carried on till near the spine of the ischium a large vein was torn. This gave rise to troublesome hemorrhage, and as it could not be picked up and tied this part of the wound was plugged with gauze. The bladder was then emptied and opened. Its walls were very thick. The opening of the diverticulum would just admit the index finger; it was about 1 inch above and to the left of the left ureter. With the finger in the opening, the wall of the sacculus was divided about half an inch from the bladder. This incision was carried round the orifice, and the diverticulum was pulled away from the bladder. This brought the ureter into view. It was about as thick as the finger and ran in a deep groove in the posterior wall of the sacculus, and then curved forwards in the cleft between the bladder and the diverticulum to its entrance into the bladder. The sacculus was now rapidly freed from some adhesions which bound it to the prostate and rectum, and was removed. The vein that was torn was picked up and ligatured above and below the tear. As the patient was now very much collapsed from loss of blood, three pints of saline were infused into his median cephalic vein, while the orifice of the diverticulum was hastily sutured. A tube was placed in his bladder, another and two gauze plugs in the space from which the sacculus had been removed, the muscles were brought together with catgut, and the skin sutured with silkworm-gut.

The patient rapidly recovered from the shock of the operation, but his convalescence was very slow, as a persistent suprapubic sinus remained. This tracked round the bladder to the opening of the diverticulum. A month after the operation the sinus was scraped under an anesthetic. It finally healed up and patient was sent to a convalescent home about three months after his operation. On leaving the hospital his stream was little more than a dribble, and he took a long time to empty his bladder. Residual urine varied from nil to half a pint.

During his stay in the home the fistula opened again, and he was readmitted to hospital on June 8 with a pinhole sinus in the suprapubic scar. This tracked down to the original opening of the diverticulum.

Operation, June 10. Trendelenburg position. The bladder was opened through an incision to the right of the old scar, the edges of the diverticular opening in the bladder-wall were freshened and brought together with catgut sutures. This was very difficult as the bladder was adherent to the lateral wall of the pelvis. As there was a very slight intravesical projection of the prostate, the gland was enucleated. The bladder was drained. Patient was discharged in a month's time with the suprapubic wound closed. He stated that his micturition was better than it ever had been, but he had 7 ounces residual urine. Cystoscopy showed a firm puckered scar at the site of the diverticular opening. Urine turbid, contained pus and colon bacilli.

He was then put on a long course of vaccine treatment. Under this his urine cleared up somewhat, but the residuum remained the same.

Early this year he was again admitted to hospital and a large ventral hernia was cured by the filigree method. At the same time a small amount of tissue was nipped out from his internal meatus by means of a Young's punch.

Present state. Frequency three to four hours by day, rises once at night. Residual urine 3 ounces. Feels perfectly well, has put on over a stone in weight.

I feel that most of this troublesome and difficult after-treatment might have been avoided if I had been able to suture the orifice more firmly in the first operation. It was unfortunate that owing to the critical state of the patient this important part of the operation had to be hurried over. I think now that the persistence of the residual urine was due more to the adhesions which formed between the bladder and the pelvic wall than to any obstruction the prostate may have offered to the evacuation of the bladder.

Case 2. Patient, a male aet. 53, was admitted to St. Peter's Hospital on March 19, 1912.

He states that he had an attack of gonorrhea about 30 years ago. About 12 years ago he was treated for stricture at one of the London hospitals. The stricture seems to have been easily dilated. He then bought a bougie and passed it on himself about twice a year. However, the second time he used it he gave himself a severe attack of cystitis. Since then his urine has always been turbid, and he had several attacks of pain and frequency of micturition. During these attacks he had to pass urine 12 or 14 times a day, and rise 10 or 12 times at night for this purpose. He had two transient attacks of hematuria, neither of them were caused by instrumentation.

Micturition. At present the frequency is almost normal, the stream is good and has been so all his life, some straining towards the end of the act. Occasionally he has noticed that he was able to pass a large quantity of urine almost immediately after apparently emptying his bladder. He has a dull suprapubic pain during micturition and when the bladder is full.

Urethra. Stricture in the bulb, which easily admits No. 17 F.; this was fully dilated in two sittings.

Residual urine. This varied very much in amount. Generally it was about 12 ounces, but has been as low as 8 ounces, and as much as 16.

Cystoscopy. Slight general cystitis. Both ureters normal, effluxes clear. Just to the left of the middle line the opening of a large sacculus is to be seen. It lies about half an inch above the interureteric bar, is oval in shape with the long axis directed vertically, and from it numerous vessels radiate just like the spokes of a wheel. The opening measures about ½ inch in its longest diameter, the shortest being perhaps ⅛ inch less. The cystoscope could be introduced into the diverticulum with ease; its walls were deep red in colour, smooth, and no vessels were visible on their surface.

Per rectum. Prostate normal; above it, a soft elastic swelling can be felt.

Urine. Acid, sp. gr. 1018, no albumin, no sugar, urea 1.9%, deposit pus and epithelial cells from the bladder.

Operation, March 22, 1912. Trendelenburg position. The bladder was washed out, emptied as much as possible, and filled with air. A median vertical incision was made from the pubis to the umbilicus. The peritoneal cavity was opened. The diverticulum appeared like an immense bleb resting on the posterior wall of the bladder and filling up the space between it and the rectum. It appeared to be absolutely adherent to the bladder over a circular area about 3 inches in diameter. From it the peritoneum passed almost directly back to the rectum, the recto-vesical pouch being filled up. I then opened the bladder, and found to my surprise that though it had been apparently emptied before the air was injected, the diverticulum was almost completely filled with a mixture of urine and lotion. This was mopped up, fortunately without soiling the peritoneum. As it was evident that the wall of the diverticulum was absolutely adherent to the bladder over a very wide area, I decided not to try to find a line of cleavage between them, but to dissect away the mucous membrane of the diverticulum, and then to remove its outer wall. To do this I split the bladder from before backwards in the middle line. My incision extended from the suprapubic opening to the orifice of the diverticulum. In making it the sacculus was widely opened. Then, commencing at the orifice of communication between the bladder and the diverticulum, I removed the entire epithelial lining of the latter cavity. This dissection was rather troublesome, especially in the lower part of the sacculus which lay behind the prostate. Ureteric catheters were previously passed up the ureters to serve as landmarks, and by this means I was able to avoid them. They passed from the bladder downwards, and then backwards under the lowest part of the diverticulum, and then upwards for a short distance along its posterior surface. The wall of the diverticulum was exceedingly thin, the muscular tissue being reduced to a very fine but continuous sheet. I removed it all except two peritoneum-covered flaps that just covered the raw area left on the posterior wall of the bladder. These were sutured in position, and the wound in the bladder closed with a through-and-through continuous suture of chromic catgut. Over this an inverting suture of the same material was inserted. A gauze wick was laid along the suture line, and the peritoneum closed, leaving only a small space for the wick. A tube was placed in the bladder, and the rest of the wound closed.

The patient bore the operation very well, and was discharged from the hospital in four weeks with his wound firmly healed. Three months later he returned with a small sinus in the suprapubic scar, through which most of his urine passed. This was excised and the opening in the bladder closed. Since then there has been no further trouble.

Present state. Patient passes urine every four hours by day, and once during the night. Micturition normal. Residual urine 2 ounces. Urine cloudy, contains pus and colon bacilli. No pain. Cystoscopy. Slight general cystitis. In the position of the old diverticular opening is a puckered scar; from this a linear ridge runs forwards to the apex of the bladder. The ureteric orifices seem rather more widely separated from each other than is usual.

THE ORIGIN OF CONGENITAL DIVERTICULA.

In this discussion I shall say nothing about the apical diverticula, which obviously arise from non-closure of the vesical end of the urachus, but will confine my remarks to the consideration of the origin of diverticula arising at or near the ureteric openings.

About two years ago it occurred to me that these diverticula might be due to the persistence and enlargement of supernumerary "ureteric buds," and since then I have endeavored to collect evidence in support of this hypothesis.

The ureter is formed from a bud that is given off from the terminal portion of the primary excretory duct (Wolffian duct). This bud springs from the duct just before it opens into the cloaca, and passes at first backwards towards the vertebral column. Soon it turns cranial-wards and comes into apposition with the rudiments of the kidney proper. In the development of the bladder from the cloaca the lower end of the primary excretory duct is absorbed into the cloacal horn. By this means the ureter acquires a separate opening into the cloaca. This opening at first lies immediately to the outer side of that of the primary excretory duct, but the part of the cloacal wall between the two openings grows rapidly, so that while the orifice of the primary excretory duct remains in its original position, that of the ureter comes to lie at a considerable distance above and to the outer side of it. In this way the trigone of the bladder is formed.

Now if two ureteric buds are developed from the primary excretory duct, one would expect that the more cranial one should come to lie with its vesical opening above and to the outer side of the lower one. This is what we do find in the case of double ureter; the opening of the upper lies above and to the outer side of that of the lower. If a line is drawn from the internal meatus to the lower opening, its prolongation should pass through the mouth of the upper ureter. For brevity I shall call this line the "ureteric line."

Now if a diverticulum is developed from a supernumerary ureteric bud that has failed to reach the kidney, its opening should lie on or near this ureteric line. I examined the records of a large number of cases to find if this was so, but was met by two difficulties in this task. The first was the multiplicity of methods that the various authors made use of in describing the position of these orifices. Also some of the descriptions were too vague, and others insufficient to determine accurately the position of the sacculus. The other difficulty was that the bladder wall is often so much distorted by the diverticulum that the true relationship of the parts is obscured. My first case illustrates this point. It seems as if the diverticulum dragged the left wall of the bladder downwards, while there was a compensatory tilting upwards of the right one. However, allowing for this, I came to the conclusion that in the vast majority of cases the openings of the diverticula that appeared to be congenital lay on or very near the ureteric line. Another point of interest is that the smaller the diverticulum, the closer does its orifice lie to this line. In the case of the very small congenital diverticula occasionally found in the routine examination of bladders, the openings, I believe, invariably lie on the ureteric line.

Again, since the diverticular openings almost invariably lie above that of the true ureter, it follows that if they are derived from embryonic ureteric buds, they must be developed from the more cranial, and the ureter from the more caudal of the two buds. Keibel and Mall [2] confirm this in a striking manner. Speaking of malformations of the kidney and ureter, these authors say: "I . . . shall only point out here that they (double or triple ureters) arise as two or three ureteric buds from the primary excretory ducts, and that these multiple ureteric buds no not develop equally, the most caudal one showing the strongest development, not only as regards the expansion of its ureteric tree, but also as regards the height that it reaches in its development. It represents the normal ureteric bud and always reaches a more cranial level than the other two buds."

Again, the frequency with which congenital diverticula of the bladder are bilateral, and the occasional finding of a diverticula on one side and double ureters on the other, are both in favor of this view.

The next question to be considered is: Have we any evidence that a blind ureteric bud can become transformed into one of these enormous diverticula? Is there any case on record in which a structure, which one must admit is a blind ureter, has become dilated so as to simulate a true diverticulum? Owing to the kindness of Mr. H. J. Stiles, of Edinburgh, I am able to answer this question in the affirmative. He has generously given me the notes of, and allowed me to publish, a case on which he operated, and which, I think, fills the gap in the evidence.

Mr. Stiles's case.

Patient, a male, aet. 2¼ years, was admitted to the Children's Hospital, Edinburgh, on March 21, 1911, with a swelling in the abdomen and difficulty in passing water.

Six months previously his water had become thick during a febrile attack. Nine days before admission micturition was noticed to be difficult, and the stream dribbling. A week later he seemed to lose control of his urine. Pain during micturition, none apart from the act. Urine only comes in drops.

Examination. Abdomen protuberant. An elastic, tensely fluctuating tumor extending almost to the umbilicus, and projecting rather more to the left of the middle line, was felt on palpation. To the right of this again there was some fullness and deep induration. A rubber catheter was passed easily, and a considerable quantity of clear urine drawn off. This caused the left-sided swelling to disappear, but brought into evidence a second fluctuating tumor which lay entirely to the right of the middle line. It lay behind the right rectus, and extended up to the level of the umbilicus. It was broader at its upper end, smooth, and fairly well defined. On rectal examination a fluctuating swelling filled the right side of the recto-vesical pouch.

Operation, March 23, 1911. Mr. Stiles. Vertical incision through the right rectus, extending from the umbilicus almost to the pubis. Peritoneum opened. The right kidney was sought for, but could not be found; the left was enlarged and lobulated, but otherwise normal. In the line of the right ureter a retroperitoneal lobulated cyst-like mass was felt. It extended from the lumbar fossa down into the true pelvis, and was fully two fingers' breadth. The intestines having been packed away, the peritoneum over the tumor was incised. It was stripped upwards and outwards off the cyst until the blind upper extremity of the latter was reached. The cyst was then dissected off the posterior abdominal wall, and was followed into the pelvis. It communicated with the base of the bladder through an aperture about 3/4 inch in diameter. Here it was divided between clamps, and the stump was closed by two layers of continuous sutures. A drainage tube was passed down to the stump. The peritoneum on the posterior abdominal wall was sutured, and the abdomen closed. The patient made a rapid recovery and left the hospital four weeks after the operation.

The specimen was a muscular tube, evidently a ureter, about 3/4 inch in diameter, and about 5 3/4 inches long. This does not represent its full length, as adhesions bound together adjacent portions of the tube. The upper end was blind, the lower communicated with the bladder through an orifice 3/4 inch in diameter.

Even from this brief *résumé* it can be seen that Mr. Stiles's case is a connecting link between the blind ureteric buds and the true congenital diverticula, and shows how the one may develop into the other. What happened here to an apparently normally growing ureter that failed to meet the rudiments of the true kidney may also be conceived to occur in cases of supernumerary ureters even though a normal ureter may also be present.

My belief is that supernumerary ureteric buds not infrequently fail to reach the developing kidney; that these may remain as tiny congenital diverticula throughout life, or, from some reason at present unknown, perhaps from the inherent power of the embryonic cells to multiply, they may increase in size. Once this happens, a certain amount of urine is suddenly forced into them every time the bladder contracts. Before these repeated shocks they dilate still more, and sooner or later lose the power of emptying themselves. Still every contraction of the bladder transmits a wave of increased pressure through the vesical opening; this acts as an expansile force within the diverticulum and tends to increase its size. They resemble aneurysms in this respect, that the larger they are the greater is the pressure, which tends to increase still more their size. Once they fail to empty themselves, that is as soon as there is residual urine, it is only a matter of time till they become infected. The inflammation is most pronounced in the diverticulum, because the stagnation is at its greatest there. This causes inflammatory adhesions with the neighboring structures that limit still more their contractile power. In addition to this the inflammation causes an infiltration and sclerosis of their walls, which not only inhibits completely what little power of contraction they may have had, but also fixes the vesical orifice so that it cannot move with the rest of the bladder when it contracts. The first result of this is that the bladder is hampered in its contraction and therefore becomes hypertrophied; the second is that the amount of residual urine increases, and now exceeds the capacity of the diverticulum in its amount; that is, at the end of micturition not only is the diverticulum completely filled, but there is also some urine in the bladder. In this way I think that the well-known phenomena these interesting cases present may be explained without invoking the aid of an obstruction to the urinary outflow. I believe that the diverticulum is the cause of the retention, and not that the retention is the prime factor in their etiology.

In conclusion I beg to submit this hypothesis, knowing full well its many imperfections; I regret the scanty and fragmentary nature of the evidence I have brought forward in support of it, but I feel that it explains some at least of the phenomena connected with this condition. Whether the explanation is a true one or not, remains for future investigators to decide.

REFERENCES

1. Warren Greene.—*American Medical Times,* No. 4, p. 13.
2. Keibel and Mall.—*Manual of Human Embryology,* ii. 867

A DEVICE FOR THE TREATMENT OF PROSTATITIS.

By Charles Morgan McKenna, M.D., Chicago, Ill.

Instructor in Surgery, College of Medicine University of Illinois; Surgeon to St. Joseph's Hospital; Cystoscopist to St. Bernard's and People's Hospitals.

ALWAYS felt very keenly the lack of an appliance for the Bier treatment in inflammations of the prostate gland. The device which I am about to describe is a glass suction tube that fits into the rectum in such a way that hyperemia of the prostate and its surrounding tissue may actually be produced.

Fig. 1a shows a conical shaped tube about three and one-half inches long and one and one-eighth inches in diameter with an outlet at the large end; on one surface there is a depression with an opening in the center; from this opening a small glass tube

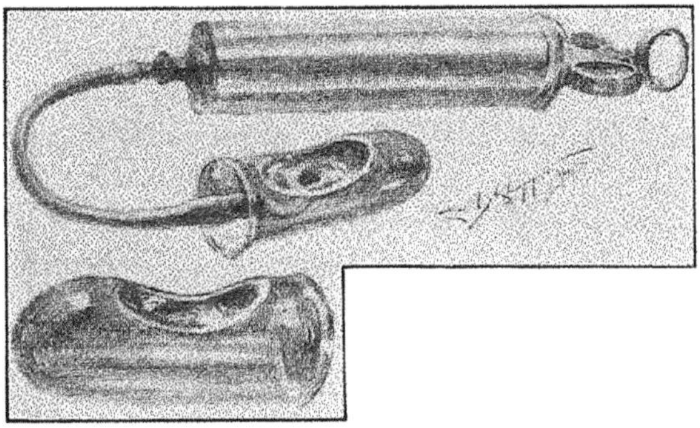

Fig. 1. Apparatus for Bier Treatment of Prostate.

extends through the lumen of the large cone where a syringe may be attached by means of a rubber tubing.

If one cystoscopes the base of the bladder while the tube is in the rectum, the prostate can be seen to move out toward the coccyx on suction of the syringe. This phenomenon furnishes the proof that the suction is effective on the base of the bladder. This, however, was done for my satisfaction only.

Fig. 1b shows a retaining tampon which is similar to No. 1 minus the opening in the depression. This depression may be filled with ichthyol and glycerine or any salt and left in the rectum for several hours at a time. The tampon is only used in case the patient can remain in bed. The suction device is left in the rectum from two to eight minutes at a time and may be released if too much pain is experienced and again used after the patient has had sufficient rest.

The following is a report of four cases in which the Bier's cup device was used:

Case 1. Referred to me by Dr. C. P. Caldwell, May 24, 1913. Mr. T., Italian, aged 34 years, contracted gonorrhea four years previously and never fully recovered. Discharge would continue three or four days at a time and then stop, usually a morning drop; smear showed no gonococci. Anterior urethra free from strictures. Patient did not drink, and had had no intercourse for months. On massaging the prostate gland a smear could be easily obtained for microscopical examination.

Treatment. Gave deep instillations of 20 per cent argyrol once a day for one week, then nitrate of silver in various strengths up to 1 per cent. in deep urethra. Patient returned ten days later unimproved. The Bier's cup device was used at sittings of three minutes at a time; each day the time was extended until ten minutes were reached. This treatment was administered every other day for three weeks and at the date of this publication the patient is free from any discharge or subjective symptoms, so that we may speak of a cure in a clinical sense. He was last seen August 12, 1913, and said that he was well; massage of the prostate did not produce any results.

Case 2. June 2, 1913. Mr. R., Irish, aged 27 years, single, occupation, street car conductor. Contracted gonorrhea three years ago. Discharge had stopped, except for the occasional appearance of a morning drop. Patient complains of a dull, heavy feeling in the rectum, and irritation on each urination. The smear showed few gonococci which appeared inactive. After eleven injections of 0.5 per cent. nitrate of silver, no gonococci could be found in the smear, although symptoms remained the same. The Bier's cup was used in the same way as in Case 1, and after three weeks symptoms had ceased.

Case 3. June 6, 1913; referred by Dr. S. McNeil. Mr. H., Scotch-Irish, aged 44 years, single, contracted gonorrhea in the years of 1898, 1903, 1909. The patient had a very long scrotum and an old hydrocele on right side. Was sent to St. Joseph's Hospital, where the scrotum was shortened, the hydrocele was operated on, and vas injected after Belfield's method. The vas was injected every day for six days with 10 per cent. argyrol and every other day for three days. Fistula was allowed to close but discharge continued without showing any gonococci. I used the above mentioned device in the office three times a week for four and a half weeks and at present the patient is symptomatically cured. The prostate gland appears to be normal to palpation.

Case 4. Mr. P., German, aged 66 years, janitor, denied ever having any venereal disease. Had an enlarged prostate which had bothered him for five years. Had used sounds on himself. Present history: could not void urine without the use of a catheter. Examination of urine showed pus with many bacteria. Patient was sent to St. Joseph's Hospital and prepared for a prostatectomy. Bier's cup device with hot irrigations used daily for ten days, at which time prostate was quite firm, and spontaneous urination was possible again under difficulty. However, owing to the size of the gland, the prostate was removed, which was followed by an uneventful recovery and complete cure as to retention.

While this device has been used only on a limited number of cases, I feel entitled to claim for it a place in the treatment of inflammatory conditions. It was noted that when the discharge was free from gonococci the pathologic condition yielded more quickly. There are a number of cases under observation at present, none of which have been treated longer than three weeks. I would be glad to see this instrument used by other men, so that reports could be compared.

I wish to thank Dr. G. Kolischer for his interest and suggestions.—*Ill. Med. Journal.*

108 North State street.

CONTRIBUTION TO DISTURBANCES OF THE URO-GENITAL FUNCTION IN DISEASES OF THE POSTERIOR URETHRA, ESPECIALLY OF THE COLLICULUS SEMINALIS

By Dr. J. Leyberg

DISEASE of the posterior urethra may cause disturbances of urination or of the sexual act or of both functions together. Hence the multitudinous manifestations of this condition, such as urgent urination, tickling or burning during micturition, cloudy urination, the presence of shreds in the urine, terminal hematuria, premature ejaculations, sticking pain during ejaculation, unsatisfactory or too frequent erections. The acute cases are of gonorrheal origin and are familiar to all, but those which are more difficult to diagnose run a more chronic course and have no direct relation or perhaps no relation whatever to gonorrhea. The ordinary examination with the air urethroscope does not give a satisfactory view of the sphincter border and of the deep portion of the posterior urethra between the sphincter and the colliculus seminalis.

On the other hand the Goldschmidt irrigation urethroscope gives an especially good view of all parts of the posterior urethra and shows off all the details of the surface of the mucosa, such as polypi, etc., by virtue of the irrigation current. Owing to the magnification brought about by this apparatus it is important to bear in mind that traumas to the mucosa produced by previous instrumentation may assume the appearance of pathological lesions. Thus the author has seen swellings of the crista urethralis, resembling post-gonorrheal infiltrations, resulting from instillations of silver and copper. These two types of tumefaction may be distinguished from each other by the fact that the former disappear spontaneously whereas the latter persist for a long time despite treatment.

The author finds that the difficulty in diagnosing large growths in the colliculus region by means of the Goldschmidt instrument can be largely overcome by introducing the sheathe or the optic in a slightly different manner or by varying the illumination. The irrigation instrument moreover is inferior to the air instrument for the study of pathological variations in circulation and changes in the color and consistency of the object to be examined. It is therefore best for the surgeon to be familiar with both instruments, not only for the purpose of examination but for therapeusis as well. The Goldschmidt instrument for the treatment of the posterior urethra is both complicated and expensive. For the simpler cases (involving local painting and galvanocauterization) the ordinary Loewenhardt or Wossidlo tube is satisfactory; for more complicated conditions the Erich Wossidlo operating urethroscope seems to be of great value.

As an illustration of the usefulness of modern endoscopy for the diagnosis and treatment of conditions of the posterior urethra, the author reports the following cases:

Case 1. Man of 32, who contracted gonorrhea 12 years ago and lues 8 years ago. For past few weeks burning and pain on urination with urgent and frequent micturition. The urine contains shreds and there is terminal hematuria. Erections are painful and there is a sticking pain at the moment of emission. Examination of the expressed prostatic fluid revealed the presence of pus and blood cells. Posterior urethroscopy revealed the presence of a soft, swollen, and bleeding colliculus, to the top of which a small cyst was attached. There were numerous polypoid excrescences in the neighborhood of the vesical sphincter. The sphincter region and the posterior urethra were painted with 20% silver nitrate which was followed by a sharp reaction. A routine of rest in bed, urotropin, and bladder irrigations again improved the patient's condition, the urine becoming clear, and the dysuria ceasing as a result. The sexual difficulties also cleared up and the patient was able to resume his occupation.

Case 2. This patient was a man of 40 who denied venereal infection. For the past 8 years he had practiced coitus interruptus without any apparent injury to his health. For the past year he had been troubled with spontaneous and very painful erections and ejaculatio precox. In addition to this, he had, for the past half year, attacks of severe dysuria and burning and tickling. A No. 18 bougie was introduced into the urethra as far as the posterior portion where a resistance was met with. Urethroscopy showed a large firm colliculus covered with a grayish white layer and with numerous polypoid excrescences projecting from its summit. The growths were then cauterized in successive sittings with the galvanocautery and with 20% silver nitrate, the patient also receiving weak silver nitrate irrigations in the intervals.

Eight weeks after the final treatment the patient was free from his urinary disturbances and his painful erections, and coitus was normal and satisfactory.

Leyberg points out that in general ejaculatio precox and painful erections can be regarded as "irritable weaknesses" only when they appear in the sexual life not as occasional phenomena but as systematically developed and regularly appearing symptoms. In the past history of such patients we find long standing masturbation, coitus interruptus, or other sexual perversion associated with abnormal functioning of the colliculus seminalis. Such sexual "irritable weaknesses," when long continued, and especially in neurasthenic individuals, can doubtlessly lead to psychic impotence, and local treatment alone may not effect a cure. For this reason many neurologists have regarded local treatment as useless. The author, however, believes that the treatment of just such cases is primarily urologic and that very satisfactory and permanent results can be obtained by first explaining to the patient the nature of his weakness and then treating the local condition in an appropriate manner.

Case 3. Patient 28 years of age. Denied venereal disease. Began sexual relations at 18 and continued them in normal fashion for 3 years. During the next 4 years while in the army he avoided coitus for fear of infection. He began to masturbate and allowed himself to become sexually excited in the presence of decent women. This excitement would lead to ejaculation at first with a complete erection and then with incomplete erections. When coitus was subsequently resumed the patient found that libido was weak, erections were poor, and ejaculation was delayed or had to be brought on by manual help. For the past 2 years impotence was complete and for the past year the patient suffered from frequent nocturnal pollutions. Examination revealed a clear urine with shreds, and a somewhat tender prostate. The introduction of a bougie caused pain at the posterior urethra. Urethroscopy, which was repeatedly performed, showed an inflammatory proliferation of the mucosa in the region of the colliculus. The granulation mass was touched, on three successive sittings, with the galvanocautery and painted with 20% silver nitrate. Six months after his discharge the patient reported that he had regained his sexual power completely.

Case 4. Man of 30, several attacks of gonorrhea. For the past few years patient had suffered from typical ejaculatio precox and incomplete erections. Urethroscopic examination revealed old infiltrations of the anterior urethra and a very greatly hypertrophied colliculus. This latter was treated with two applications of the galvanocautery followed by painting with 20% silver nitrate solution. The symptoms disappeared completely despite the fact that all previous treatment had been absolutely fruitless.

THE "WATER-ERROR" IN SALVARSAN INJECTIONS.

By Prof. Rudolf Matzenauer and Dr. Max Hesse

WECHSELMANN was the first to suggest that the presence in the water used for salvarsan injections of bacteria or of their protein metabolic products (toxins and endotoxins), either as a result of transferal during distillation or of development during standing, was the cause of the untoward effects in the intravenous administration of the drug. This suggestion was accepted by many, including Ehrlich, and numerous directions were offered for the preparation of a satistorily pure water.

Wischo, the pharmacist of the University Clinic for Dermatology and Syphilis in Gratz has worked out a method of preparing distilled water so pure that one cubic centimeter contains only from 80 to 320 organisms and that only if examined by the Müller method. This latter is a microscopic procedure by which both living and dead organisms are demonstrable. By the ordinary plate counting method it is only the living organisms which are counted, and of these only those which can develop on gelatin at room temperature. Thus, on examining a water which had been pronounced sterile by the plate method, Wischo was able to estimate 200 organisms per cubic centimeter by the microscopic method. That the water used at the university clinic is of exceptional purity can readily be seen by comparing its bacterial content (as above given) with that of sixteen samples of distilled water obtained from various drugstores in Gratz. In the latter cases the bacterial content varied between 63,000 and 6,050,000 per c.c. About 3000 intravenous injections are given annually at the clinic with only occasional slight rises in temperature. The authors ask: Are these reactions really due to the water injected? Ehrlich and others assume in defense of their position that although the introduction of a moderate number of organisms will not cause trouble in the majority of cases, a certain number of very sensitive individuals will nevertheless react under such circumstances.

Accordingly, the authors began their research with the purpose of finding out just how great a bacterial count the water must have in order to bring out a reaction following a salvarsan injection. They therefore adopted the following standard procedure, in order to rule out all interfering factors: Every injection was made with 0.3 gm. Salvarsan dissolved in 200 c.c. of a 0.5% saline solution. Only such patients were selected as had already received one or two salvarsan injections without reaction, and only those whose syphilitic manifestations were already receding in order that a Herxheimer reaction might be avoided.

The first test was in the nature of a preliminary experiment. The authors wished to determine whether it was really necessary to use freshly prepared water at each injection. Accordingly they preserved their pure water in closed flasks under sterile precautions, first for days, then for weeks, and finally for months, and found that there was absolutely no untoward effect from the use of such solutions. The knowledge of this fact will do much to prevent needless expense and trouble in giving salvarsan injections. The authors were now ready to proceed with their original problem. They began with a water containing 4800 organisms per c.c. and allowed it to stand in an open vessel in the laboratory, for one week at room temperature. At the end of this time its bacterial count was found to be 58,600 per c.c. The water was then sterilized and diluted in various strengths with a bacteria-poor (240 per c.c.) water. Twelve patients were injected with the various dilutions as well as with the full strength (58,600 per c.c.) water, with practically no reactions whatever. Next, a "stronger" water was prepared by exposing it for a month in an open vessel. This specimen contained 427,000 organisms per c.c. Two dilutions were used for injection, and then the original solution, without causing any reactions whatever. The same water was then exposed for a month longer when its bacterial content was found to have reached 1,700,000 per c.c. A dilution containing 850,000 bacteria per c.c., and then the full strength, were used without reaction. The sterile strong solution was then kept for a third month, this time under sterile precautions, in order to see whether the protein decomposition products of so great a number of organisms might bring forth a reaction. This test also proved negative.

How can the above facts be brought in harmony with the theories of Ehrlich and Wechselmann? In the first place they may object that the number of the above experiments is too small to controvert an impression gained from a much larger material. They may again point out that even a water of very great bacterial content does not of necessity *have to*, but merely *may*, bring about a reaction and that conversely it may require a relatively bacteria-poor water to cause untoward results in highly susceptible individuals. Furthermore it may be objected that the water used in the above experiments contained too few organisms, or that these were not of the kind required to bring out a reaction.

In reply to the last objection it may again be pointed out that the water was exposed for weeks at a time in a laboratory where people were constantly working so that it had the best opportunity to serve as a culture medium for every conceivable air and dust bacterium. Similarly it is very unlikely that a bacteria content greater than 1,700,000 per c.c. would ever result from any ordinarily painstaking method of water distillation. Such "strong" waters always contain numerous flocculi.

As regards the objection that the above experiments are too few in number for the establishment of definite conclusions, the authors point out that at the beginning of the salvarsan era they (as well as others) very frequently obtained reactions of such severity that the patients had to be kept in bed after the injection. Surely it is not very likely that at that period waters of a concentration greater than 1,700,000 bacteria per c.c. were used for injection. Indeed, the authors have every reason to assume that the water used at that time was practically as pure as that employed subsequently. When therefore one contrasts the original severe reactions following injections with bacteria-poor waters with the absence of reaction following the injections with bacteria-rich waters made during the above experiments, the contrast is striking though the cases are few, and the conclusion is only natural that the original reactions were not due to the water employed. In the authors' opinion it is equally clear that the toxic effects produced at that time were due to the salvarsan itself and that the dose employed was either absolutely too large, or relatively too large for the case in question.

SPECIAL ABSTRACTS.

BLENORRHAGIC INFLAMMATIONS CAUSED BY THE DIPHTHERIA BACILLUS WITH SPECIAL REFERENCE TO INFECTIONS OF THE VAGINA IN CHILDREN.

By ERWIN KOBRAK, M.D., *Medizinische Klinik, Mar. 8, 1914.*

IT is a well-known fact that a membrane is not always present in inflammations caused by the Klebs-Loeffler bacillus. Thus a typical phlegmonous angina may be caused by this organism and the condition cured by injections of diphtheria antitoxin. The author reports just such a case in a woman whose daughter came down subsequently with a characteristic membranous diphtheria.

Furthermore a diphtherial infection of the nasal mucosa may be manifested only by a thick purulent discharge, no membrane being present, and the clinical picture resemble that of a severe influenza. A similar process may develop in the middle ear. The author also describes a severe and fatal case of non-membranous laryngeal diphtheria which was tracheotomized with the escape of much foul pus. In this family, as in the one previously mentioned, other members were subsequently attacked with typical membranous throat lesions.

It was such observations as these which led Kobrak to study cases of vaginitis in children which clinically resembled gonorrhea, but in which no gonococci were demonstrable in the discharge. These cases are not to be confused with the well-known severe membranous and ulcerating diphtherias of the female genitalia. They are simply fever-free blenorrhagias which do not in any way affect the general condition and occur in children who have no throat or nasal diphtheria.

The author reports two cases in point. The first was that of a nine year old girl who complained of a painful vaginal discharge of three days' duration. There was no fever and only slightly increased pulse rate. The hymen and visible vaginal mucosa were swollen and injected and covered with a yellow discharge. There was no membrane or ulceration. Smears from the discharge showed many pus cells, a few bacilli and cocci, but no gonococci. Cultures revealed the presence of diphtheria baccili. Two thousand units of antitoxin were injected subcutaneously and in three days the discharge had almost ceased, and in ten days the parts had returned to normal. The second case was similar to the first. Smears showed the presence of Klebs-Loeffler bacilli which were recovered in cultures in great numbers. In this case also there was no disturbance in the general condition, but there was pain on urination. All symptoms subsided in two weeks after injection of 2000 units and local treatment with bichloride douches.

The author is convinced that in all such cases of vaginitis where gonococci cannot be demonstrated in the discharge material should be taken for culture. In this way not only may the individual case be rapidly cured by specific treatment, but the infection of susceptible subjects may be prevented as well. The author also points out that the production of pus in response to infection with the diphtheria bacillus does not depend upon the infecting agent so much as it does on a special disposition on the part of the patient. In this way alone—unless we blame it on a mixed infection—can we explain those cases in which the same organism produces an anginal or a purulent form of diphtheria in one member and a typically membranous form in another member of the same family.

THE TREATMENT OF GONORRHEAL COMPLICATIONS WITH GONARGIN.

By JOHANNES HERMANS, M.D., *Medizinische Klinik, Mar. 8, 1914.*

THE author has treated 25 cases of epididymitis, 3 cases of prostatitis, and 3 cases of arthritis with this new preparation of gonococcus vaccine. He gave intragluteal injections and began with doses of 10 million organisms, increasing the dose first to 25 million and then to 50 million after three days' intervals. A fourth dose was given after 3 or 4 days and usually sufficed in the epididymitis cases, but in arthritis one or two more doses were occasionally required. In none of the cases was a local or focal reaction observed. Hermans did not hesitate to inject during the febrile stage as the result was generally a diminution of the fever. In such cases the dose did not exceed 10 million.

The most striking effect of the gonargin injections was a disappearance of the pain. This was especially striking in the epididymitis cases where the swelling also rapidly subsided. The results in the prostatitis cases were not especially striking, but in those of arthritis a rapid improvement was obtained under this treatment. Although the author has not tried it, he suggests that gonargin may be of value in the treatment of cases of chronic gonorrhea with deep infiltrations.

REVIEW OF CURRENT UROLOGIC LITERATURE

JOURNAL D' UROLOGIE

Vol. V, No. 5, May 15, 1914

1. A Case of Pneumaturia.

In general pneumaturia may be due to introduction of air into the bladder during catheterization or injection, or to fistulous communication between the bladder or the intestine, or to spontaneous development of gas in the bladder from glucose fermentation in diabetics, or to gaseous decomposition of blood clots, or finally to the gas producing action of certain bacteria in the bladder.

The case described by the authors is that of a man of 32, who entered the hospital complaining of difficulty in micturition and of expulsion of air at the end of urination. The patient was in good general condition, but was very constipated. When asked to urinate under observation the patient succeeded only with great difficulty and in the squatting posture, the last drops being passed with a very loud gurgling noise. The urine in the glass was mixed with air bubbles. The urine was acid in reaction, containing much indican and leucocytes, and some albumen and red cells (previous gonorrhea and epididymitis). Cystoscopy showed that the vesical mucosa was a little infected, especially at the neck. A specimen of the urine was obtained under sterile precautions and carefully studied. Smears showed the presence of a polymorphous gram-negative bacillus which grew readily on the ordinary culture media with the formation of gas (nature of gas not mentioned.—Ed.). Injections of cultures of the organism as well as of the urine into animals caused death in a few hours. The original bacillus was recovered from cultures from the various body fluids.

The organism did not agglutinate with the patient's serum, although the same bacillus was recovered from the stools. The treatment of the case consisted in disinfection of the urine with urotropin and of the bladder locally with silver nitrate instillations on the one hand, and of thorough catharsis on the other. In less than a month the patient left the hospital, cured. A year later he was still free from pneumaturia. The authors believe that in their case the organism originated in the intestinal tract.

2. End-results of Circular Urethrorrhaphies, etc.

Marion believes that the best treatment for ruptures of the urethra is a circular urethrorrhaphy supplemented by a suprapubic cystostomy for deviation of the urinary current. This procedure ensures a rapid cicatrization and a persistence of the canal of the urethra. In addition to urethral ruptures, traumatic and inflammatory strictures and perineal fistulæ may be treated in this manner. Marion outlines the procedure in the following steps:

1. Suprapubic cystostomy. 2. Introduction of a Béniqué sound through the cystostomy wound into the neck of the bladder. 3. Perineal section. 4. Determination of the urethral ends with the aid of a sound introduced through the meatus as well as the one from the bladder. 5. Freshening the two ends of the canal. 6. Union of the two ends about a large size catheter. Two supporting sutures may be placed on the anterior end if necessary. 7. Closure of the perineal wound, deep tissues; skin left open. 8. Introduction of supra-pubic drainage tube and withdrawal of urethral catheter about which suture was effected.

The author next emphasizes certain features in the technic which he regards as important and then reports ten cases which have been successfully treated. In very extensive contusions of the urethra a perfect approximation of the torn ends should not be attempted, for the amount of resection necessary to arrive at healthy tissues would be too great for a perfect technical result. Also in ruptures of the membranous urethra associated with fractures of the pelvis a circular urethrorrhaphy should not be attempted, first, because of the great difficulty of its accomplishment and secondly, because such ruptures rarely lead to stricture and are always readily dilatable. In such cases therefore it is much better to let the urethra reconstruct itself as best it can about a permanent catheter, and if a stricture or fistula should result to deal with that later in the best manner available.

3. Treatment of Acute Gonorrhea with Atoxic Vaccine.

Jungano has attempted to duplicate the results of Nicolle and Blaizot who claim to have cured acute gonorrheas with 5 to 6 injections of their vaccine, given every other day. The author divided his cases into 3 series. In the first the vaccine treatment was employed alone. There was no improvement in any of the cases after 7 injections. In the second series the vaccine was used together with permanganate irrigations. The cases were cured in from 16 to 24 days. In the third series permanganate injections were used alone. The cases were cured in from 5 to 20 days.

The author next takes up the entire question of antigonorrheal vaccine therapy and shows that despite the source of the vaccine, whether heterogenous, autogenous, or polyvalent, and despite its dosage, whether one million or several billion, it has given but very questionable results. In fact it seems to be the consensus of opinion that vaccines are useless unless supplemented by local treatment. The author is not prejudiced against vaccine therapy as such but believes that we should be more prudent than to offer our patients, especially our genito-urinary cases, a remedy which, after a short period of enthusiasm, renders them still more neurasthenic and still more skeptical.

4. Regional and Local Anesthesia in Urology.

Lemoine takes up in detail the innervation of the pelvic organs as well as the technic of regional and local anesthesia of the parts under consideration. He describes in full the manner of injecting the dorsal and lumbar nerves (method of Sellheim-Kappis), of the sacral nerves (method of Danis), of barrier infiltration (method of Hacken Bruch) and of epidural injection (method of Cathelin-Läwen).

He concludes that the injection of the dorsal and lumbar nerves at the emergence through the intervertebral foramina (after Sellheim-Kappis) is simple and free from danger. Anesthesia of the first, and second lumbar nerves however may be replaced by infiltration of their terminal branches in the inguinal canal in case of operations on the testicle. For anesthesia of the pelvis the method of Danis of Brussels (injection into the sacral foramina) is unquestionably the most elegant, the most simple and the freest from danger. Epidural injections have not given good results in the author's hands.

5. Intravesical Extirpation of Extensive Papillomata of Peri-ureteral Origin.

The author reports two cases in which the tumor was so large that even after the bladder was opened and the growth lifted off the surrounding mucosa no ureteral orifice could be identified on the corresponding side. Rolando therefore suggests that in similar cases the procedure should be as follows: After opening and inspecting the bladder if no ureteric meatus is visible the surgeon should ligate the tumor above its implantation and remove it distal to the ligature. The removal may be done with the thermo- or electro cautery, or if the ligature is trustworthy, with the scissors. The curved clamp of Guyon should not be used, as by its size, it interferes with the inspection of the bladder. Having removed the bulk of the tumor and controlled hemorrhage the ureteric orifice is easily identified no matter what its position. The operation is then completed by excising the pedicle (e.g., by an elliptical incision) taking care not to involve the ureter in the subsequent hemostasis and mucosal suture.

6. Renal Tuberculosis and the Constant of Ambard.

The patient had a left renal tuberculosis and a severe tuberculous cystitis. Cystoscopy was first attempted but only the right ureter could be catheterized. Comparison of the urine obtained through the catheter with that obtained from the bladder (representing the left kidney urine) showed that the left kidney excreted pus but it also excreted more urea and more chlorides than did the right kidney. The coefficient of Ambard was 0.130, showing a bilateral renal involvement. In order to avoid all doubt as to the findings a cystostomy was performed and both ureters catheterized through the open bladder. The same result was obtained as in the first case. The author then decided, in spite of the high coefficient, and the paradoxical urea excretion to remove the left kidney. However a preliminary exploration of the right kidney was done which was found to be normal in all respects save that it was somewhat smaller than the average. The left kidney of course showed tuberculosis.

Determination of the blood urea after the operation showed that this substance kept increasing under superalimentation, but as soon as the patient was put on a low-nitrogen diet the urea values diminished to normal. Effectual diuresis was established after the operation and the patient did well despite the persistence of a suprapubic fistula.

7. Renal Tuberculosis in Abnormal Form.

A woman of 39 complained of attacks of left lumbar pain radiating to the groin. There was marked pyuria. The left kidney was not palpable but there was tenderness in the left costovertebral angle and along the course of the ureter. Cystoscopy revealed a diffuse redness of the bas-fond and a bullous edema about the left ureteral orifice. Catheterization of the ureters showed that the left kidney urine contained pus and less urea than that from the right side. The diagnosis was then made of a left pyelitis of intestinal origin with or without a complicating stone. The general condition of the patient was excellent. On the other hand the fact that the patient had never menstruated rendered possible the existence of a horse-shoe kidney. However an X-ray taken with X-ray catheters in place showed that the ureters were normal on both sides. In addition the plate revealed a row of irregular shadows alongside the spinal column on the left side and a mass of shadows in the left kidney region.

At this stage, when the diagnosis was by no means certain, the inoculation test came back positive. A left nephrectomy was done. The surface of the kidney was found studded with hard granules which proved to be calcified tubercles. There were similar granules on the cut surface as well as two abscess cavities filled with cheesy material. Radiography of the fresh specimen again showed the shadows seen in the original photograph. These were therefore calcified tubercles and the chain along the spinal column, calcified lymph nodes.

8. Expulsion of a Ureteral Calculus after Injection of Glycerin.

In July, 1909, the patient began to complain of marked pollakiuria. At the end of that month he suffered a short attack of appendicitis which was repeated about 15 times up to the day of his admission to the hospital in October. Examination revealed tenderness at McBurney's point and a cord like structure resembling the appendix could be rolled under the fingers. The urine was negative. At the operation the appendix was found adherent and distinctly hyperemic. Pathological examination revealed an acute process engrafted upon a chronic appendicitis. Recovery was normal except that nine days post operative there was an attack of pain in the right iliac fossa and smarting in the urethra on urination. The urine however showed no sediment.

Nevertheless the patient remained well until September, 1913, when he began again to have pain in the right loin. These attacks began in the right lumbar region, radiated to the right loin and to the end of the penis. During the crisis the patient would urinate very frequently, as often as every ten minutes. The urine was negative, but from the very first attack there were alternations of constipation and diarrhea. On examination the right kidney was thought to be a little enlarged and somewhat tender to pressure. The urine was again negative. X-ray examination revealed a small shadow in the pelvis which might have been a calculus in the ureter. Cystoscopy showed the right ureteric orifice to be a little red and edematous. Indigocarmine was eliminated from the left side after seven minutes, from the right side after eleven minutes and then but poorly. An X-ray catheter was introduced into the right ureter for a distance of 20 centimeters and a radiograph taken which proved that the shadow was actually in relation to the ureter.

A few days later the same side was again catheterized and 12 c.c. of glycerine injected into the pelvis and along the ureter. Forty-eight hours later the patient experienced a peculiar sensation in the right iliac fossa and subsequently passed a calculus while urinating. The stone was of the form and size of two rice kernels stuck together at an obtuse angle and covered with sharp points. The symptoms ceased at once after its expulsion. The author believes that the extrusion of the calculus was greatly facilitated by the previous introduction of the X-ray catheter and its retention in situ for several hours while the pictures were being taken.

9. Operative Intervention in Cystic Disease of the Kidney.

From his studies of the question the author concludes that, cystic disease of the kidney being most often bilateral, treatment should not be regarded as curative but merely as palliative. The indications for intervention are: 1. Intolerable pain. 2. Suppuration in the cysts. 3. Persistent hematurias. 4. Hydronephrosis. 5. Displacement of the kidney. 6. Anuria. 7. Intestinal obstruction.

Before operating it is essential to be assured of the function of the supposedly healthy kidney by examination of the separate kidney urines. If one kidney functions well a nephrectomy on the other side is justifiable in the presence of the indications enumerated above and the impossibility of any other procedure. If the presumably healthy kidney is found to be incapable of carrying on uropoiesis, or both kidneys are simply polycystic, conservative operations are indicated.

In the case of a suppurating kidney nephrotomy may be performed if absolutely necessary, but this should never be attempted in the case of anuria as has been recommended. If we are dealing with a large, displaced, and movable polycystic kidney which is tender, nephropexy may be done together with decapsulation and excision of the cysts.

In all other cases we should reject the method of puncture and excision of the cysts with marsupialization and carry out if possible either a partial nephrectomy, or better still, decapsulation with excision of all the cysts. The author feels that much good can be accomplished by rational surgery in this heretofore baffling disease.

10. The Three Glass Test in Urology.

In carrying out the ordinary three glass test the patient has to stop the stream of urine while the glasses are being changed. It goes without saying that this is a very disagreeable feature and that oftentimes, owing to the patient's awkwardness the test has to be repeated several times before the proper results are obtained. As a matter of fact the sudden stoppage of the urinary current causes a wave of back pressure into the bladder which disturbs the previous sedimentation in the bas-fond and introduces a source of error into the test. In order to perfect the technic the author suggests the following procedure: The three glasses are set on a table at the height of the patient's pelvis in such a way that their walls almost touch each other and while the patient urinates naturally and continuously they are passed in turn under the stream.

MISCELLANEOUS ABSTRACTS.

Prolonged Priapism treated by Drainage of the Corpora Cavernosa.

A Chalier and J. Gaté (*Lyon Médical,* Apr. 12, p. 805).— A man, aged 22, was admitted to hospital for priapism which had lasted 8 days. Three years previously in the course of an attack of typhoid fever he had suffered from severe phlebitis of the veins of the left lower limb, which remained swollen for several months. Since that time the superficial veins of the abdominal wall in the hypogastrium and left iliac fossa had been dilated. There was no history of venereal disease and the patient was in good health and fond of athletics.

Three weeks before he had a fatiguing day, hill climbing. During the night an erection occurred, persisted for 48 hours, and ceased spontaneously. After another excursion a fortnight later he had gone to bed late after drinking more wine than usual. During the night he was awakened by the desire to urinate and there was an erection. He passed urine without difficulty but the erection, which was not accompanied by any sexual desire, did not subside and the organ became increasingly painful. He did not seek advice for 3 days. He was then treated with bromide of potassium, chloral and syrup of codeine and ordered a hot bath every 3 hours with hip baths during the intervals. These measures were continued for 5 days without success. The local condition was unchanged, the pain increased, and he was unable to sleep.

After admission the baths and sedatives were continued for 2 days but without improvement. Next day a puncture was made with a large trocar at the base of the penis on the left side, and 3 or 4 c.c. of blackish tarry blood escaped. This gave some relief and the penis diminished in size and consistence but did not become normal. In the evening it resumed its former condition and the pain returned with all its previous severity. During the following 3 days a further unsuccessful attempt was made to treat the patient by drugs. The condition having then persisted for 14 days it was decided to operate. The penis was in complete erection but the glans and corpus spongiosum were not involved. The corpora cavernosa were hard and distended, with fluctuation at some points and extremely tender throughout. The perineum was slightly red and the patient had considerable difficulty in urinating, which he accomplished most easily in the genupectoral position. There was severe pain and the temperature had risen to 103°.

Under anesthesia the corpus carvernosum on each side was incised in the perineum, a small quantity of dark tarry blood escaped, and the rigidity of the organ diminished. An incision was made at the base of the penis which opened the urethra, and showed that the corpus spongiosum was slightly swollen but filled with blood, which was normal in color. The urethra was closed by 3 catgut sutures and a catheter was easily inserted into the bladder. A second incision was then made in each corpus cavernosum just behind the prepuce and a considerable quantity of dark blood evacuated. Drains were then passed by means of a pair of forceps from these anterior incisions to the perineal openings on each side so as to drain both corpora cavernosa in their whole extent. Some dark blood escaped but no further hemorrhage occurred.

On the following day the temperature had fallen to 100° and the patient was much relieved. A large quantity of dark fluid had escaped into the dressings and the penis was reduced in size and much softer in consistence. Rapid improvement followed and the drains were removed at the end of a week. He left hospital 16 days after the operation. The dilated veins on the abdominal wall were no longer visible. The other organs were healthy and there was no enlargement of the spleen or other sign of leukemia, with which priapism is frequently associated. During the time he remained in hospital and for at least a month after the operation no erections occurred. Seven months after the operation he was reported to be in good health and about to be married.

There was no sexual excess which many writers have regarded as the exciting cause in cases of this kind. The writer considers the priapism due to thrombosis, to which the patient was subject, after unusual fatigue and slight alcoholic excess. While spontaneous recovery under sedatives is possible in the majority of cases of priapism, a fatal result may follow in the absence of efficient treatment. Spontaneous recovery is very gradual, requiring weeks or even months, during which the patient may suffer severely. Incision and drainage of the corpora cavernosa give immediate relief and usually speedy recovery, but restoration of the functional power of the penis is slowly regained and often remains absent. In this respect the results of operation appear to compare favorably with that in cases treated medically. Of 48 cases collected by Terrier and Dujarier only 10 were treated surgically with 3 excellent functional results while of the remaining 38 cases in only 3 is functional recovery noted. Operation is therefore advisable when improvement has not followed the usual treatment in a few days.

Plaut-Vincent's Ulcerative Stomatitis Mistaken for Syphilis.

Tièche (*Corr.-Bl. f. Schweizer Aerzte,* Dec. 20, p. 1698).— This condition is on simple inspection of the buccal cavity, uncontrolled by a Wassermann test and bacteriological examination, liable to be mistaken for secondary or tertiary syphilis. The serious nature of such a mistake renders this comparatively rare disease important.

Case 1.—A man, aged 27, of loose sexual habits, noticed early in January an inflammatory condition of the gums. There was profuse purulent discharge which in a short time subsided. About the same time a redness appeared near the last molar tooth; this gradually developed into a dirty, yellowish ulcer. Various mouth washes and the application of silver nitrate and other caustics failed to promote healing. The ulcer became more and more painful, and both the attending practitioner and his dentist advised an antisyphilitic course. The writer saw him on Mar. 27.

There was an ulcer with an irregular edge, and a yellowish green slimy base, which appeared to be formed by the coalescence of several smaller circular ulcers. It was about 1⅕ in. long, and ⅘ in. wide, and in places was deep. The edges were not raised and were surrounded by diffuse redness. It extended from the angle of the jaw on to the mucous membrane of the cheek. In its immediate neighborhood were 2 smaller ulcers. The consistence of the ulcers did not differ from that of the surrounding normal tissues. On pressure the surface readily bled. There were no enlarged lymphatic glands and the mouth and pharynx were otherwise normal. A smear preparation showed numerous Plaut-Vincent bacilli and spirochetes. The same organisms were seen in preparations made by removal of fragments of tissue with the sharp spoon and compressing them between two coverslips. Wassermann's reaction was negative.

He was treated by an intravenous injection of 0.3 gm. of neo-salvarsan and local applications of a 3 per cent. solution of peroxide of hydrogen and a solution (1 in 10) of old salvarsan. Eight days later the ulcer had healed. But several relapses occurred, and the Plaut-Vincent bacillus and spirochetes were found in a small ulcer on July 8. Wassermann remained negative. He was then lost sight of.

Case 2.—A single woman, aged 20, noticed a painful swelling of the glands in the left submaxillary region 3 days after a visit to the dentist. There was a dirty ulcer, which extended from the left angle of the jaw on to the mucous membrane of the cheek. A practitioner diagnosed primary syphilis, and after a consultation with two confrères, early in July, began an energetic anti-syphilitic course. After 5 mercurial injections there was no improvement, and on Aug. 12 the girl consulted the writer.

There was an ulcer at the angle of the jaw ⅘ in. long and ⅗ in. wide of the same character as that in Case 1. The base was covered with grayish-green pus, which contained numerous spirochetes and fusiform bacilli. The surface bled readily and was soft. The neighboring mucosa was intensely red. Wassermann negative. The ulcer was treated by mopping with a 3 per cent. solution of hydrogen peroxide and painting with a solution of old salvarsan (0.1 gm. to 10 of water). Healing was complete in a few days, and there has been no relapse. Wassermann on Sept. 17 and again on Oct. 20 was negative.

The spirochetes in both cases stained deeply with Giemsa's solution. There was no such close resemblance to the spirocheta pallida as is alleged in the case of spirocheta microdentium. It was impossible to decide whether the spirocheta dentium, Vincenti, or buccalis was the one involved, because some specimens had 8 spirals and some only 5 or even 3. But as most authorities consider the spirochetes in these cases to be of secondary significance, the question was not of great importance. The long fusiform bacilli found in the mouth are distinct from the shorter forms with rounded but not pointed ends present in balanitis erosiva circinata, though some authorities consider the differences to depend on differences of soil rather than species. On this view the variety of balanitis in question would be caused by contact with saliva.

Neither patient had had tonsillitis. Possibly in Case 1 the ulcer was preceded by and due to pyorrhea alveolaris. In the second case the infection was probably contracted during dental operations or the buccal mucosa was so injured that the bacteria of the mouth produced the ulcer. The diagnosis is complicated by the fact that ulcers due to malignant growths or tuberculosis may become secondarily infected with the Plaut-Vincent bacillus. If primary syphilis is suspected, as in Case 2, it would not be justifiable to wait until a Wassermann test gave a positive reaction before beginning treatment, as the chances of permanent cure would be thereby reduced. Repeated examination for the spirocheta pallida should be made, and treatment begun as soon as it is found.

What is the Value of a Positive Wassermann Reaction?

Nicolas and Gate found the Wassermann reaction positive in 39 per cent. of the non-syphilitics examined, and draw the following conclusions (*Ann. de Derm. et de Syph.*, April, 1914): — Wassermann's reaction is positive in syphilis with more or less frequency. In no case does a negative reaction allow the denial of the existence of the disease or show a cure. It is influenced very irregularly by antisyphilitic treatment to which it can in no case serve as a guide. The reactivations of Wassermann's reaction by treatment are likewise irregular and inconstant. The reaction is positive without doubt in persons who present no sign of syphilis, and have no specific history, in whom the reaction is an isolated symptom. By reference to the table which the authors put at the end of their paper, it will be seen that in a number of cases the test was made twice on non-syphilitics; the reaction was positive at one time and negative at another, sometimes very positive at first and then negative; sometimes very negative at first and later positive.

Amebic Cystitis.

W. Fischer (*Münch. Med. Woch.*, Mar. 3, p. 473).—A Chinaman, aged 30, consulted the writer in Shanghai, for strangury, dribbling of urine, and pain in the region of the bladder. Three years previously he had had gonorrhea. There was no history of dysentery and when seen there were no intestinal symptoms. The urine, whether passed spontaneously or obtained by catheter, was turbid. In the sediment were a number of polymorphonuclear neutrophile leucocytes. No cocci or bacilli were present, but there were a large number of amebæ. These, morphologically, resembled the ameba tetragena commonly found in cases of dysentery in China and contained numerous vacuoles. There was no urethral stricture. Evidently the purulent cystitis was of amebic origin. How the amebæ gained access to the bladder could not be ascertained, as the man was seen only once. Most probably he had previously had an attack of dysentery or was an amebae-carrier.

Amebæ have only rarely been observed in the bladder. Bâlz, in 1883, published a case of a tuberculous Japanese woman, aged 23, who suffered with strangury and hematuria. The bladder contained large amebæ. It was assumed they had entered the urethra during bathing. Posner, in 1893, described a case in which a man, aged 37, who had never been out of Germany, was seized with a rigor and hematuria. The urine contained leucocytes, erythrocytes, and numerous amebæ. The disease persisted for over a year with several acute exacerbations. Posner believed the amebæ had entered the renal pelves. Morphologically they resembled dysentery amebæ. Kartulis also found amebæ in the bladder of a man, aged 58, with a vesical tumor.

THE AMERICAN JOURNAL OF UROLOGY, VENEREAL AND SEXUAL DISEASES
WILLIAM J. ROBINSON, M.D., EDITOR

VOL. X DECEMBER, 1914 No. 12

THE DANGERS CONNECTED WITH REMOVAL OF THE SEMINAL VESICLES

By CHARLES GREENE CUMSTON, M.D., Geneva, Switzerland.
Privat-docent at the Faculty of Medicine; Honorary Member of the Urological Society of Belgium; Corresponding Member of the Urological Association of France, etc.

THE removal of the seminal vesicles is not the simple operation that certain enthusiastic members of the profession would have us believe, and if the truth be plainly stated it most usually results in operative complications which, occasionally, may really be of serious import. These complications are of two kinds, viz.: those arising during the operation itself, such as rupture of the vas deferens; and the post-operative complications, as suppuration and fistulæ. Undoubtedly, those complications vary according to the technique employed, and in what is to follow I shall consider the anterior, inferior and posterior routes in turn.

One word relative to the surgical anatomy of the seminal vesicles. When the inguinal route is chosen for their ablation one should be careful to spare the epigastric artery, which will be found at the internal inguinal ring after the canal has been incised. Then the fascia transversalis is brought to view and inwardly, Hesselbach's ligament. This fascia is split and then the vas deferens is seen lying against the peritoneum and holding up a triangular layer of cellular tissue. The vas must be carefully freed and one should avoid the pelvic walls against which the vesicular space lies. Below the vas one finds in the following order, the obturator vessels, the fibrous cord representing the débris of the umbilical artery, and the ureter. These structures are to be avoided by drawing the vas upwards and inwardly. By this means a transversal layer is exposed which covers the genital space and this is incised on the outer aspect, at the same time ligating the vessels which are in the direct neighborhood of the incision.

By the perineal route the skin and subcutaneous fat are incised and then the superficial perineal aponeurosis, and one thus exposes the urethral bulb covered by the fibers of the bulbocavernosus muscle and on to the anorectal septum. Then come the superficial and deep transversalis, while on the inner boundaries lie the levator ani. Between the latter the membranous urethra lies in front and the rectum in the back, united by the rectourethral muscle. When this muscle is cut close to the urethra, one enters into the proper area, the so-called retroprostatic space, which is normally a virtual cavity between the prostate and posterior periprostatic aponeurosis. One should avoid keeping too far back, because in this case one will enter behind the posterior periprostatic aponeurosis into an improper space which will be created artificially and corresponds to the detachable prerectal space of Quénu and Hartmann. By following the above description the genital space is reached and one proceeds to break down the existing adhesions, bearing in mind that the peritoneum lies above and to the back, the ureter above and forwards, the vascular pedicle outwardly.

The ischiorectal route leads one directly into the ischiorectal space whose upper and internal wall, formed by the levator ani, is incised. One then comes upon the lateral aponeurosis of the prostate, then the organ itself and the genital space is reached below and outwardly.

In the coccyperineal route the bony landmarks of the ischium and coccyx must first be found. There under the skin one finds the fibers of the gluteus major, the levator ani and the left ischiococcygeal and outwardly the lower end of the sacrum and the coccyx. Lastly, farther on, the deep perineal aponeurosis must be incised on its outer aspect in order to avoid the rectum. In most subjects this is deviated to the right and surrounded by loose cellular tissue which can be easily detached by the finger. Below, the hard cord formed by the middle hemorrhoidal artery is recognized, while the posterior periprostatic aponeurosis forms the posterior wall of the genital space.

In the sacral and parasacral routes one incises successively the skin and fat, the aponeurosis, the sacrum; then the rectum is pushed aside and the posterior periprostatic aponeurosis is exposed.

Let us now consider the difficulties and dangers of the anterior route, and in the first place let me say that the suprapubic technique is extremely dangerous and should be discarded completely. Of three cases operated by this way, two died from shock on account of the length of time required to remove the vesicles. Then, in this operation, there is always danger of injuring the bladder.

Now, although the inguinal route does not give place to so much disturbance as do the posterior routes, it however offers serious operative difficulties, which in order of frequency are: (1) rupture of the vas deferens. This accident occurs so frequently that it alone condemns this technique and out of a total of seven instances published by Burcker (Trése, Paris, 1910) in three this accident occurred. Let me add, however, that in two the vas could be got hold of and the operation carried to a successful end. Weir commenced the removal of the vesicles by the inguinal route but was obliged to complete the operation through the perineum, and if I am rightly informed, even Fuller, expert as he is in this matter, was unable to remove the vesicles by this route. Others have been equally unsuccessful. It requires only slight traction on the vas to cause its rupture.

Two contingencies are to be considered according to whether the rupture occurs before or after the opening of the genital space. If the latter has not been opened the rupture arises at most any point on the vas, due to conditions quite impossible to explain. The experiments of Platon and Belosoroff on the cadaver show that in eight the vas ruptured at a point between 30 and 40 centimetres, and in seven between 20 and 30 centimetres of its length. If, on the other hand, the genital space has been opened and the adhesions are broken down while drawing on the vas near its end, a more or less considerable portion of the ampulla may be torn away and even part of the vesicle along with it, this circumstance varying according to the amount of the dissection at the time of rupture. Consequently, it would seem that in the living subject the vas ruptures a few centimetres from or at its junction with the vesicle, tearing away with it a portion of the latter, because very dense adhesions attach these organs to the neighboring viscera, particularly the rectum. The terminal portion of the vas and the vesicle form a point of resistance and it is the undissected portion which is torn away. The tuberculous lesions are more intense at this point, rendering it more fragile, thus predisposing the structure to rupture.

Tearing the peritoneum, although infrequent, has been reported by Weir, Baudet and Villard, but in each instance an immediate suture obviated the dangers of infection. Such an accident could result in most serious consequences because the perivesicular tissues would be most propitious for the diffusion of infection. In one instance, reported by Robinson, this surgeon was compelled to open the peritoneum in order to completely isolate the vas.

Wounds of the ureter would seem to be the most serious operative accident, but I am aware of only one case where this happened, that reported by Villard. The ureter was at once sutured with no untoward result. Tears of the vesicle are very common and are all the more troublesome because it is not an easy matter to ligate the vessels, so that gauze packing must be resorted to, which does not always control the oozing, which greatly hinders the completion of the operation. The oozing is not dangerous, however, except that it may result in a suppurating hematoma.

Suppuration is frequent because at the time of removing the vesicles other foci may require treatment and no matter how careful the surgeon may be in his asepsis it is most difficult to eliminate the chance of infection. Drainage after this technique is difficult and the suppuration continues. Wounds of the bladder should not occur if the operator is careful.

The complications that may accrue by the *perineal route* are of two kinds, viz.: those of the inguinal, and those pertaining to the perineal stage of the operation. The inguinal stage presents the same complications as in the inguinal route already considered. However, if the operation is begun by the perineum, the vas is more easily detached and less strong traction upon it is necessary than when it is still adherent to the vesicle. Thus, the danger of its rupture is much less than by the inguinal method. The other complications, such as opening the peritoneum, are in direct relation to the depth at which the section of the vas is made. The perineal stage is the most fertile for accidents of all kinds which are the result of the numerous operative difficulties presented. The field of operation is deep and even prostatectomy is not always an easy matter by the perineum, as all well know, and it is far more complicated in vesiculectomy, particularly with that portion of the vas which has not been removed by the inguinal route.

According to Fiolle, the base of the vesicles is seated at

from six to seven centimetres from the most elevated portion of the prostate and thus it is readily conceived at what depth one operates. It is to these technical difficulties that are due the rather large number of operative complications.

Isolation of the vesicle is the most difficult step in the technique and the organ may only be removed piecemeal, so that there is considerable chance of its incomplete ablation, and Gueillot is of opinion that morcellation is necessary in most cases. Rupture of the vas during the perineal stage is uncommon but in a case reported by Roux a portion of the vas was left in the pelvis. Although no unfortunate result arose the danger of possible inflammatory complications in such a case is only too clear. Hemorrhage is quite frequent and all the more unfortunate because it is almost an impossibility to ligate the deep seated vessels. It is more frequent when the vesicles have been completely dissected out and the amount of blood lost may be considerable because the terminal branches of the vesicular artery are torn. Gauze packing seems the most rational way of controlling the hemorrhage because, as has been pointed out, it is quite impossible to ligate the offending vessels. I have had my own little experience in vesiculotomy and removal of the vesicles by the perineal route, and although no disaster has ever befallen me, I am free to confess that it is one of the most difficult operations in surgery, no matter what may be said to the contrary.

Urinary fistulæ, resulting from wounds to the ureter, is a frequent complication. Out of a total of thirty cases collected by Baudet and Kendirdjy there were nine instances of this complication. According to these writers the accident takes place at the time the prostate is freed from the rectum, particularly when the prerectal tissue is indurated and fibrous. These fistulæ are usually very long in closing. Baudet points out that these fistulæ may also be due to section of the ejaculatory ducts, as occurred in his case.

Although drainage is more easily obtained through the perineum, the great depth of the operative field and the so frequent lesions of perivesiculitis from which pus escapes, make suppuration quite as frequent in the perineal, as in the inguinal route.

Among the more uncommon complications may be mentioned opening the rectum. This usually is the result of the perivesiculitis giving rise to many adhesions with the surrounding viscera, thus preventing separation of the intestine. All these operative possibilities naturally darken the prognosis and has caused the perineal route to be rejected by many surgeons who have preferred methods of access to the vesicles which cause much more traumatism; I refer to the sacral and para-sacral methods which I shall now consider under the heading of posterior routes.

The considerable anatomical destruction produced by these procedures, which in itself is quite enough to reject these operations, which give rise to about the same surgical accidents. These are so certain to occur in the sacral route that it would seem that the coccyperineal technique should give better results but is not free from danger. In spite of the similarity of the complications I have thought best, in order to be perfectly clear, to divide what is to follow according to the type of intervention employed, and first the sacral method will be considered.

In sections of bone so considerable as those necessitated in this method, hemostasis is naturally particularly difficult. Then there is the difficulty of removing the seminal vesicles themselves, the object of the operation. This difficulty, which is also inherent to the anterior and inferior routes and which made some surgeons resort to the sacral route for this very reason, is not avoided. Rupture of the ureter likewise occurs, usually at the time of, or just after the vesicle has been freed from the adhesions and dissected out of its bed. Extirpation of a portion of the prostate along with the vesicle, so as not to be obliged to separate the two organs by dissection, has also been recommended.

Urinary fistulæ are common sequels on account of the great frequency of injuries to the ureter. They are long in closing and frequently compromise the results of the operation. As to suppuration, it is also the rule. The parasacral route has not been employed to any extent and the number of interventions is small but, generally speaking, it presents no advantages over the sacral route. The coccyperineal route, without presenting any advantages, offers the same difficulties in reaching the vesicles and the same operative accidents, but it would seem that fistulæ are particularly frequent. Then too, this route has the added disadvantage of the proximity of the anus which may result in infection of the wound. As a conclusion, it may be said that these routes should never be employed, excepting, perhaps, in very exceptional cases. The removal of the vas and vesicles should be considered as a treatment rarely to be employed other than in a limited number of selected cases, otherwise simple vasoepididymectomy is the operation of choice.

PROGRESS IN THE DIAGNOSIS AND TREATMENT OF SYPHILIS*

By John H. Cunningham, Jr., M.D., Boston.

IF modern thought has any new truths to contribute to the inherited stock of medical wisdom, it is because we are in a position to study more exactly the forces and conditions.

Until within the past few years our knowledge of syphilis has not been of a scientific character; the parasite causing the disease was unknown and the personal equation in the establishment of the diagnosis was too often an important factor in the recognition of this disease, and treatment was conducted in a most arbitrary and unreliable manner. We did not possess much inherited knowledge in regard to this disease based upon physical observation; the opportunity for which has been great, syphilis being one of the most universal diseases, and no organ in the body being exempt from its effects.

Syphilis has been recognized by the modern world since about 1494, at which time it appeared among the soldiers in the army of Charles VIII, then King of France. It spread rapidly over Europe and has become one of the common diseases in all civilized countries. The weight of evidence seems to be that the disease was introduced into civilization by Christopher Columbus's men, and that it was acquired by them on the Island of Hayti.

Syphilis, gonorrhea, and chancroid were considered as the same disease until about 100 years ago, when Phillippe Ricord proved that syphilis and gonorrhea were distinct diseases and established the theory for primary, secondary and tertiary syphilis. The discovery of the gonococcus by Neisser and Bassereau's work, differentiating true chancre from chancroid, established these three diseases as distinct, and from that time they have been clearly separated. Since syphilis has been considered as an entity observations have established the facts that syphilis is an infectious disease, acquired by contagion or heredity, chronic in its cause, intermittent in its character, and may involve any structure of the body. We have inherited the knowledge that the acquired disease begins as in the eroded, indurated papule, at the point of inocu-

* Read before the Worcester District Medical Society, Nov. 12, 1913.

lation,' within a few weeks (usually three) after contact with the virus, the lesion being known as the chancre, and that accompanying the chancre there are associated changes in the adjacent lymph nodes, characteristic inasmuch as they are small, shotty, hard and discrete, except when the chancre is secondarily infected with pyogenic organism. We have the knowledge that within a few weeks following the appearance of the chancre (usually six) there is a general infection manifested by characteristic exanthemata, upon the skin and mucous membrane, a characteristic general glandular involvement, and perhaps an iritis or a periostitis. We have been aware that after all symptoms and lesions have disappeared, that the disease may again manifest itself in a variety of forms which we have termed tertiary lesions, and that a group of symptoms may appear which are really syphilitic in origin but which may not be clearly correlated with syphilis and are termed the parasyphilides, as, for example, tabes and general paralysis.

We have been well informed that a child born of syphilitic parents may inherit the disease, and that the disease may manifest itself in one way or another at any period of subsequent life, and that the majority of miscarriages are due to infection by this disease. Also that the disease may remain latent in the offspring of syphilitic parents and manifest itself in future generations.

All medical men have been aware of these general facts relative to the disease for many years; also that the lesions of this disease may usually be controlled by mercury and by the iodides. Clinical experience has proven it advisable to continue the administration of these drugs for many months after the secession of all symptoms in an attempt to prevent a reappearance of the lesions which experience has likewise taught us to anticipate. We know that the reappearance of lesions and the development of the parasyphilides in those considered well treated has left us without any certainty as to the effectiveness of our treatment. And so we have been aware for years that our inherited knowledge has not given us in this disease all that we have had in many other diseases.

New facts of primary importance have developed, which new truths added to our inherited stock of knowledge furnish us with an intelligent foundation for the treatment of this disease equalled by few and surpassed by none.

The investigations as to the etiological factors in the causation of syphilis, which have been conducted for years, terminated with the discovery of the Treponema pallidum or Spirocheta pallida by Schaudinn and Hoffmann in 1905. The importance of this discovery and the subsequent work proving the Treponema pallidum to be the etiological factor of syphilis has been great. As a direct result of this discovery we were given within two years the Wassermann test, which no longer leaves the diagnosis of syphilis in doubt, and makes the treatment of this disease no longer a matter of guess work. The establishment of the fact that syphilis was due to a spirillosis led Ehrlich, who was studying the effect of arsenic preparations on animals infected with different spirilla, to apply his new principle of chemotherapy to animals infected with the spirilla of syphilis and later to syphilis in the human. So it has come about since 1905 that we have learned to recognize the parasite of this widespread and important disease; to have been given a sero-diagnostic test which establishes the presence or absence of the disease in doubtful cases; and a new therapeutic measure which controls the disease far better than any measure heretofore known.

This remarkable sequence of scientific events following rapidly upon one another has aroused an unusual interest in the minds of the medical profession of the world, and has engaged the thought of the laity in one of the most important diseases to which the human race is heir. Before this interest was aroused among the medical profession syphilis often escaped detection in its later stages, and in the early stages the diagnosis depended mainly upon the development of the secondary rash, or in other words, waiting until the individual gave evidence of the general infection before treatment was begun. The old teaching that treatment should not be instituted until the diagnosis was established remains true to-day, but the diagnosis may be made earlier and treatment begun before the system is saturated with the virus of the infecting organisms. This is brought about by finding the spirocheta in the earliest of all lesions, the chancre. The finding of the organism in the chancre establishes the diagnosis and indicates that treatment should be instituted at once, and with the new form of treatment it is often possible to prevent the general infection from progressing to the point of producing general manifestations, or in other words, checking or aborting the disease without the appearance of the usual secondary signs. The spirocheta pallida is also found in mucous patches, and its demonstration in such lesions, especially when mucous patches are the only questionable lesions present, makes clear what was previously often confusing;

doubt arising whether the disturbances on the mucous membrane were due to the disease, mercurial treatment, or other affections, such, for example, as leucoplacia. The organism can also be demonstrated in the papules of the secondary eruption and in the lymph nodes, which, however, from a diagnostic standpoint, is seldom important; but their demonstration in tertiary lesions, such as ulcerations, and in condylomata, furnishes evidence that the disease is communicable through lesions of this nature. It is of scientific interest to know that the parasites may be found in nearly all of the tissues of the syphilitic fetus, even the bones, and also in the placenta and cord.

While the diagnosis of syphilis may be made by demonstrating the organism in any open lesion of syphilis, the chancre, mucous patches, ulcerations and condylomata, the patient is not always observed with these clinical manifestations of the disease, but without demonstrable lesions other than a general glandular enlargement, and even this may escape detection. In the event of a suspicion of syphilis being entertained by a questionable history, or indefinite and not absolutely characteristic symptoms, such as nocturnal headaches, rheumatism, and pain in the long bones, tumor masses which might be gummata, or nerve disturbances of nearly any variety, we must have recourse to the Wassermann reaction as applied to the blood or the spinal fluid to aid us in the diagnosis. As far as the diagnosis is concerned, therefore, we now have little excuse for not recognizing syphilis in the early or late forms. In the primary stage we are not to wait until the secondary eruption appears to begin treatment, but should demonstrate the organism in the chancre, or establish the diagnosis by a Wassermann reaction, which is sometimes, but not always present before the eruption appears. In the later stages the organism may be demonstrated in all open lesions, and a positive Wassermann reaction may be considered evidence of the disease. In the spinal cord affections fluid obtained from the spinal canal by lumbar puncture for a Wassermann test is indicated in order that the diseased condition of the cord may be decided as syphilitic or otherwise.

The demonstration of the spirocheta is not difficult and any practitioner who is capable of making an examination of urinary sediment is capable of recognizing the spirillum of syphilis. The technic is simple, the parasite being detectable in the living state by the dark field illuminator, or in dry smears by staining with different reagents. The dark field illuminator is a rapid and effective method of diagnosis, and one may observe the organisms in a living state, noting their movements and manner of reproduction, but its use must be limited as it is a special and expensive equipment.

The detection of the parasite in smears is simple, quite as satisfactory for practical purposes of diagnosis and may be carried out by the practitioner in his office, without special apparatus or devices. The preparation is made as follows: The lesion from which the smear is to be made is cleaned with water or soap and water, if necessary to remove crusts, pus, or any coagulated masses, from the real surface of the ulceration. With gauze or a small curet the lesion should be curetted at a point where the sound and ulcerated tissue approximate one another, that is, at the margin of the ulceration. Bleeding will result, and as only serum is desired for the smear, the blood is wiped away, and the curetted area is compressed firmly with gauze until the hemorrhage is checked. With the removal of the compression, a flow of serum will take place. One or two drops of this is collected by a sterilized platinum loop, and placed on a slide. Many different methods of staining have been tried, the Giemsa stain, essentially an anilin stain, was the one originally employed by Schaudinn and Hoffman, but cannot be recommended for practical purposes of diagnosis, as it requires from 18 to 24 hours to complete. To those interested in the various methods of staining the parasite, this method and that of Schereschewsky, the method of Romanowski, Hastings' stain and Stearn's silver method, will all be found satisfactory, but, as it is my desire to make the method of detecting the parasite one of simplicity and for practical purposes only, I will describe the method of staining with India ink. This method, first brought forth by Burri in 1909, and later proven to be accurate by Hecht and Wilenko and by Fruehwald, Cohen and others, consists of placing a loopful of the serum on an absolutely clean slide (washed with soap and water, placed in alcohol for one minute, and dried by passing through a flame), and mixing with one loopful of commercial India ink. After mixing these two fluids, spread the mixture over the slide by drawing the edge of another clean slide over the first, as in making a blood smear. The film dries in less than a minute without heat, and is then dark brown or black in color. Nothing further is necessary except to apply to the film a drop of oil and to make the examination with an oil immersion lens. The field is observed as a homogeneous black or brown color, with the blood cells, extraneous matter and spirochetæ shining through as colorless refractal bodies. The spirochetæ are readily differentiated from anything else. They appear as an extremely slender refractile thread from 7 to 21 microns long, which is from one to three times the diameter of a red blood corpuscle, closely wound in a corkscrew form, the windings being absolutely regular, and from 5 to 20 in number. There is one spirocheta which often appears in the smears together with the spirocheta pallida, the spirocheta refringens. This spirocheta, which grows on the surface of ulcerations, has no points in common with the spirocheta pallida. It is much thicker, has but four or five convolutions, which are more drawn out and wavy. In making smears from questionable ulcerations in the mouth, the spirocheta buccalis and dentata may appear in the smear; it cannot be confused with the spirocheta pallida because they are both thick spirilla with relatively few convolutions, and never have the closely wound corkscrew form of the spirocheta pallida. There is only one other spirillum which requires mention, which is known as Vincent's spirillum. This resembles closely the spirocheta refringens, and always is associated with a fusiform bacillus.

Just a word about the India ink for use in this method of staining. The best kind is Chinchin, made by Gunther and Wagner. Barach criticized the India ink method on the ground that India ink might contain bodies resembling spirochetæ, but this does not apply to the ink referred to above, and as Cohen and others have pointed out, is referable especially to Higgins' India ink. So much for the establishment of the diagnosis by demonstrating the infecting organism in syphilitic lesions. We will next consider the newer method of diagnosis of the disease after general infection has taken place.

Without describing the technic of performing the Wassermann reaction, which is distinctly a technical procedure, only to be carried out by trained laboratory workers to be reliable, I desire to speak of how the test is of practical value to the practitioner as an aid to diagnosis.

One is only required to know certain things to avail himself of the valuable information furnished by the Wassermann and allied tests. In the first place, the Wassermann reaction may not take place in the individual before the secondary eruption appears. I have repeatedly found it negative three weeks after the appearance of the chancre, but have frequently found it positive five weeks after the appearance of the primary sore, but even at this date it may be negative. At this stage of the disease the demonstration of the spirocheta pallida is the more reliable evidence in establishing the diagnosis. The Wassermann test should never be expected to be positive in those under mercurial treatment, and a period of at least four weeks, and better six to eight weeks, absence from mercury should elapse before a negative Wassermann finding may be considered reliable. It is a well established fact that mercury renders the Wassermann reaction temporarily negative. In the parasyphilitic affections, tabes and general paralysis, for example, the Wassermann test as applied to the blood may be negative, while the spinal fluid shows a positive reaction.

As regards the diagnostic importance of the Wassermann reaction, there has been much discussion. All information in regard to this matter, except that expressed by those who have all the facilities and the ability to make correct examinations, is worthless. The tests will, in all probability, remain limited to well equipped laboratories, and to those workers who have made the test a special study.

The Wassermann reaction must be considered a test for a systemic infection, and cannot be expected to be positive before systemic infection takes place. When the unmistakable lesions of syphilis are present, the reaction is only confirmatory evidence in the diagnosis, and of no real diagnostic value after the spirochetæ have been found. The great value of the test is in those conditions where the symptoms suggest a specific causation without sufficient clinical evidence, for example, in the inherited forms of the disease, in the female parent of the syphilitic offspring, cerebral and spinal syphilis, syphilis of the bones and internal organs, gland changes and certain tumor masses. In such conditions much weight must be given to the result of the Wassermann test in establishing the causation as syphilitic or otherwise. A negative Wassermann finding may occur in some syphilitics where the spirochetæ are few or encysted in tissue poorly supplied with blood, and repeated examinations at varying intervals are indicated when the lesions continue to excite the suspicion of a specific causation. Repeated examinations are absolutely indicated in all cases treated with salvarsan, for there is a considerable percentage of reactions negative two to three months after such treatment, that will later become positive.

No case of syphilis can be considered intelligently treated except when the Wassermann reaction is employed, as a control to decide whether the case is progressing favorably or unfavorably, and it is the information furnished by this test that enables us to decide when to stop treatment and when we should allow such patients to marry.

The blood for a Wassermann reaction is collected in the following manner. The left arm is bared if the patient is right handed, and vice versa if left handed; an area about the anterior aspect of the elbow joint is made surgically clean by scrubbing with soap and water and alcohol. A rubber tourniquet is lightly applied over the upper part of the biceps, and the fist clinched tightly. The veins thus become prominent unless the tourniquet is so tightly applied as to cut off the arterial circulation. If the arm is particularly fat, the veins may not be visible, and must be located by palpation. A vein being selected, the skin is made tense by the thumb and forefinger of the left hand of the operator, and a 17-gauge needle made sterile by boiling for at least two minutes in an ordinary tablespoon or otherwise, is plunged through the skin by the right hand of the operator, entering the vein in the direction of the course of the vein, with the point of the needle directed upward toward the shoulder. The blood is collected in a test tube, which may be made sterile by boiling, or as I prefer, a sterile 10 c.c. pill vial, which may be more easily closed by a tight fitting cork stopper. At least 8 c.c. must be collected and the vial laid on its side at an angle of 45 degrees, so as to allow the serum to separate more readily. The tourniquet is removed, and the puncture covered with a small bit of sterile gauze held in position by a strip of adhesive plaster. This dressing may be removed in eight to ten hours. To obtain the best results, the blood should not be over 24 hours old before testing.

In regard to the new method of treating syphilis much may be said. To put it briefly, the exact place which salvarsan occupies in the treatment of syphilis is not absolutely settled as yet, but there is little question that the disease is best treated by intravenous injections of this drug, alone or combined with any of the various forms of mercury.

The medical literature upon this subject has been most extensive, but after considering much that has been written, one is impressed with the variation in the ideas in regard to methods and results. It is really a difficult matter, even to-day, to know just where we stand in the rules to be followed in the treatment of syphilis by salvarsan, and statistics for and against the value of this drug serve chiefly to confuse the casual reader of medical literature.

Some authors record series of cases treated by a large initial dose of this drug, followed by two or more comparatively large doses, repeated at various intervals, some a few days, and some, weeks; with or without combined mercury treatment. Others advise small, often-repeated doses, with or without mercury as an adjuvant, while some feel that the best results are obtained by a course of mercury before salvarsan is administered at all. Beside the variations of opinion regarding the most efficacious method to employ, most reports are incomplete, inasmuch as the cases are from hospital or dispensary practice, and disappear altogether with the secession of symptoms, or are not continually observed by one observer, and in most instances the cases are not checked by repeated Wassermann reactions over a sufficient period of time to give us the hard and fast rules to guide us in outlining the best course of treatment to pursue. In other words, there is to-day no unanimity of opinion in regard to the best manner of conducting the treatment of syphilis by salvarsan.

Nevertheless, even with this confusion of ideas, based upon the variations in the individual ideas of those who have been particularly interested in this subject, certain fundamental deductions may be fairly made. In the first place, the worth of this new drug has been clearly established upon whatever basis it is administered, and it is unquestionable that the intravenous method gives the best results.

There are two important points of caution: The drug must be prepared according to directions, and asepsis must be absolute in all particulars.

In the past it was felt that patients suffering from circulatory disturbances might not receive the drug without considerable danger. This fear has passed out of my mind, for I have often given the drug to patients suffering from almost all forms of circulatory disturbances, but in all such individuals with high blood pressure, considerable blood has been drawn off before the injection was made. I have given the drug several times to patients with diabetes, and improvement rather than otherwise has taken place in those suffering from diseases of the optic nerve, the disease in these cases usually being syphilitic in character. One patient, a doctor, who was absolutely blind, received five large doses of the drug (three of .9 gms. and two of .6 gms.) with the result that the eyesight is now such that he can read and walk about the city streets without assistance. While it may not be important to bleed patients with high blood pressure at the time of making the injection, there can be no harm in so doing, and the fear of serious effects which might be caused by increasing the intravascular pressure in such individuals is minimized.

I have never in my own experience observed any permanent untoward effects from the use of this drug. In two early cases some of the drug infiltrated the subcutaneous tissue. In both of these patients, and in others that I have observed, occurring in the practice of other men, there was a slow necrosis of subcutaneous tissue and fascia, resulting in a very slow sloughing and repair process. I am familiar with two cases of death following general sepsis depending upon faulty and unclean technic. One of these patients had a septic meningitis. I believe there are unquestionably many serious results depending upon faulty technic, of which we are unfamiliar because no mention is made of them. It may be fairly said, however, that those who have given this form of treatment careful attention may carry out this new treatment with safety. As I have repeatedly said, however, this treatment should not be employed by any one who has not first seen the details of its administration, and who cannot for whatever reason carry out the details absolutely.

Beginning in November, 1910, while the drug was considered by Ehrlich as in the experimental stage, I have continued to employ it in nearly every case of syphilis which has come under my care, both in private and charity clinics. My observations are similar to those made by others who have had much experience with the treatment of this disease by salvarsan, both in regard to the impossibility of curing all syphilitics by a single dose of the drug, and the advisability and necessity of sometimes combining mercury with this new remedy in an attempt to free the individual of the infecting parasite. Indeed, it has occasionally been impossible, after repeated injections of salvarsan and energetic mercury treatment, to prevent the recurrence of a positive Wassermann reaction. I have repeatedly, in fact usually, seen all visible lesions of the disease rapidly disappear with a single dose of the drug, which was responsible more than anything else for the early belief that a single dose of this new drug resulted in a cure. The period of time that this belief could be reasonably entertained was of short duration, for the lesions often recurred, a negative Wassermann reaction was not always found even in the absence of all symptoms, and even repeated negative Wassermann reactions at intervals of months after the administration of the drug sometimes again became positive without recurring symptoms. On the other hand, I have under observation many patients in which a single dose of the drug has apparently destroyed all the parasites and repeated negative Wassermann reactions and absence of clinical signs must lead to the belief that these patients have been cured. I think that it is a fair assumption that patients who have gone two years with repeated negative tests and no clinical symptoms, may be considered cured, and I have had two patients again acquire the disease, which is to my mind the best proof of the truth of these conclusions.

It was to take care of the cases in which lesions recurred and a Wassermann reaction either remained positive or becoming negative, again became positive, that the hope of a cure in all cases by a single dose was lost, and that treatment was energetically pushed beyond the ordinary clinical and laboratory requirements by rapid repetition of injections of salvarsan, with or without mercury, in order to do too much rather than too little. How much relapses have been favorably circumvented by such energetic measures is not certain by any means, for it is well known that even under this "gunshot" method, that a recurrence and a positive Wassermann reaction and recurrence of lesions is not materially changed by such a procedure. It is impossible to accurately determine the percentage of cases benefited by over-treatment as compared with those who are treated in a more conservative manner. It is felt by certain observers that if one or two closely repeated doses of salvarsan failed to effect the desired result, that many closely repeated injections failed also. So it is in this confusion of methods that it is impossible to give to the practitioner any precise course to pursue with promise of a definite cure for his patient.

Disregarding statistics and the diverse opinions of others and considering the subject from the viewpoint of personal observation based upon a considerable experience, I have come to certain definite conclusions, the most important of which is that syphilitic patients must continue now, as in early days, to remain under observation for years.

It is urged that a conservative policy be pursued until the future offers a solution of this confusion of opinions, and for the reason that it is more prudent at this time to rely upon clinical signs and laboratory control than to impose a haphazard, hit-or-miss and most miscellaneous form of treatment, which is a tremendous inconvenience to the patient while promise of distinct advantages cannot be offered.

THE SWIFT-ELLIS INTRADURAL TREATMENT OF GENERAL PARESIS.

IN a careful study, with exhaustive histories, of the treatment of paresis by intraspinal injections of salvarsanized serum, A. Myerson, clinical director and pathologist of the Taunton State Hospital, summarizes (*Boston Med. and Surg. Jour.*, May 7, 1914) his cases and conclusions as follows:

Of eight cases, all undoubted paretics, mostly under forty and only one over fifty, the following has been the fate:

Two died.[1] Of these, one received five doses of intradural therapy, and the other three doses. The course of both was steadily "down hill," and there is nothing in their clinical histories to indicate that their treatment had the slightest effect upon the disease. In these two cases it is to be noted that there was no change in the Wassermann reaction.

[1] Since this paper was written another of these cases has died, making a total of three deaths. This is a larger ratio of mortality than is usual in the first year of paresis.

A third, altho not definitely a paretic patient on onset of treatment, and having no definite physical signs during treatment, developed in its course the Argyll-Robertson pupils and differences in his tendon reflexes. The case is a critical one for the therapy because this patient was young, robust and received treatment very early in his disease. Far more important than the fluctuation of the Wassermann reactions in his history is the appearance of these ominous physical changes. They mark a distinct progress in the lesions of paresis. Despite the clearing up of the mental signs, his case can be said to have advanced steadily, despite intensified treatment. Moreover, the disappearance of the mental signs has to be considered more in the light of a remission than as due to treatment. It is to be noted that at the onset of his disease the Wassermann reaction in spinal fluid was negative. At the present time, it is positive, so that in this respect, too, he is worse than he was. Moreover, the patient, while maintaining a robust appearance, has a pallor which William N. Graves, of St. Louis, describes as cachectic, that is, a sickly look with no apparent loss of hemoglobin. He looks distinctly sicker than on entrance to the hospital and before the beginning of his treatment.

Another case was discharged unimproved. He received only three doses of salvarsanized serum intradurally, and four doses of salvarsan. His case may be dismissed as being indifferent in its application to the question whether or not salvarsanized serum is of benefit to paresis. It is true that the spinal fluid showed changes, but how far these are related to definite improvement is one of the points at issue.

The fifth case showed very definite serological changes. Wassermann reaction early became negative and remained negative, but it is to be remarked remained negative, altho the intradural treatments had been discontinued and only neosalvarsan intravenously administered. There was no definite clinical improvement manifested. Patient said that the pains were less, but as a matter of fact this seems to have been due rather to euphoria than to actual diminution of the symptom, for at different times it was noted that he was suffering from pain. The salvarsan probably caused an enteritis in his case, for a bloody diarrhea was noted several times. After the treatment was discontinued the deterioration and downward progress became marked. Nevertheless, the Wassermann reaction in blood at present is negative.

In a general way what has been said of the above case will apply to the next two cases. In both of these cases the Wassermann reaction was exceedingly variable, in general favorably influenced by the treatment. Moreover, the cell count, the globulin and albumen all were reduced at various times by this treatment. There was, however, no abatement in physical or mental signs. The patients did not look better, feel better or act better. Following the discontinuance of the treatment, the progress downward was marked, showing that the treatment in no wise stopped the disease, although it may have checked it for a time. It would almost seem as if its discontinuance accelerated the normal progress, if such a term can be employed, of the disease. At any rate one cannot claim much for a treatment which when employed as consistently and frequently as in these cases, after it has been discontinued for three months, finds the patients far worse off than when the treatment was initiated.

The last case has shown what might seem to be the most favorable results of the treatment. A maniacal patient, deluded and hallucinated, all the reactions present in blood and spinal fluid, for a time showed a complete remission, and following the discontinuance of the treatment developed only a few hypochondriacal ideas. Wassermann reaction at the present time is doubtful, cells and globulin almost vanished, albumen greatly reduced. At first glance this would seem to be a splendid recommendation for the treatment, but it is to be noted against this view that the remission started before the treatment was instituted and was almost complete when the first dose of neosalvarsan was administered. In a disease so eminently one of remissions, one must be exceedingly careful in interpreting what one finds as the result of treatment. There are cases on record in the Taunton State Hospital where the remission had lasted two and more years, and undoubtedly such histories can be more than duplicated by any other hospital. Moreover, the patient looks worse than he did when treatment was first started. His color is not so good—it is more yellowish than formerly. He is more listless and despondent.

CONCLUSIONS.

1. Patients receiving this form of treatment show changes probably as the result of it. These changes are mostly limited to the disappearance of the Wassermann reaction and alterations in chemical-cytological composition of the spinal fluid. On the whole, no clinical improvement can be recorded which cannot otherwise be accounted for.

2. As has been stated in a previous paper, the order of changes is somewhat as follows: The Wassermann reaction seems to be the most variable—the first to disappear, the least stable. The difficulty in evaluating the Wassermann reaction lies mostly in the fact that the results obtained by various laboratories vary according to the ability of the technician and serologist. In the case of these patients, all the work was done in one laboratory, the same method used throughout, and thus a fairly standard Wassermann reaction can be recorded.

The cell count seems to have been the next most variable constituent. It seems to be profoundly affected by the treatment, but a reduction must not be taken too optimistically. It will be noted that in the case of H. N. the cell count was 50 after treatment was discontinued. Later on, without treatment, it dropped to 0 for no well defined reason. Since the examiner was the same in both cases and used the same technic and care, it is probable that the record is faithful to the facts at each time.

The globulin is perhaps a little less variable than the cell count, that is it does not diminish so much under treatment, and it rarely completely disappears.

Finally, the albumen content is the most constant of all, and is least affected by treatment.

Homer Swift, in a discussion before the New York Society of Neurology, stated that in his opinion the cell count was the most variable of the reactions, and the Wassermann next, both differing, however, very little from each other in their constancy. Next in permanency he found the globulin test. He does not record the albumen content. It will be seen that his results differ but little from my own, there being merely a transposition in relation between Wassermann reaction and cell count. Since the difference between the two is not very great, his findings and mine are essentially the same, except that I have added to the test recorded the total albumen content.

3. The Wassermann reaction probably is not nearly so important a criterion of improvement or recovery as it is frequently held to be. This statement is substantiated by the following facts:

First, It seems to be capricious in its appearance and disappearance. That is to say, there is no ascertainable relationship between it and the clinical conditions of the patient.

Second, As is shown in No. 4 and No. 5 of this series, the patients' condition may gradually grow worse both physically and mentally and the Wassermann reaction remain negative. This fact is perhaps the most important of those disclosed in the investigation of the treatment.

Third, It is generally assumed that a change for the better is accompanied by a Wassermann negative—a change for the worse, by a Wassermann positive. Whatever the Wassermann reaction may mean, it does not measure the full scope of the paretic process. It represents a diagnostic feature of great importance, but we must learn to separate the diagnostic facts from the pathogenetic facts. The treatment here recorded changes the process of the disease in that part of it from which originates the alterations leading to the appearance of the Wassermann reaction, but unfortunately these alterations are but a part of those occurring in the total disease process.

4. What has been said of the Wassermann reaction applies in a lesser degree to the chemical and cytological changes. It is

probably true that the criterion of recovery or progress at present must be in the field of the clinical manifestations.

5. Finally, it must be stated that the theoretical grounds upon which this treatment is based do not seem to me to be valid. It is assumed that because the Wassermann reaction is most constant an hour after the administration of salvarsan, therefore the blood at that time contains more anti-bodies. This, of course, is by no means certain, for the meaning of the Wassermann reaction is unknown. Furthermore, it seems to be the opinion, shared by Swift and Ellis, that the nervous system is inaccessible to medicament administered in the usual channels. One hears the term "inaccessibility of the nervous system" quite frequently, yet a little reflection shows there is no such thing. The effects of opium, chloral, bromide, alcohol, strychnia, and certain of the toxins of infectious diseases seem notably to affect the brain and nervous system, and to do this through the blood stream. The appearance of headache following all kinds of bodily disorders contradicts the assertion of the inaccessibility of the nervous system most emphatically. Further, it is assumed that the introduction of medicament into the cerebro-spinal space can affect the brain favorably and locally. Undoubtedly such administration does affect those local conditions, which are largely meningeal, as, for example, cerebro-spinal meningitis, cerebro-spinal syphilis, gummatous conditions, etc. But in paresis the bulk of the lesions are deep and spirochetes have been discovered only in the cortical substance itself. Now the current of the spinal fluid, if there be a current, is not into the cortical substance or brain tissue. Whatever be the origin of this fluid, whether secreted by the choroid plexus, whether dialyzed from the blood stream as claimed by Metrazat, or the product of the pial endothelium, its direction is from the cortical substance and the brain tissue in general, rather than towards it. So that logically intradural treatment for paresis would fail, and the only reason that the salvarsan does not cure in the case of paresis is because there is either a lack of some intermediary substance to unite it with the spirochete or else because the spirochete has acquired new resistance by reason of its long stay in the body of its host.

Moreover, despite the discovery of Noguchi, that the spirocheta pallida is present in the brain of paretics, it is probable that the sum total of the paretic process is something more than chronic syphilis, or at least a degenerative process has been added, which it is difficult to stay.

There seems to be another reason for the failure of salvarsanized serum in this treatment. Granted that its theoretical basis be correct, and that the introduction into the intradural spaces can locally and favorably influence general paresis, the amount introduced seems utterly insufficient. Of all the blood in the body, 50 c.c. are removed one hour after salvarsan has been administered. Such an insignificant fraction of the total amount of the blood present can contain only a very small amount of salvarsan. Its introduction seems *a priori* to be adding but little of local treatment to that of the salvarsanized blood stream itself.

However, the treatment merits further trial. It should not be administered to every paretic in the hospital, as some men seem to feel, but should be used on selected groups of cases. It would be very wise not to hold out hopes to the relatives or to the patient, because the result will probably be disappointment. Experience with this treatment teaches much about paresis and leads to the hope that there is a cure for the disease since we now know that it can be profoundly affected, but as far as my experience goes, the Swift-Ellis method is not the looked-for cure.

THE DIAGNOSTIC VALUE OF CYSTOSCOPY AND URETERAL CATHETERIZATION [1]

By John W. Price, Jr., M.D., Louisville, Kentucky.

When there exists disease of either the kidneys, the ureters, or the bladder, the history of the onset and the symptoms may in all cases be so similar that a definite diagnosis may oftentimes be impossible without the aid of the cystoscope, the ureteral catheter, the indigo-carmine test, and the x-ray. Another difficulty in making the diagnosis is that there may be disease of not only one but all these organs at the same time; in fact, this is of common occurrence.

The usual symptoms of disease implicating the organs mentioned are, frequent and painful urination, pyuria and hematuria. These symptoms taken in connection with the history may suffice to warrant a diagnosis of cystitis, but with the aid of the cystoscope one may determine the extent and degree of the involvement, whether the disease be acute or chronic, and there be present hemorrhagic foci, erosions, necrosis, ulcerations or gangrene, the presence of benign or malignant neoplasms, calculi or parasites.

Because cystitis is so frequently associated with renal and ureteric affections, the latter must be confirmed or eliminated by continuing investigation after establishing the diagnosis of cystitis, which can only be done by collecting urine from both kidneys by ureteral catheterization. The urine must then be examined and injected into guinea pigs. If the kidneys be found implicated, the next problem is to ascertain the extent of the involvement, which may be done by the indigo-carmine functional test and radiograms taken with impregnated catheters in the ureters. In some instances in the presence of a violent cystitis it is impossible to catheterize both ureters, but one can obtain definite information as to the functional ability of the kidneys, and also examine the urine from the side which can be catheterized, which will be of especial importance in suspected tuberculous lesions. To obtain such information would be impossible without the aid of the cystoscope and the ureteral catheter.

There is no positive method of making a diagnosis of a benign or malignant tumor of the bladder without visual inspection,

[1] Read before the Louisville Surgical Society, February 20, 1914.

and the cystoscope furnishes the easiest way. The location and extent of the neoplasm, its operability and best method of approach, can be determined by employment of the cystoscope, therefore unnecessary exploratory operations may be avoided; by using the operative cystoscope and Young's punch, sections of a doubtful tumor may be removed for microscopic examination.

The presence of a calculus in the bladder may be proven by a searcher. By employing the cystoscope one can determine if more than a single calculus is present, whether the stone (or stones) be free or imbedded, and the best method by which removal may be accomplished.

There is no better way of studying the prostate than with the cystoscope, although accurate diagnosis cannot always be made without microscopical sections. The cystoscope is especially valuable in determining the diagnosis in suspected prostatic disease when the symptoms are due to vesical calculi, polypi or tumors.

By the cystoscope and ureteral catheter the condition of the ureter may be noted, i. e., whether there are strictures, wounds, dilatations, obstructions; also the character and size of the lesion, whether due to blood vessels, tumors or calculi. Radiograms made with the catheter in the ureter will confirm the diagnosis of calculi. Radiograms made without a catheter in the ureter are misleading, because coproliths in the appendix or intestine, phleboliths and caseating glands in the region of the ureter, will present shadows which may be easily mistaken for calculi.

The functional activity of the kidney may be more accurately studied by cystoscopy, ureteroscopy, and ureteral catheterization, after the injection of indigo-carmine or phenolsulphonephthalein than by any other method, and almost all surgical lesions can be correctly diagnosed if urinalysis and proper skiagrams be made in addition. Thomas says that chromo-ureteroscopy based on the employment of indigo-carmine is the most valuable single test for renal sufficiency or insufficiency that we possess, because it is the most practical. With this we heartily agree.

In suspected hydronephrosis if the ureteral catheter passes the obstruction and drains an abnormal amount of urine from the kidney pelvis, the diagnosis is practically certain; if in addition to this collargol is injected into the renal pelvis via the ureteral catheter, and the radiogram shows an enlarged pelvis, the diagnosis is doubly sure.

Pyelitis cannot be positively diagnosed without the cystoscope, ureteral catheter and examination of the urine obtained by the latter. The ureteral orifice is dilated, edematous, and congested; the urine flows by a steady drip instead of the normal jet; the kidney pelvis contains residual urine mixed with pus. In pyelonephritis the cystoscope shows cystitis, especially of the trigone, the urine is ejected slowly from the ureter, and when collected by the catheter is found to contain pus, casts, blood, and epithelial cells. The functional activity is markedly impaired.

The bladder is involved mostly about the ureteral ortifice on the affected side when there is a pyonephrosis. The urine from the affected kidney is shown by the cystoscope to contain pus, and drops constantly. The ureteral catheter obtains residual urine containing pus. The indigo-carmine test will demonstrate that function is impaired.

In the presence of renal tuberculosis, the cystoscope will show the bladder inflamed, and it may contain tubercles and ulcers. The orifice of the ureter on the affected side is congested, swollen, edematous, the degree depending upon the amount of kidney involvement. The urinary efflux (or jet) will be affected by the amount of implication of the ureter. The urine obtained by the ureteral catheter should be injected into a guinea pig. When it is impossible to pass a catheter into the ureter on the affected side, the indigo-carmine test is most valuable and will show either impaired functional activity or complete obstruction of the ureter. Complete obstruction was noticed in one of our cases. A guinea pig test was made of urine obtained from the other side and found to be negative, after which nephrectomy was performed on the affected side and the kidney showed an early tubercular process. It is self evident that this patient should not have been operated upon without first determining the soundness of one kidney.

Renal calculi can be positively diagnosed if we use the cystoscope and make a radiogram with the catheter in the ureter. With the cystoscope the condition of the bladder contents, the ureteral orifice and the ejected urine can be noted. Pilcher first described the urinary efflux as dribbling on the diseased side. After injection of indigo-carmine the functional activity of each kidney can be noted. By the cystoscope, ureteral catheter and x-ray one may determine the relation of a stone to the renal pelvis. Pilcher says tumors of the kidney are to be diagnosed by exclusion, and it is of importance to determine the functional activity of the uninvolved kidney. The indigo-carmine test with the cystoscope is practical.

In conclusion I wish to draw attention to the fact that the cystoscope and ureteral catheter are not only of importance in aiding one to diagnose disease, but are of equal importance in determining the absence of disease.

DISCUSSION.

Dr. J. T. Windell:

From the literature and discussions before medical societies one might infer that cystoscopy and ureteral catheterization represented very easy and simple procedures, but in actual application they have been found more difficult of execution than we have hitherto been led to believe. In my opinion these procedures are of the greatest value when executed by an expert, and one can only become proficient after a great deal of experience.

In regard to the diagnosis of vesical calculi, a recent observation of mine may be of interest. A patient was examined with the cystoscope on several occasions with the bladder filled with boric acid solution and once with urine, and we failed to recognize the presence of a stone. Finally an examination was made without fluid in the bladder, and the calculus was readily detected. Therefore, in attempting to discover vesical calculi, if the patient be examined without any fluid in the bladder we may be successful, whereas otherwise we may fail as fluid sometimes serves to so obscure the view that the stone cannot be located.

Dr. H. H. Grant:

Every surgeon appreciates the necessity of using care in the diagnosis of obscure vesical and renal lesions, and the methods mentioned by Dr. Price are highly valuable. Often a positive diagnosis would be impossible without utilization of the methods he has described. There has hitherto been some hesitation about recommending the use of the cystoscope and ureteral catheter in the hands of those unfamiliar with these instruments, where perhaps their intelligent application would have afforded valuable information, but the present status of such work is most satisfactory.

Personally I have had little experience with either the cystoscope or the ureteral catheter, excepting to avail myself of the many benefits derived from careful examinations in the hands of those capable of using them. We all appreciate the importance of satisfactory information concerning the kidneys, the ureters and bladder which may be obtained by employment of these instruments, and also the significance of Dr. Windell's criticism that they must be used by experts, otherwise the information thereby afforded will likely be worthless.

Dr. W. L. Rodman:

While, like Dr. Grant, I am personally rather unfamiliar with the actual application of the cystoscope and ureteral catheter, yet in recent years I have depended upon them as diagnostic aids more than formerly, particularly as my son, Dr. Stuart Rodman, is very much interested in this kind of work and has provided himself with the most modern instruments. I believe we should always avail ourselves of the valuable knowledge to be gained especially by the use of the cystoscope, and it is one of the modern instruments which has come to stay. The instrument now used has been so perfected that it is more easily applied than those in use ten or fifteen years ago.

The remark made by the essayist that vesical calculi can always be detected by the searcher recalls a recent observation of mine where a man had marked symptoms of vesical calculus and was carefully examined with the searcher without locating the stone. It seemed certain, however, that a calculus was present, because it had been shown by the x-ray, but careful use of the searcher with the patient under ether failed to detect it. This is the first time in my experience that I have failed to locate a vesical calculus with the searcher when one was demonstrably present.

Dr. H. Bronner:

Cystoscopy is not always an easy procedure, and in my experience it is especially difficult in certain cases of tuberculosis of the genito-urinary tract. Even in the hands of the most expert cystoscopy is sometimes unsuccessful in tuberculous cases unless the patient be under a general anesthesia. I believe it is conceded that satisfactory genito-urinary surgery is at present impossible without the aid of the cystoscope and ureteral catheter, the symtoms of the various lesions being often so similar that an accurate diagnosis cannot be made without the employment of these instruments.

In the diagnosis of renal lesions, in addition to the cystoscope and ureteral catheter, the injection of collargol is sometimes a valuable aid. At the present time we are using collargol injections in the early diagnosis of renal tumors. Quite frequently the diagnosis of kidney tumor is only made after the condition of the patient has become practically hopeless, and any method by which early diagnosis can be made is therefore of great importance. Those who have extensively studied the question of collargol injections in renal tumors have found that frequently early in the history of such cases there is a decided change in the outline of the kidney pelvis. This change should always be regarded with suspicion, especially if a renal function test shows a decided deficiency on that side. While I am aware that Thomas, of Philadelphia, favors the indigo-carmine test, I believe phenolsulphonephthalein is much superior. The method of making this test depends largely upon the information it is desired to obtain. If we simply wish to ascertain the total kidney function, we employ intra-muscular injections; to determine the function of one kidney intravenous injections should be made.

Dr. I. N. Bloom:

Although the essayist made no reference to fulguration, it may be interesting to note that Young has quite recently reported nineteen cases of vesical lesions successfully treated by this method.

Like Dr. Rodman, until quite recently I had supposed it was a relatively simple matter with an ordinary searcher to locate a vesical calculus. Not long ago, however, a patient came to me for examination giving a clear history of bladder stone, stating that a prominent surgeon in another city had failed to locate the calculus. After several unsuccessful attempts with the searcher, I finally located the stone by using the Brown-Buerger cystoscope. The patient was later operated upon and the calculus removed. Therefore even in the hands of experts it may sometimes be impossible to detect a small stone by means of the ordinary searcher. However, with the Brown-Buerger cystoscope it is a comparatively easy matter, and the water system seems to be a great improvement over the air dilatation in the majority of cases. Of course cystoscopy has been greatly simplified within the last ten years.

Dr. J. W. Price, Jr. (closing):

My paper was not intended to present anything original, it was simply a brief review of the observations of others. It was made as concise as possible and referred only to the diagnostic value of cystoscopy and ureteral catheterization.

The cystoscope and ureteral catheter should be used by those who not only possess the requisite manual dexterity in the introduction and manipulation of these instruments to produce the minimum amount of trauma, but experience in living pathology is also of the greatest assistance. That is, the man who is accustomed to the study of pathological lesions in the living subject is better equipped to successfully employ these instruments than one who has had less pathological training.

MY VIEWS ON HOMOSEXUALITY

By William J. Robinson, M.D., New York.

Editor of The American Journal of Urology, Venereal and Sexual Diseases; Editor of the Critic and Guide; Chief of Department of Genito-Urinary Diseases and Dermatology, Bronx Hospital and Dispensary.

IT is the same old story over again. Extremes in one direction lead to extremes in the opposite direction. Our ignorant attitude towards any sexual abnormality, our brutal treatment of any man found guilty of homosexuality or of any other sexual perversion, has led a number of earnest students to investigate the entire subject of sexual abnormalities, and they have reached conclusions greatly or entirely at variance with the popular notions. Thus for instance the notion about homosexuality that prevailed up to a short time ago was that the homosexuals are a low degraded type of men, depraved mentally, morally and physically, and deserving of the severest punishment for their "crime." Those who investigated the question in a calm unbiased manner, particularly those who had to deal with homosexuals as patients, soon discovered that this notion was radically wrong, that the homosexuals were not necessarily degenerates or morally depraved. They found that there were among them people of high intellectual attainments, and even of a high moral calibre. It was but right therefore that those sexologists urged that the vulgar notion about homosexuals be changed, and demanded that the brutal punishments inflicted upon them when discovered be abolished or modified.

So far so good, and so far I am in full agreement. But some sexologists thought it necessary to go further. Some boldly say that homosexuality is not a crime, not a vice, not a sign of degeneracy, not even a sexual abnormality, merely a sexual variation. To such an opinion, which does credit to the heart but not to the head of its promulgators, I must enter an emphatic protest. It is *not* a crime; we will agree not to call it a vice; we might even argue as to whether it is a sign of degeneracy, tho I would maintain that it is; but there can be no question whatever that it is a serious abnormality, a sad, deplorable, pathological phenomenon. Every sexual deviation or disorder which has for its result an inability to perpetuate the race is *ipso facto* pathologic, *ipso facto* an abnormality, and this is pre-eminently true of true homosexuality. It is sufficient to state that the entire human race would die out very quickly if all its members showed homosexual tendencies, to become aware of the fact that we are dealing here with an abnormality or a perversion. I do not mean to imply that all homosexuals are physically impotent or suffer with *impotentia generandi*, but of course all true homosexuals loathe the opposite sex, and the result is therefore practically the same.

And the very fact that the homosexuals are not satisfied with their condition, and would give a good deal to be rid of it, is proof that they themselves are aware that there is something wrong with them, that they are abnormal. For I deny that there are many or any homosexuals that are as satisfied with their condition as healthy heterosexuals are. I judge of course from my personal experience. My homosexual patients are all of the cultured, intellectual type, and I have not had one who did not deplore his condition most deeply, and who was not willing to bring every possible sacrifice in time, money, etc., in order to be rid of what they considered their great misfortune. I know the objection that is apt to be interposed here, that it is only homosexuals who wish to get rid of their abnormality who go to the physician, while those who are satisfied with their condition do not invoke medical aid. But I have treated homosexuals who came to me, not to be treated for their homosexuality, but for other conditions, and I have also known homosexuals who were not patients at all, and without exception they considered their condition a great punishment, tho some of them were resigned to it.

There is another tendency on the part of certain sexologists which we must oppose, that is the tendency to idealize the homosexual, the tendency to present him not only as a perfectly normal individual but even as something superior to normal, as some kind of superman. This is all bosh, and merely illustrates the tendency of some enthusiasts to become extremists, the tendency of some well meaning people to become over-zealous in the defence of their cause and thus do it more harm than good. The true homosexual is not a normal individual. There are some sweet types among them, there are some capable artists, writers, poets, but I have yet to see a great or even a capable thinker among them, and when examined into they will all show one or more points of distinct inferiority to the normal man. They are not men that are doing something of large, permanent value; and I fear, cruel as it may be to say it, that the world could get along very well without these step-children of nature.

Let us demand the abolition of all stupid laws against the homosexuals, laws which do no good but only breed disgrace and foster blackmail. Let us work for a humane, intelligent attitude towards them, but let us not minimize their faults, let us not exaggerate their virtues, in short let us not falsely idealize them. *Ne quid nimis.*

REVIEW OF CURRENT UROLOGIC LITERATURE

ZEITSCHRIFT FUR UROLOGIE

Vol. VIII, No. 6, 1914.

On the Third International Urological Congress in Berlin.
The Limitations of Nephrectomy. By Prof. Legueu.
The Surgical Treatment of Hypospadias. By Prof. Pousson.
4. Two New Points of View in the Question of Nephrectomy for Renal Tuberculosis. By Frank Kidd.
5. The Diagnosis of Enuresis Nocturna. By A. Alexeieff.
6. Lipoma of the Epididymis. By H. Wildbolz.
7. A Case of Obscure Renal Infection. By Hans v. Haberer.
8. A Case of Separation of a Horseshoe Kidney. By H. Brongersma.
9. Hyperalgetic Zones and Herpes Zoster in Diseases of the Kidneys. By C. Adrian.

2. The Limitations of Nephrectomy.

Legueu takes up three methods, corresponding to three successive epochs, of determining the sufficiency of the kidney function. According to the first method the urea-concentration of any given specimen of urine was determined. If this was found to be 15–20% the corresponding kidney was pronounced functionally sufficient. Similarly if the concentration was below 10% the kidney was declared functionally incompetent. This point of view has been shown by Legueu to be wrong, for the figure 20% can be regarded as satisfactory only when it expresses the average urea concentration for an individual, the normal maximum concentration being 50–54%. Moreover higher values may be unfavorable, pointing to hydropic nephritis, whereas lower values may very well go with functionally normal kidneys.

The second method is that of Albarran, and calls for the determination of the urea output during two successive hours. According to this authority, the normal figures are 0.7–1.0 for women and 1.2–1.5 g. for men. Again Legueu points out that these limits do not hold for all cases and declares that if one were to follow these figures to the letter he would fail to operate on many patients who would need operation and who would be cured by nephrectomy.

The third method is that suggested by the author in which the fluid excretion and the maximum concentration are studied together. His procedure is as follows: The fluid output is determined with the aid of the experimental polyuria procedure but it is not the total 2 hour output which is measured but rather the greatest output in any one half hour. If, for example, a kidney excretes 86 cc. in the third half hour, it can theoretically put out 86 x 48 = 4128 cc. in one day. Similarly the maximum urea concentration is determined for any one half hour. Say this is 18.4 gm. per mille. In this case therefore the kidney is theoretically capable of excreting 4128 x 18.4 = 76 gm. urea in one day. The margin between this figure and the actual necessary amount (25–30 g.) is wide and a nephrectomy can be successfully carried out in this case. This method is of considerable accuracy and is the only one available when the entire urine output cannot be obtained as in nephrostomy cases. In some instances, however, even this procedure stamps the kidney as insufficient when such is not the case and this can be demonstrated by the employment of:

A fourth method, namely, the estimation of the ureo-secretory coefficient of Ambard. This procedure depends upon the quality as well as the quantity of the secreting parenchyma, whereas the maximum concentration method depends only on the quality of the kidney tissue. When both methods are used to check each other the most reliable results are obtained. Thus so long as the constant (of Ambard) is under 0.100 the kidneys are little affected for the patient still possesses 50% of his kidney function and it is very probable that the loss of function is limited to the diseased kidney. If the constant is greater than 0.120 the problem is more complicated, for although the patient will probably survive nephrectomy he would have only one-third his kidney substance and it would still be an open question whether this third would belong exclusively to the healthy kidney. In such doubtful cases Legueu cautions that we must not rely too much on figures but above all remain clinicians and size up our cases rather from that point of view.

3. The Surgical Treatment of Hypospadias.

Pousson has not had good results with the tunnelization method of treating hypospadias, but has fallen back entirely upon urethroplasty by skin flaps. He believes that the main point in the surgical treatment of this condition is the straightening of the penis by destroying the band which holds that organ bent toward the scrotum. Only after the penis has become entirely straight and the scar tissue supple, should the restoration of the canal be attempted. This implies an interval of two to four months.

Pousson points out that when a hypospadic penis is looked at from the side an angle is formed by the glans with the body of the organ. This condition is distinct in the relaxed state but is much more marked in the state of erection owing to the enlargement (from the increased blood flow) of the corpora cavernosa and the sinking down of the glans. The latter can no longer be supported from below, so to speak, by the short and rudimentary corpus spongiosum in which the circulation is correspondingly insufficient. In case the separation of the ligament holding the glans down is not done it is easy to imagine under what unfavorable conditions (as regard conception) ejaculation will take place after restoration of the canal.

The semen will be deposited against the posterior vaginal wall where no ciliated epithelium is present, and should the vaginal secretions be unfavorable the chances of the spermatozoa reaching the uterine neck by their own exertions are very slim indeed.

Technic of straightening the glans.— The frenulum under the glans may be cut either before or after this stage of the operation is carried out. The straightening proper is carried out as follows: A soft rubber catheter is tied around the base of the penis to control hemorrhage. An incision is then made with a bistouri in the balano-preputial fold separating the glans from both corpora cavernosa. The cut is carried down halfway between the dorsum of the penis and the urethra. The knife is then placed 1 cm. posterior to the first incision and a cut made obliquely downward and forward meeting the first incision at its bottom and thus removing a wedge-shaped piece of tissue. The glans is then sewed on to the cut ends of the corpora cavernosa, using a deep suture, such as is employed in the operation for hare-lip, to insure hemostasis. As a result of this procedure, of course, the glans is brought into a line with the rest of the organ. During the first few days following the operation the glans appears flaccid and its sensibility is diminished but soon its normal appearance and sensation are restored.

Technic of reconstruction of the urethra.— The improvement embodied in the author's technic consists in supplying the urethra with a skin covering containing partially erectile tissue, by making use of traces of corpus spongiosum which may be found around the hypospadic groove. The technic of outlining and freeing the flaps is as follows: A longitudinal incision is made on one side of the hypospadic groove, at 8 mm. distance, beginning at the glans and extending back to the level of the abnormal orificium urethræ. At either end of this incision two short cuts are made at right angles to the original incision, for 6 mm. in an outward direction. A flap, embracing the entire thickness of the penis wall, is thus outlined and freed. This flap differs from that advocated by Duplay and Marion in that its free border begins further out from the median line thus permitting of the outlining of a small median flap of 4-5 mm. thickness which can be turned inward to form the inner wall of the reconstructed urethra. This inner flap is outlined externally by the longitudinal incision, and at either end by two short transverse incisions and contains within it, of course, the remains of the corpus spongiosum.

On the opposite side of the hypospadic groove two similar flaps are formed with this difference, however, that the intervening longitudinal incision is brought nearer the median line, at a distance of about 5 cm. so that the median flap on this side will be narrower than was the corresponding one on the opposite aspect of the organ. This unevenness in the width of the two inner flaps will bring their line of approximation over to one side so that it will not correspond to the suture line of the overlying skin flaps. Accordingly a catheter is placed in the future urethra and the inner flaps united about it with a catgut glover's suture. The outer flaps are then approximated over the former in such a way that the raw surfaces of the latter are approximated. They are then united by a cuneiform suture. In order to insure the union of the suture lines and to prevent their contamination by the urine the author institutes a deviation of the urinary current either by introducing a catheter into the bladder through the hypospadias opening or by making a perineal urethrostomy behind this opening.

4. **Two New Points of View in the Question of Nephrectomy for Renal Tuberculosis.**

Nephrectomy is indicated when ureteral catheterization shows that the tuberculous process is unilateral. The operation is subject to the following disadvantages. In the first place, the bladder is in many cases so irritable that the surgeon has to delay a long time before he can carry out the procedures of cystoscopy and ureteral catheterization. In the second place, in many patients the nephrectomy wound becomes infected with tubercle bacilli and breaks open with the formation of a local fistula which may prevent ultimate recovery.

The remedies for these conditions, as proposed by the author, are as follows: (1) When cystoscopy and ureteral catheterization is impossible the laying bare of one or both ureters in their pelvic course will show which is the infected kidney. (2) The secret of obtaining healing by primary union after nephrectomy lies in the removal of the kidney as a whole with its perirenal fat and fascia as well.

5. **The Diagnosis of Enuresis Nocturna.**

When the cystoscope is introduced carefully without exerting undue pressure on the sphincter, Alexeieff obtains the following picture: Instead of a sharply circumscribed sphincter there is an oblique sloping of the bladder neck in which the connective tissue bundles are seen to taper off gradually forwards. Often three prominent bundles are visible over which the verumontanum is seen to project with the utriculus masculinus at its apex. If the beak of the cystoscope is allowed to remain in place for a longer time and to press upon the bladder neck the fan shaped muscle bundles of the sphincter are seen to draw together, the colliculus increases in size and the corpora cavernosa of the penis begin to swell. The cystoscopic field darkens and soon only the colliculus and two lateral striæ remain visible. The above picture, according to the author, is characteristic of enuresis.

6. **Lipoma of the Epididymis.**

In January, 1910, Wildbolz was consulted by a colleague in regard to a swelling of the epididymis. As there was no previous gonorrheal infection, and no family history of tuberculosis, the patient feared that the condition might be a sarcoma and requested early operation. There was no pain or any local symptom whatever. The general condition was excellent. In the head of the left epididymis two irregular swellings were palpable. These were the size of a small berry and contained several small firm nodules. Similar tumors were felt in the right epididymis as well. Every other examination was negative.

A left epididymectomy was performed under local anesthesia. The wound healed well. During the next four years there was no change whatever in the condition of the right testicle. Pathological examination of the removed specimen showed that the nodules were composed of fatty tissue surrounded by an inflammatory infiltration of leucocytes. Wildbolz points out that under normal circumstances there is no fatty tissue between the tubules of the epididymis. On the other hand there is always some to be found in the tunica of that organ. The lipoma described in the above preparation must therefore have arisen from this source. Just why this rare lipoma formation should occur within the tissue of the epididymis is hard to say. The presence of the leucocytic infiltration might suggest an inflammatory origin, but such an etiology for lipoma finds no analogy in pathology. It is much more likely, therefore, that the lipoma was the cause of the inflammation. Clinically the palpatory findings might have suggested tuberculosis and even the histological picture might speak in that direction but this possibility cannot be accepted in view of the fact that no typical tubercles were found and that the clinical course of the disease showed no symptoms whatever characteristic of tuberculous infection.

7. **A Case of Obscure Renal Infection.**

The patient was a woman of 41, who for several years past had felt occasional pains in the right loin associated with slight rises in temperature. The author examined her during an attack of fever and found the right kidney and ureter sensitive on pressure. Cystoscopic examination revealed merely a slight inflammation of the vertex of the bladder. The indigocarmine test showed a slightly delayed excretion on the part of the right kidney. A probable diagnosis of multiple abscesses (hematogenous) of the right kidney was made. This was confirmed at operation where a nephrotomy was performed.

This operation was followed in three days by a rise in temperature and uremic symptoms and as there was no evidence that the split kidney was functioning a secondary nephrectomy was done. As a result, the general condition improved but three weeks later there was a chill, the temperature and pulse went up, there was headache and vomiting and the urine diminished in amount. Coincidently the left kidney became palpable and sensitive. A blood culture was negative but culture of the urine showed the presence of cocci, which appeared to be intracellular in smears. This attack lasted but four days but recurred in the same manner twelve days later.

Following this there was a free period of six days, and then again a third attack of remittent fever with the same symptoms. By this time the pathological report was available and this showed the presence of the same diplococci in the abscesses as had been recovered from the urine previously A pyelitic process was now suspected in the remaining kidney and a second cystoscopy performed. The urine obtained from the left side, however, was perfectly clear and the indigocarmine excretion found to be even more rapid than on the original examination. Bacteriological examination of the urine was negative. These findings, of course, ruled out the possibility of a pyelitis. An autogenous vaccine was now prepared from the diplococcus above described and vaccinetherapy instituted. Twelve injections were given in all during the next 2½ months, beginning with a dose of 25 millions and ending with a dose of 90 millions. Despite two rather severe recrudescences during the early part of this treatment, recovery was on the whole steady and the patient seemed absolutely cured at the time of writing.

The author concludes that the second kidney was affected in the same way as the first, the infection being here also hematogenous in nature.

8. A Case of Separation of a Horseshoe Kidney.

The patient was a woman who from childhood on had been complaining of pains in both loins, more marked on the left side. Later, these pains extended more to the lower abdomen, became colicky at times, and were associated with fever and prostration. Each of three pregnancies was very stormy and delivery was always instrumental. It was during the first pregnancy that albumen was discovered in the urine. The patient had had six curettages for menorrhagia. In May, 1907, her appendix was removed without any relief from her pains. In July, 1908, the diagnosis of stone in the left kidney was made because of the localization of the pains to the left and the presence of albumen and pus in the urine. At operation no stone was found but the existence of a horseshoe kidney was established. From then until September, 1912, when she was first seen by the author, the patient became steadily worse, the pains increased in severity, requiring morphine injections, and there were frequent attacks of cardiac collapse which seemed almost terminal in their severity.

Examination showed that the patient was weak, pale, and flabby. There was much tenderness on pressure over the lower abdomen and rigidity as well. The catheterized bladder urine contained albumen, pus and red cells, but no casts or tubercle bacilli. Cystoscopy showed that the ureter orifices were normal but that indigocarmine was excreted late from both sides, more so on the left. Both kidney pelves were dilated, the left more so. The 24 hour urine measured 1500 cc., with good urea content. X-ray failed to show stone. The diagnosis was made of bilateral pyelitis in a horseshoe kidney and ureteral irrigations were begun. Under this treatment the pyelitis cleared up completely although the pains were unaffected and for this reason an operation for the separation of the connecting bridge between the two kidneys was suggested.

Before this was undertaken, however, an attempt was made to localize exactly the situation of the bridge. For this purpose an X-ray picture was taken with both pelves injected with argyrol. As the left pelvis was found to lie much further away from the spinal column than the right it was clear that the connecting bridge was to be found on the left side of the abdomen. A left rectus incision was therefore made and the bridge located as expected, tied, cut and the kidneys allowed to sink back into their natural positions. The result of the operation was in every way excellent, the pains completely disappearing and the urine becoming normal.

9. Hyperalgetic Zones and Herpes Zoster.

Head has shown that disease or irritation of a viscus is accompanied by a disturbance in the skin segments which are supplied by sensory fibers emerging from the same cord level as the nerves supplying the viscus. The skin disturbances result in the appreciation of ordinary touch or temperature stimuli as pain. The suspected skin area may be tested by pinching or by stroking with a pin or by test-tubes containing warm water.

The skin areas for the kidney and ureter are supplied chiefly by the X dorsal and to a less extent by the XI and XII dorsal and I lumbar segments of the cord. Not only does the area of disturbed sensation vary in extent but the sensitiveness of certain points is greater than that of others. Such points have been called "puncta maxima" by Head. Kidney conditions in which "Head zones" have been described are nephrolithiasis and floating kidney.

Herpes zoster has also been described in various skin conditions such as nephritis, nephrolithiasis, intermittent hydronephrosis, pyonephrosis, floating kidney, kidney trauma. The author gives protocols of cases described in the literature and reports one of his own. The patient was a sufferer from typical left sided kidney colics with hematuria. X-ray showed a calculus in the left pelvis. In 1911 the patient had a herpetic eruption similar to the one subsequently observed by the author and *not* associated with hematuria or colic. The attack described by the author occurred in 1912. This was a typical herpes zoster of the left dorso-abdominal and lumbo-inguinal regions. The areas involved corresponded to the X to XII dorsal segments with a partial extension to the I lumbar. The rash occurred during the recession period of a typical left sided renal colic. The patient never presented a Head zone.

As regards the etiology of the herpes Head has presented autopsy evidence showing the presence of a lesion (hemorrhage, inflammation) of the posterior root ganglia supplying the skin areas involved. In general the lesions are caused by an infection (meningitis, influenza) but this can explain only a few of the kidney cases. As regards the rest,— especially aseptic stone cases,— a toxic element must be invoked to explain them. This is more readily understood when we recall that herpetic eruptions have been described in the medicinal use of potassium iodid, arsenic (lately salvarsan), in carbon monoxid poisoning, and finally in uremia.

MISCELLANEOUS ABSTRACT

A New Sign of Syphilis.

Beck (*Munch. med. Woch.*) has found one of the earliest signs of constitutional syphilis to be a diminution in the bone conduction of sound, coexisting with otherwise normal hearing. An apparently healthy man, with normal hearing but impaired bone conduction, should be suspected of being syphilitic. A tuning fork is struck and placed on the patient's mastoid process. When he no longer hears it, the fork is placed upon the physician's mastoid region. If the fork is still audible to the physician, the test is positive, provided the patient's hearing was otherwise acute. This reaction, which is apparently due to increased intracranial pressure, disappears for a few days after lumbar puncture. It is positive, besides syphilis, in brain tumors, hydrocephalus, epilepsy, and tetany.

Lightning Source UK Ltd.
Milton Keynes UK
UKHW02f0746230918
329386UK00013B/759/P

9 781527 941151